Prevention of Complications in Obstetrics

Yariv Yogev • Asma Khalil
Editors

Prevention of Complications in Obstetrics

Springer

Editors
Yariv Yogev
Obstetrics and Gynecology
Lis Hospital for Women's Health Tel,
Aviv Sourasky Medical Center,
Associate Dean for Clinical Affairs,
Gray Faculty of Medicine and Health
Science
Tel Aviv, Israel

Asma Khalil
Department of Obstetrics and
Gynaecology
City St George's University of
London,
London, UK

ISBN 978-3-032-23478-0 ISBN 978-3-032-23479-7 (eBook)
https://doi.org/10.1007/978-3-032-23479-7

This Springer imprint is published by the registered company Springer Nature Switzerland AG
The registered company address is: Gewerbestrasse 11, 6330 Cham, Switzerland

Contents

IV Neonatal Care

Contributors

Eran Ashwal Division of Maternal-Fetal Medicine, Department of Obstetrics and Gynecology, McMaster University, Hamilton, ON, Canada

Elizabeth Asztalos Department of Newborn & Developmental Pediatrics, Sunnybrook Health Sciences Centre, University of Toronto, Toronto, ON, Canada

Emmanuel Attali Tel Aviv Sourasky University Medical Center (Ichilov), Gray Faculty of Medical and Health Sciences, Tel Aviv University, Tel Aviv, Israel

Amir Aviram Division of Maternal-Fetal Medicine, Dan Women and Babies Program, Sunnybrook Health Sciences Center, Toronto, ON, Canada

Department of Obstetrics and Gynecology, Temerty Faculty of Medicine, University of Toronto, Toronto, ON, Canada

Tomer Avnon Department of Obstetrics and Gynecology, Soroka University Medical Center, Beer-Sheva, Israel

Işıl Ayhan Department of Obstetrics and Gynecology, Division of Perinatology, Antalya City Hospital, Antalya, Türkiye

Matitiahu Berkovitch Clinical Pharmacology and Toxicology Unit, Shamir Medical Center, Zerifin, Israel

The Andy-Lebach Chair of Clinical Pharmacology and Toxicology, Gray Faculty of Medical and Health Sciences, Tel-Aviv University, Tel Aviv, Israel

Roy Bitan Lis Hospital for Women's Health, Tel Aviv Sourasky Medical Center, Gray Faculty of Medicine and Health Science, Tel Aviv University, Tel Aviv, Israel

Piya Chaemsaithong Maternal Fetal Medicine Division, Department of Obstetrics and Gynecology, Faculty of Medicine, Ramathibodi Hospital, Mahidol University, Bangkok, Thailand

Daniel Crankshaw Liverpool Women's Hospital, Liverpool, UK

Chen Ben David Department of Obstetrics and Gynecology, Rambam Health Care Campus, Haifa, Israel

Ruth & Bruce Rappaport Faculty of Medicine, Technion Institute of Technology, Haifa, Israel

Chloe De Souza North Bristol NHS Trust, Bristol, UK

Andrew Demetri University of Bristol, Bristol, UK

Chris Dewhurst Liverpool Women's Hospital, Liverpool, UK

Zakaria Doughan McGovern Medical School at the University of Texas Health Science Center at Houston, Department of Obstetrics, Gynecology and Reproductive Sciences, Division of Maternal-Fetal Medicine, Department of Obstetrics, Gynecology and Reproductive Sciences, University of Texas Health Science Center at Houston, Houston, TX, USA

Tim Draycott North Bristol NHS Trust and Royal College of Obstetricians and Gynaecologists, Bristol, UK

Abdullatif Elfituri St George's, Epsom and St Helier Group (GESH), St Helier University Hospital, Sutton, UK

Yuval Fouks Lis Maternity and Women's Hospital, Tel Aviv Sourasky Medical Center, Tel Aviv University, Tel Aviv, Israel

Daniel Gabbai Lis Hospital for Women's Health, Tel Aviv Sourasky Medical Center, Faculty of Medicine and Health Science, Tel Aviv University, Tel Aviv, Israel

Rinat Gabbay-Benziv Department of Obstetrics and Gynecology, Hillel Yaffe Medical Center, Hadera, Israel

Itamar Gilboa Lis Hospital for Women's Health, Tel Aviv Sourasky Medical Center, Tel Aviv, Israel

Gray Faculty of Medicine and Health Science, Tel Aviv University, Tel Aviv, Israel

Liran Hiersch Tel Aviv Sourasky University Medical Center (Ichilov), Gray Faculty of Medical and Health Sciences, Tel Aviv University, Tel Aviv, Israel

Naphtali Justman Department of Obstetrics and Gynecology, Rambam Health Care Campus, Haifa, Israel

Ruth & Bruce Rappaport Faculty of Medicine, Technion Institute of Technology, Haifa, Israel

Yannay Khaikin Division of Maternal-Fetal Medicine, Dan Women and Babies Program, Sunnybrook Health Sciences Center, Toronto, ON, Canada

Department of Obstetrics and Gynecology, Temerty Faculty of Medicine, University of Toronto, Toronto, ON, Canada

Asma Khalil Fetal Medicine Unit, St George's University Hospitals NHS Foundation Trust, London, UK

Vascular Biology Research Centre, Molecular and Clinical Sciences Research Institute, City St George's University of London, London, UK

Fetal Medicine Unit, Liverpool Women's Hospital, Liverpool, UK

Dror Mandel Department of Neonatology, Dana Dwek Children's Hospital, Tel Aviv Sourasky University Medical Center, Tel Aviv, Israel

Gray Faculty of Medical and Health Science, Tel Aviv University, Tel Aviv, Israel

Esther Maor-Sagie Hillel Yaffe Medical Center, Hadera, Israel

Anastasia Martin Department of Women and Children's Health, Kings College London, London, UK

Nir Melamed Division of Maternal-Fetal Medicine, Department of Obstetrics and Gynecology, Sunnybrook Health Sciences Centre, University of Toronto, Toronto, ON, Canada

Rafael Mendelsohn Tel Aviv Medical Center and Gray Faculty of Medicine Tel Aviv University, Tel Aviv, Israel

Sharon Morag Department of Neonatology, Dana Dwek Children's Hospital, Tel Aviv Sourasky University Medical Center, Tel Aviv, Israel

Nicole Moriarty Division of Women's Health, King's College London, Women's Health Academic Centre, London, UK

Amir Naeh Department of Obstetrics and Gynecology, Hillel Yaffe Medical Center, Hadera, Israel

Nicola Adanna Okeahialam St Mary's Hospital, Manchester, UK

Brunel University of London, London, UK

Liona C. Poon Department of Obstetrics and Gynaecology, Prince of Wales Hospital, The Chinese University of Hong Kong, Sha Tin, Hong Kong

Lee Reicher Department of Computer Science and Applied Mathematics, Weizmann Institute of Science, Rehovot, Israel

Department of Molecular Cell Biology, Weizmann Institute of Science, Rehovot, Israel

Lis Maternity and Women's Hospital, Tel Aviv Sourasky Medical Center, Tel Aviv University, Tel Aviv, Israel

Faculty of Medical and Health Sciences, Tel Aviv University, Tel Aviv, Israel

Misgav Rottenstreich Department of Obstetrics & Gynecology, Shamir Medical Center (Assaf Harofeh), Affiliated to Gray Faculty of Medicine, Tel Aviv University, Tel Aviv, Israel

Eran Segal Department of Computer Science and Applied Mathematics, Weizmann Institute of Science, Rehovot, Israel

Department of Molecular Cell Biology, Weizmann Institute of Science, Rehovot, Israel

Mohamed bin Zayed University of Artificial Intelligence, Abu Dhabi, UAE

Hassan Shehata Centre of Reproductive Immunology and Pregnancy, Epsom, Surrey, UK

St George's, Epsom and St Helier Group (GESH), St Helier University Hospital, Sutton, UK

Andrew Shennan Division of Women's Health, King's College London, Women's Health Academic Centre, London, UK

Department of Women and Children's Health, Kings College London, London, UK

Baha M. Sibai McGovern Medical School at the University of Texas Health Science Center at Houston, Department of Obstetrics, Gynecology and Reproductive Sciences, Division of Maternal-Fetal Medicine, Department of Obstetrics, Gynecology and Reproductive Sciences, University of Texas Health Science Center at Houston, Houston, TX, USA

Mariane Silva-Edge Centre of Reproductive Immunology and Pregnancy, Epsom, Surrey, UK

Ido Solt Department of Obstetrics and Gynecology, Rambam Health Care Campus, Haifa, Israel

Ruth & Bruce Rappaport Faculty of Medicine, Technion Institute of Technology, Haifa, Israel

P. J. Steer Imperial College London, Academic Department of Obstetrics and Gynaecology, Chelsea and Westminster Hospital, London, UK

Abdul H. Sultan Croydon University Hospital, Thornton Heath, UK

Brunel University of London, London, UK

St George's, University of London, London, UK

Ranee Thakar Croydon University Hospital, Thornton Heath, UK

University of Liverpool, Liverpool, UK

St George's, University of London, London, UK

Violeta Torres-Sanchez Liverpool Women's Hospital, Liverpool, UK

Laura van der Krogt Division of Women's Health, King's College London, Women's Health Academic Centre, London, UK

Yariv Yogev Lis Hospital for Women's Health, Tel Aviv Sourasky Medical Center, Gray Faculty of Medicine and Health Science, Tel Aviv University, Tel Aviv, Israel

Faculty of Medicine and Health Science, Tel Aviv University, Tel Aviv, Israel

Sackler Faculty of Medicine, Tel Aviv University, Tel Aviv, Israel

Gray Faculty of Medicine and Health Science, Tel Aviv University, Tel Aviv, Israel

Liron Zahavi Department of Computer Science and Applied Mathematics, Weizmann Institute of Science, Rehovot, Israel

Department of Molecular Cell Biology, Weizmann Institute of Science, Rehovot, Israel

The Role of Prevention in Obstetrics

Yariv Yogev and Asma Khalil

Contents

Y. Yogev, A. Khalil (eds.), *Prevention of Complications in Obstetrics*,
https://doi.org/10.1007/978-3-032-23479-7_1

1.1 Introduction

Preventive care is a fundamental aspect of modern medicine, with a significant impact on patient outcomes and healthcare systems. In the field of obstetrics and gynecology, prevention is particularly crucial due to the potential for serious complications during pregnancy and childbirth and throughout a woman's reproductive life.

This chapter delves into the essential role of prevention in obstetrics, discussing various strategies employed at different levels of prevention and the challenges faced in implementation and providing real-world examples to illustrate these concepts.

The prevention of overtreatment is substantial and multifaceted. Preventive care, such as routine prenatal visits, screenings, and health education, significantly reduces the incidence of pregnancy-related complications that can lead to costly interventions and extended hospital stays. For example, early detection and management of conditions like gestational diabetes and preeclampsia can avert more serious health issues that may result in intensive medical care or emergency interventions, thus saving healthcare systems both direct costs and resources. Additionally, healthy pregnancies with fewer complications are associated with a reduced need for neonatal intensive care, which is often financially burdensome. By investing in preventive programs and services, healthcare systems can enhance maternal and infant health outcomes while simultaneously decreasing healthcare spending. A proactive approach not only alleviates financial strain on families and health systems but also promotes a healthier population, ultimately leading to lower healthcare costs over the long term. Investing in prevention is, therefore, not just a moral imperative but also a sound economic strategy that benefits society as a whole.

1.2 General Role of Prevention in Medicine

Preventive health strategies can be categorized into three primary levels: primary, secondary, and tertiary prevention. Understanding these levels is vital for the effective implementation of preventive measures in obstetrics and gynecology.

- **Primary Prevention**
  - *Definition*: Primary prevention aims to prevent the occurrence of disease or injury before it happens.
  - *Examples*: Vaccinations, health education, and counseling that promote a healthy lifestyle.
- **Secondary Prevention**
  - *Definition*: Secondary prevention focuses on early detection of disease and intervention to halt its progression.
  - *Examples*: Screening tests, regular health checkups, and monitoring of high-risk patients.
- **Tertiary Prevention**
  - *Definition*: Tertiary prevention aims to reduce complications and improve the quality of life among patients with established diseases.
  - *Examples*: Rehabilitation, ongoing management of chronic conditions, and support groups.

The historical focus in medicine often emphasized treatment rather than prevention. However, a shift toward preventive healthcare has shown that prioritizing prevention can significantly reduce disease burden, enhance quality of life, and result in substantial cost savings for healthcare systems.

1.3 Primary Prevention in Obstetrics

Primary prevention encompasses various strategies aimed at maintaining optimal health and preventing complications.

Early identification of risk factors is paramount in preventing complications in obstetrics.

Risk assessment begins at the first prenatal visit, where healthcare providers evaluate various factors, including:

- **Maternal History**: Previous pregnancy complications, chronic health conditions (e.g., diabetes and hypertension), and family history of genetic disorders.
- **Socioeconomic Factors**: Access to healthcare, financial stability, and education play vital roles in a woman's ability to engage in recommended prenatal practices.
- **Demographic Factors**: Maternal age, either very young (adolescents) or older (generally above 35), can increase the likelihood of complications during pregnancy.

Based on these evaluations, healthcare providers can tailor a preventive care plan that includes closer monitoring, referrals to specialists when necessary, and appropriate lifestyle modifications.

Screening for specific conditions can help identify issues early on. For example, blood pressure checks can reveal gestational hypertension, while glucose tolerance tests assess the risk of gestational diabetes. Other vital screenings include prepregnancy genetic screening and screening for infectious diseases.

1.4 Nutritional Counseling and Lifestyle Interventions

Nutrition plays a pivotal role in a healthy pregnancy. Based on established guidelines, healthcare providers should engage expectant mothers in **nutritional counseling**. Key components include:

- **Folic Acid Intake**: Adequate folic acid consumption before conception and during early pregnancy is essential for preventing neural tube defects within the developing fetus.
- **Balanced Diet**: A nutrient-rich diet, including whole grains, fruits, vegetables, lean proteins, and healthy fats, supports healthy fetal growth and development. Monitoring weight gain during pregnancy is equally important; both excessive and inadequate weight gain can lead to complications. Additionally, prevention of excessive weight gain and even weight loss in obese women during pregnancy is recommended.

1.5 Barriers to Effective Prevention in Obstetrics

Despite the clear benefits of preventive care in obstetrics, several barriers hinder the implementation and effectiveness of these strategies. Understanding these challenges is crucial for healthcare providers and policymakers who aim to promote optimal maternal and fetal health.

1. **Access to Care**: One of the most significant barriers to effective prevention in obstetrics is limited access to healthcare services. Geographic location plays a crucial role, particularly in rural areas where healthcare facilities may be scarce. Women in these regions often face difficulties in accessing routine prenatal care, leading to delayed or missed screenings and assessments. Additionally, socioeconomic factors can impede access; women with lower incomes or those lacking health insurance may be unable to afford prenatal visits, preventive screenings, or necessary medications, resulting in increased risk of complications during pregnancy.
2. **Educational Gaps and Health Literacy**: Low health literacy among pregnant women can impede their understanding of the importance of preventive care.

Comprehensive education regarding pregnancy health, nutrition, and the significance of prenatal visits is essential for empowering women to take charge of their health. However, without effective communication and educational resources, many women may not recognize the necessity of engaging in preventive practices. This lack of awareness can lead to inadequate prenatal care and unaddressed health concerns.

3. **Cultural and Social Influences**: Cultural beliefs and social norms can also impact a woman's willingness or ability to seek preventive care during pregnancy. In some communities, traditional practices or mistrust of the healthcare system might deter women from attending scheduled prenatal visits or accepting preventive advice. Educators and healthcare providers must tailor interventions to respect and integrate cultural perspectives while effectively communicating the benefits of preventive healthcare.
4. **Provider-Related Factors**: Healthcare providers also face barriers that can hinder the delivery of preventive care. Time constraints during patient visits may limit thorough assessments and discussions about preventive measures. Additionally, varying levels of awareness and adherence to clinical guidelines among providers can lead to inconsistencies in care. Some healthcare professionals may not prioritize preventive measures due to their focus on treatment, particularly in high-pressure environments where immediate clinical issues dominate discussions.
5. **Fragmented Healthcare Systems**: A lack of coordination among different healthcare providers can hinder effective preventive care. Expectant mothers often navigate a complex healthcare landscape with multiple providers, including obstetricians, primary care physicians, nutritionists, and mental health professionals. Fragmentation among these services can lead to missed opportunities for comprehensive care, inadequate follow-up, and disjointed communication regarding patients' health needs. Improving integration within healthcare systems can facilitate a more holistic approach to preventive care.
6. **Financial Constraints**: The costs associated with preventive services can also pose significant barriers. Many women may prioritize other household expenditures over healthcare, particularly if they face financial instability. Furthermore, insufficient insurance coverage for preventive services or high out-of-pocket expenses can discourage women from seeking necessary care. Addressing these financial barriers through policy interventions and expanded coverage options is vital to promoting access to effective preventive care.
7. **Mental Health Considerations**: Mental health challenges, such as anxiety and depression, can also hinder a woman's engagement in preventive care during pregnancy. Women experiencing mental health issues may have difficulties prioritizing their physical health or may feel overwhelmed by their circumstances, leading to decreased motivation to attend prenatal appointments or adhere to recommended screenings.

Addressing the barriers to effective prevention in obstetrics requires a multifaceted approach. Initiatives that improve access to care, enhance health literacy, acknowledge cultural differences, and promote provider coordination will contribute to a more effective preventive care framework. By working collaboratively to overcome these challenges, healthcare systems can significantly improve maternal and fetal health outcomes and ultimately reduce the burden of pregnancy-related complications.

1.6 Future Directions in Preventive Practices in Obstetrics

The future of preventive practices in obstetrics holds great promise, driven by advancements in technology, evolving healthcare paradigms, and a growing emphasis on personalized medicine. One significant direction is the increasing integration of **telemedicine**, which has the potential to enhance access to prenatal care for women in underserved or remote areas. This approach allows for virtual consultations, remote monitoring, and timely interventions, making it easier for expectant mothers to engage in routine care without the barriers of transportation and time constraints. Additionally, the use of **artificial intelligence and data analytics** in predicting pregnancy complications based on individual health profiles can lead to more tailored preventive strategies, enabling healthcare providers to address risk factors more effectively. Furthermore, there is a push toward expanding educational programs that emphasize health literacy and the importance of preventive care from preconception through postpartum. Community outreach initiatives that focus on culturally sensitive education can empower women to take control of their health and make informed decisions. As research continues to evolve, exploring areas such as nutrition, mental health, and environmental influences will bolster our understanding of their impact on pregnancy outcomes. Overall, the integration of innovative technology, enhanced educational outreach, and a focus on personalized care will be pivotal in transforming preventive practices in obstetrics, ultimately leading to healthier pregnancies and improved maternal and infant health outcomes.

Antenatal Care

Contents

Prevention of Miscarriage

Mariane Silva-Edge, Abdullatif Elfituri, and Hassan Shehata

Contents

Y. Yogev, A. Khalil (eds.), *Prevention of Complications in Obstetrics*,
https://doi.org/10.1007/978-3-032-23479-7_2

Key Topics Covered in This Chapter

- Classification and epidemiology of sporadic and recurrent miscarriage
- Common and emerging risk factors contributing to pregnancy loss
- Diagnostic workup, including genetic, hormonal, immunological, and anatomical assessments
- Evidence-based preventive strategies and management approaches
- Psychological impact of miscarriage and the importance of patient-centred supportive care

Learning Objectives

By the end of this chapter, readers will be able to:

1. **Understand the epidemiology and impact of miscarriage**: Recognize its prevalence, risk factors, and psychological consequences.
2. **Conduct a comprehensive history-taking process**: Systematically assess obstetric, gynaecological, medical, lifestyle, and family history to identify potential underlying causes.
3. **Evaluate modifiable and non-modifiable risk factors**: Distinguish between genetic, hormonal, immunological, environmental, and lifestyle factors contributing to pregnancy loss.
4. **Interpret relevant investigations**: Identify appropriate laboratory, imaging, and genetic tests for assessing couples with recurrent miscarriage.
5. **Discuss evidence-based preventive strategies**: Understand preconception care, lifestyle modifications, and medical interventions to improve pregnancy outcomes.
6. **Apply a multidisciplinary approach to management**: Recognize the role of different specialists in optimizing care for affected couples.
7. **Provide patient-centred counselling**: Effectively communicate risks, prognosis, and management options while offering emotional support.

This chapter will critically review the available literature, highlight best practice recommendations, and discuss evolving evidence and controversies in miscarriage prevention. By providing a structured approach to diagnosis and management, it aims to equip clinicians with the knowledge to enhance pregnancy outcomes and improve patient care.

Learning Objectives

- Explain mechanisms and classifications of miscarriage and recurrent miscarriage.
- Identify evidence-based investigations, and avoid unnecessary testing.
- Apply preventive strategies targeting modifiable medical and lifestyle factors.
- Describe appropriate therapeutic options (thyroid, progesterone, metformin, and APS management).
- Integrate psychological care into miscarriage management.

2.1 Introduction

Pregnancy loss is a common and distressing complication that affects many couples trying to conceive. While a single miscarriage is often attributed to chance, recurrent miscarriage (RM) requires a thorough evaluation to identify and address underlying causes. This chapter explores the risk factors, diagnostic approach, and preventive strategies for miscarriage, with a focus on evidence-based interventions that may improve pregnancy outcomes.

This chapter is integral to the broader theme of preventing complications in pregnancy by emphasizing early identification and targeted management of factors contributing to miscarriage. It provides clinicians with a structured approach to recognizing high-risk individuals, optimizing preconception care, and applying medical and lifestyle interventions to enhance reproductive success.

2.2 Definitions

Miscarriage is defined as the spontaneous loss of pregnancy before 24 weeks of gestation, the threshold for foetal viability. It is a common occurrence, affecting approximately 10–20% of clinically recognized pregnancies, with the majority occurring in the first trimester [1]. While many cases are isolated incidents, some individuals experience recurrent pregnancy loss, which requires further investigation and targeted management.

Miscarriages are categorized into sporadic and recurrent. Sporadic miscarriage is a singular pregnancy loss, often attributed to random foetal chromosomal abnormalities [2]. The incidence of sporadic miscarriage increases with maternal age, ranging from approximately 10% in women under 30 to over 50% in women aged 45 and older [3]. It is also increased in men aged 45 and older. In contrast, recurrent miscarriage (RM) refers to the loss of two or more pregnancies, though historically, it was defined as three or more consecutive losses. The prevalence of RM is estimated to be between 1% and 5% of couples trying to conceive [4]. However, this figure varies due to differences in definitions, reporting, population studies, and inconsistencies in reporting methods.

While early miscarriages are frequently associated with chromosomal abnormalities (sporadic), late miscarriages account for approximately 1% of all pregnancies and are less commonly linked to genetic causes [5]. Instead, late pregnancy losses are often due to uterine anomalies, cervical insufficiency, or infection or immune issues and require distinct diagnostic and management approaches.

Several features distinguish recurrent miscarriage from sporadic pregnancy loss. Unlike isolated miscarriages that occur randomly, RM is increasingly recognized as a distinct clinical entity, often involving underlying maternal, paternal, or embryonic factors [6, 7]. Genetic abnormalities are observed less frequently in RM, and the risk of future pregnancy loss rises with each additional miscarriage, highlighting the need for a comprehensive evaluation.

The emotional and psychological impact of RM is profound, with affected couples experiencing heightened levels of stress, anxiety, and grief [8–10]. As such, an integrated approach that combines medical, psychological, and supportive care is essential. The management of RM remains challenging due to variations in clinical practice, guideline recommendations, and evolving evidence regarding investigations and therapeutic interventions.

This chapter aims to provide a comprehensive overview of the prevention of miscarriage, addressing established and emerging risk factors, diagnostic strategies, and evidence-based management approaches.

2.3 Detailed History Taking in the Evaluation of Miscarriage

A comprehensive and systematic history-taking process is fundamental in the assessment and management of miscarriage in general and RM in particular. An accurate clinical history not only aids in identifying underlying aetiologies but also directs the need for targeted investigations and tailored interventions. Given the multifactorial nature of miscarriage, history taking should encompass various domains, including obstetric, gynaecological, medical, surgical, pharmacological, lifestyle, and familial factors.

2.3.1 Pregnancy Loss History

A meticulous pregnancy loss history is critical in distinguishing between different types of miscarriage. The gestational age at which a miscarriage occurs provides key diagnostic insights. Early pregnancy losses <6 weeks of gestation, such as biochemical pregnancies, often indicate the strength of the pathological cause, whereas losses occurring between 6 and 8 weeks of gestation occur most commonly but do not indicate the cause. In contrast, second-trimester losses may signal cervical insufficiency, infection, uterine anomalies, or underlying maternal medical conditions.

Understanding the specific circumstances of a late miscarriage, including foetal viability at the time of loss, associated symptoms, and the presence of infection or thrombotic events, is essential for guiding future management.

2.3.2 Obstetric History

A thorough obstetric history provides crucial information regarding previous pregnancies, deliveries, and neonatal outcomes. A history of pre-eclampsia, intrauterine growth restriction, or stillbirth may suggest an underlying immunological or vascular pathology, such as chronic histiocytic intervillositis or antiphospholipid syndrome (APS) [11–13]. In such cases, prolonged treatment strategies may be warranted beyond the first trimester. Additionally, a history of prior successful pregnancies with subsequent RM may indicate acquired pathology rather than an inherent reproductive abnormality.

2.3.3 Gynaecological History

A detailed gynaecological history, including menstrual cycle regularity and previous cervical or uterine procedures, is crucial in planning investigations and management strategies. Menstrual irregularities may indicate polycystic ovarian syndrome (PCOS) or luteal phase defects, both of which have been implicated in RM. A history of multiple uterine surgeries, such as dilation and curettage (D&C), myomectomy, or caesarean section, raises the possibility of intrauterine adhesions or endometrial dysfunction, necessitating further anatomical assessment through hysteroscopy or sonohysterography.

2.3.4 Medical History

Pre-existing medical conditions, particularly autoimmune and endocrine disorders, are well-established contributors to pregnancy loss. Conditions such as systemic lupus erythematosus, APS, and thyroid dysfunction require targeted investigations, including autoantibody screening and thyroid function tests. Endocrine disorders, such as poorly controlled diabetes mellitus and hyperprolactinaemia, may also impair implantation and early placental development, necessitating optimized metabolic control prior to conception.

2.3.5 Surgical History

A history of prior pelvic or abdominal surgery can provide insights into potential anatomical factors contributing to recurrent miscarriage. Previous myomectomy or uterine septoplasty may predispose to intrauterine adhesions, whereas surgeries involving the cervix, such as loop electrosurgical excision procedures or cone biopsy, may compromise cervical competence.

2.3.6 Drug History

While most prescribed medications do not have a strong association with recurrent miscarriage, certain drugs warrant careful consideration. High-dose nonsteroidal anti-inflammatory drugs have been implicated in early pregnancy loss due to their inhibitory effects on prostaglandin synthesis and implantation. However, there is currently no conclusive evidence linking routine medication use to recurrent miscarriage. A thorough review of prescribed and over-the-counter medications should be undertaken, with discontinuation or substitution considered when necessary.

2.3.7 Lifestyle History

Lifestyle factors, including smoking, obesity, and alcohol consumption, have been implicated in adverse pregnancy outcomes, although their direct impact on recurrent miscarriage remains inconclusive. Smoking is strongly associated with an increased risk of stillbirth, preterm birth, and foetal growth restriction. While studies on the association between smoking and recurrent miscarriage are limited [14, 15], heavy paternal smoking has been shown to contribute to increased risk, likely due to sperm DNA damage [16]. Obesity is another significant modifiable risk factor affecting female reproductive health. Women with a high body mass index (BMI) have been found to have an increased prevalence of RM, likely due to disrupted hormonal balance, inflammation, and endometrial dysfunction [17–19]. Conversely, there is no clear evidence linking low BMI to RM [20]. While the impact of male obesity on RM remains unexplored, sperm DNA fragmentation may contribute to early pregnancy loss indirectly. Alcohol consumption has well-established adverse effects on foetal development, and although evidence regarding RM is inconsistent, excessive alcohol intake during pregnancy has been associated with an increased risk of miscarriage [21, 22]. The use of recreational drugs, such as cannabis, lacks definitive evidence in RM, but general avoidance is recommended.

2.3.8 Family History

A thorough assessment of family history is essential in evaluating RM, as emerging evidence suggests a potential genetic and immunological predisposition. Some studies have reported an increased risk among first-degree relatives of affected individuals compared to controls, indicating a possible hereditary component [14, 23]. Additionally, a family history of thrombotic or autoimmune disorders, such as APS or systemic lupus erythematosus, may suggest an underlying predisposition to pregnancy loss. However, further research is needed to explain the precise heritability patterns and their clinical implications (Table 2.1).

Table 2.1 Preconception management recommendations for couples with recurrent first-trimester miscarriage

Recommendation	Quality of evidence	Strength of recommendation
A holistic approach is highly recommended and should include psychological and mental health support	⊕⊕⊕⊕	Strong
When managing couples with recurrent first-trimester miscarriage, it is important to consider a thorough and in-depth assessment of both partners. This includes detailed history taking of each of the pregnancy losses, obstetric, gynaecological, medical, surgical, drug, lifestyle, and family history	⊕⊕⊕⊕	Strong
Preconception counselling and care are recommended, including the opportunity to address bodyweight, smoking, substance abuse, alcohol consumption, and diet, particularly intake of micronutrients, such as the appropriate dose of folic acid and vitamin D	⊕⊕⊕⊕	Strong
Females should be advised to avoid alcohol consumption and substance abuse when planning a pregnancy and during pregnancy	⊕⊕⊕⊕	Strong
Females should be advised to avoid smoking when planning a pregnancy and during pregnancy. Obese women should be advised to reduce their weight	⊕⊕⊕	Weak
Male partners should be advised to stop or reduce alcohol consumption and substance abuse when planning a pregnancy and during pregnancy	⊕⊕	Weak
Male partners should be advised to avoid smoking when planning a pregnancy and during pregnancy. Obese men should be advised to reduce their weight	⊕⊕	Weak

Adapted from Ali et al. [24]

2

2.4 Causes

2.4.1 Chromosomal Abnormalities

Chromosomal abnormalities arise due to errors during gametogenesis, when sperm or oocytes undergo meiosis, or in early embryonic development due to mitotic errors after fertilization. They can be classified into numerical abnormalities, structural abnormalities such as microdeletions or translocations, and mosaicism.

Numerical chromosomal abnormalities result from errors in chromosomal segregation, commonly due to nondisjunction, where homologous chromosomes fail to separate during meiosis. This leads to aneuploidy, where an individual has an extra or missing chromosome. Trisomy, the presence of an additional chromosome, is seen in conditions such as Down syndrome (trisomy 21). Monosomy, the loss of a chromosome, occurs in conditions like Turner syndrome (45,X). In some cases, an entire extra set of chromosomes is inherited, known as polyploidy, often caused by fertilization by two sperm (dispermy) or a diploid gamete. Triploidy, for example, results in 69 chromosomes instead of 46 and is usually incompatible with life.

Structural chromosomal abnormalities occur when a chromosome undergoes breakage and is improperly repaired, leading to deletions, duplications, or rearrangements. Microdeletions and microduplications involve the loss or gain of small segments of genetic material, often due to non-allelic homologous recombination or errors in DNA double-strand break repair. A well-known example is the 22q11.2 deletion syndrome (DiGeorge syndrome), which causes congenital heart defects, immune deficiencies, and developmental delays.

Translocations occur when segments of two non-homologous chromosomes exchange places. Balanced translocations do not result in genetic loss or gain and may leave carriers asymptomatic but at risk of producing unbalanced gametes. Unbalanced translocations, however, lead to genetic duplications or deletions, often causing pregnancy loss or congenital disorders. A common example is Robertsonian translocation, where two acrocentric chromosomes fuse at the centromere, as seen in some cases of familial Down syndrome. Reciprocal translocations, where segments of two different chromosomes are exchanged, can lead to RM due to abnormal chromosomal segregation in gametes.

Mosaicism occurs when an individual has two or more genetically distinct cell populations due to a mitotic error after fertilization. It can be somatic, affecting only specific tissues, or germline, confined to reproductive cells and potentially transmissible to offspring despite a normal parental karyotype.

Chromosomal abnormalities are the leading cause of sporadic miscarriage, accounting for 50–59.4% of cases. The exact percentage varies depending on the detection method (conventional karyotyping, array comparative genomic hybridization, single nucleotide polymorphism array, or next-generation sequencing) [25, 26].

In RM, chromosomal abnormalities are less prevalent than in sporadic losses, with aneuploidy detected in about 40% of cases [27]. This suggests that non-genetic factors, such as uterine abnormalities, immune dysfunction, and hormonal imbalances, may play a larger role in repeated pregnancy loss. Moreover, multiple euploid miscarriages indicate an increased risk of subsequent pregnancy loss [28], suggesting an underlying medical condition yet to be identified or treated.

Trisomy 16 is a ► chromosomal abnormality in which there are three copies of ► chromosome 16 rather than 2. It is the most common autosomal trisomy leading to ► miscarriage and the second most common chromosomal cause (closely following ► X-chromosome monosomy) [29]. About 6% of miscarriages have trisomy 16 [30].

Balanced translocations in one parent increase the risk of passing an unbalanced chromosomal complement to offspring [31, 32]. In such cases, genetic counselling can help couples understand reproductive options, including preimplantation genetic testing

(PGT) during IVF to select chromosomally normal embryos or the use of donor gametes.

Parental karyotyping may be recommended in specific cases, such as when there is a history of congenital abnormalities, a family history of chromosomal rearrangements, or the identification of a chromosomal translocation in foetal tissue following a miscarriage [33]. However, the likelihood of a parental translocation causing RM is relatively low [34], especially in couples without a family history of chromosomal abnormalities, women over 39, and those with fewer than three pregnancy losses. Therefore, routine genetic testing is not recommended for all RM cases. Although sporadic chromosomal abnormalities occur in about one in five pregnancies, particularly with advancing maternal age, they are not the primary cause of RM. A comprehensive evaluation of uterine, immune, and endocrine factors is often necessary to identify and address potential causes of pregnancy loss.

2.5 Hormonal

2.5.1 Polycystic Ovary Syndrome (PCOS)

PCOS is a complex hormonal disorder that affects reproductive, metabolic, and endocrine function. It is one of the most common causes of infertility, impacting up to 10% of reproductive-aged women [35]. PCOS is characterized by hyperandrogenism, irregular or absent ovulation, and polycystic ovarian morphology on ultrasound. The underlying hormonal imbalance often involves dysregulation of the hypothalamic–pituitary–ovarian (HPO) axis, leading to increased luteinizing hormone (LH) secretion relative to follicle-stimulating hormone (FSH). This LH dominance can result in excessive androgen production by the ovaries, contributing to symptoms such as acne, hirsutism, and hair thinning. Additionally, insulin resistance plays a central role in PCOS, even in lean individuals. Elevated insulin levels stimulate the ovaries to produce more androgens, exacerbating hormonal disturbances and disrupting normal follicular development. Insulin resistance is also linked to metabolic complications, including an increased risk of type 2 diabetes, cardiovascular disease, and obesity. The combination of ovulatory dysfunction, hormonal imbalances, and metabolic disturbances can negatively impact fertility and pregnancy outcomes.

Studies investigating the relationship between PCOS and miscarriage have produced inconsistent findings. Some research indicates that PCOS patients may have a higher risk of miscarriage [36, 37], whereas other studies have not established a clear association [38]. The prevalence of PCOS among individuals experiencing recurrent miscarriage appears to be greater than in the general population, although reported rates vary considerably [39]. Several factors associated with PCOS, including increased luteinizing hormone levels, androgen excess, insulin resistance, and reduced endometrial blood flow, have been suggested as potential contributors to miscarriage risk [36, 38]. A matched-pair study observed that lean individuals with PCOS had a significantly higher rate of early miscarriage and a lower live birth rate compared to non-PCOS controls, even when embryo karyotype was accounted for [37]. While these findings suggest that PCOS may independently influence miscarriage risk, further research is required to better define this connection.

2.6 Progesterone

2.6.1 Luteal Phase Insufficiency and Its Impact on Pregnancy

Luteal phase insufficiency refers to inadequate progesterone production, which can impair the secretory transformation of the endometrium, potentially affecting embryo implantation and early pregnancy maintenance [40]. It has been linked to endocrine disorders such as stress, PCOS, and prolactin imbalances [41].

Diagnosing luteal phase insufficiency is challenging due to the pulsatile nature of progesterone secretion and the limited reliability of available tests. While mid-luteal serum progesterone levels below a certain threshold are commonly used as a diagnostic criterion, studies have shown significant variability [42]. Other diagnostic methods, such as endometrial biopsy and basal body temperature tracking [43, 44], have also demonstrated inconsistent sensitivity and specificity.

Research on the connection between luteal phase insufficiency and RM has produced mixed results. Some studies have reported a higher prevalence of luteal phase defects in women with RM compared to controls [45, 46], while others have failed to establish a significant association [43, 47, 48]. Additionally, luteal phase insufficiency does not appear to reliably predict pregnancy outcomes [48].

A large randomized controlled trial [49] found no significant difference in live birth rates between women with unexplained recurrent miscarriage who received vaginal progesterone from a positive pregnancy test and those who received a placebo. Similarly, a systematic review and meta-analysis suggested that synthetic progestogens might offer some benefit over natural progesterone, but the evidence is limited due to the inclusion of older, lower-quality studies with small sample sizes [50].

Most studies on progesterone supplementation have started treatment only after pregnancy confirmation, leaving uncertainty about whether earlier administration during the luteal phase could be more effective [51]. While synthetic progestogens may have a potential role in reducing pregnancy loss, further high-quality trials are needed to determine the optimal type, timing, and dosage [51].

2.7 Thyroid Dysfunction

Thyroid disorders can impact pregnancy outcomes, with both hyperthyroidism and hypothyroidism potentially contributing to complications.

2.7.1 Hyperthyroidism

Hyperthyroidism, most commonly caused by Graves' disease, affects 0.1–0.4% of pregnant women [52]. It has been linked to various pregnancy complications, including miscarriage [53], pre-eclampsia, preterm birth, and heart failure. However, no conclusive evidence directly associates hyperthyroidism with RM.

2.7.2 Hypothyroidism

Research on the relationship between overt hypothyroidism and RM is limited, and high-quality studies demonstrating a direct link are lacking. Some studies have reported a higher prevalence of hypothyroidism in women with RM compared to those without a history of pregnancy loss. However, when comparing pregnancy outcomes between hypothyroid and euthyroid women, no significant differences in miscarriage rates have been consistently observed [54, 55].

Studies investigating subclinical hypothyroidism (SCH), defined by elevated thyroid-stimulating hormone (TSH) levels with normal thyroid hormone levels, show no association with pregnancy loss. One study reported that SCH was present in 27% of 100 pregnant women with a history of RM, a prevalence similar to that observed in a control group of 100 pregnant women without prior pregnancy loss (24%) [56]. Other studies identified SCH in only 2.4% of 848 women with RM and found no significant differences in miscarriage rates or live birth rates between those with SCH and euthyroid women [57].

Pre-gestational diabetes has been associated with an increased risk of sporadic early pregnancy losses, though the exact mechanisms remain unclear [58, 59]. It is hypothesized that hyperglycaemia may have a detrimental effect on the developing yolk sac, leading to disturbances such as increased free oxygen radicals, deficiencies in essential compounds like myoinositol and arachidonic acid, and disruptions in cellular signal transduction [60–64]. These imbalances could result in genotoxic effects, potentially causing morphological damage to the foetus. However, current scientific evidence does not support uncontrolled hyperglycaemia in diabetes as a causative factor for RM.

2.8 Immune Factors

Pregnancy is a complex immunological process that requires precise regulation of maternal immune responses across various stages, from implantation and placentation to foetal growth and parturition. The maternal immune system must adapt dynamically to tolerate the semi-allogeneic foetus while preserving its ability to respond to potential threats. A fine-tuned balance between immune tolerance and surveillance at the maternal–foetal interface is essential for a successful pregnancy. Dysregulation of these immune processes can contribute to implantation failure, pregnancy loss, and complications such as preterm birth, pre-eclampsia, and placental insufficiency, all of which negatively impact foetal development.

▪▪ The Immune System and Pregnancy:

The human immune system consists of two primary components: the innate and adaptive immune systems. Both play critical roles in establishing immune tolerance and ensuring a successful pregnancy.

▪▪ Innate Immune System:

The innate immune system serves as the first line of defence, rapidly recognizing pathogens through pattern recognition receptors (PRRs) and activating antigen-presenting cells. Key innate immune cells include macrophages, dendritic cells (DCs), and natural killer (NK) cells, all of which are present in the reproductive tract and contribute to immune regulation at the maternal–foetal interface [65].

One of the most abundant immune cell populations in the uterine environment is the NK cell subset [66, 67]. Unlike peripheral NK cells, which are primarily cytotoxic, uterine NK (uNK) cells play a supportive role in pregnancy by facilitating embryo implantation, trophoblast invasion, and vascular remodelling to ensure adequate placental perfusion [68]. Women with RM often exhibit higher levels and increased activity of peripheral NK cells [69, 70], with an elevated percentage of CD56+ cells and a disrupted CD56+^{bright}:CD56+^{dim} ratio [70, 71]. Additionally, heightened activation of uNK cells and increased production of pro-inflammatory cytokines have been observed, potentially impairing implantation and early placental development [72, 73].

Toll-like receptors (TLRs), a subset of PRRs, play a crucial role in immune modulation during pregnancy by recognizing microbial components and regulating inflammation. TLRs are expressed in the placenta, decidua, and foetal membranes, helping balance immune responses. However, excessive activation of TLRs—particularly TLR2, TLR3, TLR4, and TLR9 has been implicated in pregnancy complications, including RM [74, 75]

▪▪ Adaptive Immune System:

The adaptive immune system, characterized by antigen specificity and immunological memory, consists of T and B lymphocytes. For a pregnancy to be successful, the maternal adaptive immune system must develop tolerance toward the foetus, which expresses paternal antigens.

A long-standing hypothesis in reproductive immunology suggests that pregnancy favours a shift toward a T helper type 2 (Th2) cytokine profile over a T helper type 1 (Th1) profile to prevent foetal rejection [76, 77]. Regulatory T cells (Tregs) also play a crucial role in maintaining immune tolerance and suppressing excessive maternal immune responses against foetal antigens [78, 79].

Elevated levels of Th1-associated cytokines, particularly tumour necrosis factor-alpha (TNF-α) and interferon-gamma (IFN-γ), have been detected in the decidual tissue of women experiencing RM [80]. Murine studies have further demonstrated that the administration of TNF-α can induce foetal loss, supporting the hypothesis that excessive Th1 activity contributes to pregnancy failure [81, 82]. Additionally, an imbalance between T helper 17 (Th17) cells and Tregs has been implicated in RM and other pregnancy-related complications [83, 84].

Despite these findings, the clinical utility of NK cell testing and other immunological markers in RM remains uncertain due to conflicting evidence and limited study sizes.

2.9 Autoantibodies

A number of studies identified significant associations between autoantibodies and adverse pregnancy outcomes.

▪▪ Thyroid Autoantibodies:

These have been linked to an increased risk of miscarriage and preterm birth. A meta-analysis found that the presence of thyroid autoantibodies nearly quadruples the odds of miscarriage and doubles the risk of preterm birth, suggesting an underlying immune-mediated mechanism [85].

▪▪ Antinuclear Antibodies (ANA):

ANA positivity has been associated with RM, with meta-analyses demonstrating a higher prevalence of ANA in RM patients compared to controls [86, 87]. Studies have reported an ANA positivity rate of 22% in RM groups versus 8.3% in controls, with higher ANA titres (≥1:160) showing a stronger correlation with RM [86]. However, lower ANA titres (1:40–1:80) have not demonstrated a significant association [88]. Additionally, a homogeneous ANA pattern appears more frequent in RM patients, though the most strongly associated pattern remains uncertain [88].

While research has provided valuable insights into the role of the immune system in pregnancy loss, clinical translation remains a challenge due to inconsistent findings. Further well-designed studies are required to refine diagnostic tools and develop targeted immune-modulatory therapies for women with RM.

2.10 Thrombophilias

The term thrombophilia is used to describe inherited or acquired disorders of the haemostatic mechanism that predispose to thrombosis. Thrombophilia has long been implicated in recurrent pregnancy loss, based on the hypothesis that an increased tendency toward thrombosis could impair placental circulation, leading to foetal loss [89, 90]. Historically, both inherited and acquired thrombophilias were thought to contribute to miscarriage risk, prompting widespread anticoagulant therapy in affected individuals. However, recent large-scale studies challenge this paradigm, suggesting a weaker association between thrombophilia and miscarriage than previously believed.

2.11 Inherited Thrombophilias

Inherited thrombophilias, such as factor V Leiden (FVL) mutation, protein C and S deficiencies, antithrombin deficiency, and prothrombin gene mutation, are well-known causes of systemic thrombosis. They have also been investigated as potential contributors to RM and late pregnancy complications, with the presumed mechanism involving thrombosis of the uteroplacental circulation.

2.12 Protein S Deficiency

Protein S is a vitamin K–dependent glycoprotein that acts as a cofactor for activated protein C, helping inactivate clotting factors Va and VIIIa, reduce thrombin generation, and promote fibrinolysis. Its deficiency disrupts these anticoagulant mechanisms, increasing thrombotic risk [91].

The prevalence of protein S deficiency is challenging to determine due to variations in levels, testing methods, and diagnostic criteria [92]. Its link to pregnancy loss remains unclear. While some studies suggest an association with second-trimester losses and complications like intrauterine foetal death and placental abruption, others find no significant connection, particularly for first-trimester losses or subsequent live birth rates [93–95].

2.13 Protein C Deficiency

Protein C is a vitamin K–dependent anticoagulant protein that, once activated, inactivates clotting factors Va and VIIIa, reducing thrombin generation. It also has anti-inflammatory and cytoprotective properties. Protein S acts as a cofactor, enhancing its anticoagulant effects [96].

Inherited protein C deficiency is found in approximately 0.2–0.5% of the general population and in 2–5% of individuals with venous thromboembolism (VTE). There is no consistent evidence linking protein C deficiency to RM [93, 94].

2.14 Factor V Leiden (FVL)

Factor V Leiden is the most common inherited thrombophilia, particularly among individuals of European descent. It results from a mutation in the F5 gene that prevents activated protein C (aPC) from effectively inactivating factor Va, leading to increased thrombin production and a higher risk of thrombosis. However, many carriers never experience a clotting event [97].

The prevalence of factor V Leiden varies by population, being highest in parts of Europe and absent in some African and Asian groups [98–102]. It is the most common thrombophilia among individuals with venous thromboembolism (VTE), though its associated risk is lower than that of protein C, protein S, or antithrombin deficiencies.

While early research suggested a link between factor V Leiden and miscarriage, more recent studies indicate no significant link between this inherited thrombophilia and pregnancy loss [103].

2.15 Prothrombin G20210A Mutation (PGM)

Prothrombin G20210A is the second most common inherited thrombophilia after factor V Leiden. It results from a G-to-A substitution at position 20210 in the prothrombin (F2) gene, leading to increased prothrombin production and a higher risk of venous thromboembolism (VTE) [104]. Most individuals with this mutation are heterozygous, experiencing a three- to fourfold increased VTE risk, while homozygosity is rare and associated with even higher thrombotic risk [105, 106].

The mutation is most prevalent in white populations, affecting 1–6% of individuals. While some studies suggest a potential association between PGM and miscarriages [93, 107], current evidence does not strongly support a link, especially in the absence of other risk factors [103].

2.16 Antithrombin III Deficiency

Antithrombin III is a non-vitamin K–dependent serine protease inhibitor that regulates coagulation by inhibiting thrombin and other clotting factors. Its function is greatly enhanced by heparin, making it crucial for the anticoagulant effects of unfractionated and low-molecular-weight heparin [108].

Deficiency of antithrombin III leads to a hypercoagulable state, increasing the risk of venous thrombosis and thromboembolism [109]. It can be inherited (autosomal dominant) or acquired due to conditions such as nephrotic syndrome (urinary loss), liver disease (reduced production), or disseminated intravascular coagulation (increased consumption).

While some studies have suggested a possible link between antithrombin III deficiency and miscarriage, a meta-analysis found no strong association [93].

2.17 Other Conditions: Methylenetetrahydrofolate Reductase (MTHFR) and PAI-1 Polymorphisms

Current research on MTHFR and PAI-1 polymorphisms in relation to pregnancy complications remains inconclusive. There is no substantial evidence to support routine genetic testing for these polymorphisms in patients with a history of miscarriage or adverse pregnancy outcomes, nor is there evidence to justify altering clinical management based on these results.

MTHFR polymorphisms (C677T and A1298C) are relatively common and may lead to mildly elevated homocysteine levels, particularly in individuals with low-normal folate levels. However, large epidemiological studies have not demonstrated a clear link between these polymorphisms and venous thromboembolism (VTE) or pregnancy loss [93, 110].

PAI-1 4G/5G polymorphism is prevalent in about 50% of the population, with 20–25% being homozygous (4G/4G), a genotype linked to higher PAI-1 levels. While some studies suggest a potential association with thrombosis and pregnancy complications, meta-analyses found no association between PAI-1 4G/5G polymorphism and recurrent pregnancy loss [111].

Overall, genetic testing for MTHFR and PAI-1 is not recommended, as current evidence does not support a strong role in recurrent miscarriage or other adverse pregnancy outcomes.

2.18 Acquired Thrombophilia

Antiphospholipid syndrome (APS) is a systemic autoimmune disorder characterized by recurrent thrombosis and obstetric morbidity. Beyond clinical manifestations, the diagnosis of APS requires two positive tests at least 12 weeks apart (and at least six weeks post-miscarriage) for either lupus anticoagulant or anticardiolipin (aCL) antibodies of immunoglobulin G (IgG) and/or IgM class present in medium or high titre (i.e. more than 40 GPL or MPL or more than the 99th percentile). For anti-beta-2-glycoprotein-I antibody, IgG and/or IgM class in high titre (i.e. more than the 99th percentile) can be used [112]. For detecting lupus anticoagulant, the dilute Russell's viper venom time (dRVVT) test, combined with a platelet neutralization procedure, offers greater sensitivity and specificity compared to the activated partial thromboplastin time (aPTT) or kaolin clotting time (KCT) tests [113].

Historically, the impairment of foetal–maternal exchange caused by intervillous thrombosis was assumed to be the main driver of pregnancy morbidity in APS. However, thrombosis is not reliably detected in the placentae of antiphospholipid antibody (aPL)–positive pregnancies [114, 115] Rather, clinical and experimental observations suggest that obstetric complications in APS are mediated primarily by trophoblast dysfunction and complement activation [116, 117].

The mechanisms underlying first-trimester pregnancy loss and late pregnancy complications in APS appear to be distinct. First-trimester losses are typically attributed to direct inhibitory effects of aPL on trophoblast viability, proliferation, and invasion, preventing proper placental anchorage [118]. aPL antibodies can also induce a pro-inflammatory trophoblast phenotype [119]. Late pregnancy complications have been linked to antibody-mediated complement activation, which may disrupt trophoblast proliferation and differentiation, impair spiral artery development, and trigger a localized inflammatory response. This process can result in placental fibrin deposition, placental infarctions, and overall placental dysfunction [117, 120–122].

Mouse models have demonstrated that aPL-induced foetal damage involves neutrophil activation, C5a receptor–dependent inflammation, and TNF-alpha and tissue factor amplification [123]. Studies in human pregnancies have shown higher circulating complement markers, such as Bb and soluble C5b-9, in APS pregnancies, correlating with adverse pregnancy outcomes [124]. The therapeutic effect of heparin in APS may be partly explained by its ability to inhibit placental complement activation.

A frequently cited study reported a prevalence of antiphospholipid antibodies in women with recurrent miscarriage as high as 15% [113]. However, this estimate was based on data collected before the publication of the original Sapporo criteria in 1999. The study included patients with antiphospholipid antibody levels even lower than 10 U/mL—below the threshold for laboratory diagnosis—and did not adhere to the now-standard 12-week interval between confirmatory tests. These factors likely led to an overestimation of prevalence.

When the revised Sapporo criteria (2006) are retrospectively applied to this study, incorporating the stricter laboratory threshold of 40 U/mL, the number of patients with raised aCL IgG antibodies decreases from 15 to four women, and the number of raised IgM antibodies drops from nine to three out of a total of 500 patients. This yields a revised prevalence of raised aCL antibodies at just 1.4% (7/500), compared to the original study's estimate of 5.5% (24/500). Similarly, for lupus anticoagulant, the updated criteria specify that the dRVVT ratio should be ≥1.2 to qualify as positive. Applying this threshold to the same study reduces the number of patients with positive lupus anticoagulant from 46 to 9, revising the prevalence from 9.6% (46/500) to just 1.8% (9/500).

Taken together, these revisions adjust the study's total estimated prevalence from 15% to a maximum of 3.2%. However, this figure likely remains an overestimation, as applying the full Sapporo criteria—including the requirement for a persistent positive result after 12 weeks—would reduce the numbers further [103]. More recent studies that have used the revised Sapporo criteria from the outset consistently report a much lower prevalence of APS in RM, typically ranging between 1 and 2% [125, 126]. This aligns with the updated estimates derived from reanalysing older data under current diagnostic standards and underscores the importance of strict adherence to standardized criteria when assessing APS prevalence in recurrent miscarriage populations.

The most recent 2023 American College of Rheumatology (ACR)/The European Alliance of Associations for Rheumatology (EULAR) APS diagnosis criteria state ≥3 points from clinical domains and ≥3 points from laboratory domains. A history of three or more miscarriages before 10 weeks of gestation scores only 1 point in the clinical domain. As a result, recurrent miscarriage (RM) alone is not sufficient to justify testing for antiphospholipid syndrome (APS). Testing should only be considered if there are additional clinical features suggestive of APS, such as livedo reticularis or a history of thromboembolic events (e.g., pulmonary embolism or deep vein thrombosis) [127].

2.19 Uterine Factors

Congenital and acquired uterine abnormalities have been implicated in RM. Congenital uterine malformations are documented risk factors for miscarriage, potentially leading to pregnancy loss due to impaired uterine distention, abnormal implantation from reduced vascularity in a septum, increased inflammation, or altered endometrial responsiveness to steroid hormones [128]. Acquired uterine abnormalities, including submucosal fibroids, endometrial polyps, and intrauterine adhesions, are frequently observed in women with RM. However, their precise impact on miscarriage risk is less clearly established.

Congenital uterine anomalies (CUAs) result from the incomplete development, fusion, or resorption of the Müllerian ducts during embryogenesis. While many CUAs are asymptomatic and do not impact fertility, some have been associated with adverse reproductive outcomes, including RM. The female reproductive tract forms from two Müllerian ducts during the first six weeks of foetal life. In the absence of anti-Müllerian hormone (AMH), these ducts fuse caudally to form the uterus and the upper third of the vagina, remain unfused at the top to form the fallopian tubes, and undergo resorption, allowing the central septum to dissolve and create a single uterine cavity. The lower fused part connects with the urogenital sinus to form the vaginal plate, which later develops into the vagina. CUAs arise when errors occur at any of these three stages of Müllerian duct development: formation (uterine aplasia/agenesis or unicornuate uterus), fusion (bicornuate uterus, uterus didelphys, transverse vaginal septum, or imperforate hymen), or resorption (septate uterus or arcuate uterus).

There are multiple classification systems for congenital uterine anomalies, each with its own criteria and limitations. The European Society of Human Reproduction and Embryology (ESHRE)/European Society for Gynaecological Endoscopy (ESGE) classification [129] aimed to improve objectivity, particularly in defining a septate uterus, but has been criticized for potentially overestimating the diagnosis compared to previous systems. In contrast, the American Society for Reproductive Medicine (ASRM) classification has been suggested to underestimate the prevalence of a septate uterus [130]. Despite efforts to refine classification, no single system has achieved universal acceptance. CUAs have been linked to various adverse reproductive outcomes, including infertility, RM, preterm birth, foetal malpresentation, increased caesarean delivery rates, and foetal growth restriction. Additionally, affected women may have a higher risk of complications, such as placental abruption, pre-eclampsia, and stillbirth [131, 132]. The impact of CUAs varies depending on the type of anomaly [133]. A systematic review found that resorption defects, such as septate and partial septate uteri, are associated with the poorest reproductive outcomes, including lower conception rates and increased risks of first-trimester miscarriage, preterm birth, and foetal malpresentation [132]. Bicornuate and unicornuate uteri increase the risk of first-trimester miscarriage, preterm birth, and foetal malpresentation, while uterus didelphys is primarily linked to preterm labour and foetal malpresentation [133].

Acquired uterine malformations, including submucous myomas, endometrial polyps, and intrauterine adhesions, are frequently found in women who experience pregnancy loss. However, their precise role in infertility and RM remains uncertain [134]. Some studies suggest that these anomalies may interfere with implantation and foetal development, while others indicate that their impact may be overstated due to confounding factors. Additionally, chronic endometritis has been increasingly recognized as a potential contributor to pregnancy complications.

Uterine fibroids are a common finding in reproductive-aged women and are, in the majority, asymptomatic and do not affect pregnancy outcomes. A large meta-analysis of an obstetric population found no significant increase in overall miscarriage risk. In a study of women with RM, myomas were found in 8.2% of cases, which is comparable to the general population [135, 136].

Endometrial polyps are localized overgrowths of the endometrial tissue, often found incidentally during fertility evaluations. While polyps have been associated with implantation failure and reduced pregnancy rates, there is a lack of data specifically examining their impact on miscarriage risk, either in sporadic miscarriage or RM. Given the uncertainty, the management of polyps in women with RM is typically guided by general recommendations, which suggest hysteroscopic removal of symptomatic or large (>1.5 cm) polyps that may interfere with implantation.

Intrauterine adhesions (IUAs), also known as Asherman's syndrome, are bands of fibrous scar tissue that form within the uterine cavity, often following uterine surgery, infections, or surgical management of miscarriages. Although IUAs have been linked to RM, definitive evidence remains limited, and only small cohort studies suggest that women with IUAs and an endometrial thickness of less than 5 mm have a significantly higher miscarriage rate [137]. Larger prospective studies are required to confirm these findings.

Chronic endometritis is a persistent inflammatory condition of the endometrial mucosa, characterized by abnormal infiltration of plasmacytes within the stromal tissue [138]. Diagnosing chronic endometritis remains complex due to the absence of universally accepted criteria [139]. Histopathological analysis, particularly the identification of CD138-positive plasma cells, is considered the gold standard for diagnosis. However, the precise threshold for a definitive diagnosis is still under debate [139].

2.20 Emerging Factors

2.20.1 Sperm DNA Fragmentation

Sperm DNA fragmentation (SDF) refers to breaks or damage within the DNA strands, which can impair embryonic development and increase the risk of implantation failure, miscarriage, and RM.

A growing body of evidence suggests that elevated SDF levels are associated with adverse reproductive outcomes. A systematic review and meta-analysis reported that high levels of sperm DNA damage were significantly linked to increased miscarriage [140]. Research on IVF outcomes further demonstrated that SDF levels exceeding 13% correlated with increased miscarriage rates [141]. Additionally, a study of couples with RM revealed that, despite normal conventional semen parameters, men in RM-affected couples had significantly higher sperm DNA fragmentation values than controls, with levels positively correlated with paternal age and the number of miscarriages [142].

2.20.2 Microbiome

Emerging research suggests a link between both the vaginal and uterine microbiome and the risk of miscarriage. Vaginal dysbiosis, characterized by a reduced abundance of *Lactobacillus* species, has been associated with an increased risk of adverse pregnancy outcomes, including preterm birth and miscarriage [143, 144]. Women with non-*Lactobacillus*-dominant vaginal microbiomes appear to have a higher likelihood of early miscarriage compared to those with *Lactobacillus crispatus* dominance, suggesting that vaginal microbial composition may influence pregnancy viability [144, 145]. The vaginal microbiome contributes to immune regulation and infection prevention, both of which are essential for implantation and placental development [143, 146].

Similarly, while a healthy endometrial microbiome is typically dominated by Lactobacilli, an imbalance favouring non-*Lactobacillus* species has been observed in patients with early pregnancy loss [145]. Uterine dysbiosis has been linked to recurrent implantation failure and miscarriage, with specific bacterial species, such as *Ureaplasma*, identified as independent risk factors for pregnancy loss with a normal karyotype [147].

2.21 Recommended Investigations

A comprehensive investigative approach is essential for the evaluation of couples experiencing RM, as it aids in identifying potential underlying causes and guiding management. The current recommended investigations encompass general health assessments, hormonal and immunological profiling, thrombophilia screening, genetic testing, and advanced reproductive evaluations.

2.21.1 General Investigations

Routine blood tests are recommended for both partners to assess their overall health and detect potential metabolic or nutritional deficiencies that could impact pregnancy outcomes. These include a full blood count to evaluate for anaemia or infection, renal and liver function tests to identify systemic disorders and the ability of the body to metabolize any intended medications, and vitamin D levels, given the emerging evidence suggesting an association between vitamin D deficiency and pregnancy loss.

2.21.2 Hormonal Profile

Endocrine abnormalities can contribute to pregnancy loss, necessitating an assessment of thyroid function (thyroid-stimulating hormone and free thyroxine), serum prolactin levels, and ovarian reserve markers such as anti-Müllerian hormone and follicle-stimulating hormone. Thyroid dysfunction, particularly hypothyroidism and the presence of thyroid antibodies, has been implicated in RM, while hyperprolactinaemia may indicate an underlying pituitary disorder affecting ovulation and implantation. Ovarian reserve assessment is essential to help anticipate conception chances.

2.21.3 Immunological Investigations

Dysregulation of the maternal immune system has been proposed as a contributory factor in some cases of recurrent miscarriage. Therefore, immunological assessments, including antinuclear antibody, thyroid peroxidase antibody, gliadin antibody, cytokine profiling, natural killer cell, cytokine, and TLR testing, may be considered if available, particularly in women with a history of autoimmune disorders.

2.21.4 Thrombophilia Screening

Routine testing for inherited thrombophilia is not recommended in RM unless there is a personal or family history of thromboembolic events [148]. Studies have demonstrated that the prevalence of inherited thrombophilia in women with recurrent miscarriage is comparable to that in the general population, and there is insufficient evidence supporting a causal relationship. Acquired thrombophilia, particularly APS, has been considered a well-established cause of recurrent miscarriage. Recent evidence showed that the prevalence of acquired thrombophilia, using the revised Sapporo criteria, in the cohort of RMs is like that in the general population [103]. Most recent changes in the classification of APS have yielded testing for the condition redundant. The new 2023 ACR/EULAR APS classification criteria state that APS diagnosis when a patient has ≥3 points from clinical domains AND ≥3 points from laboratory domains and having ≥3 consecutive pre-foetal (<10 w) and/or early foetal (10 w 0 d–15 w 6 d) deaths gives a score of only 1. Therefore, testing for antiphospholipid antibodies (lupus anticoagulant, anticardiolipin antibodies, and β2-glycoprotein I antibodies) should be reserved for when there is clinical evidence of antiphospholipid disease, e.g. livedo reticularis, and should follow internationally recognized diagnostic criteria with appropriate confirmatory testing intervals [103].

2.21.5 Parental Genetic Testing

Routine genetic testing in couples with recurrent miscarriage is not currently supported by evidence, as sporadic chromosomal abnormalities, although common in early pregnancy losses, do not typically account for recurrent miscarriage [149]. However, parental karyotyping may be indicated in specific clinical scenarios, such as a family history of chromosomal abnormalities, a previous child with congenital anomalies, or when unbalanced translocations have been detected in pregnancy tissue. The likelihood of a balanced chromosomal translocation in couples with recurrent miscarriage is low, particularly in those with no prior affected offspring, maternal age over 39 years, and fewer than three pregnancy losses [34].

2.22 Additional Investigations

Emerging evidence suggests that sperm DNA fragmentation may contribute to recurrent miscarriage, warranting further investigation in selected cases [150]. Although increased DNA fragmentation has been associated with an increased risk of miscarriage, the clinical utility of interventions aimed at reducing fragmentation remains uncertain, with limited data on whether such measures improve live birth rates.

A detailed uterine and ovarian assessment is a critical component of recurrent miscarriage evaluation. Two-dimensional (2D) ultrasound is the initial modality of choice, but in cases requiring higher diagnostic accuracy, three-dimensional (3D) pelvic ultrasound, saline infusion sonography, or hysteroscopy may be considered. The selection of an imaging modality should be guided by the clinical presentation, clinician expertise, and available resources.

2.23 Monitoring in Subsequent Pregnancies

Psychological distress is a common concern among couples who have experienced RM, necessitating a supportive and accessible approach to care in subsequent pregnancies. Early pregnancy reassurance scans, typically between six and ten weeks of gestation, can provide psychological support and allow for early detection of pregnancy complications, such as subchorionic haematomas, which may necessitate tailored management. While there is no standardized recommendation regarding the frequency of scans, good clinical practice suggests offering two or three ultrasound assessments before the routine 12-week scan, depending on the availability of resources (Table 2.2). Mental health support should also be integrated into RM care, as anxiety

Table 2.2 Investigations and monitoring in couples with recurrent first-trimester miscarriage

Recommendation	Quality of evidence	Strength of recommendation
Blood investigations tailored to each couple's requirements and background history are recommended	⊕⊕⊕⊕	**Strong**
It is recommended to offer general blood investigations, including well-being tests, such as blood count, kidney and liver function tests, and vitamin D level for both partners	⊕⊕⊕	**Weak**
It is recommended to offer hormonal profile investigations, such as thyroid function and serum prolactin, and check for polycystic ovary syndrome and baseline ovarian reserve tests for the woman	⊕⊕⊕	**Weak**
Thorough and detailed immunological investigations, such as antinuclear antibodies panel (ANA), thyroid antibodies, gliadin antibodies, NK cells, and cytokine tests, are to be considered if available	⊕⊕⊕	**Weak**
Thrombophilia screening is no longer recommended unless there is evidence of previous associated disorders, such as thromboembolic disease and livedo reticularis	⊕⊕⊕⊕	**Strong**
Parental genetic testing is not recommended for couples with RM	⊕⊕⊕⊕	**Strong**
A detailed anatomy scan of the uterus and ovaries is recommended. A higher level of assessment accuracy may be required for some selected patients; this may include 3D pelvic ultrasound with or without saline and hysteroscopy	⊕⊕⊕	**Weak**
It is recommended to give support to the couple in the form of easy accessibility to the early pregnancy services for reassurance scan and queries, as well as mental health support	⊕⊕⊕	**Weak**
Despite thorough investigations, there may be no cause for the miscarriages, with the only advice being to try again. It is the authors' view that empirical treatment may prove helpful in some cases	⊕	**Weak**
Regular scans are recommended. There is currently no guidance on the frequency or the benefit of regular early foetal scans. It is assumed good practice to offer two or three scans prior to the 12-week prenatal scan	⊕⊕	**Weak**

Adapted from Ali et al. [24]

and depression are prevalent among affected couples. Providing a multidisciplinary approach with access to early pregnancy services and psychological support can significantly improve the overall well-being of patients navigating recurrent miscarriage.

2.24 Pharmacological and Therapeutic Strategies for Miscarriage Prevention

2.24.1 Management of Thyroid Dysfunction

Thyroid dysfunction has been identified as a significant contributor to miscarriage risk. A systematic review by Quenby et al. [151] found that the presence of maternal thyroid autoantibodies more than doubled the miscarriage risk, irrespective of clinical thyroid status. Additionally, subclinical hypothyroidism was associated with an increase in miscarriage risk compared to euthyroid individuals [151].

The Royal College of Obstetricians and Gynaecologists advises that women with subfertility and positive thyroid peroxidase antibodies who are asymptomatic do not derive benefit from levothyroxine therapy [152]. However, these individuals should undergo baseline thyroid function assessment at 7–9 weeks' gestation, with subsequent trimesterly monitoring, as 8% may progress to subclinical hypothyroidism [153]. In cases where mildly elevated thyroid-stimulating hormone levels are detected in asymptomatic women, The Royal College of Obstetricians and Gynaecologists (RCOG) guidelines recommend initiating levothyroxine therapy preconceptionally [152].

2.24.2 Progesterone Treatment

Progesterone is widely recognized as a key hormone in early pregnancy, facilitating endometrial receptivity for embryo implantation and modulating maternal immune responses [154–157]. However, its precise role in sustaining pregnancy remains incompletely understood [51]. Despite its physiological importance, current evidence suggests that progesterone supplementation does not significantly improve live birth rates compared to placebo in women with recurrent miscarriage [51].

The International Federation of Gynaecology and Obstetrics (FIGO) Good Practice Recommendations on the Use of Progesterone in the Management of Recurrent First-Trimester Miscarriage acknowledge emerging evidence supporting the use of synthetic oral progesterone, although definitive conclusions regarding its efficacy are yet to be established [51]. Most clinical trials investigating progesterone therapy have employed similar study designs in terms of the route and timing of administration. However, alternative approaches such as the use of oral progesterone formulations or initiating treatment in the luteal phase rather than upon pregnancy confirmation may offer improved outcomes.

Further research is required to determine the optimal progesterone regimen, including the most effective formulation, dosage, and timing of administration. Large, well-powered randomized controlled trials with standardized outcome measures are essential to clarify its clinical utility. Additionally, investigating the role of progesterone in specific patient subgroups, such as those with endometrial dysfunction, may provide insights into targeted therapeutic strategies.

While progesterone remains a promising intervention, current evidence emphasizes the need for more rigorous evaluation before widespread implementation in clinical practice.

2.24.3 Metformin Therapy in PCOS

PCOS affects 10–15% of reproductive-aged women [158] and has been found to increase first-trimester miscarriage risk [151]. Its pathophysiology involves obesity, hyperinsulinaemia, hormonal dysregulation, and inflammation [158]. Metformin, an insulin-sensitizing agent that inhibits glucagon and hepatic gluconeogenesis [159], has been explored for miscarriage prevention, with a meta-analysis suggesting a reduction in late miscarriage [160]. However, no standardized regimen exists. Gastrointestinal side effects are common, and modified-release formulations may improve tolerance.

2.24.4 Anticoagulant Therapy

Thrombophilic disorders, both inherited (e.g. factor V Leiden mutation and protein C/S deficiency) and acquired (e.g. APS), do not contribute to RM [161, 162]. Meta-analyses show that treatment with low-dose aspirin and heparin reduces miscarriage risk and improves live birth rates in certain groups, but the reasons remain unclear. However, anticoagulation with Low-Molecular-Weight Heparin (LMWH) is not recommended for miscarriage prevention [103, 148, 163].

2.24.5 Antioxidant Therapies

Oxidative stress is implicated in miscarriage pathophysiology, affecting intrauterine conditions and increasing aneuploidy risk [164]. Despite this, a Cochrane review (2016) found no significant miscarriage reduction with vitamin supplementation, though a potential protective effect against stillbirth was noted [165]. Another review in subfertile women similarly reported minimal impact on miscarriage risk [166].

Sperm DNA fragmentation is also linked to miscarriage, with a systematic review of 16 studies showing a significant association [151]. However, few RCTs have assessed interventions to reduce DNA fragmentation and miscarriage risk [167]. A Cochrane review of 90 RCTs found that antioxidant therapy may increase live birth rates but did not significantly reduce miscarriage rates [168].

2.24.6 Surgical Management of Uterine Anomalies

Congenital and acquired uterine abnormalities, including Müllerian anomalies (e.g. septate and bicornuate uteri) and intrauterine pathology (e.g. fibroids and polyps), increase miscarriage risk. Women with septate and bicornuate uteri may have a higher risk of first-trimester loss, whereas arcuate, didelphic, and unicornuate uteri show no clear association [169]. While septate uterus resection is common, a recent RCT found no significant improvement in live birth rates post-surgery [170].

2.24.7 Psychological Support

Recurrent miscarriage has profound emotional and psychological consequences for the affected women and their partners (◘ Table 2.2). While much of the existing research has focused on the psychological impact on women, there remains a paucity of studies addressing the experiences of partners despite emerging evidence suggesting that they also experience significant distress [171–173]. The emotional burden of recurrent miscarriage emphasizes the need for a structured and compassionate approach to psychological support within clinical care.

A comprehensive psychological support strategy should encompass several key elements. Firstly, clinicians should acknowledge and discuss the emotional impact of recurrent miscarriage, providing a safe space for couples to express their concerns and grief. This should be accompanied by the provision of clear, timely, and detailed medical information regarding the causes, prognosis, and potential management options. In cases where additional psychological support is required, referral to a mental health professional, ideally one with expertise in perinatal mental health, is recommended.

The role of psychotherapeutic interventions in recurrent miscarriage is not well-established; however, certain approaches have been associated with improved live birth outcomes. These include the implementation of continuity of care models, regular follow-up appointments, structured patient education, and psychological counselling when necessary. A systematic review has suggested that psychological interventions, particularly those providing emotional support and structured counselling, may enhance psychological well-being in women following miscarriage, thereby potentially mitigating adverse pregnancy-related outcomes in subsequent pregnancies [14].

It is crucial to recognize that couples' psychological needs vary considerably, and an individualized approach should be adopted. Clinicians should facilitate open discussions, allowing patients and their partners the opportunity to ask questions and express their concerns. Sensitivity in communication is paramount, requiring the use of clear, honest, and empathetic language. Providing realistic expectations regarding future pregnancy outcomes, while simultaneously offering reassurance based on individual prognostic factors, enables couples to make informed decisions regarding future pregnancy attempts [174].

Ultimately, psychological support should be embedded within the broader multidisciplinary management of RM, integrating medical, emotional, and psychosocial care to optimize outcomes for affected couples.

2.25 Pearls and Pitfalls in Investigations and Treatment of Recurrent Miscarriages

2.25.1 Investigations

- **Comprehensive history taking is key**: A detailed obstetric, medical, lifestyle, and family history helps identify modifiable and non-modifiable risk factors.
- **Thorough evaluation of pregnancy loss history**: Gestational age at loss provides diagnostic insights (early losses suggest chromosomal factors, while late losses indicate anatomical or immunological causes).
- **Routine blood investigations are essential**: Complete blood count, renal/liver function tests, and vitamin D levels should be part of the initial workup.
- **Hormonal assessment is necessary**: Thyroid function, serum prolactin, and ovarian reserve markers should be evaluated.
- **Immunological testing should be considered selectively**: Testing for antinuclear antibodies, thyroid antibodies, NK cells, and cytokines may be relevant in some cases.
- **Thrombophilia screening is not recommended routinely**: Only indicated if there is a history of thromboembolic events or associated conditions (e.g. livedo reticularis).
- **Parental karyotyping is not routinely required**: Should only be considered in cases with a previous child with congenital anomalies or suspected chromosomal translocations.
- **Advanced imaging for uterine assessment**: 3D pelvic ultrasound, saline infusion sonography, or hysteroscopy may be needed for suspected uterine anomalies.
- **Sperm DNA fragmentation testing has potential but lacks standardized guidelines**: Emerging evidence suggests an association with miscarriage, but interventions remain unclear.
- **Avoid unnecessary over-testing**: Many investigations lack strong evidence in recurrent miscarriage management and may lead to undue patient anxiety and financial burden.

2.25.2 Treatment

- **Preconception care is crucial**: Women should optimize body weight, quit smoking, reduce alcohol consumption, and manage chronic conditions before conception.
- **Thyroid dysfunction must be addressed**: Women with subclinical hypothyroidism may benefit from levothyroxine therapy to reduce miscarriage risk.
- **Progesterone therapy may be beneficial in selected cases**: Oral progesterone has shown promise for women with recurrent miscarriage, but more studies are needed to evaluate the timing of start of treatment, e.g. luteal phase.
- **Metformin has potential benefits in PCOS**: May reduce late miscarriage risk in insulin-resistant women.

- **Anticoagulation therapy is not recommended for unexplained miscarriage**: Low-dose aspirin and LMWH are **only** beneficial in cases of diagnosed antiphospholipid syndrome in the presence of other clinical associations, such as livedo reticularis or a history of thromboembolic disease.
- **Oxidative stress reduction may be useful**: While vitamin and antioxidant supplementation has limited direct evidence, optimizing overall health is beneficial.
- **Surgical correction of uterine anomalies should be individualized**: Septate uterus correction may improve outcomes, but other anomalies (e.g. arcuate and bicornuate uterus) require case-by-case assessment.
- **Psychological support is an essential part of care**: Emotional distress is common, and structured counselling improves psychological well-being and future pregnancy success.
- **Avoid empirical treatments without evidence**: Unproven therapies, such as immunoglobulin therapy or routine antibiotics, do not improve pregnancy outcomes and should not be used outside clinical trials.
- **Do not delay referral to a specialist**: Couples with unexplained RM loss should be managed in a specialized setting for optimal assessment and care.

By focusing on evidence-based investigations and treatments while avoiding unnecessary interventions, clinicians can provide effective, patient-centred care to couples experiencing recurrent miscarriage.

2.25.3 Summary

Miscarriage is a common yet often distressing experience, affecting approximately 10–20% of clinically recognized pregnancies. While many cases result from chromosomal abnormalities, a range of modifiable and non-modifiable risk factors can contribute to pregnancy loss. A thorough evaluation of a patient's medical, obstetric, genetic, and lifestyle history is essential in identifying potential causes and guiding appropriate interventions.

Key Prevention Strategies:

Preventing miscarriage requires a proactive approach to addressing modifiable risk factors, including:

- **Lifestyle factors:** Reducing smoking, alcohol consumption, and obesity can lower the risk of pregnancy loss.
- **Medical conditions:** Optimizing the management of diabetes, thyroid disorders, lupus, and other autoimmune diseases is crucial in preventing complications.
- **Targeted medical interventions:** Endocrine profiling, reproductive immune testing, and personalized treatment strategies may be beneficial, particularly for women with recurrent pregnancy loss.

A Multidisciplinary Approach to Care:

Managing miscarriage risk requires collaboration across specialties to ensure comprehensive and individualized care. Obstetricians, reproductive endocrinologists, immunologists, and mental health professionals play a vital role in supporting both the physical and emotional well-being of affected individuals. Patient-centred counselling is essential, as pregnancy loss often leads to significant psychological distress for couples.

Optimizing Pregnancy Outcomes:

While not all miscarriages can be prevented, early identification of risk factors, personalized preconception care, and evidence-based interventions can significantly improve pregnancy outcomes. A multidisciplinary, patient-focused approach ensures that women receive both medical and emotional support, ultimately enhancing reproductive health and overall well-being.

A structured tool for history taking, investigations, and treatment options for recurrent miscarriage is provided below. It can be used as a clinical decision support tool to guide efficient assessment and management. This can be used as a clinical decision support tool for efficient assessment and management.

2.26 Recurrent Miscarriage Clinical Assessment and Management Tool

Step 1: Comprehensive History-Taking Checklist

Use this structured approach to identify potential risk factors.

Category	Key questions/factors to assess
Pregnancy loss history	Number of losses, gestational age at loss, ultrasound findings, foetal heart activity, symptoms (bleeding or pain), need for intervention (D&C or medical management)
Obstetric history	Prior live births, stillbirths, preterm deliveries, foetal growth restriction (FGR), hypertensive disorders, gestational diabetes, mode of delivery
Gynaecological history	Menstrual cycle regularity, prior uterine surgeries (D&C, myomectomy, or caesarean section), fibroids, endometriosis, congenital anomalies
Medical history	Autoimmune diseases (Systemic Lupus Erythematosus (SLE) or APS), endocrine disorders (thyroid, PCOS, or diabetes), renal disease, chronic hypertension
Surgical history	Previous abdominal or pelvic surgery, cervical procedures (Large loop excision of the transformation zone (LLETZ) or cone biopsy)
Drug history	Current medications, Nonsteroidal Anti-inflammatory Drugs (NSAIDs), anticoagulants, illicit drugs, supplements
Lifestyle factors	Smoking, alcohol intake, BMI, diet, physical activity, exposure to environmental toxins
Family history	Recurrent pregnancy loss, thromboembolic events, autoimmune disorders, genetic syndromes

Step 2: Recommended Investigations

Investigations should be **tailored** based on history and clinical suspicion.

Category	Tests	Indications
General health panel	Full Blood Count (FBC), renal and liver function, vitamin D	Routine for overall health assessment
Hormonal profile	TSH, free T4, serum prolactin, FSH, LH, AMH	Assess thyroid function, ovarian reserve, and endocrine disorders
Immunological tests	ANA, thyroid antibodies, NK cell assay, cytokine profile, and TLRs	For suspected autoimmune causes
Thrombophilia screening	**Only if indicated**: APS panel (lupus anticoagulant, anticardiolipin, and β2-glycoprotein-I antibodies)	Consider only the history of thrombosis, late pregnancy loss, livedo reticularis
Parental genetic testing	Karyotyping	Only if history of congenital anomalies or a suspected chromosomal translocation
Uterine and ovarian imaging	**First line:** Transvaginal ultrasound (2D/3D) **Second line:** Hysteroscopy, MRI, saline infusion sonography	Assess structural abnormalities, adhesions, septate uterus
Sperm quality (if indicated)	Sperm DNA fragmentation index	If suspected male factor (poor semen quality or history of infertility)

Step 3: Treatment Options Based on Results

Findings	Recommended treatment	Evidence strength
Unexplained recurrent miscarriage	Early pregnancy surveillance, supportive care, progesterone in selected cases	Moderate
Thyroid dysfunction (TSH >2.5 in pregnancy)	Levothyroxine to maintain TSH <2.5	Strong
PCOS or insulin resistance	Metformin in women with insulin resistance	Moderate
Obesity (BMI >30)	Preconception weight loss, lifestyle modification	Strong
APS (diagnosed by clinical and lab criteria): only in the presence of other clinical manifestations such as livedo reticularis and a history of thromboembolic disease	Low-dose aspirin + LMWH	Strong
Structural uterine abnormality	Consider surgical correction (e.g. hysteroscopic metroplasty for a septate uterus)	Moderate
Sperm DNA fragmentation >30%	Antioxidants, lifestyle changes, and consider assisted reproductive techniques	Weak
Psychological impact	Referral for counselling, early pregnancy reassurance scans	Strong

Step 4: Follow-Up and Pregnancy Monitor ing

Preconception Care

- Optimize weight, nutrition, and vitamin D levels.
- Manage modifiable lifestyle factors (smoking, alcohol, and caffeine).
- Address pre-existing medical conditions.

During Pregnancy:

- Early scans (6–10 weeks) for reassurance
- Close monitoring if APS or thyroid disorder is present
- Individualized approach based on past pregnancy losses

Post-pregnancy loss Counselling

- Supportive discussion of results and next steps
- Psychological support and bereavement care if needed

Summary and Implementation

- Use this tool to streamline history taking, investigations, and management.
- Apply evidence-based treatments tailored to each case.
- Offer preconception counselling and psychological support as standard care.

Chapter Key Points

- Miscarriage affects 10–20% of pregnancies; recurrent miscarriage warrants structured evaluation.
- Risk factors span genetic, endocrine, immune, anatomical, and lifestyle domains.
- Routine thrombophilia testing is not recommended unless clinically indicated.

2

- Preconception optimization (weight, smoking, alcohol, and thyroid control) is one of the strongest preventive measures.
- Psychological support and early pregnancy monitoring significantly improve patient well-being and outcomes.

Chapter-End Summary

Miscarriage is a multifactorial condition requiring a comprehensive approach to history taking, investigations, and prevention. While many sporadic miscarriages arise from chromosomal abnormalities, recurrent cases often reflect underlying endocrine, immune, or anatomical contributors. Evidence-based prevention focuses on preconception care, appropriate investigations, management of thyroid disease and PCOS, selective use of anticoagulation (only for confirmed APS with other clinical signs), and tailored surgical or medical interventions. Psychological distress is highly prevalent and necessitates structured emotional support. A multidisciplinary model offers the best chance of improving live birth outcomes while minimizing unnecessary treatments.

References

1. Hardy K, Hardy PJ. 1(st) trimester miscarriage: four decades of study. Transl Pediatr. 2015;4(2):189–200. PubMed PMID: 26835373. Pubmed Central PMCID: PMC4729087. Epub 2016/02/03. eng
2. Evaluation and treatment of recurrent pregnancy loss: a committee opinion. Fertil Steril. 2012;98(5):1103–11. PubMed PMID: 22835448. Epub 2012/07/28. eng
3. Magnus MC, Wilcox AJ, Morken NH, Weinberg CR, Håberg SE. Role of maternal age and pregnancy history in risk of miscarriage: prospective register based study. BMJ (Clin Res Ed). 2019;364:l869. PubMed PMID: 30894356. Pubmed Central PMCID: PMC6425455 at www.icmje.org/coi_disclosure.pdf and declare: no support from any organisation for the submitted work; no financial relationships with any organisations that might have an interest in the submitted work in the previous three years; no other relationships or activities that could appear to have influenced the submitted work. Epub 2019/03/22. eng
4. Turesheva A, Aimagambetova G, Ukybassova T, Marat A, Kanabekova P, Kaldygulova L, et al. Recurrent Pregnancy Loss Etiology, Risk Factors, Diagnosis, and Management. Fresh Look into a Full Box. J Clin Med. 2023;12(12) PubMed PMID: 37373766. Pubmed Central PMCID: PMC10298962. Epub 2023/06/28. eng
5. Wyatt PR, Owolabi T, Meier C, Huang T. Age-specific risk of fetal loss observed in a second trimester serum screening population. Am J Obstet Gynecol. 2005;192(1):240–6. PubMed PMID: 15672031. Epub 2005/01/27. eng
6. Rai R, Regan L. Recurrent miscarriage. Lancet (London, England). 2006;368(9535):601–11. PubMed PMID: 16905025. Epub 2006/08/15. eng
7. Saravelos SH, Regan L. Unexplained recurrent pregnancy loss. Obstet Gynecol Clin N Am. 2014;41(1):157–66. PubMed PMID: 24491990. Epub 2014/02/05. eng
8. Frost M, Condon JT. The psychological sequelae of miscarriage: a critical review of the literature. Aust N Z J Psychiatry. 1996;30(1):54–62. PubMed PMID: 8724327. Epub 1996/02/01. eng
9. Johnson MP, Puddifoot JE. The grief response in the partners of women who miscarry. Br J Med Psychol. 1996;69(4):313–27. PubMed PMID: 8989980. Epub 1996/12/01. eng
10. Volgsten H, Jansson C, Svanberg AS, Darj E, Stavreus-Evers A. Longitudinal study of emotional experiences, grief and depressive symptoms in women and men after miscarriage. Midwifery. 2018;64:23–8. PubMed PMID: 29864578. Epub 2018/06/05. eng
11. Reus AD, van Besouw NM, Molenaar NM, Steegers EA, Visser W, de Kuiper RP, et al. An immunological basis for chronic histiocytic intervillositis in recurrent fetal loss. Am J Rep Immunol (New York, NY: 1989). 2013;70(3):230–7. PubMed PMID: 23611029. Epub 2013/04/25. eng
12. Abou-Nassar K, Carrier M, Ramsay T, Rodger MA. The association between antiphospholipid antibodies and placenta mediated complications: a systematic review and meta-analysis. Thromb Res. 2011;128(1):77–85. PubMed PMID: 21420151. Epub 2011/03/23. eng
13. Esplin MS. Management of antiphospholipid syndrome during pregnancy. Clin Obstet Gynecol. 2001;44(1):20–8. PubMed PMID: 11219243. Epub 2001/02/24. eng
14. Zhang BY, Wei YS, Niu JM, Li Y, Miao ZL, Wang ZN. Risk factors for unexplained recurrent spontaneous abortion in a population from

southern China. Int J Gynaecol Obstet. 2010;108(2):135–8. PubMed PMID: 19897189. Epub 2009/11/10. eng
15. Wilcox AJ, Weinberg CR, Baird DD. Risk factors for early pregnancy loss. Epidemiology (Cambridge, MA). 1990;1(5):382–5. PubMed PMID: 2078614. Epub 1990/09/01. eng
16. Venners SA, Wang X, Chen C, Wang L, Chen D, Guang W, et al. Paternal smoking and pregnancy loss: a prospective study using a biomarker of pregnancy. Am J Epidemiol. 2004;159(10):993–1001. PubMed PMID: 15128612. Epub 2004/05/07. eng
17. Metwally M, Saravelos SH, Ledger WL, Li TC. Body mass index and risk of miscarriage in women with recurrent miscarriage. Fertil Steril. 2010;94(1):290–5. PubMed PMID: 19439294. Epub 2009/05/15. eng
18. Pandey S, Pandey S, Maheshwari A, Bhattacharya S. The impact of female obesity on the outcome of fertility treatment. J Human Reprod Sci. 2010;3(2):62–7. PubMed PMID: 21209748. Pubmed Central PMCID: PMC2970793. Epub 2011/01/07. eng
19. Lashen H, Fear K, Sturdee DW. Obesity is associated with increased risk of first trimester and recurrent miscarriage: matched case-control study. Hum Rep (Oxford, England). 2004;19(7):1644–6. PubMed PMID: 15142995. Epub 2004/05/15. eng
20. Lo W, Rai R, Hameed A, Brailsford SR, Al-Ghamdi AA, Regan L. The effect of body mass index on the outcome of pregnancy in women with recurrent miscarriage. J Fam Community Med. 2012;19(3):167–71. PubMed PMID: 23230382. Pubmed Central PMCID: PMC3515955. Epub 2012/12/12. eng
21. Andersen AM, Andersen PK, Olsen J, Grønbæk M, Strandberg-Larsen K. Moderate alcohol intake during pregnancy and risk of fetal death. Int J Epidemiol. 2012;41(2):405–13. PubMed PMID: 22253313. Epub 2012/01/19. eng
22. Avalos LA, Roberts SC, Kaskutas LA, Block G, Li DK. Volume and type of alcohol during early pregnancy and the risk of miscarriage. Subst Use Misuse. 2014;49(11):1437–45. PubMed PMID: 24810392. Pubmed Central PMCID: PMC4183196. Epub 2014/05/09. eng
23. Kolte AM, Nielsen HS, Moltke I, Degn B, Pedersen B, Sunde L, et al. A genome-wide scan in affected sibling pairs with idiopathic recurrent miscarriage suggests genetic linkage. Mol Hum Reprod. 2011;17(6):379–85. PubMed PMID: 21257601. Epub 2011/01/25. eng
24. Ali A, Elfituri A, Doumouchtsis SK, Zini ME, Jan H, Ganapathy R, et al. Managing couples with recurrent miscarriage: A narrative review and practice recommendations. Int J Gynaecol Obstet. 2024;164(2):499–503. PubMed PMID: 37431204. Epub 2023/07/11. eng
25. Zhu X, Li J, Zhu Y, Wang W, Wu X, Yang Y, et al. Application of chromosomal microarray analysis in products of miscarriage. Mol Cytogenet. 2018;11:44. PubMed PMID: 30140311. Pubmed Central PMCID: PMC6098645. Epub 2018/08/25. eng
26. Levy B, Sigurjonsson S, Pettersen B, Maisenbacher MK, Hall MP, Demko Z, et al. Genomic imbalance in products of conception: single-nucleotide polymorphism chromosomal microarray analysis. Obstet Gynecol. 2014;124(2 Pt 1):202–9. PubMed PMID: 25004334. Epub 2014/07/09. eng
27. Zhang T, Sun Y, Chen Z, Li T. Traditional and molecular chromosomal abnormality analysis of products of conception in spontaneous and recurrent miscarriage. BJOG. 2018;125(4):414–20. PubMed PMID: 29220118. Epub 2017/12/09. eng
28. Ogasawara M, Aoki K, Okada S, Suzumori K. Embryonic karyotype of abortuses in relation to the number of previous miscarriages. Fertil Steril. 2000;73(2):300–4. PubMed PMID: 10685533. Epub 2000/02/24. eng
29. DeCherney AN, L. Current Diagnosis & Treatment Obstetrics & Gynecology, Tenth Edition Current Diagnosis & Treatment Obstetric & Gynecologic LANGE CURRENT Series Lange medical book, ISSN 0197-582X. illustrated ed 2007.
30. Benn P. Trisomy 16 and trisomy 16 Mosaicism: a review. Am J Med Genet. 1998;79(2):121–33. PubMed PMID: 9741470. Epub 1998/09/19. eng
31. Barisić I, Zergollern L, Muzinić D, Hitrec V. Risk estimates for balanced reciprocal translocation carriers – prenatal diagnosis experience. Clin Genet. 1996;49(3):145–51. PubMed PMID: 8737980. Epub 1996/03/01. eng
32. Neri G, Serra A, Campana M, Tedeschi B. Reproductive risks for translocation carriers: cytogenetic study and analysis of pregnancy outcome in 58 families. Am J Med Genet. 1983;16(4):535–61. Epub 1983/12/01. eng
33. Barber JC, Cockwell AE, Grant E, Williams S, Dunn R, Ogilvie CM. Is karyotyping couples experiencing recurrent miscarriage worth the cost? BJOG. 2010;117(7):885–8. PubMed PMID: 20482539. Epub 2010/05/21. eng
34. Franssen MT, Korevaar JC, Leschot NJ, Bossuyt PM, Knegt AC, Gerssen-Schoorl KB, et al. Selective chromosome analysis in couples with two or more miscarriages: case-control study. BMJ (Clin Res Ed). 2005;331(7509):137–41. PubMed PMID: 15985440. Pubmed Central PMCID: PMC558698. Epub 2005/06/30. eng
35. Bozdag G, Mumusoglu S, Zengin D, Karabulut E, Yildiz BO. The prevalence and phenotypic features of polycystic ovary syndrome: a systematic review and meta-analysis. Hum Rep (Oxford, England). 2016;31(12):2841–55. PubMed PMID: 27664216. Epub 2016/09/25. eng

36. Banu J, Fatima P, Sultana P, Chowdhury MA, Begum N, Anwary SA, et al. Association of infertile patients having polycystic ovarian syndrome with recurrent miscarriage. MMJ. 2014;23(4):770–3. PubMed PMID: 25481599. Epub 2014/12/08. eng
37. Luo L, Gu F, Jie H, Ding C, Zhao Q, Wang Q, et al. Early miscarriage rate in lean polycystic ovary syndrome women after euploid embryo transfer – a matched-pair study. Reprod Biomed Online. 2017;35(5):576–82. PubMed PMID: 28802704. Epub 2017/08/15. eng
38. Truelsen MK, Clausen HV. Polycystic ovary syndrome and miscarriage. Ugeskr Laeger. 2011;173(6):425–30. PubMed PMID: 21299936. Epub 2011/02/09. Polycystisk ovariesyndrom og spontan abort. dan
39. Wartena R, Matjila M. Polycystic ovary syndrome and recurrent pregnancy loss, a review of literature. Front Endocrinol. 2023;14:1183060. PubMed PMID: 38027110. Pubmed Central PMCID: PMC10643146. Epub 2023/11/29. eng
40. Palomba S, Santagni S, La Sala GB. Progesterone administration for luteal phase deficiency in human reproduction: an old or new issue? J Ovarian Res. 2015;8:77. PubMed PMID: 26585269. Pubmed Central PMCID: PMC4653859. Epub 2015/11/21. eng
41. Smith ML, Schust DJ. Endocrinology and recurrent early pregnancy loss. Semin Reprod Med. 2011;29(6):482–90. PubMed PMID: 22161461. Epub 2011/12/14. eng
42. Thomsen LH, Kesmodel US, Andersen CY, Humaidan P. Daytime Variation in Serum Progesterone During the Mid-Luteal Phase in Women Undergoing In Vitro Fertilization Treatment. Front Endocrinol. 2018;9:92. PubMed PMID: 29615975. Pubmed Central PMCID: PMC5867298. Epub 2018/04/05. eng
43. Annos T, Thompson IE, Taymor ML. Luteal phase deficiency and infertility: difficulties encountered in diagnosis and treatment. Obstet Gynecol. 1980;55(6):705–10. PubMed PMID: 7383457. Epub 1980/06/01. eng
44. Jordan J, Craig K, Clifton DK, Soules MR. Luteal phase defect: the sensitivity and specificity of diagnostic methods in common clinical use. Fertil Steril. 1994;62(1):54–62. PubMed PMID: 8005304. Epub 1994/07/01. eng
45. Balasch J, Vanrell JA. Luteal phase deficiency: an inadequate endometrial response to normal hormone stimulation. Int J Fertil. 1986;31(5):368–71. PubMed PMID: 2898441. Epub 1986/11/01. eng
46. Daya S, Ward S, Burrows E. Progesterone profiles in luteal phase defect cycles and outcome of progesterone treatment in patients with recurrent spontaneous abortion. Am J Obstet Gynecol. 1988;158(2):225–32. PubMed PMID: 3341399. Epub 1988/02/01. eng
47. Baird DD, Weinberg CR, Wilcox AJ, McConnaughey DR, Musey PI, Collins DC. Hormonal profiles of natural conception cycles ending in early, unrecognized pregnancy loss. J Clin Endocrinol Metab. 1991;72(4):793–800. PubMed PMID: 2005203. Epub 1991/04/01. eng
48. Ogasawara M, Kajiura S, Katano K, Aoyama T, Aoki K. Are serum progesterone levels predictive of recurrent miscarriage in future pregnancies? Fertil Steril. 1997;68(5):806–9. PubMed PMID: 9389806. Epub 1997/12/09. eng
49. Coomarasamy A, Williams H, Truchanowicz E, Seed PT, Small R, Quenby S, et al. A Randomized Trial of Progesterone in Women with Recurrent Miscarriages. N Engl J Med. 2015;373(22):2141–8. PubMed PMID: 26605928. Epub 2015/11/26. eng
50. Saccone G, Schoen C, Franasiak JM, Scott RT Jr, Berghella V. Supplementation with progestogens in the first trimester of pregnancy to prevent miscarriage in women with unexplained recurrent miscarriage: a systematic review and meta-analysis of randomized, controlled trials. Fertil Steril. 2017;107(2):430–8 e3. PubMed PMID: 27887710. Epub 2016/11/27. eng
51. Shehata H, Elfituri A, Doumouchtsis SK, Zini ME, Ali A, Jan H, et al. FIGO Good Practice Recommendations on the use of progesterone in the management of recurrent first-trimester miscarriage. Int J Gynaecol Obstet. 2023;161(Suppl 1):3–16. PubMed PMID: 36958854. Epub 2023/03/24. eng
52. Bahn Chair RS, Burch HB, Cooper DS, Garber JR, Greenlee MC, Klein I, et al. Hyperthyroidism and other causes of thyrotoxicosis: management guidelines of the American Thyroid Association and American Association of Clinical Endocrinologists. Thyroid. 2011;21(6):593–646. PubMed PMID: 21510801. Epub 2011/04/23. eng
53. Andersen SL, Olsen J, Wu CS, Laurberg P. Spontaneous abortion, stillbirth and hyperthyroidism: a Danish population-based study. Eur Thyroid J. 2014;3(3):164–72. PubMed PMID: 25538898. Pubmed Central PMCID: PMC4224233. Epub 2014/12/30. eng
54. Rao VR, Lakshmi A, Sadhnani MD. Prevalence of hypothyroidism in recurrent pregnancy loss in first trimester. Indian J Med Sci. 2008;62(9):357–61. PubMed PMID: 18923214. Epub 2008/10/17. eng
55. van den Boogaard E, Vissenberg R, Land JA, van Wely M, van der Post JA, Goddijn M, et al. Significance of (sub)clinical thyroid dysfunction and thyroid autoimmunity before conception and in early pregnancy: a systematic review. Hum Reprod Update. 2011;17(5):605–19. PubMed PMID: 21622978. Epub 2011/05/31. eng
56. Lata K, Dutta P, Sridhar S, Rohilla M, Srinivasan A, Prashad GR, et al. Thyroid autoimmunity and obstetric outcomes in women with recurrent miscarriage: a case-control study. Endocr Connect. 2013;2(2):118–24. PubMed PMID: 23802061.

Pubmed Central PMCID: PMC3691574. Epub 2013/06/27. eng
57. van Dijk MM, Vissenberg R, Bisschop PH, Dawood F, van Wely M, Goddijn M, et al. Is subclinical hypothyroidism associated with lower live birth rates in women who have experienced unexplained recurrent miscarriage? Reprod Biomed Online. 2016;33(6):745–51. PubMed PMID: 27720162. Epub 2016/10/11. eng
58. Miodovnik M, Skillman C, Holroyde JC, Butler JB, Wendel JS, Siddiqi TA. Elevated maternal glycohemoglobin in early pregnancy and spontaneous abortion among insulin-dependent diabetic women. Am J Obstet Gynecol. 1985;153(4):439–42. PubMed PMID: 4050917. Epub 1985/10/15. eng
59. Greene MF, Hare JW, Cloherty JP, Benacerraf BR, Soeldner JS. First-trimester hemoglobin A1 and risk for major malformation and spontaneous abortion in diabetic pregnancy. Teratology. 1989;39(3):225–31. PubMed PMID: 2727930. Epub 1989/03/01. eng
60. Reece EA, Homko CJ. Why do diabetic women deliver malformed infants? Clin Obstet Gynecol. 2000;43(1):32–45. PubMed PMID: 10694986. Epub 2000/03/01. eng
61. Hod M. Advances in the understanding of diabetic embryopathy: signal transduction. Early Pregnancy Biol Med. 1996;2(2):121–8. PubMed PMID: 9363209. Epub 1996/06/01. eng
62. Sadler TW, Hunter ES 3rd, Wynn RE, Phillips LS. Evidence for multifactorial origin of diabetes-induced embryopathies. Diabetes. 1989;38(1):70–4. PubMed PMID: 2909414. Epub 1989/01/01. eng
63. Eriksson UJ, Borg LA. Diabetes and embryonic malformations. Role of substrate-induced free-oxygen radical production for dysmorphogenesis in cultured rat embryos. Diabetes. 1993;42(3):411–9. PubMed PMID: 8432412. Epub 1993/03/01. eng
64. Reece EA, Homko CJ, Wu YK. Multifactorial basis of the syndrome of diabetic embryopathy. Teratology. 1996;54(4):171–82. PubMed PMID: 9122886. Epub 1996/10/01. eng
65. Weng J, Couture C, Girard S. Innate and Adaptive Immune Systems in Physiological and Pathological Pregnancy. Biology. 2023;12(3) PubMed PMID: 36979094. Pubmed Central PMCID: PMC10045867. Epub 2023/03/30. eng
66. Trundley A, Moffett A. Human uterine leukocytes and pregnancy. Tissue Antigens. 2004;63(1):1–12. PubMed PMID: 14651517. Epub 2003/12/04. eng
67. King A. Uterine leukocytes and decidualization. Hum Reprod Update. 2000;6(1):28–36. PubMed PMID: 10711827. Epub 2000/03/11. eng
68. Dosiou C, Giudice LC. Natural killer cells in pregnancy and recurrent pregnancy loss: endocrine and immunologic perspectives. Endocr Rev. 2005;26(1):44–62. PubMed PMID: 15689572. Epub 2005/02/04. eng
69. Seshadri S, Sunkara SK. Natural killer cells in female infertility and recurrent miscarriage: a systematic review and meta-analysis. Hum Reprod Update. 2014;20(3):429–38. PubMed PMID: 24285824. Epub 2013/11/29. eng
70. King K, Smith S, Chapman M, Sacks G. Detailed analysis of peripheral blood natural killer (NK) cells in women with recurrent miscarriage. Hum Rep (Oxford, England). 2010;25(1):52–8. PubMed PMID: 19819893. Epub 2009/10/13. eng
71. Beer AE, Kwak JY, Ruiz JE. Immunophenotypic profiles of peripheral blood lymphocytes in women with recurrent pregnancy losses and in infertile women with multiple failed in vitro fertilization cycles. Am J Rep Immunol (New York, NY: 1989). 1996;35(4):376–82. PubMed PMID: 8739457. Epub 1996/04/01. eng
72. Guerrero B, Hassouneh F, Delgado E, Casado JG, Tarazona R. Natural killer cells in recurrent miscarriage: an overview. J Reprod Immunol. 2020;142:103209. PubMed PMID: 32992208. Epub 2020/09/30. eng
73. Kuon RJ, Vomstein K, Weber M, Müller F, Seitz C, Wallwiener S, et al. The "killer cell story" in recurrent miscarriage: Association between activated peripheral lymphocytes and uterine natural killer cells. J Reprod Immunol. 2017;119:9–14. PubMed PMID: 27865124. Epub 2016/11/20. eng
74. Bao SH, Shuai W, Tong J, Wang L, Chen P, Sun J. Increased expression of Toll-like receptor 3 in decidual natural killer cells of patients with unexplained recurrent spontaneous miscarriage. Eur J Obstet Gynecol Reprod Biol. 2012;165(2):326–30. PubMed PMID: 22944378. Epub 2012/09/05. eng
75. Xu L, Qiu T, Wang Y, Chen Y, Cheng W. Expression of C-type lectin receptors and Toll-like receptors in decidua of patients with unexplained recurrent spontaneous abortion. Reprod Fertil Dev. 2017;29(8):1613–24. PubMed PMID: 29482715. Epub 2018/02/28. eng
76. Piccinni MP, Giudizi MG, Biagiotti R, Beloni L, Giannarini L, Sampognaro S, et al. Progesterone favors the development of human T helper cells producing Th2-type cytokines and promotes both IL-4 production and membrane CD30 expression in established Th1 cell clones. J Immunol (Baltimore, MD: 1950). 1995;155(1):128–33. PubMed PMID: 7541410. Epub 1995/07/01. eng
77. Marzi M, Vigano A, Trabattoni D, Villa ML, Salvaggio A, Clerici E, et al. Characterization of type 1 and type 2 cytokine production profile in physiologic and pathologic human pregnancy. Clin Exp Immunol. 1996;106(1):127–33. PubMed PMID: 8870710. Pubmed Central PMCID: PMC2200555. Epub 1996/10/01. eng
78. Sakaguchi S, Yamaguchi T, Nomura T, Ono M. Regulatory T cells and immune tolerance.

2

Cell. 2008;133(5):775–87. PubMed PMID: 18510923. Epub 2008/05/31. eng
79. Mold JE, Michaëlsson J, Burt TD, Muench MO, Beckerman KP, Busch MP, et al. Maternal alloantigens promote the development of tolerogenic fetal regulatory T cells in utero. Science (New York, NY). 2008;322(5907):1562–5. PubMed PMID: 19056990. Pubmed Central PMCID: PMC2648820. Epub 2008/12/06. eng
80. Laird SM, Tuckerman EM, Cork BA, Linjawi S, Blakemore AI, Li TC. A review of immune cells and molecules in women with recurrent miscarriage. Hum Reprod Update. 2003;9(2):163–74. PubMed PMID: 12751778. Epub 2003/05/20. eng
81. Berman J, Girardi G, Salmon JE. TNF-alpha is a critical effector and a target for therapy in antiphospholipid antibody-induced pregnancy loss. J Immunol (Baltimore, MD: 1950). 2005;174(1):485–90. PubMed PMID: 15611274. Epub 2004/12/22. eng
82. Silver RM, Lohner WS, Daynes RA, Mitchell MD, Branch DW. Lipopolysaccharide-induced fetal death: the role of tumor-necrosis factor alpha. Biol Reprod. 1994;50(5):1108–12. PubMed PMID: 8025168. Epub 1994/05/01. eng
83. Wang WJ, Hao CF, Yi L, Yin GJ, Bao SH, Qiu LH, et al. Increased prevalence of T helper 17 (Th17) cells in peripheral blood and decidua in unexplained recurrent spontaneous abortion patients. J Reprod Immunol. 2010;84(2):164–70. PubMed PMID: 20106535. Epub 2010/01/29. eng
84. Figueiredo AS, Schumacher A. The T helper type 17/regulatory T cell paradigm in pregnancy. Immunology. 2016;148(1):13–21. PubMed PMID: 26855005. Pubmed Central PMCID: PMC4819144. Epub 2016/02/09. eng
85. Thangaratinam S, Tan A, Knox E, Kilby MD, Franklyn J, Coomarasamy A. Association between thyroid autoantibodies and miscarriage and preterm birth: meta-analysis of evidence. BMJ (Clin Res Ed). 2011;342:d2616. PubMed PMID: 21558126. Pubmed Central PMCID: PMC3089879 form at www.icmje.org/coi_disclosure.pdf (available on request from the corresponding author) and declare: no support from any organisation for the submitted work; no financial relationships with any organisations that might have an interest in the submitted work in the previous three years; no other relationships or activities that could appear to have influenced the submitted work. The authors have been funded by the NIHR (National Institute of Health Research, UK) EME Programme (09-100-10) to conduct a multicentre placebo-controlled randomised trial on the pregnancy effects of levothyroxine treatment in thyroid antibody positive women with normal thyroid function (the TABLET trial). Epub 2011/05/12. eng
86. Cavalcante MB, Cavalcante C, Sarno M, da Silva ACB, Barini R. Antinuclear antibodies and recurrent miscarriage: Systematic review and meta-analysis. Am J Rep Immunol (New York, NY: 1989). 2020;83(3):e13215. PubMed PMID: 31821640. Epub 2019/12/11. eng
87. Ticconi C, Inversetti A, Logruosso E, Ghio M, Casadei L, Selmi C, et al. Antinuclear antibodies positivity in women in reproductive age: from infertility to adverse obstetrical outcomes – A meta-analysis. J Reprod Immunol. 2023;155:103794. PubMed PMID: 36621091. Epub 2023/01/10. eng
88. Chen S, Yang G, Wu P, Sun Y, Dai F, He Y, et al. Antinuclear antibodies positivity is a risk factor of recurrent pregnancy loss: A meta-analysis. Semin Arthritis Rheum. 2020;50(4):534–43. PubMed PMID: 32442739. Epub 2020/05/23. eng
89. Brenner B. Inherited thrombophilia and pregnancy loss. Thromb Haemost. 1999;82(2):634–40. PubMed PMID: 10605761. Epub 1999/12/22. eng
90. Kutteh WH, Triplett DA. Thrombophilias and recurrent pregnancy loss. Semin Reprod Med. 2006;24(1):54–66. PubMed PMID: 16418978. Epub 2006/01/19. eng
91. Esmon CT. Protein-C: biochemistry, physiology, and clinical implications. Blood. 1983;62(6):1155–8. PubMed PMID: 6315112. Epub 1983/12/01. eng
92. Puri S, Grover AK, Narula AK, Choudhry PN, Gupta AP. Atypical presentation of pulmonary embolism and deep vein thrombosis due to protein S deficiency in a young female with chest pain. The Egyptian. J Intern Med. 2022;34(1):37.
93. Rey E, Kahn SR, David M, Shrier I. Thrombophilic disorders and fetal loss: a meta-analysis. Lancet (London, England). 2003;361(9361):901–8. PubMed PMID: 12648968. Epub 2003/03/22. eng
94. Preston FE, Rosendaal FR, Walker ID, Briët E, Berntorp E, Conard J, et al. Increased fetal loss in women with heritable thrombophilia. Lancet (London, England). 1996;348(9032):913–6. PubMed PMID: 8843809. Epub 1996/10/05. eng
95. Alfirevic Z, Roberts D, Martlew V. How strong is the association between maternal thrombophilia and adverse pregnancy outcome? A systematic review. Eur J Obstet Gynecol Reprod Biol. 2002;101(1):6–14. PubMed PMID: 11803092. Epub 2002/01/23. eng
96. Clouse LH, Comp PC. The regulation of hemostasis: the protein C system. N Engl J Med. 1986;314(20):1298–304. PubMed PMID: 3010107. Epub 1986/05/15. eng
97. Cramer TJ, Gale AJ. The anticoagulant function of coagulation factor V. Thromb Haemost. 2012;107(1):15–21. PubMed PMID: 22116556. Epub 2011/11/26. eng
98. Rees DC, Cox M, Clegg JB. World distribution of factor V Leiden. Lancet (London, England). 1995;346(8983):1133–4. PubMed PMID: 7475606. Epub 1995/10/28. eng

99. Ridker PM, Miletich JP, Hennekens CH, Buring JE. Ethnic distribution of factor V Leiden in 4047 men and women. Implications for venous thromboembolism screening. JAMA. 1997;277(16):1305–7. PubMed PMID: 9109469. Epub 1997/04/23. eng
100. Awidi A, Shannak M, Bseiso A, Kailani MA, Kailani MA, Omar N, et al. High prevalence of factor V Leiden in healthy Jordanian Arabs. Thromb Haemost. 1999;81(4):582–4. PubMed PMID: 10235443. Epub 1999/05/11. eng
101. Irani-Hakime N, Tamim H, Kreidy R, Almawi WY. The prevalence of factor V R506Q mutation-Leiden among apparently healthy Lebanese. Am J Hematol. 2000;65(1):45–9. PubMed PMID: 10936863. Epub 2000/08/11. eng
102. Taher A, Khalil I, Shamseddine A, El-Ahdab F, Bazarbachi A. High prevalence of Factor V Leiden mutation among healthy individuals and patients with deep venous thrombosis in Lebanon: is the eastern Mediterranean region the area of origin of this mutation? Thromb Haemost. 2001;86(2):723–4. PubMed PMID: 11522037. Epub 2001/08/28. eng
103. Shehata H, Ali A, Silva-Edge M, Haroon S, Elfituri A, Viswanatha R, et al. Thrombophilia screening in women with recurrent first trimester miscarriage: is it time to stop testing? – a cohort study and systematic review of the literature. BMJ Open. 2022;12(7):e059519. PubMed PMID: 35831047. Pubmed Central PMCID: PMC9280906. Epub 2022/07/14. eng
104. Meeks SL, Abshire TC. Abnormalities of prothrombin: a review of the pathophysiology, diagnosis, and treatment. Haemophilia. 2008;14(6):1159–63. PubMed PMID: 19141155. Epub 2009/01/15. eng
105. Margaglione M, Brancaccio V, Giuliani N, D'Andrea G, Cappucci G, Iannaccone L, et al. Increased risk for venous thrombosis in carriers of the prothrombin G-->A20210 gene variant. Ann Intern Med. 1998;129(2):89–93. PubMed PMID: 9669991. Epub 1998/07/21. eng
106. Lim MY, Deal AM, Kim S, Musty MD, Conard J, Simioni P, et al. Thrombophilic risk of individuals with rare compound factor V Leiden and prothrombin G20210A polymorphisms: an international case series of 100 individuals. Eur J Haematol. 2016;97(4):353–60. PubMed PMID: 26773706. Epub 2016/01/17. eng
107. Bradley LA, Palomaki GE, Bienstock J, Varga E, Scott JA. Can Factor V Leiden and prothrombin G20210A testing in women with recurrent pregnancy loss result in improved pregnancy outcomes?: Results from a targeted evidence-based review. Genet Med. 2012;14(1):39–50. PubMed PMID: 22237430. Epub 2012/01/13. eng
108. Büller HR, ten Cate JW. Acquired antithrombin III deficiency: laboratory diagnosis, incidence, clinical implications, and treatment with antithrombin III concentrate. Am J Med. 1989;87(3B):44S–8S. PubMed PMID: 2679070. Epub 1989/09/11. eng
109. Demers C, Ginsberg JS, Hirsh J, Henderson P, Blajchman MA. Thrombosis in antithrombin-III-deficient persons. Report of a large kindred and literature review. Ann Intern Med. 1992;116(9):754–61. Epub 1992/05/01. eng
110. Hickey SE, Curry CJ, Toriello HV. ACMG Practice Guideline: lack of evidence for MTHFR polymorphism testing. Genet Med. 2013;15(2):153–6. PubMed PMID: 23288205. Epub 2013/01/05. eng
111. Su MT, Lin SH, Chen YC, Kuo PL. Genetic association studies of ACE and PAI-1 genes in women with recurrent pregnancy loss: a systematic review and meta-analysis. Thromb Haemost. 2013;109(1):8–15. PubMed PMID: 23179239. PubMed PMID: 1489375. Epub 2012/11/28. eng
112. Arachchillage DJ, Platton S, Hickey K, Chu J, Pickering M, Sommerville P, et al. Guidelines on the investigation and management of antiphospholipid syndrome. Br J Haematol. 2024;205(3):855–80. PubMed PMID: 39031476. Epub 2024/07/20 20:46. eng
113. Rai RS, Regan L, Clifford K, Pickering W, Dave M, Mackie I, et al. Antiphospholipid antibodies and beta 2-glycoprotein-I in 500 women with recurrent miscarriage: results of a comprehensive screening approach. Hum Rep (Oxford, England). 1995;10(8):2001–5. PubMed PMID: 8567830. Epub 1995/08/01. eng
114. Viall CA, Chamley LW. Histopathology in the placentae of women with antiphospholipid antibodies: a systematic review of the literature. Autoimmun Rev. 2015;14(5):446–71. PubMed PMID: 25620498. Epub 2015/01/27. eng
115. Levy RA, Avvad E, Oliveira J, Porto LC. Placental pathology in antiphospholipid syndrome. Lupus. 1998;7(Suppl 2):S81–5. PubMed PMID: 9814679. Epub 1998/11/14. eng
116. Pierangeli SS, Chen PP, Raschi E, Scurati S, Grossi C, Borghi MO, et al. Antiphospholipid antibodies and the antiphospholipid syndrome: pathogenic mechanisms. Semin Thromb Hemost. 2008;34(3):236–50. PubMed PMID: 18720303. Epub 2008/08/23. eng
117. Alijotas-Reig J, Esteve-Valverde E, Anunciación-Llunell A, Marques-Soares J, Pardos-Gea J, Miró-Mur F. Pathogenesis, diagnosis and management of obstetric antiphospholipid syndrome: a comprehensive review. J Clin Med. 2022;11(3) PubMed PMID: 35160128. Pubmed Central PMCID: PMC8836886. Epub 2022/02/16. eng
118. Pantham P, Abrahams VM, Chamley LW. The role of anti-phospholipid antibodies in autoimmune reproductive failure. Reproduction (Cambridge, England). 2016;151(5):R79–90. PubMed PMID: 26884418. Epub 2016/02/18. eng
119. Mulla MJ, Pasternak MC, Salmon JE, Chamley LW, Abrahams VM. Role of NOD2 in antiphos-

pholipid antibody-induced and bacterial MDP amplification of trophoblast inflammation. J Autoimmun. 2019;98:103–12. PubMed PMID: 30594350. Epub 2018/12/31. eng

2

120. Knight JS, Branch DW, Ortel TL. Antiphospholipid syndrome: advances in diagnosis, pathogenesis, and management. BMJ (Clin Res Ed). 2023;380:e069717. PubMed PMID: 36849186. Epub 2023/02/28. eng
121. Tripodi A. Laboratory testing for lupus anticoagulants: a review of issues affecting results. Clin Chem. 2007;53(9):1629–35. PubMed PMID: 17712001. Epub 2007/08/23. eng
122. Andreoli L, Chighizola CB, Iaccarino L, Botta A, Gerosa M, Ramoni V, et al. Immunology of pregnancy and reproductive health in autoimmune rheumatic diseases. Update from the 11(th) International Conference on Reproduction, Pregnancy and Rheumatic Diseases. Autoimmun Rev. 2023;22(3):103259. PubMed PMID: 36549355. Epub 2022/12/23. eng
123. Girardi G. Complement inhibition keeps mothers calm and avoids fetal rejection. Immunol Investig. 2008;37(5):645–59. PubMed PMID: 18716942. Epub 2008/08/22. eng
124. Kim MY, Guerra MM, Kaplowitz E, Laskin CA, Petri M, Branch DW, et al. Complement activation predicts adverse pregnancy outcome in patients with systemic lupus erythematosus and/or antiphospholipid antibodies. Ann Rheum Dis. 2018;77(4):549–55. PubMed PMID: 29371202. Pubmed Central PMCID: PMC6037302. Epub 2018/01/27. eng
125. Clark CA, Davidovits J, Spitzer KA, Laskin CA. The lupus anticoagulant: results from 2257 patients attending a high-risk pregnancy clinic. Blood. 2013;122(3):341–7. quiz 466. PubMed PMID: 23649468. Epub 2013/05/08. eng
126. Bowman ZS, Wünsche V, Porter TF, Silver RM, Branch DW. Prevalence of antiphospholipid antibodies and risk of subsequent adverse obstetric outcomes in women with prior pregnancy loss. J Reprod Immunol. 2015;107:59–63. PubMed PMID: 25453202. Epub 2014/12/03. eng
127. Barbhaiya M, Zuily S, Naden R, Hendry A, Manneville F, Amigo MC, et al. 2023 ACR/EULAR antiphospholipid syndrome classification criteria. Ann Rheum Dis. 2023;82(10):1258–70. PubMed PMID: 37640450. Epub 2023/08/29. eng
128. Propst AM, Hill JA 3rd. Anatomic factors associated with recurrent pregnancy loss. Semin Reprod Med. 2000;18(4):341–50. PubMed PMID: 11355792. Epub 2001/05/18. eng
129. Grimbizis GF, Gordts S, Di Spiezio SA, Brucker S, De Angelis C, Gergolet M, et al. The ESHRE/ESGE consensus on the classification of female genital tract congenital anomalies. Hum Reprod (Oxford, England). 2013;28(8):2032–44. PubMed PMID: 23771171. Pubmed Central PMCID: PMC3712660. Epub 2013/06/19. eng
130. Pfeifer S, Butts S, Dumesic D, Gracia C, Vernon M, Fossum G, et al. Uterine septum: a guideline. Fertil Steril. 2016;106(3):530–40.
131. Fox NS, Roman AS, Stern EM, Gerber RS, Saltzman DH, Rebarber A. Type of congenital uterine anomaly and adverse pregnancy outcomes. J Matern Fetal Neonatal Med. 2014;27(9):949–53. PubMed PMID: 24050215. Epub 2013/09/21. eng
132. Kim MA, Kim HS, Kim YH. Reproductive, Obstetric and Neonatal Outcomes in Women with Congenital Uterine Anomalies: A Systematic Review and Meta-Analysis. J Clin Med. 2021;10(21) PubMed PMID: 34768344. Pubmed Central PMCID: PMC8584292. Epub 2021/11/14. eng
133. Chan YY, Jayaprakasan K, Tan A, Thornton JG, Coomarasamy A, Raine-Fenning NJ. Reproductive outcomes in women with congenital uterine anomalies: a systematic review. Ultrasound Obstet Gynecol. 2011;38(4):371–82. PubMed PMID: 21830244. Epub 2011/08/11. eng
134. Hooker AB, Lemmers M, Thurkow AL, Heymans MW, Opmeer BC, Brölmann HA, et al. Systematic review and meta-analysis of intrauterine adhesions after miscarriage: prevalence, risk factors and long-term reproductive outcome. Hum Reprod Update. 2014;20(2):262–78. PubMed PMID: 24082042. Epub 2013/10/02. eng
135. Hartmann KE, Velez Edwards DR, Savitz DA, Jonsson-Funk ML, Wu P, Sundermann AC, et al. Prospective Cohort Study of Uterine Fibroids and Miscarriage Risk. Am J Epidemiol. 2017;186(10):1140–8. PubMed PMID: 28591761. Pubmed Central PMCID: PMC5860279. Epub 2017/06/08. eng
136. Saravelos SH, Yan J, Rehmani H, Li TC. The prevalence and impact of fibroids and their treatment on the outcome of pregnancy in women with recurrent miscarriage. Hum Rep (Oxford, England). 2011;26(12):3274–9. PubMed PMID: 21954281. Epub 2011/09/29. eng
137. Baradwan S, Shafi D, Baradwan A, Bashir MS, Al-Jaroudi D. The effect of endometrial thickness on pregnancy outcome in patients with Asherman's syndrome post-hysteroscopic adhesiolysis. Int J Women's Health. 2018;10:77–82. PubMed PMID: 29483785. Pubmed Central PMCID: PMC5813766. Epub 2018/02/28. eng
138. Kitaya K, Matsubayashi H, Yamaguchi K, Nishiyama R, Takaya Y, Ishikawa T, et al. Chronic endometritis: potential cause of infertility and obstetric and neonatal complications. Am J Rep Immunol (New York, NY: 1989). 2016;75(1):13–22. PubMed PMID: 26478517. Epub 2015/10/20. eng
139. Kitaya K, Ishikawa T. Chronic endometritis: simple can be harder than complex? Fertil Steril. 2021;115(6):1443–4. PubMed PMID: 33892957. Epub 2021/04/25. eng
140. Robinson L, Gallos ID, Conner SJ, Rajkhowa M, Miller D, Lewis S, et al. The effect of sperm DNA

fragmentation on miscarriage rates: a systematic review and meta-analysis. Hum Rep (Oxford, England). 2012;27(10):2908–17. PubMed PMID: 22791753. Epub 2012/07/14. eng
141. Choi HY, Kim SK, Kim SH, Choi YM, Jee BC. Impact of sperm DNA fragmentation on clinical in vitro fertilization outcomes. Clin Exp Reprod Med. 2017;44(4):224–31. PubMed PMID: 29376020. Pubmed Central PMCID: PMC5783920. Epub 2018/01/30. eng
142. Carlini T, Paoli D, Pelloni M, Faja F, Dal Lago A, Lombardo F, et al. Sperm DNA fragmentation in Italian couples with recurrent pregnancy loss. Reprod Biomed Online. 2017;34(1):58–65. PubMed PMID: 27838218. Epub 2016/11/14. eng
143. Saadaoui M, Singh P, Ortashi O, Al Khodor S. Role of the vaginal microbiome in miscarriage: exploring the relationship. Front Cell Infect Microbiol. 2023;13:1232825. PubMed PMID: 37780845. Pubmed Central PMCID: PMC10533927. Epub 2023/10/02. eng
144. Gudnadottir U, Debelius JW, Du J, Hugerth LW, Danielsson H, Schuppe-Koistinen I, et al. The vaginal microbiome and the risk of preterm birth: a systematic review and network meta-analysis. Sci Rep. 2022;12(1):7926. PubMed PMID: 35562576. Pubmed Central PMCID: PMC9106729. Epub 2022/05/14. eng
145. Lebedeva OP, Popov VN, Syromyatnikov MY, Starkova NN, Maslov AY, Kozarenko ON, et al. Female reproductive tract microbiome and early miscarriages. APMIS. 2023;131(2):61–76. PubMed PMID: 36511842. Pubmed Central PMCID: PMC10107729. Epub 2022/12/14. eng
146. Taylor BD, Wise LA. Understanding the impact of the vaginal microbiota on miscarriage: Are we there yet? Paediatr Perinat Epidemiol. 2024;38(7):612–4. PubMed PMID: 39109608. Pubmed Central PMCID: PMC11567085. Epub 2024/08/07. eng
147. Shi Y, Yamada H, Sasagawa Y, Tanimura K, Deguchi M. Uterine endometrium microbiota and pregnancy outcome in women with recurrent pregnancy loss. J Reprod Immunol. 2022;152:103653. PubMed PMID: 35717684. Epub 2022/06/20. eng
148. Quenby S, Booth K, Hiller L, Coomarasamy A, de Jong PG, Hamulyák EN, et al. Heparin for women with recurrent miscarriage and inherited thrombophilia (ALIFE2): an international open-label, randomised controlled trial. Lancet. 2023;402(10395):54–61.
149. Franssen MT, Korevaar JC, van der Veen F, Leschot NJ, Bossuyt PM, Goddijn M. Reproductive outcome after chromosome analysis in couples with two or more miscarriages: index [corrected]-control study. BMJ (Clin Res Ed). 2006;332(7544):759–63. PubMed PMID: 16495333. Pubmed Central PMCID: PMC1420685. Epub 2006/02/24. eng
150. Haddock L, Gordon S, Lewis SEM, Larsen P, Shehata A, Shehata H. Sperm DNA fragmentation is a novel biomarker for early pregnancy loss. Reprod Biomed Online. 2021;42(1):175–84. PubMed PMID: 33082108. Epub 2020/10/22. eng
151. Quenby S, Gallos ID, Dhillon-Smith RK, Podesek M, Stephenson MD, Fisher J, et al. Miscarriage matters: the epidemiological, physical, psychological, and economic costs of early pregnancy loss. Lancet (London, England). 2021;397(10285):1658–67. PubMed PMID: 33915094. Epub 2021/04/30. eng
152. Dhillon-Smith RK, Boelaert K, Jeve YB, Maheshwari A, Coomarasamy A. Subclinical hypothyroidism and antithyroid autoantibodies in women with subfertility or recurrent pregnancy loss: Scientific Impact Paper No. 70 June 2022: Scientific Impact Paper No. 70 June 2022. BJOG. 2022;129(12):e75–88. PubMed PMID: 35765760. Epub 2022/06/30. eng
153. Dhillon-Smith RK, Middleton LJ, Sunner KK, Cheed V, Baker K, Farrell-Carver S, et al. Levothyroxine in Women with Thyroid Peroxidase Antibodies before Conception. N Engl J Med. 2019;380(14):1316–25. PubMed PMID: 30907987. Epub 2019/03/26. eng
154. Swyer GI, Daley D. Progesterone implantation in habitual abortion. Br Med J. 1953;1(4819):1073–7. PubMed PMID: 13042138. Pubmed Central PMCID: PMC2016475. Epub 1953/05/16. eng
155. Society for Maternal-Fetal Medicine Publications Committee waoVB. Progesterone and preterm birth prevention: translating clinical trials data into clinical practice. Am J Obstet Gynecol. 2012;206(5):376–86. PubMed PMID: 22542113. Epub 2012/05/01. eng
156. Meis PJ, Klebanoff M, Thom E, Dombrowski MP, Sibai B, Moawad AH, et al. Prevention of recurrent preterm delivery by 17 alpha-hydroxyprogesterone caproate. N Engl J Med. 2003;348(24):2379–85. PubMed PMID: 12802023. Epub 2003/06/13. eng
157. Szekeres-Bartho J, Par G, Dombay G, Smart YC, Volgyi Z. The antiabortive effect of progesterone-induced blocking factor in mice is manifested by modulating NK activity. Cell Immunol. 1997;177(2):194–9. PubMed PMID: 9178647. Epub 1997/05/01. eng
158. Teede HJ, Tay CT, Laven JJE, Dokras A, Moran LJ, Piltonen TT, et al. Recommendations From the 2023 International Evidence-based Guideline for the Assessment and Management of Polycystic Ovary Syndrome. J Clin Endocrinol Metab. 2023;108(10):2447–69. PubMed PMID: 37580314. Pubmed Central PMCID: PMC10505534. Epub 2023/08/15. eng
159. Notaro ALG, Neto FTL. The use of metformin in women with polycystic ovary syndrome: an updated review. J Assist Reprod Genet. 2022;39(3):573–9. PubMed PMID: 35156149.

Pubmed Central PMCID: PMC8995234. Epub 2022/02/15. eng
160. Løvvik TS, Carlsen SM, Salvesen Ø, Steffensen B, Bixo M, Gómez-Real F, et al. Use of metformin to treat pregnant women with polycystic ovary syndrome (PregMet2): a randomised, double-blind, placebo-controlled trial. Lancet Diabetes Endocrinol. 2019;7(4):256–66. PubMed PMID: 30792154. Epub 2019/02/23. eng
161. Vomstein K, Herzog A, Voss P, Feil K, Goeggl T, Strowitzki T, et al. Recurrent miscarriage is not associated with a higher prevalence of inherited and acquired thrombophilia. Am J Rep Immunol (New York, NY: 1989). 2021;85(1):e13327. PubMed PMID: 32860294. Epub 2020/08/30. eng
162. van Dijk MM, Kolte AM, Limpens J, Kirk E, Quenby S, van Wely M, et al. Recurrent pregnancy loss: diagnostic workup after two or three pregnancy losses? A systematic review of the literature and meta-analysis. Hum Reprod Update. 2020;26(3):356–67. PubMed PMID: 32103270. Pubmed Central PMCID: PMC7161667. Epub 2020/02/28. eng
163. Skeith L, Carrier M, Kaaja R, Martinelli I, Petroff D, Schleußner E, et al. A meta-analysis of low-molecular-weight heparin to prevent pregnancy loss in women with inherited thrombophilia. Blood. 2016;127(13):1650–5. PubMed PMID: 26837697. Epub 2016/02/04. eng
164. Sasaki H, Hamatani T, Kamijo S, Iwai M, Kobanawa M, Ogawa S, et al. Impact of Oxidative Stress on Age-Associated Decline in Oocyte Developmental Competence. Front Endocrinol. 2019;10:811. PubMed PMID: 31824426. Pubmed Central PMCID: PMC6882737. Epub 2019/12/12. eng
165. Balogun OO, da Silva Lopes K, Ota E, Takemoto Y, Rumbold A, Takegata M, et al. Vitamin supplementation for preventing miscarriage. Cochrane Database Syst Rev. 2016;2016(5):CD004073. PubMed PMID: 27150280. Pubmed Central PMCID: PMC7104220 Supplements with vitamin C and vitamin E for the prevention of pre-eclampsia (Rumbold 2006). This trial is included in this review but its eligibility for inclusion, trial quality assessments and data extraction were carried out independently by two of the review authors not involved in the original trial. Erika Ota: none known. Olukunmi O Balogun: none known. Katharina da Silva Lopes: none known. Yo Takemoto: none known. Mizuki Takegata: none known. Rintaro Mori's institution receives government funding from the Clinical Research Program for Child Health and Development, AMED, Japan to provide support for the PCG Satellite in Japan. Epub 2016/05/07. eng
166. Showell MG, Mackenzie-Proctor R, Jordan V, Hart RJ. Antioxidants for female subfertility. Cochrane Database Syst Rev. 2020;8(8):CD007807. PubMed PMID: 32851663. Pubmed Central PMCID: PMC8094745 shareholder in Western IVF. He has received educational sponsorship from Merck Serono and Ferring pharmaceuticals, and is on the medical advisory board of MSD and Ferring Pharmaceuticals. Rebecca Mackenzie-Proctor: no conflict of interest to declare Vanessa Jordan: no conflict of interest to declare Marian Showell: no conflict of interest to declare. Epub 2020/08/28. eng
167. Romano M, Cirillo F, Spadaro D, Busnelli A, Castellano S, Albani E, et al. High sperm DNA fragmentation: do we have robust evidence to support antioxidants and testicular sperm extraction to improve fertility outcomes? A narrative review. Front Endocrinol. 2023;14:1150951. PubMed PMID: 37867514. Pubmed Central PMCID: PMC10585152. Epub 2023/10/23. eng
168. de Ligny W, Smits RM, Mackenzie-Proctor R, Jordan V, Fleischer K, de Bruin JP, et al. Antioxidants for male subfertility. Cochrane Database Syst Rev. 2022;5(5):CD007411. PubMed PMID: 35506389. Pubmed Central PMCID: PMC9066298 unrestricted grant for conducting the trial NCT03337360, to cover the salary of the trial co-ordinators Wiep R de Ligny and Roos M Smits. This trial (NCT03337360) started in April 2018. No data have been extracted from this study. The trial NCT03337360 is submitted to 'Ongoing studies'. This matter was referred to Cochrane's Funding Arbiters who have confirmed that Dr de Ligny's and Dr Smits' declared interest does not constitute a COI under the current policy. The following author has reported financial activities outside the submitted work: KF has received travel and conference support from Ferring. JdB, VJ, MGS and RM-P have no conflicts to declare. Epub 2022/05/05. eng
169. Regan L, Rai R, Saravelos S, Li TC. Recurrent MiscarriageGreen-top Guideline No. 17. BJOG. 2023;130(12):e9–e39. PubMed PMID: 37334488. Epub 2023/06/19. eng
170. Rikken JFW, Kowalik CR, Emanuel MH, Bongers MY, Spinder T, Jansen FW, et al. Septum resection versus expectant management in women with a septate uterus: an international multicentre open-label randomized controlled trial. Hum Rep (Oxford, England). 2021;36(5):1260–7. PubMed PMID: 33793794. Pubmed Central PMCID: PMC8058590. Epub 2021/04/02. eng
171. Kolte AM, Olsen LR, Mikkelsen EM, Christiansen OB, Nielsen HS. Depression and emotional stress is highly prevalent among women with recurrent pregnancy loss. Hum Rep (Oxford, England). 2015;30(4):777–82. PubMed PMID: 25662810. Pubmed Central PMCID: PMC4359400. Epub 2015/02/11. eng
172. San Lazaro Campillo I, Meaney S, McNamara K, O'Donoghue K. Psychological and support interventions to reduce levels of stress, anxiety or depression on women's subsequent pregnancy

with a history of miscarriage: an empty systematic review. BMJ Open. 2017;7(9):e017802. PubMed PMID: 28882928. Pubmed Central PMCID: PMC5595175. Epub 2017/09/09. eng
173. Mevorach-Zussman N, Bolotin A, Shalev H, Bilenko N, Mazor M, Bashiri A. Anxiety and deterioration of quality of life factors associated with recurrent miscarriage in an observational study. J Perinat Med. 2012;40(5):495–501. PubMed PMID: 23120756. Epub 2012/11/03. eng
174. Lund M, Kamper-Jørgensen M, Nielsen HS, Lidegaard Ø, Andersen AM, Christiansen OB. Prognosis for live birth in women with recurrent miscarriage: what is the best measure of success? Obstet Gynecol. 2012;119(1):37–43. PubMed PMID: 22183209. Epub 2011/12/21.eng

Prevention of Fetal Malformation: The Role of Folic Acid

Matitiahu Berkovitch

Contents

Y. Yogev, A. Khalil (eds.), *Prevention of Complications in Obstetrics*,
https://doi.org/10.1007/978-3-032-23479-7_3

3

Introduction in Brief

- Folic acid—vitamin B9—is important for the prevention of neural tube defects (NTDs).
- Most cases of NTDs—70%—are of a genetic origin.
- In many countries, a spontaneous decrease in the prevalence of NTD was observed before any intervention to improve the folate status of pregnant women was implemented.
- The mechanism of NTD prevention by folic acid is unknown.
- There is probably a "ceiling effect" of 25%–35% prevention of NTDs with folic acid.
- The recommended dose of folic acid supplementation is 0.4 mg per day, starting one month before pregnancy and continued until the end of the first trimester.
- Folic acid supplementation does not reduce the risk of other major malformations.
- A daily dose of 4–5 mg of folic acid should be recommended for women with a previous NTD pregnancy, women with diabetes, or those with anticonvulsant treatment.
- There is no evidence to support the administration of high-dose folic acid (4–5 mg daily) to women with obesity (BMI $\geq$ 30).
- Lipomyelomeningocele is not prevented by folic acid.
- There is controversy about whether the administration of folic acid during pregnancy is associated with atopic diseases later in the life of children.
- Studies are showing an association between folic acid use during pregnancy and increased risk of autism, while others are showing a protective effect.
- Deficiency of folic acid during pregnancy may result in macrocytic (megaloblastic) anemia.

Learning Objectives

- Explain the biological role and metabolism of folic acid
- Describe the etiology and epidemiology of neural tube defects
- Evaluate evidence for folic acid supplementation effectiveness and limitations
- Identify recommended folic acid doses for various risk groups
- Assess controversies and potential adverse associations of folic acid exposure

3.1 Introduction

Folic acid—vitamin B9—is a vitamin B essential for nucleoprotein synthesis and erythropoiesis.

The term "folic acid" comes from the Latin word "*folium*," which means "leaf."

Folate, the natural form of vitamin B9, is found mainly in green leafy vegetables, citrus fruits, yeast extracts, liver, and kidney. Moderate sources include whole wheat bread, potatoes, and dairy products. Tomatoes and cucumbers are other sources of folic acid.

The absorption of folic acid occurs in the small intestine. There is a controversy about whether natural forms of folate are less bioavailable than synthetic folic acid. Natural forms of folate are generally less bioavailable than synthetic folic acid. This is due to the greater stability of oxidized folic acid, compared with the polyglutamate conjugation of food folate. However, both forms are beneficial.

Folic acid is metabolized in the liver to tetrahydrofolate (THF). THF is involved in purine and thymidine monophosphate (dTMP) synthesis, mitochondrial protein translation, and methionine regeneration. Folate metabolism is important for DNA and RNA synthesis, homocysteine, and protein metabolism.

3.2 Neural Tube Defects (NTDs)

The failure of neural closure during early embryogenesis may result in a spectrum of neural tube defects (NTDs). Folding of the neural walls and closure of the neural tube (neural tube formation) occur between 21 and 28 days post-conception. NTDs affect 0.5–2 per 1000 pregnancies and, after congenital heart defects, are the second most common group of birth defects.

NTD includes several malformations: myelomeningocele (open spina bifida), anencephaly, and encephalocele.

3.3 What Causes NTDs?

The pathogenesis of the various NTDs is diverse, with multifactorial etiology, genetic in 70% and mostly unknown for individual cases [1].

Most cases of infants born with NTDs are not born to mothers with clinical folate deficiency. At least 70% of the variance in the prevalence of NTDs is due to genetic factors. Evidence for genetic causation includes the high recurrence risk for siblings of index cases (2–5%), approximately 50-fold more than in the general population, together with a gradually decreasing risk in more distant relatives [1]. Women with two or more affected pregnancies have a very high risk (around 10%) of further recurrence [2].

In many countries worldwide, a spontaneous decrease in the prevalence of NTDs was observed before any intervention to improve the folate status of pregnant women was implemented. In the United States, the prevalence of NTDs decreased from 5.9 cases per 10,000 births in 1984 to 3.2 cases per 10,000 births in 1990 before the publication of the Centers for Disease Control's (CDC) recommendation on folic acid (published in September 1992) and before implementation of mandatory food fortification in 1998 [3]. Also, in other countries, such as the UK, Ireland, Sweden, the Netherlands, Portugal, and Israel, a spontaneous decline in the prevalence of NTDs was observed before issuing recommendations on folic acid supplementation [4–8]. In Israel, a decline of 18% in the rate of spina bifida and a 35% decline in anencephaly were observed before the recommendations on folic acid supplementation were published [9].

- **A woman asks, "I am planning a pregnancy. What can I do to reduce the possibility of NTDs in my fetus?"**

Answer: On September 11, 1992, the Centers for Disease Control (CDC) in the United States published recommendations for the use of folic acid to reduce the number of cases of spina bifida and other neural tube defects [10]. In this publication, it was stated that "There are three potential approaches for delivery of folic acid to the general population in the dosage recommended: (a) improvement of dietary habits, (b) fortification of the US food supply, and (c) use of dietary supplements."

One of the main studies quoted by the CDC was a randomized controlled trial sponsored by the British Medical Council (MRC) [11].

The MRC study was a randomized double-blind prevention trial with a factorial design, conducted at 33 centers in seven countries, to determine whether supplementation with folic acid or a mixture of seven other vitamins (A, D, B1, B2, B6, C, and nicotinamide) "around the time of conception" can prevent neural tube defects (anencephaly, spina bifida, and encephalocele). A total of 1817 women at a high risk of having a pregnancy with neural tube defects because of a previously affected pregnancy were allocated at random to one of four groups: folic acid, other vitamins, both, or neither. One thousand one hundred and ninety-five had a completed pregnancy in which the fetus or infant was known to have or not have a neural tube defect; 27 of these had a known neural tube defect, six in the folic acid group and 21 in the other two groups, a 72% protective effect (relative risk: 0.28; 95% confidence interval (CI): 0.12–0.71) The other vitamins group showed no significant protective effect (relative risk: 0.8; 95% CI: 0.32–1.72).

Women in this study were asked to take a single capsule each day from the date of randomization until 12 weeks of pregnancy (estimated from the first day of the last menstrual period). Capsules for those in the folic acid group contained 4 mg of folic acid. However, it was not clear from the protocol of the study how long before conception the supplementation was taken by the mothers [12].

In another study, by Czeizel AE and Dudas I [13], women planning a pregnancy (in most cases, their first) were randomly assigned to receive a single tablet of a vitamin supplement (containing 12 vitamins, including 0.8 mg of folic acid; four minerals; and three trace elements) or a trace element supplement (containing copper, manganese, and zinc and a very low dose of vitamin C) daily for at least one month before conception and until the date of the second missed menstrual period or later. Two thousand one hundred and four women received the vitamin supplement, and 2052 received the trace element supplement. There were six cases of neural tube defects in the group receiving the trace element supplement, as compared with none in the vitamin supplement group ($P = 0.029$). However, the dose of folic acid administered in this study was 0.8 mg, higher than that used in many other countries. Furthermore, the prevalence of NTDs in Hungary was 2.8 cases per 1000 live births. However, in the study, the prevalence of NTDs in the control group was 5.7 cases per 1000 live births. Therefore, in this study, there was probably a selection bias in the control group since the risk of NTDs in the control group was higher than that in the general Hungarian population.

Mills JL et al. published in 1989 the results of a study performed in the United States. Three groups of women were included in the study: 571 women who had a fetus with NTD and two control groups—573 women who delivered a normal child and 546 women who had a stillbirth or an infant with another defect. NTDs included in this study were anencephaly, meningocele, myelomeningocele, encephalocele, rachischisis, iniencephaly, and lipomeningocele. The periconceptional use of multivitamins, both in terms of vitamin supplements only and when combined with fortified cereals, was evaluated for each group. The results of this study showed that the use of either multivitamins or folate supplements does not reduce the frequency of NTDs [14].

A study from Japan, published in 2019, compared a cohort of 92269 women who were adequate users of folic acid supplements and had started before conception with inadequate users who began after pregnancy recognition or those with a nonuse of folic acid supplements. Neural tube defect outcomes included spina bifida, anencephaly, and encephalocele. No statistically significant differences associated with folic acid supplementation were reported [15].

- **A woman asks, "If I take folic acid according to the recommendations, to what extent can it reduce the risk of NTDs?"**

Answer: Several publications have shown that folic acid may prevent around 30% of NTDs. Six years after the mandatory food fortification with folic acid (mandatory fortification of cereal grain products went into effect in January 1998), the CDC reported a spina bifida decline by 31%, and the prevalence of anencephaly declined by 16% [15]. Of note, in 2004, women in the United States were exposed to folic acid through dietary supplements containing folic acid and through fortification of food with folic acid. In this issue of the morbidity and mortality weekly report (MMWR) the CDC has stated that "The observed decrease in NTD-affected pregnancies of approximately 26% is less than what was estimated from the research trials" [16].

The decline in the NTD rate did not change a decade later. The CDC reported in January 2015 a reduction of 28% [17]. According to the CDC, "The birth prevalence of anencephaly and spina bifida during the pre-fortification (1995–1996) and post-fortification periods (biennial from 1998–2008, last 3 years of available data from 2009–2011, and all years from 1999–2011) for programs with and without prenatal ascertainment were estimated. Overall, a 28% reduction in prevalence was observed for anencephaly and spina bifida using data from all participating programs; a greater reduction (35%) was observed among programs with prenatal ascertainment than for programs without prenatal ascertainment (21%)" [17].

3.4 There Is Probably of "Ceiling Effect" of 25%–35% Prevention of NTDs with Folic Acid

In 2009, Heseker HB et al. published a review titled "Not all cases of neural-tube defects can be prevented by increasing the intake of folic acid" [18]. The objective of the review by Heseker HB et al. was to evaluate the beneficial effects of different levels of folic acid administration on the prevalence of NTDs. The authors have concluded that countries with mandatory fortification and recommendations for supplementation achieved an increase in folate intake and a decrease in the prevalence of NTDs. However, they claimed that the prevalence of NTDs at birth declined to approximately five cases per 10,000 births and seven to eight cases at birth or abortion per 10,000 births. The decline observed was independent of the amount of folic acid administered, and apparently, there is a "floor effect" for folic acid–preventable NTDs. According to the CDC, the prevalence of NTDs has fallen only by 26% in the United States after food fortification with folic acid [19].

Another study, by Mosley BS et al. [19], used data from the National Birth Defects Prevention Study between the years 1998 and 2003. The authors' objective was to evaluate the association between neural tube defects and maternal folic acid intake among pregnancies conceived after folic acid fortification of the food supply in the United States. Periconceptional supplement use did not reduce the risk of having a pregnancy affected by a neural tube defect. The authors hypothesized that "… it is possible that we failed to find an association because of a 'ceiling effect'. Folate intake among the US childbearing population may have reached levels where nearly all folate-sensitive neural tube defects have been prevented" [20].

In an editorial by Mitchell LE on the US Preventive Services Task Force (USPSTF) Statement on Folic Acid Supplementation in the Era of Mandatory Folic Acid Fortification, the author stated that "In the United States, mandatory folic acid fortification was initiated in January 1998 and was followed by a 35% decline in the prevalence of neural tube defects" [21].

3.4.1 What Is the Mechanism of Folic Acid in Preventing NTDs?

The exact mechanism of action of folic acid in preventing NTDs is not fully understood. Teratogenic drugs like valproic acid and carbamazepine carry an NTD risk of 1–2% when taken during pregnancy. The mode of action of valproic acid and carbamazepine is thought to be carried out by the inhibition of histone deacetylase, which may affect gene methylation, while folate itself has a major role in securing normal methylation patterns [22]; however, limited data so far suggest that this risk cannot be lowered by periconceptional folic acid supplementation. On the other hand, there are folate antagonists like methotrexate, which are teratogenic, but NTD is not a typical feature of its embryopathy.

- **A woman asks, "If I take folic acid according to the recommendations, would it prevent other congenital malformations?"**

Answer: Despite some hypotheses, folic acid supplementation did not significantly decrease the risk of major malformations beyond NTDs [23].

A systematic review and meta-analysis also found no strong evidence that folate alone is associated with oral cleft etiology [24].

- **A woman asks, "I am planning a pregnancy; how much folic acid should I take?"**

Answer: In most European countries, the recommendation is that women planning a pregnancy should take a daily dose of 0.4 mg of folic acid from one month before conception until the end of the first trimester [25].

The US Preventive Services Task Force (USPSTF) suggested that the dose of folic acid should be 0.4 mg–0.8 mg. The supplementation starts at least one month before conception and continues through the first 2–3 months of pregnancy [26].

- **A woman asks, "I have struggled with high weight for years without success. Now that I am planning a pregnancy, how much folic acid should I take?"**

Answer: No published studies show that a high dose of folic acid (5 mg) is better than the regular recommended dose of 0.4 mg. Additionally, no published studies show that a high dose of folic acid (4 or 5 mg) decreases the risk of neural tube defects in children born to women with obesity.

In a review of European guidelines on periconceptional folic acid supplementation, an online search of country-specific folic acid guidelines was performed between November and December 2014. Eleven European countries make no specific folic acid recommendations for obesity: Austria, the Netherlands, Switzerland, Spain, Germany, Belgium, Portugal, Malta, Poland, Hungary, and Croatia. Denmark and Finland also do not recommend high-dose folic acid for obesity. The recommendation in these countries is to use 0.4 mg daily of folic acid. Italy recommends 4–5 mg daily for obese women with diabetes mellitus but does not recommend it for obese women who do not have diabetes [25, 26].

The WHO also does not recommend high-dose folic acid for women with obesity. A high dose of folic acid, according to the WHO, is recommended for women who have previously had a baby with NTD, who have diabetes, or who receive anticonvulsant treatment [27].

- **A woman asks, "I have a seizure disorder and am treated with antiepileptic medications. What dose of folic acid should I take?"**

Answer: High doses, 4–5 mg daily of folic acid, are recommended for women with risk factors. The evidence for the use of 4 mg of folic acid per day comes from the MRC trial [11]. This study observed a 72% protective effect (relative risk: 0.28; 95% confidence interval: 0.12–0.71) for neural tube defect recurrence with a 4 mg daily dose of folic acid compared with a multivitamin without folic acid [11]. The choice of a folic acid dose of 4 mg was arbitrary [11]. It is unknown if a lower dose would also be effective and protective.

Most European countries recommend a supplement dose of 4 mg daily of folic acid to prevent the recurrence of NTD [25].

According to the World Health Organization (WHO), a daily dose of 5 mg and increased folate intake should be recommended to women with previous NTD pregnancy, women with diabetes, or those receiving anticonvulsant treatment [27].

The American College of Obstetricians and Gynecologists in the United States is recommending 4 mg per day of folic acid for women with a previous NTD pregnancy or those with epilepsy [28].

The UK National Institute for Health and Care Excellence recommended 5 mg per day of folic acid when planning a pregnancy or in the early stages of pregnancy for personal or partner history of NTD, previous newborn with NTD, individual or partner family history of NTDs, and type 1 or type 2 diabetes and when taking an antiepileptic drug [28, 29].

No trials compare a 4–5 mg dose to the standard 0.4 mg daily dose of folic acid to prevent NTDs. There is no evidence to suggest that women with type 1 or type 2 diabetes would benefit from higher doses. Women with preexisting diabetes have higher rates of neural tube defects than women in the general population (2.4% vs. 0.57%, 4.2 times increased risk (95% CI: 2.0–7.8)) [30].

There is no evidence supporting the use of high-dose folic acid for women taking antiepileptic medications or other folate antagonists [31].

Not all European countries recommend high-dose folic acid for women with epilepsy or diabetes mellitus [25]. Austria, Portugal, Poland, the Netherlands, Malta, Switzerland, Spain, Hungary, Germany, Belgium, and Croatia make no specific recommendations for epilepsy or diabetes mellitus [25]. Denmark and Finland recommend the usual 0.4-mg daily dose in these circumstances [25].

In a recent review on periconceptional folic acid supplementation for women with epilepsy, it was shown that the risk of major congenital malformations was relatively higher in those with periconceptional folic acid supplementation (17,463 pregnancies; OR: 1.34; 95% CI: 1.12–1.6) and was similar between those with and without a folic acid supplementation of ≥4 mg (3822 pregnancies; OR: 0.9; 95% CI: 0.65–1.24). Results showed that periconceptional folic acid supplementation may be beneficial for neurodevelopment, but the evidence was limited [32].

3.4.2 Lipomyelomeningocele and Other Conditions Not Dependent on Folic Acid

Lipomyelomeningocele is a type of spinal dysraphism where an abnormal growth of fat attaches to the spinal cord and its membranes. Unlike some other forms of spinal dysraphism, lipomyelomeningocele is not prevented by folic acid administration [33, 34].

Other spinal dysraphisms not prevented by folic acid are spina bifida occulta, thickened filum terminale, diastematomyelia, caudal regression syndrome, intradural lipoma, lipomeningocele, split notochord, and other forms of myelodysplasia. This category of mainly caudal defects may be embryologically distinct from myelomeningocele [33, 34].

- **A woman asks, "I am taking folic acid according to the recommendations. Are there any adverse effects associated with folic acid supplementation in the offspring?"**

Answer: There are some reports on an increased risk incidence of atopic allergy in infants. The risk is probably small. A large study in Norway involving almost 40,000 women and children showed that 1901 children had a diagnosis of asthma. Maternal intake of folate from supplements and food was evaluated at 22 weeks of pregnancy. Asthma at the age of 7 years was diagnosed from a national prescription database. There was a 23% increased risk of asthma in children whose mothers fell into the top quintile of total folate intake (risk ratio: 1.23; 95% CI: 1.06–1.44) [35].

In a review by McStay et al., the authors discussed how folic acid acts as a methyl donor, potentially altering DNA methylation. In animal studies, folic acid has been shown to modify gene expression, which is linked to the development of allergic diseases in offspring. These findings, alongside several human population studies, raise questions about the role of folic acid exposure in late pregnancy concerning allergic disease development in children, especially after the critical period for preventing neural tube defects. However, results from epidemiological cohort studies are conflicting, and there is a notable lack of conclusive human trials, particularly in populations with adequate folate levels [36].

- **A woman asks, "Can folic acid supplementation during pregnancy increase the risk of autism in my child?"**

Answer: Folic acid during pregnancy has been the subject of various studies regarding its potential impact on the risk of autism in children. Some research suggests that adequate folic acid intake before conception and during early pregnancy may have protective effects against developmental disorders, including autism spectrum disorders (ASDs) [37].

However, there are epidemiological studies that reported a possible association between maternal folate supplementation and an increased risk of autism in offspring [38].

3.5 Other Potential Implications for Public Health

Folic acid can mask a vitamin B12 deficiency. High levels of folic acid can prevent the symptoms of B12 deficiency from appearing, which can lead to potential neurological damage if the deficiency remains unaddressed [39, 40].

3.6 Macrocytic (Megaloblastic) Anemia

3

The most common phenomenon of maternal folic acid deficiency is megaloblastic anemia. The pathogenesis of megaloblastic anemia in pregnancy involves inadequate maternal intake of folic acid, depletion of maternal folic acid stores by the fetus, and decreased absorption [41]. Other factors such as multiple pregnancies, hemorrhage, and hemolytic anemia may further decrease maternal levels [41].

Pancytopenia as a result of folate deficiency during pregnancy was also rarely reported [42].

3.7 Conclusions

Folic acid should not be promoted as a teratologic panacea. While folic acid prevents NTDs, it does not prevent other malformations. A woman who has a child with NTD should not feel guilty for not taking folic acid supplementation before and during pregnancy.

Most cases of NTD—70%—are of a genetic origin. There is probably a "ceiling effect" of 25%–35% prevention of NTDs with folic acid. The recommended dose of folic acid supplementation is 0.4 mg per day, starting one month before pregnancy and continued until the end of the first trimester.

A daily dose of 4–5 mg of folic acid should be recommended for women with a previous NTD pregnancy, women with diabetes, or those receiving anticonvulsant treatment. There is no evidence to support the administration of high-dose folic acid (4–5 mg daily) to women with obesity (BMI $\geq$ 30).

Lipomyelomeningocele is not prevented by folic acid.

Deficiency of folic acid during pregnancy may result in macrocytic (megaloblastic) anemia.

Chapter Key Points

- Genetic and multifactorial origins of neural tube defects (NTDs)
- Observed spontaneous declines in NTD prevalence prior to folic acid interventions
- Evidence on folic acid's preventive effect and its estimated ceiling of 25–35%
- Recommended supplementation regimens for the general population and high-risk groups
- Limitations of folic acid in preventing non-NTD malformations

Chapter-End Summary

This chapter explores the role of folic acid in the prevention of neural tube defects, highlighting its metabolic functions, relevant epidemiological trends, and evidence base. While folic acid supplementation reduces a proportion of NTDs, its preventive capacity appears limited by a ceiling effect, and most cases remain genetically determined. The chapter outlines recommended supplementation strategies for the general population and high-risk groups and clarifies conditions not responsive to folate. Emerging debates regarding associations with allergic disease and autism are summarized to support balanced counseling. Together, these elements provide a comprehensive overview that reinforces and expands upon the introductory context.

References

1. Copp AJ, Green ND. Neural tube defects- disorders of neurulation and related embryonic processes. Wiley Interdiscip Rev Dev Biol. 2013;2(2):213–27.

2. Rampersaud E, Melvin EC, Speer MC. Nonsyndromic neural tube defects: genetic basis and genetic investigations. In: Wszynski DF, editor. Neural tube defects: from origin to treatment. Oxford: Oxford University Press; 2006. p. 165–75.
3. CDC- Centers for Disease Control and Prevention. Morbidity and mortality weekly report (MMWR). 1992;41(27):497.
4. Romijn JA, Treffers PE. Anencephaly in the Netherlands: a remarkable decline. Lancet. 1983;1(8314–5):64–5.
5. Kallen B, Lofkvist E. Time trends of spina bifida in Sweden 1947–81. J Epidemiol Community Health. 1984;38(2):103–7.
6. Kadir RA, Sabin C, Whitlow B, Brockbank E, Economides D. Neural tube defects and periconceptional folic acid in England and Wales: retrospective study. BMJ. 1999;319(7202):92–3.
7. Botto LD, Lisi A, Bower C, Canfield MA, Dattani N, De VC, et al. Trends of selected malformations about folic acid recommendations and fortification: an international assessment. Birth Defects Res A Clin Mol Teratol. 2006;76(10):693–705.
8. Botto LD, Lisi A, Robert-Gnansia E, Erickson JD, Vollset SE, Mastroiacovo P, et al. International retrospective cohort study of neural tube defects about folic acid recommendations: are the recommendations working? BMJ. 2005;330(7491):571.
9. Zlotogora J, Amitai Y, Levental A. Surveillance of neural tube defects in Israel: the effect of the recommendation for periconceptional folic acid. IMAJ. 2006;8:601–4.
10. CDC- Centers for Disease Control and Prevention. Morbidity and mortality weekly report (MMWR). MMWR. 1992;41(RR-14):001.
11. MRC Vitamin Study Research Group. Prevention of neural tube defects: results of the Medical Research Council Vitamin Study. The Lancet. 1991;338:131–7.
12. Anonymous. Folic acid and neural tube defects. Lancet. 1991;338:153–4.
13. Czeizel AE, Dudas I. Prevention of the first occurrence of neural tube defects by periconceptional vitamin supplementation. N Engl J Med. 1992;327:1832–5.
14. Mills JL, Rhoads GG, Simpson JL, et al. The absence of a relation between the periconceptional use of vitamins and neural-tube defects. N Engl J Med. 1989;321:430–5.
15. Nishigori H, Obara T, Nishigori T, et al. Japan Environment & Children's study group. Preconception folic acid supplementation use and the occurrence of neural tube defects in Japan: a nationwide birth cohort study of the Japan Environment and Children's Study. Congenital Anomalies (Kyoto). 2019;59(4):11–117.
16. CDC- Centers for Disease Control and Prevention. Morbidity and Mortality Weekly Report (MMWR). MMWR. 2004;53:362–5.
17. CDC- Centers for Disease Control and Prevention. Morbidity and Mortality Weekly Report (MMWR). MMWR. 2015;64(1):1–5.
18. Heseker HB, Mason JB, Selhub J, Rosenberg IH, Jacques PF. Not all cases of neural tube defects can be prevented by increasing the intake of folic acid. Br J Nutr. 2009;102:173–80.
19. Williams LJ, Rasmussen SA, Flores A, et al. Decline in the prevalence of spina bifida and anencephaly by race/ethnicity: 1995–2002. Pediatrics. 2005;116:580–6.
20. Mosley BS, Cleves MA, Siega-Riz AM, et al. Neural tube defects and maternal folate intake among pregnancies conceived after folic acid fortification in the United States. Am J Epidemiol. 2009;169(1):9–17.
21. Mitchell LA. Folic Acid for the prevention of Neural Tube Defects – The US Preventive Services Task Force Statement on Folic acid supplementation in the era of mandatory folic acid fortification. JAMA. 2017;317(2):E1-E.
22. Irwin RE, Pentieva K, Cassidy T, Lees-Murdock DJ, McLaughlin M, Prasad G, McNulty H, Walsh CP. The interplay between DNA methylation, folate and neurocognitive development. Epigenomics. 2016;8(6):863–79.
23. Canfield MA, Collins JS, Botto LD, et al. Changes in the birth prevalence of selected birth defects after grain fortification with folic acid in the United States: findings from a multi-state population-based study. Birth Defects Res A Clin Mol Teratol. 2005;73:679–89.
24. Johnson CY, Little J. Folate intake, markers of folate status and oral clefts: is the evidence converging? Int J Epidemiol. 2008;26:1–18.
25. Cawley S, Mullaney L, McKeating A, Farren M, McCartney D, Turner MJ. A review of European guidelines on periconceptional folic acid supplementation. Eur J Clin Nutr. 2016;70:143–54.
26. US Preventive Services Task Force. Folic acid supplementation to prevent neural tube defects. US Preventive Services Task Force Reaffirmation Recommendation Statement. JAMA. 2023;330(5):454–9.
27. World Health Organization, Department of Making Pregnancy Safer. Integrated Management of Pregnancy and Children. Standards for maternal and neonatal care. WHO; 2007.
28. ACOG. ACOG committee opinion number 762. Pregnancy counseling. Obstetr Gynecol. 2019;133:e78–9.
29. National Institute for Health and Care Excellence. Epilepsies: diagnosis and management (clinical guideline CG137). 2021. https://www.nice.org.uk/guidance/cg137
30. Dwyer ER, Filion KB, MacFarlane AJ, Platt RW, Mehrabadi A. Who should consume high-dose folic acid supplements before and during early pregnancy for the prevention of neural tube defects? BMJ. 2022;377:e067728.

3

31. WHO. Management of epilepsy in women of childbearing age. 2012.
32. Peng A, Zhou Y, Zhu L, et al. Periconceptional folic acid supplementation for women with epilepsy: a systematic review of the literature. Epilepsy Behav. 2024;161:110064.
33. De Wals P, et al. Reduction in neural-tube defects after folic acid fortification in Canada. N Enl J Med. 2007;357:135–42.
34. McNeely PD, Howes WJ. Ineffectiveness of dietary folic acid supplementation on the incidence of lipomyelomeningocele: pathogenetic implications. J Neurosurg. 2004;100(2 Suppl Pediatrics):98–100.
35. Parr CL, Magnus MC, Karlstad O, et al. Maternal folate intake during pregnancy and childhood asthma in a population-based cohort. Am J Respir Crit Care Med. 2017;195(2):221–8.
36. McStay CL, Prescott SL, Bower C, Palmer DJ. Maternal folic acid supplementation during pregnancy and childhood allergic disease outcomes: a question of timing? Nutrients. 2017;9:123.
37. Levine SZ, Kodesh A, Viktorin A, et al. Association of maternal use of folic acid and multivitamin supplements in the periods before and during pregnancy with the risk of autism spectrum disorder in offspring. JAMA Psychiatry. 2018;75(2):176–84.
38. Wiens D, DeSoto MC. Is high folic acid intake a risk factor for autism? – a review. Brain Sci. 2017;7(11):149.
39. CDC- Centers for Disease Control and Prevention. Morbidity and Mortality Weekly Report (MMWR). Use of folic acid for prevention of spina bifida and other neural tube defects-1983–1991. MMWR. 1991;40:513–6.
40. Glanville NT, Cook HW. Folic acid and prevention of neural tube defects. Can Med Assoc J. 1992;146:39.
41. Giles C. An account of 335 cases of megaloblastic anemia of pregnancy and the puerperium. J Clin Pathol. 1966;19:1–11.
42. Solano FX Jr, Councell RB. Folate deficiency presenting as pancytopenia in pregnancy. Am J Obstet Gynecol. 1986;154:1117–8.

Fetal Anomalies: The Role of Early Anatomy Scan

Işıl Ayhan and Asma Khalil

Contents

Y. Yogev, A. Khalil (eds.), *Prevention of Complications in Obstetrics*,
https://doi.org/10.1007/978-3-032-23479-7_4

4

Learning Objectives

- Explain the clinical role and timing of the first-trimester ultrasound anatomy scan
- Identify ultrasound markers used in aneuploidy screening
- Describe structural anomalies detectable, potentially detectable, or undetectable in the first trimester
- Understand limitations and challenges in early anomaly detection
- Discuss the importance of operator skill, protocols, and follow-up imaging

4.1 Introduction

The first-trimester ultrasound plays a crucial role in the early detection of congenital anomalies, offering an opportunity for timely diagnosis and management. The primary objective of the first-trimester ultrasound is often to provide information that will enable optimal prenatal care with the best possible outcome for both the mother and the fetus. Typically performed between 11 and 14 weeks of pregnancy, a first-trimester ultrasound allows the assessment of fetal development, identification of structural abnormalities, and screening for chromosomal abnormalities. The first-trimester ultrasound examination has evolved in the past decades, expanding beyond aneuploidy screening to encompass an assessment of early anatomy. Early detection of anomalies enables parents and clinicians to make informed decisions about further testing, treatment options, or pregnancy management, improving overall prenatal care and outcomes.

4.2 Screening for Aneuploidies

In the 1990s and 2000s, the "combined test," which included fetal nuchal translucency (NT) measurement, maternal age, and serum levels of beta human chorionic gonadotropin (beta-hCG) and pregnancy-associated plasma protein-A (PAPP-A), was performed efficiently for trisomy 21 screening, with an 82–91% sensitivity and a 5% false-positive rate [1, 2]. The combined test requires an ultrasound scan during the first trimester, and attempts have been made to improve the detection rate by including other ultrasound markers such as tricuspid regurgitation, nasal bone, and ductus venosus Doppler examination. In 2011, cell-free DNA (cfDNA) screening emerged in clinical practice, leading to a fundamental shift in aneuploidy screening. If the cfDNA result is negative for aneuploidies, the Society for Maternal-Fetal Medicine (SMFM) does not recommend any additional invasive genetic testing just for the presence of soft markers of aneuploidy [3]. Nevertheless, a first-trimester ultrasound remains the most critical component of first-trimester assessment, as it is essential to ascertain the absence of significant fetal anomalies before proceeding with a "screening" test.

4.2.1 Nuchal Translucency (NT)

Nuchal translucency (NT) is the clear space at the fetal neck, seen between the spine and the edge of the skin. Lymphatic abnormalities, cardiovascular abnormalities, and variables associated with extracellular matrix synthesis have all been implicated in the pathogenesis of increased NT [4]. NT is measured between 11 and 14 weeks of gestation, and the fetal crown-rump length (CRL) must be between 45 and 84 mm. In the midsagittal section, the ultrasonic beam must be perpendicular to the NT lines to obtain a clear image of the edges, and reducing the gain of the ultrasound equipment may assist in eliminating edge artifacts within the translucency. The measurement should be performed at the thickest section of the NT, ensuring that the calipers are positioned along the lines delineating the NT (Fig. 4.1). Values ≥3 or 3.5 mm, or ≥ 95th or 99th percentile, for the CRL are considered increased (Fig. 4.2). Institutions

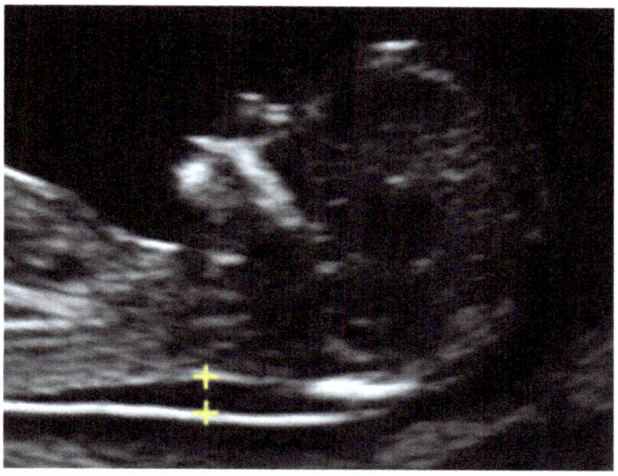

Fig. 4.1 Nuchal translucency measurement in the midsagittal view. Note that the calipers are positioned at the thickest section

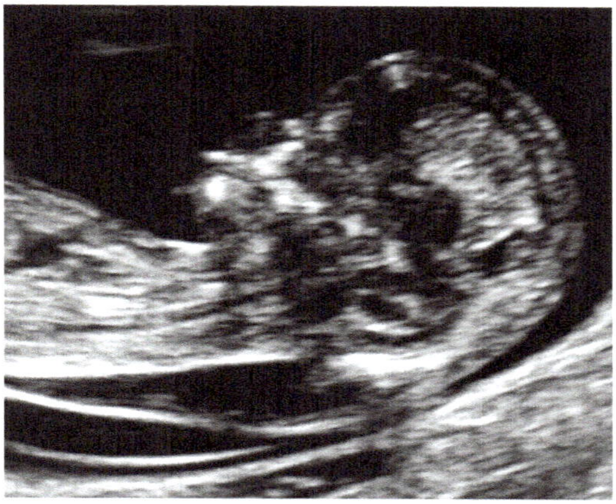

Fig. 4.2 Increased nuchal translucency. Note that the amniotic membrane and the edge of fetal skin are visualized separately

and organizations may choose different cutoff thresholds; nonetheless, it is advisable to use lower cutoffs for offering additional investigations [5].

Measurement of the NT is crucial despite the advent of cfDNA. An increased NT might indicate different structural and genetic abnormalities, even without aneuploidy. A recent, nationwide study reported that the rate of abnormalities was 21% for fetuses with NT between the 95th and 99th percentile and 62% for fetuses with NT ≥99th percentile, with prevalences of single-gene disorders and submicroscopic, chromosomal, and structural abnormalities at 2%, 2%, 30%, and 9%, respectively [6]. In fetuses with increased NT and normal karyotype, chromosomal microarray has a 5% additional yield for finding copy number variants (CNVs) [7]. Whole exome sequencing (WES) yields an extra 3.9% (95% confidence interval (CI): 1.6–7.1) pathogenic or likely pathogenic variants in fetuses with isolated increased NT and normal karyotype/microarray [8]. RASopathies (e.g., Noonan syndrome and Costello syndrome) are clinical entities to be considered in cases with NT >5 mm or >3.5 mm with other selected anomalies [9].

Aside from genetic abnormalities, an increased NT is strongly associated with structural abnormalities, mainly cardiac malformations. The causal relationship remains unclear; animal studies have identified candidate genes encoding endothelium that may regulate both cardiac and lymphatic development [10].

In conclusion, despite the widespread availability of cfDNA, NT's significance and predictive potential in aneuploidies and structural abnormalities cannot be disputed. Therefore, an early second-trimester ultrasound scan at 16 weeks may be considered if an increased NT is detected and if the first-trimester ultrasound is otherwise unremarkable [1]. Furthermore, an anatomy scan between 18 and 22 weeks of gestation and a fetal echocardiogram, as indicated, are recommended.

4.2.2 Nasal Bone

The intramembranous ossification process of the nasal bone seems to be delayed in trisomy 21, as first reported by Dr. Langdon Down in 1866. This delayed process leads to a hypoplasic nasal bone in the second-trimester scan yet an absent nasal bone in the first-trimester ultrasound scan. Approximately 68% of fetuses with chromosomal abnormalities have an absent nasal bone in the first-trimester ultrasound [11]. The midsagittal view used for evaluating the NT displays the nasal bone as two parallel lines—-"equal sign"—which indicates the nasal bone and the overlying skin (◘ Figs. 4.3 and 4.4). To define the nasal bone as "present," it must be thicker and more echogenic than the skin above it.

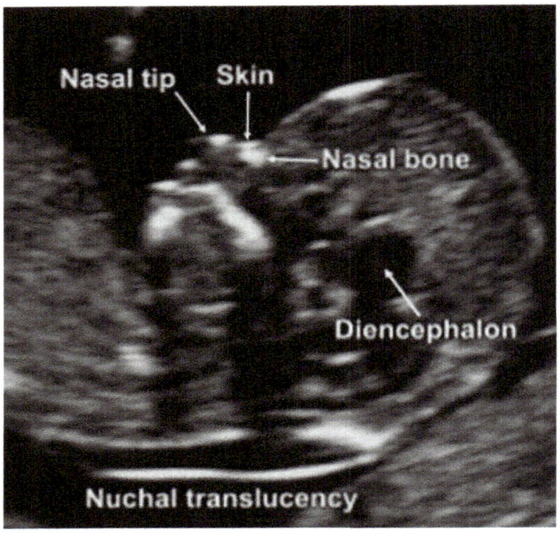

◘ **Fig. 4.3** Midsagittal view demonstrating the "equal sign"

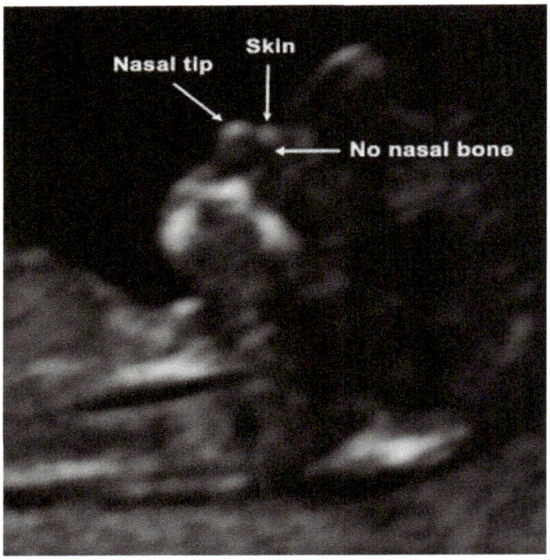

◘ **Fig. 4.4** Absent nasal bone

4.2.3 Tricuspid Valve

Evaluation of tricuspid valve regurgitation with pulsed-wave Doppler has gained attention in recent decades, as 55% of fetuses with trisomy 21 exhibit tricuspid regurgitation, but just 1% of euploid fetuses present with this condition [12]. In the four-chamber view, a pulse Doppler sample is applied on the tricuspid valve, and forward flow through the valve is assessed (◘ Fig. 4.5). A correlation exists between congenital cardiac diseases and tricuspid regurgitation during the first trimester; thus, careful monitoring and counseling in these cases are essential, even when genetic diagnostic investigations yield normal results [13].

4.2.4 Right Subclavian Artery

An aberrant right subclavian artery (ARSA) is found in 29% of aneuploid fetuses and is also considered a marker for cardiac anomalies [14]. It is also observed in 1.5% of euploid fetuses, and recent studies indicate that it should be regarded as a normal variant if isolated [15, 16].

Without advanced equipment and sufficient expertise, it might be difficult to see the right subclavian artery's usual path during a first-trimester ultrasound (◘ Figs. 4.6 and 4.7).

4.2.5 Ductus Venosus

Ductus venosus is a unique anatomic structure, vital in fetal life since it directs the oxygenated blood in the umbilical vein directly to the heart. The flow pattern of the ductus venosus is triphasic, and the "a-"wave repre-

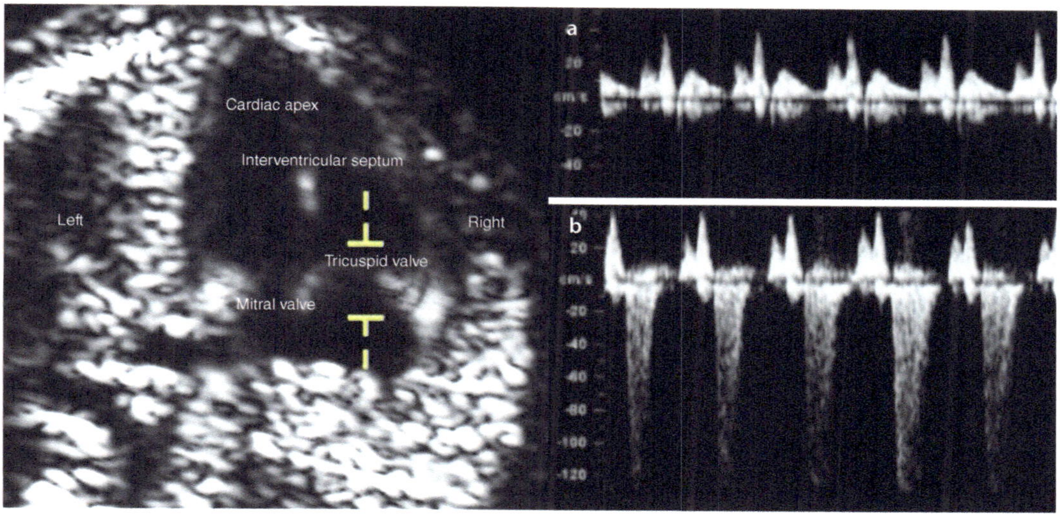

Fig. 4.5 Assessment of the tricuspid valve. **a** Normal tricuspid flow on pulsed-Doppler. **b** Pansystolic regurgitation

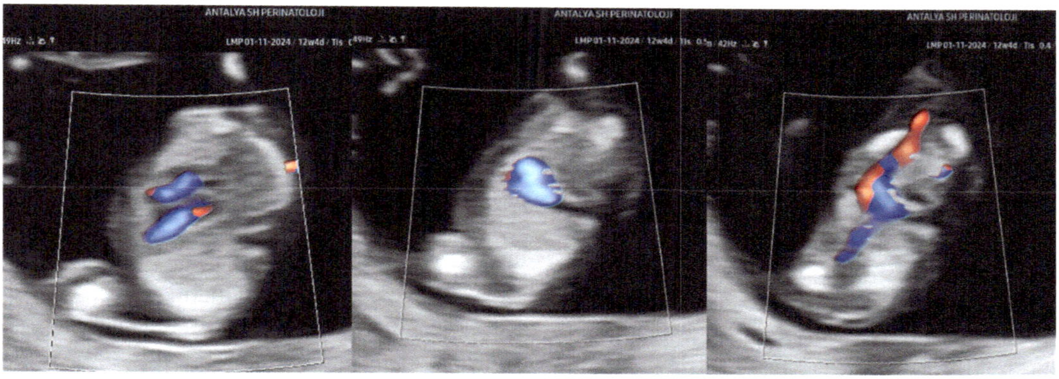

Fig. 4.6 Normal four-chamber, three-vessel, and right subclavian artery views in a 12-week fetus

Fig. 4.7 Aberrant right subclavian artery coursing behind the trachea

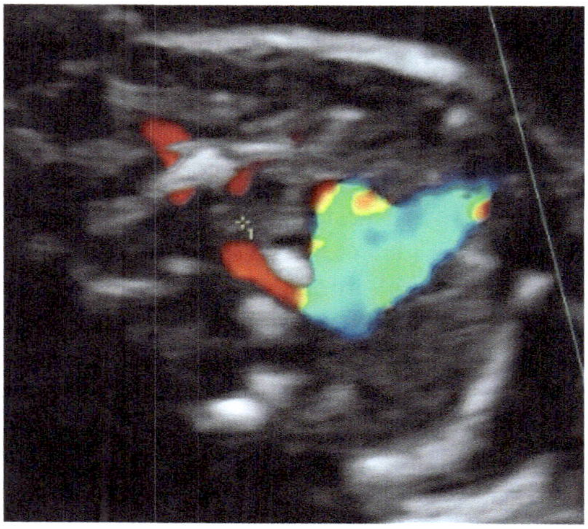

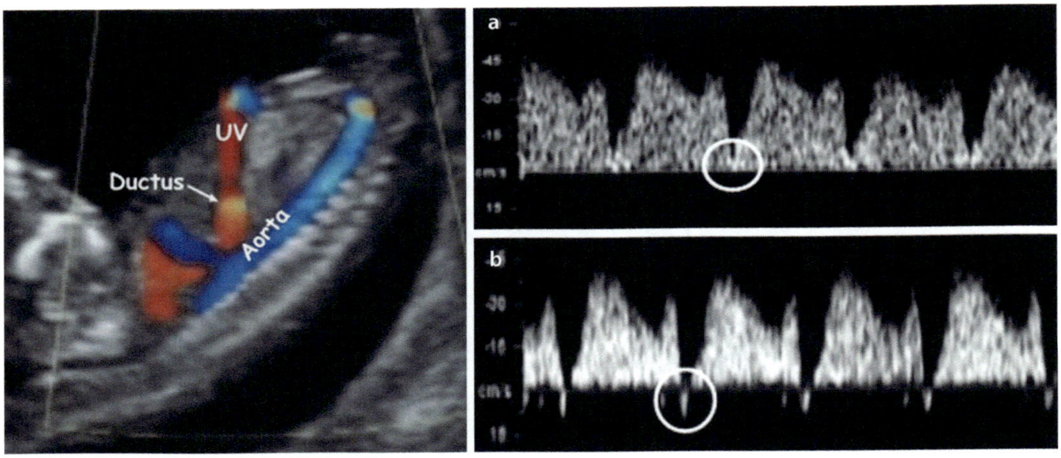

Fig. 4.8 Ductus venosus draining into the inferior vena cava via the subdiaphragmatic vestibulum. **a** Normal ductus venosus flow pattern with positive a-wave and **b** reversed a-wave

sents atrial contraction (Fig. 4.8a). A reversed a-wave in the Doppler examination of the ductus venosus can be present in fetuses with aneuploidies and cardiac anomalies (Fig. 4.8b) [17].

4.3 Screening for Fetal Anomalies

The second-trimester anatomy scan is the gold standard for evaluating fetal structural abnormalities. Nonetheless, fetal abnormalities are now possible to identify in the first trimester, thanks to advancements in ultrasound technology and enhanced training for medical personnel [18]. First-trimester ultrasound screening for fetal malformations reassures families when no structural defects are observed. Conversely, if an anomaly or abnormal finding is identified, it facilitates earlier genetic testing and, if necessary, termination of pregnancy. Yet, due to the progressive nature of phenotypic expression of fetal anomalies with gestation, not all abnormalities can be detected in the first trimester. Therefore, fetal anomalies are classified as "always detectable," "potentially detectable," and "undetectable" [4]. The abnormalities that are "always detectable" are those evident in the first-trimester ultrasound scan, such as acrania, hydrops, ectopia cordis, omphalocele, gastroschisis, megacystis, and body stalk anomalies [19]. Undetectable abnormalities typically manifest during the second or third trimester of pregnancy, such as migrational anomalies of the brain, agenesis of the corpus callosum, and congenital pulmonary airway malformation (CPAM) [19]. The sensitivity of the first-trimester ultrasound screening for fetal anomalies ranges between 32% and 61% and increases when a standardized protocol for the scan is adopted [20]. Organizations have published protocols that define the components of basic and detailed ultrasonographic examination of fetal anatomy in the first trimester [18, 21].

4.3.1 Brain and Spine

The sonographic evaluation of the fetal brain has consistently posed a significant difficulty in both screening and diagnostic contexts, owing to the complexity of the cerebral architecture and the ongoing development of cranial anatomy. Therefore, diagnosing central nervous system anomalies is not always possible in the first trimester. However, numerous defects can be detected in the first trimester by looking at specific structures, including the cisterna magna, choroid plexuses of the lateral ventricles, and falx cerebri (Fig. 4.9).

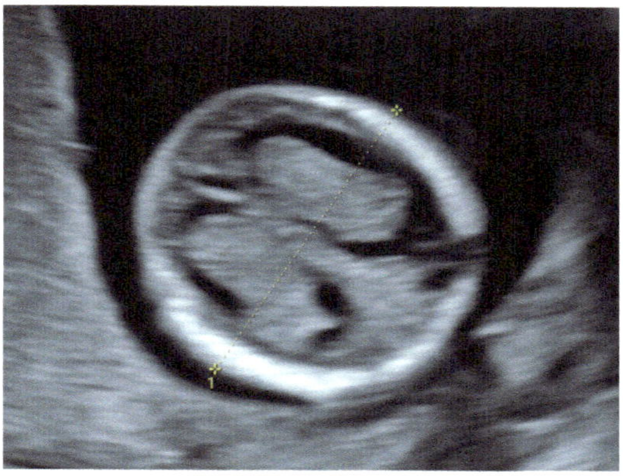

Fig. 4.9 Normal cranium with "butterfly-shaped" choroid plexuses in the first trimester

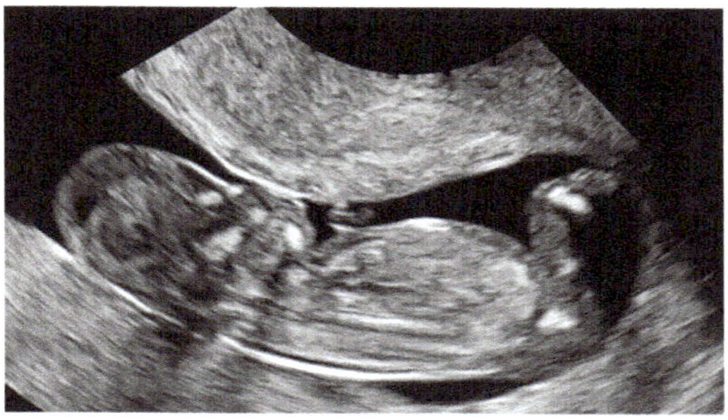

Fig. 4.10 Acrania in a 12-week fetus

"Always detectable" anomalies of the central nervous system in the first trimester are the acrania–exencephaly–anencephaly sequence, alobar and semilobar holoprosencephaly, and large cephaloceles [4]. The observation of absent cranial vault (acrania) and exposed brain tissue (exencephaly) as a result is pretty straightforward (Fig. 4.10). A cystic lesion protruding from the fetal skull (generally the occipital region) indicates a cephalocele (Fig. 4.11). Holoprosencephaly is characterized sonographically by the partial or complete absence of the midline falx and the absence of the distinctive butterfly sign of the choroid plexuses (Fig. 4.12).

Open neural tube defects and subsequent Chiari II malformations are considered to be potentially detectable in the first trimester (Fig. 4.13). Large myelomeningoceles can be diagnosed by evaluating the spine using the direct midsagittal view of the spinal column and the skin covering it, but a normal appearance during the first trimester cannot rule out open spina bifida since the defect would not be sufficiently evident at this stage. Intracranial translucency (IT) would be obliterated due to the compression of the brain stem in Chiari II malformation, which is pertinent for suspecting open neural tube defects in the first trimester [22].

Microcephaly and abnormalities of the corpus callosum and vermis (agenesis/dysgenesis) are undetectable in the first-trimester anatomic evaluation [4].

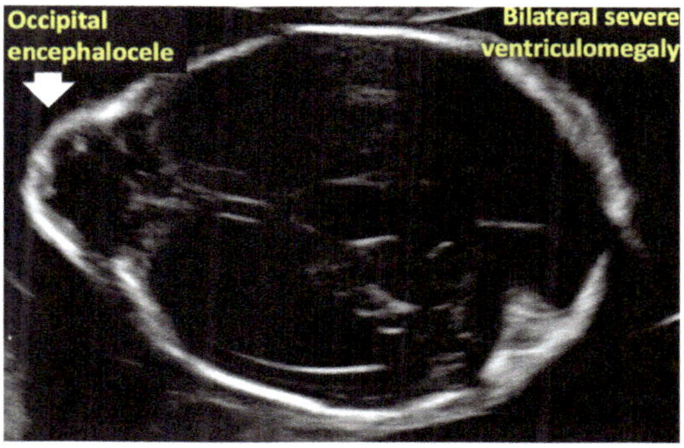

Fig. 4.11 Occipital cephalocele with accompanying bilateral ventriculomegaly

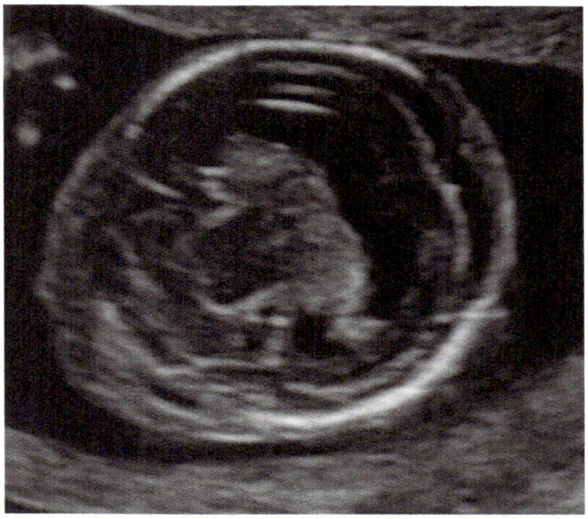

Fig. 4.12 Holoprosencephaly. Note the fused thalami, monoventricle, and the absence of falx cerebri

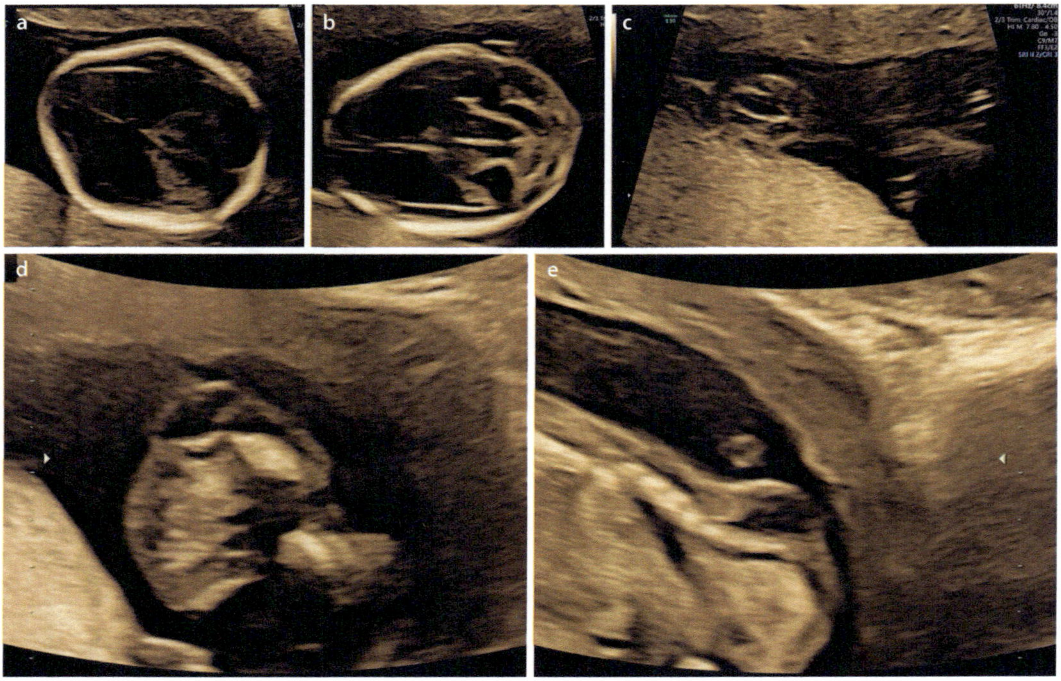

Fig. 4.13 Neural tube defect with Chiari II malformation. **a** "Lemon sign" of the frontal bone. **b** "Banana sign" of the cerebellum herniating through the foramen magnum, thereby obliterating the posterior fossa. **c** Open spinal defect in the coronal view. **d** Meningomyelocele sac in the axial view. **e** Lumbosacral meningomyelocele in the sagittal view

4.3.2 Face

Fetal face in the first trimester should be evaluated in midsagittal, transverse, and coronal views in order to visualize the profile, nasal bone, orbits, and the retronasal triangle. Still, facial abnormalities are not always detectable and offer only subtle signs in the first trimester scan. Potentially detectable anomalies of the face are micrognathia and facial clefts. Due to the often challenging visualization of the lip and the small size of these structures, only major clefts can be diagnosed in the first trimester [23].

4.3.3 Thorax

The chest typically contains the lungs of homogeneous echogenicity on the first-trimester ultrasound, without evidence of cystic or solid masses. Pulmonary masses such as CPAM or bronchopulmonary sequestration are undetectable anomalies in the first trimester. Congenital diaphragmatic hernias, on the other hand, are potentially detectable in the first trimester by carefully evaluating the position of the fetal heart and abdominal organs—mainly the stomach (Fig. 4.14). Approximately 50% of cases may be identified in the first trimester, facilitating early genetic testing and the option for pregnancy termination in this potentially fatal condition [4].

4.3.4 Heart

Cardiac anomalies are the most common type of congenital anomalies, which affect 0.8% of all fetuses, and are a significant cause of neonatal death [24]. Stillbirth may occur in up to 20–30% and neonatal death in up to 40–60% of fetal cardiac anomalies, depending on the diagnosis [25]. Prenatal detection of congenital cardiac anomalies facilitates the preparation of an ideal delivery plan, ensuring the

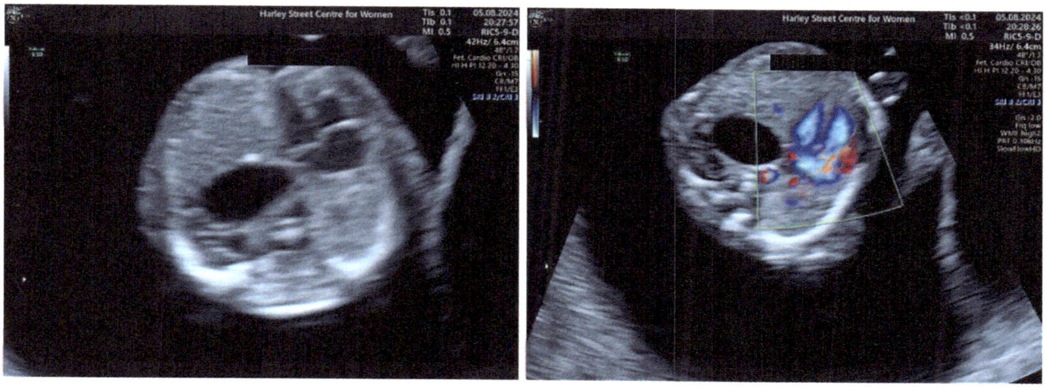

Fig. 4.14 Congenital diaphragmatic hernia in the first trimester. Note that the stomach is visible in the thorax, herniating through the defective diaphragm

presence of cardiac and neonatal teams, thus enhancing neonatal survival rates [26].

Many first-trimester markers of aneuploidy that are already being evaluated during the first-trimester scan, such as increased NT, reverse a-wave in ductus venosus and tricuspid regurgitation, are in fact indirect signs of a cardiac anomaly. Fetal echocardiography during the second trimester is typically recommended for cases of increased NT; however, advancements in ultrasound technology and the widespread application of a transvaginal approach have integrated cardiac assessment into first-trimester ultrasound protocols.

As the assessment of tricuspid inflow for regurgitation requires evaluating the cardiac four-chamber view, many sonographers are familiar with this view during the first trimester (Fig. 4.5). The use of the color Doppler in evaluating the four-chamber view helps confirm the presence of two atrioventricular inflows and two ventricles. An abnormal four-chamber view in the first trimester has a 50% detection rate for congenital cardiac anomalies and is the most specific sign [27]. However, only 30% of congenital cardiac anomalies have an abnormal four-chamber view. Therefore, the assessment of ventriculo-arterial connections and three-vessel view is crucial for conotruncal anomalies, which often require emergency intervention in the postpartum period. The outflow tracts of the great arteries cannot be easily visualized during first-trimester ultrasounds due to the very small actual size of the fetal heart at this stage. Yet the three-vessel view can be efficiently assessed with the help of color Doppler [28]. The evaluation of the four-chamber and three-vessel views is therefore included in the guidelines for the first-trimester screening of cardiac anomalies in high-risk patients (e.g., prior pregnancy with cardiac anomaly, poorly controlled diabetes, high-risk aneuploidy testing result, or increased NT) [29]. Figure 4.6 demonstrates normal cardiac views in the first trimester.

Situs anomalies are always detectable via a first-trimester ultrasound, focusing on the fetal spine and head to ascertain the fetal left side and the stomach's position. Detection of major congenital cardiac anomalies is still challenging and requires further scanning a few weeks later. Minor defects like ventricular septal defects (VSDs) and late-onset diseases are undetectable by the first-trimester cardiac evaluation [27].

A recent meta-analysis has reported that a first-trimester ultrasound for cardiac anomalies has a pooled sensitivity of 55.8% (95% CI: 45.9–65.5%), a specificity of 99.98% (95% CI: 99.97–99.99%), and a positive predictive value of 94.9% (95% CI: 91.6–97.3%) in the low-risk population [24]. But the sensitivity depends on the gestational age, with sensitivity increasing with increasing gestational age, and maternal body mass index (BMI), if conducted by a transabdominal ultrasound.

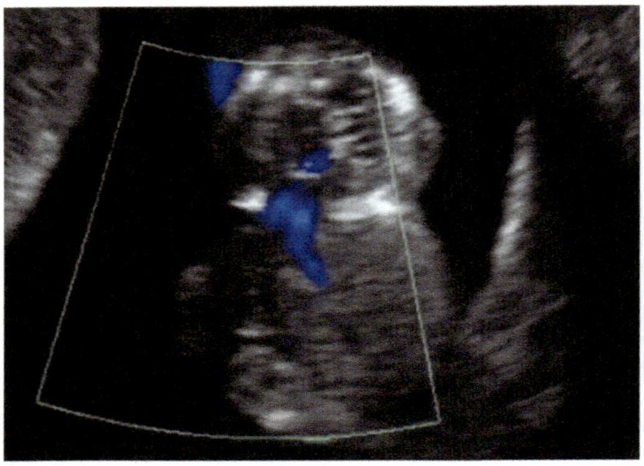

Fig. 4.15 A large exomphalos containing the fetal liver

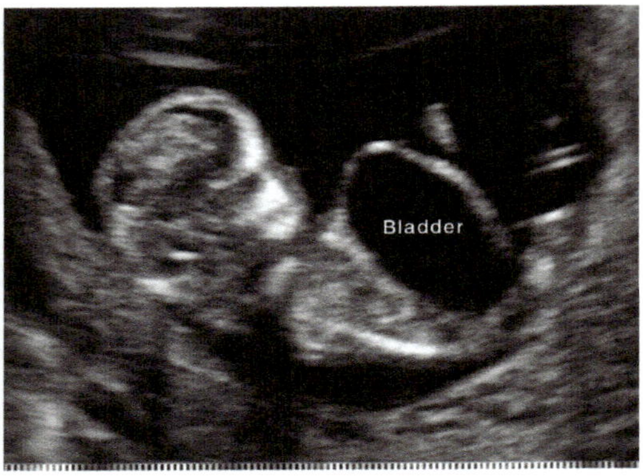

Fig. 4.16 An 11-week fetus with megacystis

4.3.5 Abdomen

The basic transverse view of the cord insertion to the fetal abdomen is enough to detect abdominal wall anomalies in the first trimester. Normal size and position of the stomach may help rule out situs anomalies and some types of congenital diaphragmatic hernias. Both omphalocele and gastroschisis are always detectable in the first-trimester ultrasound [30, 31]. Care should be taken for omphaloceles diagnosed before the 12th week since physiological bowel herniation may mimic an omphalocele. However, if the omphalocele sac contains the liver, the diagnosis can be made confidently (Fig. 4.15). Both anomalies are linked to neonatal mortality and surgical morbidity; thus, early detection ensures optimal delivery plans with the available pediatric surgical team. Also, genetic counseling and invasive diagnostic testing should be offered in omphalocele cases since it is strongly associated with aneuploidies, mainly trisomy 18 [32].

4.3.6 Urinary Tract

The fetal bladder must be seen in the transverse view in the first trimester. Bilateral kidneys are also visible, but their echogenicity is indistinguishable from the surrounding structures and, therefore, might be hard to visualize with transabdominal transducers. Renal agenesis may be detectable in the first trimester; however, it is frequently challenging to diagnose due to the lack of the most indicative sign—oligohydramnios—resulting from ultrafiltration being the primary source of amniotic fluid at that stage. Still, a transvaginal approach to identify the kidneys should be implemented if the bladder is not visible, even after waiting a certain amount of time. Conversely, the fetal bladder may be enlarged, defined as megacystis, if measured more than 7 mm in the longitudinal diameter (Fig. 4.16). Megacystis may be a clue for both aneuploidies—mainly trisomy 13 and 18—and lower urinary tract obstruction [33]. If the maximum longitudinal diameter of the fetal bladder is measured between 7 and 15 mm, megacystis is associated with aneuploidies in 24% of cases. However, if the bladder is more than 15 mm, the cause is most likely lower urinary tract obstruction—either posterior urethral valve or urethral atresia.

4.3.7 Extremities

Ultrasonographic evaluation of fetal extremities in the first trimester should aim to show the presence of all three segments of each extremity: thigh, leg, and foot in both lower extremities and arm, forearm, and hand in both upper extremities. In addition, all bones should be checked for normal appearance and mineralization. Clubfeet and transverse reduction defects may be evident in the first trimester; however, the small size of these structures and their positional variability complicate reliable diagnosis when isolated.

4.4 Pitfalls of First-Trimester Ultrasound

The first-trimester anatomic evaluation is crucial in antenatal care. With the widespread availability of cfDNA testing, patients may undergo a cfDNA test as early as the tenth gestational week and be "assured" with a negative result. However, this approach misses major structural anomalies in the first trimester, which may be easily detectable by the first-trimester ultrasound scan [34]. The first-trimester anatomy scan should be performed and interpreted by experienced sonographers and physicians. Transvaginal imaging is recommended when the transabdominal visualization of the necessary anatomic elements is inadequate, an anomaly is suspected, or an enlarged nuchal translucency is present, as it increases the detection of structural abnormalities [35]. The performance of a first-trimester anatomy scan must be followed up by a second-trimester anatomic assessment of the fetus because some anomalies may not be detected until later in gestation or even after birth [36].

The sensitivity of a first-trimester scan was 37.5% for the detection of structural anomalies overall (95% confidence interval (CI): 31.1–44.3); however, 91.3% for lethal anomalies (95% CI 83.9–95.5), with an overall specificity of 99.9% (95% CI: 99.9–100), was reported in the most recent Cochrane review regarding the diagnostic accuracy of the first-trimester ultrasound [37]. Two-stage screening with both first- and second-trimester anatomy scans had a combined sensitivity of 83.8% (95% CI: 74.7–90.1), while screening only with the second-trimester ultrasound had a sensitivity of 50.5% (95% CI: 38.5–62.4) [37]. The first-trimester ultrasound is anticipated to accurately detect 113 out of 124 fetuses with lethal anomalies (91.3%) and 665 out of 1776 fetuses with any structural abnormality (37.5%) in a hypothetical cohort of 100,000 pregnancies [37]. Nevertheless, out of 98,224 fetuses, 79 (0.08%) are expected to receive false-positive diagnoses [37]. A high (>80%) detection rate was reported for major anomalies, including acrania (98%), gastroschisis (96%), omphalocele (95%), and holoprosencephaly (88%); the detection rate was lower for open spina bifida (69%), lower urinary tract obstruction (66%), lethal skeletal dysplasias (57%), and limb reduction defects (50%); and the detection rate was below 50% for facial clefts (43%), polydactyly (40%), and congenital diaphragmatic hernia (38%) in a recent meta-analysis [38]. Anomalies with a low (<30%) detection rate included bilateral renal agenesis (25%), closed spina bifida (21%), isolated cleft lip (14%), and clubfoot (11%) [38].

The conclusions of the literature should be interpreted with caution because detection rates improve as the publication year progresses, and the screening performance is significantly affected by using established imaging protocols [38]. Many obstacles arise from concerns regarding the cost and feasibility of implementing these protocols, the sonography team training and quality control methods, and meeting the minimum requirements of ultrasound equipment. Research indicates that the first-trimester anatomy scan increases the cost of healthcare per pregnancy, while the detection of anomalies is also increased [39]. Globally, healthcare policies and guidelines and uniform access to first-trimester ultrasound are inadequate; however, organizations should highlight the significance and guide clinicians.

Chapter Key Points

- Evolution and purpose of the first-trimester anatomy scan
- Key markers for aneuploidy screening (NT, nasal bone, tricuspid valve, ductus venosus, and ARSA)
- Structures assessed for early fetal anomaly detection
- Limitations and pitfalls of the first-trimester ultrasound
- Role of standardized protocols and operator expertise

4

Chapter-End Summary

This chapter outlines the expanding role of the first-trimester anatomy scan, highlighting its dual purpose in aneuploidy screening and early structural assessment. Key sonographic markers such as nuchal translucency, nasal bone, tricuspid flow, ductus venosus, and right subclavian artery contribute to detecting chromosomal and cardiac anomalies. The chapter details which anomalies are always, potentially, or not detectable in the first trimester, emphasizing the impact of gestational development and technical limitations. Despite these challenges, standardized protocols, operator expertise, and complementary second-trimester scanning significantly enhance diagnostic accuracy and prenatal counseling, reinforcing the essential role of early ultrasound.

References

1. Le Lous M, Bouhanna P, Colmant C, Rozenberg P, Quibel T. The performance of an intermediate 16th-week ultrasound scan for the follow-up of euploid fetuses with increased nuchal translucency. Prenat Diagn. 2016;36(2):148–53.
2. Screening for Fetal Chromosomal Abnormalities: ACOG practice bulletin, number 226. Obstet Gynecol. 2020;136(4):e48–69.
3. Prabhu M, Kuller JA, Biggio JR. Society for Maternal-Fetal Medicine Consult Series #57: evaluation and management of isolated soft ultrasound markers for aneuploidy in the second trimester: (replaces consults #10, single umbilical artery, October 2010; #16, isolated echogenic bowel diagnosed on second-trimester ultrasound, august 2011; #17, evaluation and management of isolated renal pelviectasis on second-trimester ultrasound, December 2011; #25, isolated fetal choroid plexus cysts, April 2013; #27, isolated echogenic intracardiac focus, august 2013). Am J Obstet Gynecol. 2021;225(4):B2–B15.
4. Syngelaki A, Chelemen T, Dagklis T, Allan L, Nicolaides KH. Challenges in the diagnosis of fetal non-chromosomal abnormalities at 11–13 weeks. Prenat Diagn. 2011;31(1):90–102.
5. Pasquini L, Ponziani I, Spataro E, Masini G, Biancareddu E, Cordisco A, et al. Elevated nuchal translucency, is it time to discuss the cut off? Int J Gynaecol Obstet. 2023;163(2):540–6.
6. Bardi F, Bosschieter P, Verheij J, Go A, Haak M, Bekker M, et al. Is there still a role for nuchal translucency measurement in the changing paradigm of first trimester screening? Prenat Diagn. 2020;40(2):197–205.
7. Grande M, Jansen FA, Blumenfeld YJ, Fisher A, Odibo AO, Haak MC, et al. Genomic microarray in fetuses with increased nuchal translucency and normal karyotype: a systematic review and meta-analysis. Ultrasound Obstet Gynecol. 2015;46(6):650–8.
8. Di Girolamo R, Rizzo G, Khalil A, Alameddine S, Lisi G, Liberati M, et al. Whole exome sequencing in fetuses with isolated increased nuchal translucency: a systematic review and meta-analysis. J Matern Fetal Neonatal Med. 2023;36(1):2193285.
9. Sinajon P, Chitayat D, Roifman M, Wasim S, Carmona S, Ryan G, et al. Microarray and RASopathy-disorder testing in fetuses with increased nuchal translucency. Ultrasound Obstet Gynecol. 2020;55(3):383–90.
10. Burger NB, Bekker MN, de Groot CJ, Christoffels VM, Haak MC. Why increased nuchal translucency is associated with congenital heart disease: a systematic review on genetic mechanisms. Prenat Diagn. 2015;35(6):517–28.
11. Cicero S, Rembouskos G, Vandecruys H, Hogg M, Nicolaides KH. Likelihood ratio for trisomy 21 in fetuses with absent nasal bone at the 11–14-week scan. Ultrasound Obstet Gynecol. 2004;23(3):218–23.
12. Faiola S, Tsoi E, Huggon IC, Allan LD, Nicolaides KH. Likelihood ratio for trisomy 21 in fetuses with tricuspid regurgitation at the 11 to 13 + 6-week scan. Ultrasound Obstet Gynecol. 2005;26(1):22–7.
13. Kagan KO, Valencia C, Livanos P, Wright D, Nicolaides KH. Tricuspid regurgitation in screening for trisomies 21, 18 and 13 and Turner syndrome at 11+0 to 13+6 weeks of gestation. Ultrasound Obstet Gynecol. 2009;33(1):18–22.
14. Borenstein M, Minekawa R, Zidere V, Nicolaides KH, Allan LD. Aberrant right subclavian artery at 16 to 23 + 6 weeks of gestation: a marker for chromosomal abnormality. Ultrasound Obstet Gynecol. 2010;36(5):548–52.
15. Paladini D, Sglavo G, Pastore G, Masucci A, D'Armiento MR, Nappi C. Aberrant right subclavian artery: incidence and correlation with other markers of Down syndrome in second-trimester fetuses. Ultrasound Obstet Gynecol. 2012;39(2):191–5.
16. Odacılar A, Ayhan I, Karaman A, Demirci O. Aberrant right subclavian artery in the absence of other prenatal ultrasound findings: should we still be concerned? J Clin Ultrasound. 2024;52:1096.
17. Maiz N, Valencia C, Emmanuel EE, Staboulidou I, Nicolaides KH. Screening for adverse pregnancy outcome by ductus venosus Doppler at 11–13+6 weeks of gestation. Obstet Gynecol. 2008;112(3):598–605.

18. Obstetrics ISoUi, Gynecology, Bilardo CM, Chaoui R, Hyett JA, Kagan KO, et al. ISUOG practice guidelines (updated): performance of 11–14-week ultrasound scan. Ultrasound Obstet Gynecol. 2023;61(1):127–43.
19. Syngelaki A, Hammami A, Bower S, Zidere V, Akolekar R, Nicolaides KH. Diagnosis of fetal non-chromosomal abnormalities on routine ultrasound examination at 11–13 weeks' gestation. Ultrasound Obstet Gynecol. 2019;54(4):468–76.
20. Karim JN, Roberts NW, Salomon LJ, Papageorghiou AT. Systematic review of first-trimester ultrasound screening for detection of fetal structural anomalies and factors that affect screening performance. Ultrasound Obstet Gynecol. 2017;50(4):429–41.
21. Volpe N, Sen C, Turan S, Sepulveda W, Khalil A, Rolnik DL, et al. First trimester examination of fetal anatomy: clinical practice guideline by the World Association of Perinatal Medicine (WAPM) and the Perinatal Medicine Foundation (PMF). J Perinat Med. 2022;50(7):863–77.
22. Chaoui R, Benoit B, Mitkowska-Wozniak H, Heling KS, Nicolaides KH. Assessment of intracranial translucency (IT) in the detection of spina bifida at the 11–13-week scan. Ultrasound Obstet Gynecol. 2009;34(3):249–52.
23. De Robertis V, Rembouskos G, Fanelli T, Votino C, Volpe P. Cleft palate with or without cleft lip: the role of retronasal triangle view and maxillary gap at 11–14 weeks. Fetal Diagn Ther. 2019;46(6):353–9.
24. Karim JN, Bradburn E, Roberts N, Papageorghiou AT. First-trimester ultrasound detection of fetal heart anomalies: systematic review and meta-analysis. Ultrasound Obstet Gynecol. 2022;59(1):11–25.
25. Johnson B, Simpson LL. Screening for congenital heart disease: a move toward earlier echocardiography. Am J Perinatol. 2007;24(8):449–56.
26. Holland BJ, Myers JA, Woods CR Jr. Prenatal diagnosis of critical congenital heart disease reduces risk of death from cardiovascular compromise prior to planned neonatal cardiac surgery: a meta-analysis. Ultrasound Obstet Gynecol. 2015;45(6):631–8.
27. Volpe P, Ubaldo P, Volpe N, Campobasso G, De Robertis V, Tempesta A, et al. Fetal cardiac evaluation at 11–14 weeks by experienced obstetricians in a low-risk population. Prenat Diagn. 2011;31(11):1054–61.
28. De Robertis V, Rembouskos G, Fanelli T, Volpe G, Muto B, Volpe P. The three-vessel and trachea view (3VTV) in the first trimester of pregnancy: an additional tool in screening for congenital heart defects (CHD) in an unselected population. Prenat Diagn. 2017;37(7):693–8.
29. Freud LR, Simpson LL. Fetal cardiac screening: 1st trimester and beyond. Prenat Diagn. 2024;44(6–7):679–87.
30. Khalil A, Arnaoutoglou C, Pacilli M, Szabo A, David AL, Pandya P. Outcome of fetal exomphalos diagnosed at 11–14 weeks of gestation. Ultrasound Obstet Gynecol. 2012;39(4):401–6.
31. David AL, Tan A, Curry J. Gastroschisis: sonographic diagnosis, associations, management and outcome. Prenat Diagn. 2008;28(7):633–44.
32. Ayhan I, Demirci O, Uygur L, Odacilar Ş, Özbay Ayvaz OD, Karaman A, et al. An analysis of factors affecting survival in prenatally diagnosed omphalocele. J Perinat Med. 2023;51(9):1189–96.
33. Liao AW, Sebire NJ, Geerts L, Cicero S, Nicolaides KH. Megacystis at 10–14 weeks of gestation: chromosomal defects and outcome according to bladder length. Ultrasound Obstet Gynecol. 2003;21(4):338–41.
34. Bardi F, Beekhuis AM, Bakker MK, Elvan-Taşpınar A, Bilardo CM. Timing of diagnosis of fetal structural abnormalities after the introduction of universal cell-free DNA in the absence of first-trimester anatomical screening. Prenat Diagn. 2022;42(10):1242–52.
35. Bromley B, Platt LD. First-trimester ultrasound screening in routine obstetric practice. Obstet Gynecol. 2024;143(6):730–44.
36. AIUM practice parameter for the performance of standard diagnostic obstetric ultrasound. J Ultrasound Med. 2024;43(6):E20–32.
37. Buijtendijk MFJ, Bet BB, Leeflang MMG, Shah H, Reuvekamp T, Goring T, et al. Diagnostic accuracy of ultrasound screening for fetal structural abnormalities during the first and second trimester of pregnancy in low-risk and unselected populations. Cochrane Database Syst Rev. 2024;5(5):CD014715.
38. Karim JN, Di Mascio D, Roberts N, Papageorghiou AT. Detection of non-cardiac fetal abnormalities on ultrasound at 11–14 weeks: systematic review and meta-analysis. Ultrasound Obstet Gynecol. 2024;64(1):15–27.
39. Pietersma CS, Rousian M, Moolenaar L, Steegers EAP, Mulders A. Impact of first-trimester anomaly scan on health-related quality of life and healthcare costs: a scoping review. J Psychosom Obstet Gynaecol. 2024;45(1):2330414.

Prevention of Stillbirth

Işıl Ayhan and Asma Khalil

Contents

Y. Yogev, A. Khalil (eds.), *Prevention of Complications in Obstetrics*,
https://doi.org/10.1007/978-3-032-23479-7_5

Learning Objectives

- Explain the epidemiology and definitions of stillbirth across regions
- Identify major maternal, fetal, placental, and intrapartum risk factors
- Describe the main causes and classification systems used for stillbirth evaluation
- Summarize recommended diagnostic approaches, including pathology and genetic testing
- Assess the role and limitations of biomarkers and ultrasound in predicting stillbirth
- Apply prevention strategies tailored to women with and without a history of stillbirth

5.1 Introduction

Stillbirth is a devastating event with a profound emotional and psychological impact on families. Clinically, stillbirth is a complex phenomenon due to its variable etiology, as well as challenges and obstacles in diagnostic evaluation. The variable etiology may include maternal health conditions, placental abnormalities, and fetal genetic disorders. Understanding the causes and risk factors is crucial for healthcare providers to develop preventive strategies, improve prenatal care, and prevent stillbirth, which remains a critical concern in maternal–fetal medicine.

5.2 Epidemiology

The definition and classification of stillbirth vary throughout different regions of the world. Fetal mortality after the 20th week of gestation is generally considered the standard definition. However, the absence of agreement on specific criteria and classification poses challenges in obtaining precise data, ultimately leading to a lack of established guidelines on prevention methods.

The Centers for Disease Control and Prevention (CDC) classifies stillbirth into three groups based on onset: early stillbirth (20–27 completed weeks), late stillbirth (28–36 completed weeks), and term stillbirth (≥37 completed weeks) [1]. Annually, there are two million cases of late or term stillbirths worldwide [2]. The number of stillbirths has decreased by 35% over the past two decades [3]. The decrease has been linked to greater access to antenatal care, as well as an increasing awareness of the known risks of stillbirth; however, regional disparities still exist. The incidence is 3 per 1000 births in high-income countries, while it is significantly higher in low-income countries, at 22.7 per 1000 births [2]. Fifty percent of stillbirths occur during labor and delivery and are attributed to insufficient resources and staff to perform emergency caesarean sections in sub-Saharan Africa and South Asia [2].

5.3 Risk Factors

Numerous conditions are considered risk factors for stillbirth rather than direct causes, and these conditions are often found in live births as well. Advanced maternal age, obesity, and smoking are all excellent examples. Differentiating between the causes and risk factors of stillbirth poses a challenge. One approach to defining the risk factors is to classify conditions that are infrequent in live births but prevalent in stillbirths as causes, while classifying factors that are prevalent in live births but even more prevalent in stillbirths as risk factors [3].

5.3.1 Race/Ethnicity

Non-Hispanic Blacks have the highest fetal mortality rate (10.53 deaths per 1000 births), whereas non-Hispanic Whites have the lowest (4.88 deaths per 1000 births) [4]. While this difference in risk between different racial groups can be attributed to the availability and quality of antenatal care, other factors play a role, as Black pregnant individuals have a higher likelihood of stillbirth even when they get appropriate prenatal care [5]. This might be a result of a combination of genetic, behavioral, and environmental factors, yet other factors remain unclarified.

5.3.2 Extremes of Reproductive Age

A U-shaped correlation exists between maternal age and the risk of stillbirth. The stillbirth rates are more than twice as high for women under the age of 15 (15.88) and women aged 45 and older (13.76) compared to women between the ages of 30–35, who are at the lowest risk of stillbirth [4]. Despite the adjustment for other risk factors, the risk associated with advanced maternal age remains significantly elevated [6].

5.3.3 Parity

Stillbirth rates are 21% higher for nulliparous women (5.88 per 1000 births) than for women who had one prior pregnancy, 18% higher for women with two prior pregnancies, 47% higher for women with three prior pregnancies, and 134% higher for women with four or more previous pregnancies when compared with women who had one prior pregnancy [7]. Still, no preventive strategies would be available regarding parity, as this is not a modifiable risk factor.

5.3.4 Previous Stillbirth

Research has shown an increased risk up to tenfold for women with a history of stillbirth [8]. This is understandable, given that the cause of the previous stillbirth might still endure in the subsequent pregnancy. The risk is greatest if the previous stillbirth was before the 28th gestational week or due to intrapartum adverse events [9].

5.3.5 Obesity

The pathophysiology of stillbirth in obesity might be attributable to intrapartum adverse events due to macrosomia but also uteroplacental insufficiency if there is maternal hypertension. However, besides increasing the risk of diabetes and hypertensive disorders, obesity is an independent risk factor for stillbirth [10]. Prepregnancy obesity is associated with a nearly fourfold increase in the risk of term stillbirth [11].

5.3.6 Smoking

The Stillbirth Collaborative Research Network (SCRN) found a correlation between the number of cigarettes smoked and the risk of stillbirth. Women who smoked ≥10 cigarettes per day had a two- to threefold increased risk [12]. The risk of stillbirth at this smoking level has been reported to be 10–15 per 1000 births [13].

5.4 Etiology

Determining the cause of fetal demise is a complex task. Multiple factors can contribute to fetal demise. Additionally, the critical nature of stillbirth cases could limit the completion of a comprehensive examination to ascertain the precise cause of death. This complicates the process of determining the cause of death, often rendering it challenging or even impossible. A major challenge in addressing stillbirths is the lack of a practical classification system for low-income countries that aligns with more complex systems used elsewhere. This gap prevents two-thirds of the world's stillbirths from being categorized in ways that inform prevention strategies. While at least 33 classification systems exist, most are designed for high-income settings, requiring laboratory and pathological examinations that are often unavailable [14]. In contrast, low-resource settings rely primarily on verbal autopsies conducted long after the loss, making these systems impractical. Yet it is essential to establish the underlying cause in order to proactively avoid future stillbirths. Therefore, classification methods have been created to assign causes of death in stillbirths,

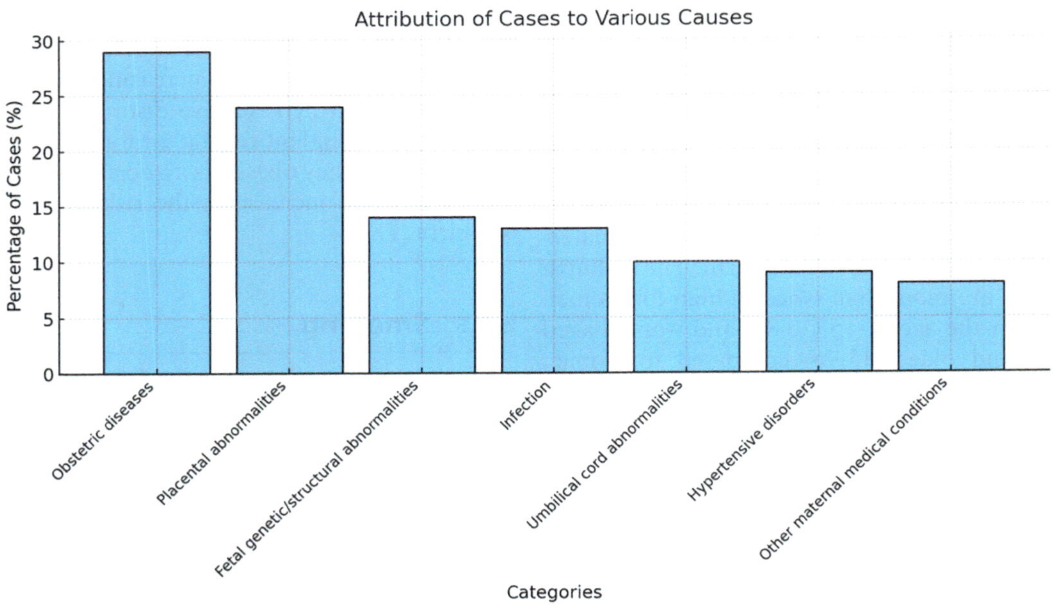

Fig. 5.1 The frequency of stillbirth causes as assigned by the INCODE system [15]

5

but a consensus has not been reached about a standardized methodology.

The SCRN developed the Initial Causes of Fetal Death (INCODE) classification system to assign a cause of death in stillbirths [15]. This system categorized the causes of stillbirth as "probable causes," "possible causes," and "condition present." In a cohort of 512 systematically evaluated stillbirths, there was a probable cause in approximately 60%, based on the INCODE system [15]. The frequency of stillbirth causes as assigned by the INCODE system is shown in Fig. 5.1 [15].

Even though the causes of stillbirth are classified differently by various studies and organizations, this chapter will examine the etiology under the following sections: infections, maternal medical conditions, fetal causes, placental causes, and intrapartum causes.

5.4.1 Infections

The relationship between maternal infection and stillbirth is generally unclear, mainly because the presence of microorganisms in the placenta or on the neonate does not establish causality. Furthermore, identifying causal organisms, including *Mycoplasma*/*Ureaplasma* and specific viruses, is not straightforward. In low- and middle-income countries, infections are responsible for approximately 50% of stillbirths, while in high-income countries, it accounts for 10–25% [16] of stillbirths. Infectious causes are frequently linked to early stillbirths [17].

Stillbirth may result from infections that directly infect the fetus, resulting in anomalies or fetal sepsis. Fetal infection may ascend from the lower genital tract to the maternal decidua, eventually infecting the amniotic fluid and the fetus. Group B *Streptococcus* and *E. coli* are two pathogens that might potentially induce chorioamnionitis, funisitis, and/or fetal pneumonitis through this process. Intrauterine infections may result in stillbirth due to spontaneous preterm birth at a previable gestational age. In general, organisms like *Bacteroides*, *Gardnerella*, and *Mobiluncus* spp. have low virulence and may remain in the uterus for months before causing preterm labor, and the majority of women do not exhibit classic symptoms of infection, such as a fever, chills, or leukocytosis. Instead, the symptoms of these infections appear to be contractions and, in the end, ruptured membranes [18]. Moreover, maternal infections might spread to the fetus through the hematogenous route, resulting in villitis and typically affecting the fetal liver [19]. An example of this mechanism is *Listeria* infection.

Some pathogens cause stillbirth through placental infection and subsequent insufficiency; syphilis is a good example. *Treponema pallidum* can cross the placenta, resulting in stillbirth in 50% of infected fetuses [20]. Malaria is another cause of stillbirth that results in placental insufficiency and is one of the most prevalent etiologies in endemic regions [21].

Severe maternal infectious disease may result in stillbirth even without the transmission of microorganisms to the placenta or fetus due to factors such as fever, respiratory distress, or systemic reactions to the infection. For instance, there have been higher rates of stillbirths observed during influenza pandemics. The COVID-19 pandemic is another recent example. There is an increased risk of stillbirth in severely ill pregnant women with COVID-19, especially with the delta variant [22].

Viral infections may also cause fetal death, though they are even more difficult to show as the main cause. A positive viral serological result does not establish causation, and DNA or RNA viral identification, which has only recently become broadly available, is technically challenging. Parvovirus causes fifth disease in children, though adults may not show any symptoms when infected. Parvovirus attacks erythropoietic tissue, resulting in severe anemia and hydrops. Additionally, it can lead to myocarditis and cardiac dysfunction. Parvovirus has been found to be responsible for up to 7.5% of fetal deaths [23]. Nevertheless, the incidence is significantly reduced in more recent series, and the majority of systematically assessed cases of acute parvovirus infection do not lead to stillbirth [18, 24]. Cytomegalovirus (CMV) is the most common congenital viral infection and is associated with sporadic stillbirth [25].

5.4.2 Maternal Medical Conditions

(a) **Diabetes**

Women with diabetes have a higher risk of stillbirth, especially at or near term. Four percent of stillbirths are associated with maternal diabetes [26]. Cases followed up by diet alone have a risk of 6–10 per 1000 births, while insulin treatment is associated with a risk of 6–35 per 1000 births [13].

The main factors contributing to the risk of stillbirth in fetuses of diabetic mothers are fetal hyperglycemia and hyperinsulinemia, which increase the fetal need for oxygen. This can potentially lead to fetal hypoxemia and acidosis if the fetus does not receive enough oxygen. Additionally, maternal vasculopathy (generally seen with pregestational diabetes) and hyperglycemia can result in reduced blood flow to the uterus and placenta, potentially leading to impaired fetal growth. Pregestational diabetes can also result in stillbirth due to diabetic embryopathy; congenital heart disorders and neural tube defects are linked to poor glycemic control before conception [27, 28].

Gestational diabetes, which can result in macrosomia and polyhydramnios, can lead to stillbirth due to an increased risk of intrapartum adverse events such as shoulder dystocia, umbilical cord prolapse, and malpresentation.

Even though studies show that well-controlled maternal diabetes confers a low risk of stillbirth, quantitative measures of glycemic control and risk of stillbirth are not well-characterized [29].

(b) **Hypertensive Disorders**

Hypertensive disorders are a significant cause of stillbirth. The risk increases with the severity of hypertensive disorder, with chronic hypertension with superimposed preeclampsia posing the greatest risk [15]. The incidence of fetal death in women with chronic hypertension, preeclampsia without severe features, and preeclampsia with severe features is estimated to be 6–25 per 1000, 9–51 per 1000, and 12–29 per 1000 births, respectively [13].

(c) **Renal Disease**

Severe renal impairment with high creatinine levels is associated with stillbirth [30]. Concomitant hypertension poses a tenfold increased risk in patients with renal disease [30]. Need for dialysis during pregnancy also has a poor prognosis, with a 52% live birth rate [31].

5

(d) **Systemic Lupus Erythematosus (SLE)**

As women with SLE have a rate of stillbirth of up to 150 per 1000 births, the risk is increased only in patients with active flare, renal involvement, and antiphospholipid syndrome (APS) [13]. Approximately one-third of patients with SLE have antiphospholipid antibodies linked to a high risk of thrombosis in the placental vasculature. If the patient has anti-Ro/anti-La antibodies, which can cross the placenta and interfere with the fetal cardiac conduction system, fetal death may occur as a result of fetal heart block and subsequent hydrops [32].

(e) **Intrahepatic Cholestasis of Pregnancy (ICP)**

ICP has long been acknowledged as a potential cause of sudden fetal death in the third trimester, yet evidence from recent studies is controversial. In a large cohort of 45,000 pregnant women who were screened with serum bile acid measurement, the stillbirth rate was 0.4% in those who had bile acid levels higher than 40 micromol/L, a rate not so different from the general population [33]. However, when serum bile acid level is higher than 100 micromol/L, there's a 30-fold higher risk of stillbirth, therefore the risk depends on serum bile acid levels [34]. Another population-based study showed that the proportion of cases with increased serum bile acid levels was similar among those with stillbirths and live births [35]. Current evidence does not support routine bile acid measurement screening in pregnancy for the prevention of stillbirth.

5.4.3 Fetal Causes

(a) **Fetal Genetic/Structural Abnormalities**

Fetal structural abnormalities are associated with stillbirth. This is to be expected, as structural abnormalities indicate a higher risk of genetic disorders. However, even in the absence of genetic abnormalities, malformations may lead to fetal death as a result of heart failure and hydrops [3]. Approximately 25% of stillborn neonates have at least one detectable structural abnormality [36]. On the other hand, the prevalence data should be interpreted with care because not all fetal structural abnormalities will result in stillbirth; there must also be a biologically plausible reason for fetal death, and finally, sociodemographic factors can affect the accessibility of prenatal diagnosis and termination of pregnancy [37].

Up to 13% of all stillborn fetuses are aneuploid [38]. The rate increases to 38% in the presence of fetal structural abnormalities [38]. The majority of studies on the relevance of genetic testing in evaluating stillbirth rely on conventional karyotyping. However, with the recent broad availability of molecular genetic studies, submicroscopic genetic etiologies of stillbirth are being identified. Microarray analysis yields a genetic cause in 8.3% of stillbirths [39]. A recent study on the role of exome sequencing in otherwise structurally and genetically "normal" stillborns has reported that 6.1% of cases had genomic variants linked to stillbirth [40]. Overall, 18% of stillbirths have a genetic abnormality [40].

Confined placental mosaicism (CPM) is a condition where the fetus has a normal karyotype despite the presence of an abnormal cell line in the placenta. This has been identified as a potential cause of stillbirth. Key predictors of adverse pregnancy outcomes in patients with CPM include the specific chromosomes affected (such as 2, 3, 7, 8, 9, 16, and 22), the presence of the abnormal cell line throughout pregnancy, the proportion of aneuploid cells in the placenta, and the cell lineage that contains these cells [41, 42].

(b) **Fetal Growth Disorders**

Fetal growth restriction (FGR) is one of the greatest risk factors of stillbirth, with risk increasing as the severity increases. FGR might be a presentation of placental or genetic disorders, and the risk of stillbirth varies based on the root cause. Therefore, it might be safe to say that FGR is more like a risk factor than a cause [43]. Furthermore, it is clinically challenging to distinguish FGR from a non-pathologic, constitutionally small baby. The utilization of "customized" growth curves has been proposed to offer improved differentiation between constitutionally small babies and those who are pathologically small [43]. Nonetheless, population-based studies report that stillbirth has a significant association with small for gestational age (SGA) based on population data (odds ratio [OR]: 3.0; 95% confidence interval [CI]: 2.2–4.0), ultrasound measurements (OR: 4.7; 95% CI: 3.7–5.9), and individualized norms (OR: 4.6; 95% CI: 3.6–5.9) [44].

(c) **Multiple Pregnancies**

Multiple pregnancies are associated with increased risks of preterm birth, preeclampsia, and FGR, ultimately posing a greater risk of stillbirth. However, the higher stillbirth rate in multiple pregnancies is mainly caused by the complications of monochorionic placentation. Twin-to-twin transfusion syndrome, twin-reversed arterial perfusion, selective fetal growth restriction, twin anemia–polycythemia sequence, and cord accidents/entanglement in monoamniotic pregnancies are potential causes of single or double fetal demise.

(d) **Alloimmunization**

Hemolytic disease of the fetus causes fetal anemia and subsequent hydrops. Anti-Rhesus (RhD), anti-Rhc, and anti-Kell antibodies account for the majority of fetuses with severe disease. However, more than 50 red cell antigens have been associated with the disease. Implementing RhD immunoglobulin (Ig) into clinical practice in the past decades has decreased the rate of stillbirth caused by red cell alloimmunization. Still, no immunoglobulins for other red cell antigens are available. Therefore, red cell alloimmunization continues to be a cause of hydropic stillbirth.

Platelet alloimmunization occurs when maternal IgG antibodies against paternally inherited fetal platelet antigens cross the placenta, bind to fetal platelets, and lead to their clearance, may cause stillbirth via fetal thrombocytopenia, resulting in fetal intracranial hemorrhage.

5.4.4 Placental Causes

Placental causes of stillbirth include abruption, ruptured vasa previa, neoplasm, structural or vascular malformations, and infarction. It is often difficult to assign placental abnormalities as "the" cause of stillbirth because histopathological variations are present in live births also. Yet placental etiologies that present with fetomaternal hemorrhage, like abruption and vasa previa, have a strong association with stillbirth [45]. Small placentas are associated with growth restriction, which is also a cause of stillbirth.

5.4.5 Intrapartum

The occurrence of intrapartum stillbirth varies between 1 and 25 per 1000 births, with the prevalence being influenced by the level of resources available in the geographical region [3]. The study conducted by SCRN found that 17% of stillbirths were classified as intrapartum [15]. The majority of these cases were attributed to preterm birth occurring during the periviable gestation period. However, adverse events during labor, such as cord prolapse, shoulder dystocia, and severe birth trauma, may lead to stillbirth.

5.4.6 Unexplained Stillbirth

An unexplained stillbirth refers to the occurrence of fetal death where the cause cannot be determined based on the current level of diagnostic ability. Unfortunately, even with the contemporary approach to stillbirth, 25–60% of all fetal deaths are thought to be unaccounted for [3, 46, 47].

5.5 Evaluation

Parents are shocked and distressed when they receive a stillbirth diagnosis, so it may not always be possible to have a crucial conversation about the evaluation process for stillbirths. Parents might not opt for a workup because it would not change the end point of having a stillborn baby. The cost of genetic studies, religious beliefs, and attitudes toward autopsy can also pose challenges to the workup. However, identifying the cause of stillbirth holds important psychological and biological significance. If the cause is determined and can be modified, steps may be taken to prevent a recurrence in a future pregnancy. Considering these factors, addressing the extensive range of potential causes is challenging. Therefore, clinicians and institutions must establish protocols to ensure an optimal and comprehensive evaluation.

The most important part of the evaluation is a detailed maternal medical and obstetric history. This might reveal clues on risk factors and facilitate or shorten the diagnostic process.

Placental pathology yields the most valuable information on the cause of stillbirth [48]. Besides placental causes, placental pathological examination provides information on many other causes of stillbirth [3]. Through a careful evaluation, various conditions such as placental abruption, umbilical cord thrombosis, velamentous cord insertion, and vasa previa can be identified. Umbilical cord entanglement and knots may be seen in many live births; therefore, they should not be solely assigned as the cause of death if there is no other indication of cord occlusion and hypoxia. An autopsy following published guidelines is also recommended, which may reveal not only structural defects but also infection, anemia, and hypoxia [13, 48–50]. Unfortunately, the lack of access to qualified perinatal pathologists often hinders the crucial process of pathological examination of the placenta and fetus. Genetic testing of the fetus and placenta should be offered in all cases, with microarray analysis being the test of choice [51].

If the history or pathological examination is suspicious of placental insufficiency (recurrent stillbirth, preeclampsia, etc.), testing for APS with lupus anticoagulant and anticardiolipin–anti-beta 2 microglobulin antibodies (both IgG and IgM) is useful [52]. Hereditary thrombophilia panels are not recommended [53].

Aside from the tests above, other investigations, such as serum bile acid measures, infectious disease panels, toxicology, or testing for maternal medical conditions, provide information about the cause in less than 2% of cases [48]. Therefore, additional testing should be guided by history and clinical presentation.

5.6 Prediction

Prevention strategies for stillbirth necessitate the identification of at-risk women. Prior research has tried to develop risk models for the prediction of stillbirth. However, stillbirth prediction models are limited by the fact that risk factors found in cases of stillbirth are also seen in cases of live births. The SCRN study on identifying risk factors for stillbirths has reported that certain factors, such as maternal age over 40, multiple pregnancy, diabetes, history of stillbirth, Black race, and drug abuse, are found to be significantly more common in cases of stillbirth compared to live births [54]. Yet most pregnant women with these risk factors deliver uneventfully. On the other hand, most of the stillbirth cases do not have any of these risk factors [55]. Therefore, prediction efforts for stillbirth generally focus on ultrasound markers and laboratory tests.

There is a correlation between certain biochemical markers and the risk of stillbirth. A low level of pregnancy-associated plasma protein A (PAPP-A) in the first trimester is linked to a higher risk of stillbirth. Within a cohort of 7934 pregnancies, it was observed that a

PAPP-A level below the 5th percentile at 10 weeks was linked to a substantial 9.2-fold increase in the overall stillbirth risk and an even more pronounced 46-fold increase in the risk of stillbirth specifically attributed to placental insufficiency, such as abruption or growth restriction [56].

Studies from the late nineties have shown elevated alpha-fetoprotein (AFP) and human chorionic gonadotropin (hCG) multiples of median (MoM) levels to be associated with stillbirth [57, 58]. However, the positive predictive values of these two biomarkers are too low to take into clinical consideration [56, 58].

Lately, proteins associated with placental function, like placental growth factor (PlGF), have been studied as markers of adverse pregnancy outcomes, including stillbirth. Low levels of PlGF are associated with stillbirth, possibly through preeclampsia and FGR [59]. The risk of stillbirth was found to be 29 times higher in a study of a maternal plasma angiogenic index that was composed of PlGF, soluble endoglin, and soluble vascular endothelial growth factor receptor-1 [60]. Levels of these biomarkers differ throughout gestation, and comparisons should be made accordingly. However, the fact that these biomarkers are not readily available worldwide limits their use.

By detecting FGR and flow abnormalities in uterine and fetal vessels, ultrasound, particularly Doppler, can identify placental insufficiency and, as a result, cases at risk of stillbirth. Evidence is not strong for an increased risk of stillbirth with abnormal uterine artery Doppler in unselected populations [61, 62]. Abnormal umbilical artery indices, absent or reverse flow at the end diastole, are associated with stillbirth if the fetus is growth-restricted [63]. Yet again, the usefulness of umbilical artery Doppler studies in low-risk populations is not yet clarified.

At this point, there is no existing screening method available to assess the risk of stillbirth. Nevertheless, the possibility of biomarkers being used to identify pregnancies at a high risk of stillbirth is yet to be ascertained.

5.7 Prevention

5.7.1 For Women Who Do Not Have a History of Stillbirth

Given that stillbirth can happen in both high-risk patients with underlying conditions and low-risk patients with no known risk factors, it is challenging to determine the specific focus of preventive measures. Treatment of maternal medical conditions like diabetes, hypertension, and APS will decrease the risk. The risk can be reduced by optimizing general maternal health, such as the promotion of weight reduction in obese women and the cessation of smoking.

In addition to the overall health status, specific medical interventions are suggested to have beneficial effects by explicitly aiming to reduce inflammation or enhance blood flow in the placenta. Low-dose aspirin, which decreases the risk of several conditions associated with stillbirth, such as preeclampsia, spontaneous preterm birth, FGR, and placental insufficiency, is the most thoroughly studied. While it has proven efficacy in high-quality studies, its effect is modest [3]. In a meta-analysis of 40 trials, in women who were given low-dose aspirin, a 14% reduction in fetal or neonatal deaths (risk ratio: 0.86; 95% CI: 0.76–0.98) was found; the number needed to treat for this result was 243 [64]. Despite the lack of clarity regarding the most effective dosage, time, and target population, low-dose aspirin is a potential candidate for decreasing the rate of stillbirth. Low-molecular-weight heparin has also been used to improve placental function, but controversial data on benefits limit its use to only women with APS [65]. Prednisolone and hydroxychloroquine are theoretically useful but currently regarded as experimental treatments that aim to decrease inflammation. Nitric oxide donors, such as sildenafil, have also shown no benefit [66].

Probably the most crucial part of stillbirth prevention efforts is assessing and managing the risks associated with FGR and placental abruption. This is because research indicates that these two issues are responsible for more than

50% of fetal deaths [67]. A large cohort study of nulliparous women found that routine third-trimester ultrasound increased the detection of FGR by threefold [68]. On the other hand, placental abruption cannot be predicted accurately by ultrasound examination; therefore, a low level of suspicion in symptomatic women is the only clinical strategy we can implement.

Almost all women who experienced stillbirths have reported decreased fetal movements. Nevertheless, it is typically regarded as unreliable because it is a measure that only the patient can quantify. One study reported that providing a uniform description of decreased fetal movements to patients and improving standardized guidelines for healthcare providers in the management were associated with a reduction in stillbirth [69]. In contrast, a large randomized-controlled trial and a meta-analysis showed no significant decrease in stillbirth, with possible increases in interventions such as inductions and hospital admissions [70, 71]. Therefore, currently, there is no strong evidence to make specific recommendations for fetal kick counts [72]. However, patients should still be instructed to seek assistance from the nearest obstetric care center if they notice decreased fetal movements.

Given that the risk of stillbirth increases after the 41st gestational week, inducing labor at term has been considered a potential and successful preventive strategy. There were concerns that it would increase the rate of caesarean section [73], but those were discredited by the evidence from later studies [74, 75]. In low-risk women who are induced after the 37th week, the risk ratio for stillbirth was 0.30 (95% CI: 0.12–0.75), according to a recent meta-analysis [76]. However, the risk/benefit ratio needs to be carefully considered for women without risk factors before offering elective induction. There is currently no guideline on elective induction at term to prevent stillbirth.

5.7.2 For Women with a History of Stillbirth

Because having a stillbirth is a devastating event for the families, they generally seek reassurance and support in a subsequent pregnancy. Preconception counseling is beneficial for reassessing risk factors and implementing necessary measures. Key actions include optimization of medical conditions such as diabetes, thyroid disorders, and hypertension; encouragement for quitting substance use if needed; and optimization of BMI.

The risk of recurrence is three to four times higher if the previous event was unexplained, but the evidence is scarce, and since it was unexplained, there are no risk factors to address [77, 78].

Still, parental anxiety levels may be alleviated by more frequent prenatal visits and antenatal testing. There is little evidence that more frequent monitoring in subsequent pregnancies will make a significant difference in preventing stillbirth. However, the risk of recurrent stillbirth is as high as the risk of other medical/obstetric conditions for which antenatal testing is warranted. Moreover, women who have a history of stillbirth are at an increased risk of adverse pregnancy outcomes like preeclampsia, FGR, and preterm birth. Therefore, antenatal testing would be beneficial. For patients with a previous stillbirth after the 32nd gestational week, the American College of Obstetricians and Gynecologists (ACOG) suggests antenatal testing once or twice weekly beginning at 32^{+0} weeks or 1–2 weeks before the gestational age of the prior stillbirth [13].

If no high-risk factors are present in the current pregnancy, it is not advisable to deliver before the 39th week of gestation [78]. If the patient strongly prefers early-term delivery and suffers severe parental distress, patient-centered decision-making should prioritize the balance between the potential benefits and the risks of increased neonatal morbidity [3]. Patients may elect to proceed with early-term delivery after considering these factors.

▫ Table 5.1 lists the broad actions that can be implemented for the general population, in addition to the specialized strategies for women with or without a history of stillbirth [79].

Table 5.1 Review of interventions to reduce stillbirth in the general population [79]

	Key interventions
Periconceptional and antenatal care	Promote healthy family and community behaviors Reduce exposure to indoor air pollution and tobacco Provide antenatal care and nutritional support (supplement folic acid, iron, and micronutrients and offer vitamin A, magnesium, and balanced protein-energy support for deficiencies)
Antenatal monitoring	Identify high-risk pregnancies through screening and fetal monitoring Conduct biophysical tests and amniotic fluid assessment Provide home/hospital monitoring for high-risk cases
Enhancing training and availability in healthcare	Promote community awareness and demand for care Build capacity through training for birth attendants, midwives, and health workers Conduct obstetric drills and neonatal resuscitation training Strengthen health systems through partnerships and maternity waiting homes Encourage perinatal audits and improve delivery standards

Chapter Key Points

- Epidemiology and global burden of stillbirth
- Major risk factors, including maternal age, obesity, smoking, and previous stillbirth
- Etiological categories: infections, maternal medical conditions, fetal causes, and placental and intrapartum causes
- Key evaluation components: maternal history, placental pathology, autopsy, and genetic testing
- Challenges and limitations in stillbirth prediction and available biomarkers
- Prevention strategies for low-risk and high-risk women, including antenatal monitoring and risk-specific management

Chapter-End Summary

This chapter provides an in-depth overview of the epidemiology, risk factors, causes, and clinical management of stillbirth. It highlights the global disparities in stillbirth rates, the multifactorial nature of its etiology, and the challenges in identifying a definitive cause in many cases. Diagnostic evaluation—particularly maternal history, placental pathology, and genetic testing—remains essential for guiding prevention strategies. Although prediction tools and biomarkers offer some insight into high-risk pregnancies, their clinical utility is limited. Prevention strategies focus on optimizing maternal health, managing underlying conditions, improving antenatal surveillance, and supporting women with a prior stillbirth through tailored monitoring. The chapter ultimately reinforces the need for multidisciplinary care and improved global access to diagnostic and preventive resources.

References

1. https://www.cdc.gov/stillbirth/data-research/index.html. Data and statistics on stillbirth, CDC. 2024.
2. Hug L, You D, Blencowe H, Mishra A, Wang Z, Fix MJ, et al. Global, regional, and national estimates and trends in stillbirths from 2000 to 2019: a systematicassessment. Lancet. 2021;398(10302):772–85.
3. Silver RM, Reddy U. Stillbirth: we can do better. Am J Obstet Gynecol. 2024;231:152.

4. MacDorman MF, Gregory EC. Fetal and perinatal mortality: United States, 2013. Natl Vital Stat Rep. 2015;64(8):1–24.
5. Wingate MS, Smith RA, Petrini JR, Barfield WD. Disparities in gestational age-specific fetal mortality rates in the United States, 2009–2013. Ann Epidemiol. 2017;27(9):570–4.
6. Balayla J, Azoulay L, Assayag J, Benjamin A, Abenhaim HA. Effect of maternal age on the risk of stillbirth: a population-based cohort study on 37 million births in the United States. Am J Perinatol. 2011;28(8):643–50.
7. Macdorman MF, Kirmeyer S. The challenge of fetal mortality. NCHS Data Brief. 2009;16:1–8.
8. Black M, Shetty A, Bhattacharya S. Obstetric outcomes subsequent to intrauterine death in the first pregnancy. BJOG. 2008;115(2):269–74.
9. Sharma PP, Salihu HM, Kirby RS. Stillbirth recurrence in a population of relatively low-risk mothers. Paediatr Perinat Epidemiol. 2007;21(Suppl 1):24–30.
10. Villamor E, Cnattingius S. Interpregnancy weight change and risk of adverse pregnancy outcomes: a population-based study. Lancet. 2006;368(9542):1164–70.
11. Nohr EA, Bech BH, Davies MJ, Frydenberg M, Henriksen TB, Olsen J. Prepregnancy obesity and fetal death: a study within the Danish national birth cohort. Obstet Gynecol. 2005;106(2):250–9.
12. Varner MW, Silver RM, Rowland Hogue CJ, Willinger M, Parker CB, Thorsten VR, et al. Association between stillbirth and illicit drug use and smoking during pregnancy. Obstet Gynecol. 2014;123(1):113–25.
13. Management of stillbirth: obstetric care consensus no, 10. Obstet Gynecol. 2020;135(3):e110–32.
14. Korteweg FJ, Gordijn SJ, Timmer A, Erwich JJ, Bergman KA, Bouman K, et al. The tulip classification of perinatal mortality: introduction and multidisciplinary inter-rater agreement. BJOG. 2006;113(4):393–401.
15. Dudley DJ, Goldenberg R, Conway D, Silver RM, Saade GR, Varner MW, et al. A new system for determining the causes of stillbirth. Obstet Gynecol. 2010;116(2 Pt 1):254–60.
16. Goldenberg RL, McClure EM, Saleem S, Reddy UM. Infection-related stillbirths. Lancet. 2010;375(9724):1482–90.
17. Korteweg FJ, Erwich JJ, Timmer A, van der Meer J, Ravisé JM, Veeger NJ, et al. Evaluation of 1025 fetal deaths: proposed diagnostic workup. Am J Obstet Gynecol. 2012;206(1):53.e1–12.
18. McClure EM, Goldenberg RL. Infection and stillbirth. Semin Fetal Neonatal Med. 2009;14(4):182–9.
19. Goldenberg RL, Thompson C. The infectious origins of stillbirth. Am J Obstet Gynecol. 2003;189(3):861–73.
20. Sheffield JS, Sánchez PJ, Wendel GD Jr, Fong DW, Margraf LR, Zeray F, et al. Placental histopathology of congenital syphilis. Obstet Gynecol. 2002;100(1):126–33.
21. Newman RD, Hailemariam A, Jimma D, Degifie A, Kebede D, Rietveld AE, et al. Burden of malaria during pregnancy in areas of stable and unstable transmission in Ethiopia during a nonepidemic year. J Infect Dis. 2003;187(11):1765–72.
22. Boettcher LB, Metz TD. Maternal and neonatal outcomes following SARS-CoV-2 infection. Semin Fetal Neonatal Med. 2023;28(1):101428.
23. Skjöldebrand-Sparre L, Tolfvenstam T, Papadogiannakis N, Wahren B, Broliden K, Nyman M. Parvovirus B19 infection: association with third-trimester intrauterine fetal death. BJOG. 2000;107(4):476–80.
24. Dijkmans AC, de Jong EP, Dijkmans BA, Lopriore E, Vossen A, Walther FJ, et al. Parvovirus B19 in pregnancy: prenatal diagnosis and management of fetal complications. Curr Opin Obstet Gynecol. 2012;24(2):95–101.
25. Iwasenko JM, Howard J, Arbuckle S, Graf N, Hall B, Craig ME, et al. Human cytomegalovirus infection is detected frequently in stillbirths and is associated with fetal thrombotic vasculopathy. J Infect Dis. 2011;203(11):1526–33.
26. Causes of death among stillbirths. JAMA. 2011;306(22):2459–68.
27. Yazdy MM, Liu S, Mitchell AA, Werler MM. Maternal dietary glycemic intake and the risk of neural tube defects. Am J Epidemiol. 2010;171(4):407–14.
28. Arendt LH, Pedersen LH, Pedersen L, Ovesen PG, Henriksen TB, Lindhard MS, et al. Glycemic control in pregnancies complicated by pre-existing diabetes mellitus and congenital malformations: a Danish population-based study. Clin Epidemiol. 2021;13:615–26.
29. Syed M, Javed H, Yakoob MY, Bhutta ZA. Effect of screening and management of diabetes during pregnancy on stillbirths. BMC Public Health. 2011;11(Suppl 3):S2.
30. Fischer MJ. Chronic kidney disease and pregnancy: maternal and fetal outcomes. Adv Chronic Kidney Dis. 2007;14(2):132–45.
31. Vidaeff AC, Yeomans ER, Ramin SM. Pregnancy in women with renal disease. Part I: general principles. Am J Perinatol. 2008;25(7):385–97.
32. Breur JM, Kapusta L, Stoutenbeek P, Visser GH, van den Berg P, Meijboom EJ. Isolated congenital atrioventricular block diagnosed in utero: natural history and outcome. J Matern Fetal Neonatal Med. 2008;21(7):469–76.
33. Glantz A, Marschall HU, Mattsson LA. Intrahepatic cholestasis of pregnancy: relationships between bile acid levels and fetal complication rates. Hepatology. 2004;40(2):467–74.
34. Ovadia C, Seed PT, Sklavounos A, Geenes V, Di Ilio C, Chambers J, Kohari K, Bacq Y, Bozkurt N, Brun-Furrer R, Bull L, Estiú MC, Grymowicz M, Gunaydin B, Hague WM, Haslinger C, Hu Y, Kawakita T, Kebapcilar AG, Kebapcilar L, Kondrackienė J, Koster MPH, Kowalska-Kańka A, Kupčinskas L, Lee RH, Locatelli A, Macias

RIR, Marschall HU, Oudijk MA, Raz Y, Rimon E, Shan D, Shao Y, Tribe R, Tripodi V, Yayla Abide C, Yenidede I, Thornton JG, Chappell LC, Williamson C. Association of adverse perinatal outcomes of intrahepatic cholestasis of pregnancy with biochemical markers: results of aggregate and individual patient data meta-analyses. Lancet. 2019;393(10174):899–909. https://doi.org/10.1016/S0140-6736(18)31877-4. Epub 2019 Feb 14. Erratum in: Lancet. 2019 Mar 16;393(10176):1100.
35. Silver RM, Parker CB, Goldenberg R, Reddy UM, Dudley DJ, Saade GR, et al. Bile acids in a multicenter, population-based case-control study of stillbirth. Am J Obstet Gynecol. 2014;210(5):460.e1–9.
36. Pauli RM, Reiser CA. Wisconsin stillbirth service program: II. Analysis of diagnoses and diagnostic categories in the first 1,000 referrals. Am J Med Genet. 1994;50(2):135–53.
37. Reddy UM, Goldenberg R, Silver R, Smith GCS, Pauli RM, Wapner RJ, et al. Stillbirth classification--developing an international consensus for research: executive summary of a National Institute of Child Health and Human Development workshop. Obstet Gynecol. 2009;114(4):901–14.
38. Korteweg FJ, Bouman K, Erwich JJ, Timmer A, Veeger NJ, Ravisé JM, et al. Cytogenetic analysis after evaluation of 750 fetal deaths: proposal for diagnostic workup. Obstet Gynecol. 2008;111(4):865–74.
39. Reddy UM, Page GP, Saade GR, Silver RM, Thorsten VR, Parker CB, et al. Karyotype versus microarray testing for genetic abnormalities after stillbirth. N Engl J Med. 2012;367(23):2185–93.
40. Stanley KE, Giordano J, Thorsten V, Buchovecky C, Thomas A, Ganapathi M, et al. Causal genetic variants in stillbirth. N Engl J Med. 2020;383(12):1107–16.
41. Wolstenholme J. Confined placental mosaicism for trisomies 2, 3, 7, 8, 9, 16, and 22: their incidence, likely origins, and mechanisms for cell lineage compartmentalization. Prenat Diagn. 1996;16(6):511–24.
42. Kalousek DK. Pathogenesis of chromosomal mosaicism and its effect on early human development. Am J Med Genet. 2000;91(1):39–45.
43. Martins JG, Biggio JR, Abuhamad A. Society for Maternal-Fetal Medicine Consult Series #52: diagnosis and management of fetal growth restriction: (replaces clinical guideline number 3, April 2012). Am J Obstet Gynecol. 2020;223(4):B2–17.
44. Bukowski R, Hansen NI, Willinger M, Reddy UM, Parker CB, Pinar H, et al. Fetal growth and risk of stillbirth: a population-based case-control study. PLoS Med. 2014;11(4):e1001633.
45. Giacoia GP. Severe fetomaternal hemorrhage: a review. Obstet Gynecol Surv. 1997;52(6):372–80.
46. Huang DY, Usher RH, Kramer MS, Yang H, Morin L, Fretts RC. Determinants of unexplained antepartum fetal deaths. Obstet Gynecol. 2000;95(2):215–21.
47. Aminu M, Bar-Zeev S, van den Broek N. Cause of and factors associated with stillbirth: a systematic review of classification systems. Acta Obstet Gynecol Scand. 2017;96(5):519–28.
48. Page JM, Christiansen-Lindquist L, Thorsten V, Parker CB, Reddy UM, Dudley DJ, et al. Diagnostic tests for evaluation of stillbirth: results from the stillbirth collaborative research network. Obstet Gynecol. 2017;129(4):699–706.
49. Flenady V, Frøen JF, Pinar H, Torabi R, Saastad E, Guyon G, et al. An evaluation of classification systems for stillbirth. BMC Pregnancy Childbirth. 2009;9:24.
50. Bove KE. Practice guidelines for autopsy pathology: the perinatal and pediatric autopsy. Autopsy Committee of the College of American Pathologists. Arch Pathol Lab Med. 1997;121(4):368–76.
51. Committee opinion no.682: microarrays and next-generation sequencing technology: the use of advanced genetic diagnostic tools in obstetrics and gynecology. Obstet Gynecol. 2016;128(6):e262–8.
52. Barbhaiya M, Zuily S, Naden R, Hendry A, Manneville F, Amigo MC, et al. 2023 ACR/EULAR antiphospholipid syndrome classification criteria. Ann Rheum Dis. 2023;82(10):1258–70.
53. ACOG Practice Bulletin No. 197: inherited Thrombophilias in pregnancy. Obstet Gynecol. 2018;132(1):e18–34.
54. Association between stillbirth and risk factors known at pregnancy confirmation. JAMA. 2011;306(22):2469–79.
55. Reddy UM. Prediction and prevention of recurrent stillbirth. Obstet Gynecol. 2007;110(5):1151–64.
56. Smith GC, Crossley JA, Aitken DA, Pell JP, Cameron AD, Connor JM, et al. First-trimester placentation and the risk of antepartum stillbirth. JAMA. 2004;292(18):2249–54.
57. Waller DK, Lustig LS, Smith AH, Hook EB. Alpha-fetoprotein: a biomarker for pregnancy outcome. Epidemiology. 1993;4(5):471–6.
58. Walton DL, Norem CT, Schoen EJ, Ray GT, Colby CJ. Second-trimester serum chorionic gonadotropin concentrations and complications and outcome of pregnancy. N Engl J Med. 1999;341(27):2033–8.
59. Heazell AE, Hayes DJ, Whitworth M, Takwoingi Y, Bayliss SE, Davenport C. Biochemical tests of placental function versus ultrasound assessment of fetal size for stillbirth and small-for-gestational-age infants. Cochrane Database Syst Rev. 2019;5(5):Cd012245.
60. Chaiworapongsa T, Romero R, Erez O, Tarca AL, Conde-Agudelo A, Chaemsaithong P, et al. The prediction of fetal death with a simple maternal blood test at 20–24 weeks: a role for angiogenic index-1 (PlGF/sVEGFR-1 ratio). Am J Obstet Gynecol. 2017;217(6):682.e1–13.
61. Smith GC, Yu CK, Papageorghiou AT, Cacho AM, Nicolaides KH. Maternal uterine artery

Doppler flow velocimetry and the risk of stillbirth. Obstet Gynecol. 2007;109(1):144–51.
62. Parry S, Sciscione A, Haas DM, Grobman WA, Iams JD, Mercer BM, et al. Role of early second-trimester uterine artery Doppler screening to predict small-for-gestational-age babies in nulliparous women. Am J Obstet Gynecol. 2017;217(5):594.e1–10.
63. Caradeux J, Martinez-Portilla RJ, Basuki TR, Kiserud T, Figueras F. Risk of fetal death in growth-restricted fetuses with umbilical and/or ductus venosus absent or reversed end-diastolic velocities before 34 weeks of gestation: a systematic review and meta-analysis. Am J Obstet Gynecol. 2018;218(2s):S774–S82.e21.
64. Duley L, Henderson-Smart DJ, Meher S, King JF. Antiplatelet agents for preventing pre-eclampsia and its complications. Cochrane Database Syst Rev. 2007;2:Cd004659.
65. Hamulyák EN, Scheres LJ, Marijnen MC, Goddijn M, Middeldorp S. Aspirin or heparin or both for improving pregnancy outcomes in women with persistent antiphospholipid antibodies and recurrent pregnancy loss. Cochrane Database Syst Rev. 2020;5(5):Cd012852.
66. Pels A, Ganzevoort W, Kenny LC, Baker PN, von Dadelszen P, Gluud C, et al. Interventions affecting the nitric oxide pathway versus placebo or no therapy for fetal growth restriction in pregnancy. Cochrane Database Syst Rev. 2023;7(7):Cd014498.
67. Smulian JC, Ananth CV, Vintzileos AM, Scorza WE, Knuppel RA. Fetal deaths in the United States. Influence of high-risk conditions and implications for management. Obstet Gynecol. 2002;100(6):1183–9.
68. Sovio U, White IR, Dacey A, Pasupathy D, Smith GCS. Screening for fetal growth restriction with universal third trimester ultrasonography in nulliparous women in the Pregnancy Outcome Prediction (POP) study: a prospective cohort study. Lancet. 2015;386(10008):2089–97.
69. Tveit JV, Saastad E, Stray-Pedersen B, Børdahl PE, Flenady V, Fretts R, et al. Reduction of late stillbirth with the introduction of fetal movement information and guidelines - a clinical quality improvement. BMC Pregnancy Childbirth. 2009;9:32.
70. Norman JE, Heazell AEP, Rodriguez A, Weir CJ, Stock SJE, Calderwood CJ, et al. Awareness of fetal movements and care package to reduce fetal mortality (AFFIRM): a stepped wedge, cluster-randomised trial. Lancet. 2018;392(10158):1629–38.
71. Bellussi F, Po G, Livi A, Saccone G, De Vivo V, Oliver EA, et al. Fetal movement counting and perinatal mortality: a systematic review and meta-analysis. Obstet Gynecol. 2020;135(2):453–62.
72. Hayes DJL, Dumville JC, Walsh T, Higgins LE, Fisher M, Akselsson A, et al. Effect of encouraging awareness of reduced fetal movement and subsequent clinical management on pregnancy outcome: a systematic review and meta-analysis. Am J Obstet Gynecol MFM. 2023;5(3):100821.
73. Yeast JD, Jones A, Poskin M. Induction of labor and the relationship to cesarean delivery: a review of 7001 consecutive inductions. Am J Obstet Gynecol. 1999;180(3 Pt 1):628–33.
74. Mishanina E, Rogozinska E, Thatthi T, Uddin-Khan R, Khan KS, Meads C. Use of labour induction and risk of cesarean delivery: a systematic review and meta-analysis. CMAJ. 2014;186(9):665–73.
75. Grobman WA, Rice MM, Reddy UM, Tita ATN, Silver RM, Mallett G, et al. Labor induction versus expectant management in low-risk nulliparous women. N Engl J Med. 2018;379(6):513–23.
76. Middleton P, Shepherd E, Morris J, Crowther CA, Gomersall JC. Induction of labour at or beyond 37 weeks' gestation. Cochrane Database Syst Rev. 2020;7(7):Cd004945.
77. Gordon A, Raynes-Greenow C, McGeechan K, Morris J, Jeffery H. Stillbirth risk in a second pregnancy. Obstet Gynecol. 2012;119(3):509–17.
78. Measey MA, Tursan d'Espaignet E, Charles A, Douglass C. Unexplained fetal death: are women with a history of fetal loss at higher risk? Aust N Z J Obstet Gynaecol. 2009;49(2):151–7.
79. Lawn JE, Yakoob MY, Haws RA, Soomro T, Darmstadt GL, Bhutta ZA. 3.2 million stillbirths: epidemiology and overview of the evidence review. BMC Pregnancy Childbirth. 2009;9(1):S2.

Prevention of Preterm Birth

Contents

Cervical Length Assessment in Singleton and Multiple Pregnancies

Laura van der Krogt, Nicole Moriarty, and Andrew Shennan

Contents

Y. Yogev, A. Khalil (eds.), *Prevention of Complications in Obstetrics*,
https://doi.org/10.1007/978-3-032-23479-7_6

6.1 Introduction

Preterm birth (PTB) is a major cause of perinatal morbidity and mortality [1]. Despite advances in obstetric care, the rate of PTB is increasing, as the ability to accurately predict preterm labour remains elusive [2, 3]. This is, in part, because the aetiology of preterm labour is multifactorial [4]. Early prediction and identification of those at risk of preterm birth would provide the opportunity to target interventions to prevent preterm labour, such as progesterone and cerclage. Moreover, it would facilitate the provision of optimised care to infants born preterm, such as the timely administration of antenatal corticosteroids.

Therefore, screening tests for the prediction of preterm birth are used in clinical practice to identify women most at risk. Current screening tests for the prediction of preterm birth include risk factor assessment, cervical length measurement, and biomarker testing. Often, a combination of some, or all three is used. This chapter will focus on cervical length screening in singleton and multiple pregnancies, exploring current practice and developments for the future.

Learning Objectives

1. Understand the significance of early prediction for targeted interventions and the optimisation of outcomes for preterm infants.
2. Recognise current screening methods for preterm birth prediction, including risk factor assessment, cervical length measurement, and biomarker testing.
3. Understand the principles of how to perform a cervical length measurement.
4. Recognise the clinical application of cervical length in both singleton and multiple pregnancies.
5. Identify future directions in cervical length screening and other methods aimed at improving preterm birth prediction.

6.2 Preterm Labour and the Cervix

Preterm labour may be initiated by several different and often overlapping processes [4]. These include inflammation and infection, activation of the hypothalamic–adrenal axis in response to stress, decidual haemorrhage, uterine overdistension, and cervical weakness [4]. The multiple aetiologies of preterm labour result in the 'common pathway' of increased myometrial contractility, cervical dilatation, and rupture of the chorioamniotic membranes [4].

One of the early changes that precedes spontaneous preterm birth is the shortening of the cervix, which can be measured by transvaginal ultrasound scanning [5]. Even if the cervix shortens or dilates, the progression to delivery is variable [6]. Therefore, the finding of a short cervix is associated with sufficient time for intervention to be considered, facilitating its use as a screening test.

6.3 Principles of Screening Tests

The purpose of a screening test is to identify those at an increased risk of a condition, with a view to offer more information, further tests, or treatment as appropriate [7]. Screening should only be recommended and provided if evidence shows that the planned screening pathway, including further treatment, will do more good than harm and is provided at a reasonable cost [7]. A screening test can be offered to a whole population or can be targeted for those with a heightened risk of a condition [7]. See ► Box 6.1 for a summary of Wilson and Junger's principles of screening.

Box 6.1 Wilson & Junger's Principles of Screening

1. The condition should be an important health condition
2. There should be an accepted treatment for patients with the recognized disease

3. Facilities for diagnosis and treatment should be available
4. There should be a recognizable latent or early symptomatic phase
5. There should be a suitable test or examination
6. The test should be acceptable to the population
7. The natural history of the condition, including development from latent to declared disease should be adequately understood
8. There should be an agreed policy on whom to treat as patients
9. The cost of case-finding (including diagnosis and treatment of patients diagnosed) should be economically balanced in relation to possible expenditure on medical care as a whole
10. Case-finding should be a continuous process and not a 'once and for all' project.

6.4 Assessment of Risk Factors for Preterm Birth

There are many risk factors for spontaneous preterm birth, including previous spontaneous preterm birth, uterine anomalies, cervical surgery, and full-dilatation caesarean section; see ◘ Table 6.1 for a summary. More than 50% of women who deliver preterm do not have traditional risk factors, and two-thirds

◘ **Table 6.1** Risk factors for spontaneous preterm birth

High risk	Intermediate risk	Other factors to consider	Modifiable risk factors
Previous second-trimester loss (16–23 weeks)	History of significant cervical excision (i.e. LLETZ with >15 mm depth removed or >1 LLETZ)	Cervical dilatation procedure, especially second-trimester surgical management	Smoking
Previous spontaneous preterm birth (24–34 weeks)	Cone biopsy (knife or laser)	Short interpregnancy interval	Urinary infection
Previous PPROM (<34 weeks)	Previous caesarean section at full dilatation	Multiple pregnancy	Bacterial vaginosis
Uterine anomaly (i.e. unicornuate uterus, bicornuate uterus, or uterine septum)		IVF	Sexually transmitted infections
Intrauterine adhesions (Asherman's syndrome)		Primiparity	Periodontitis
History of trachelectomy		Maternal age <18 or >40	
		Collagen abnormalities	
		Low BMI	
		Domestic violence	
		Social deprivation	

PPROM preterm prelabour rupture of membranes, *LLETZ* large loop excision of the transformation zone, *IVF* in vitro fertilisation, *HPV* human papilloma virus, *BMI* body mass index of women with traditional risk factors deliver at term [8–10].

It is recommended that all women be assessed for risk factors for preterm birth at booking [11]. Population-based and modifiable risk factors should be addressed, for example, by referral to smoking cessation services and involvement of adolescent pregnancy teams. Women should have routine testing for urinary infections and vaginal infections where appropriate [11].

Those pregnant women identified to have 'intermediate' and 'high' risk factors benefit from onwards referral and management in a preterm birth prevention clinic where further tests, including cervical length, may be offered on the surveillance pathway [11].

6.5 Cervical Length

As cervical shortening is one of the early changes that precede spontaneous preterm birth, detection by ultrasound is one of the most used tools for the prediction of preterm birth [12]. The risk of preterm birth is inversely proportional to cervical length, with women with both a history of a preterm birth and a short cervix being at the highest risk [5, 13].

6.5.1 How to Perform a Cervical Length Measurement

The gold standard for cervical length measurement is transvaginal ultrasound [14]. Transvaginal measurements are highly reproducible, and measurements are unaffected by maternal position, obesity, and shadowing from foetal parts [14, 15].

A cervical length should be performed by a sonographer or clinician with specific training in cervical length scanning. There is good intra- and inter-observer agreement for cervical length assessment performed with a standardised technique, although variation does occur [16].

The patient should empty their bladder prior to the examination, ideally 20 min prior to the scan to avoid isthmic contractions [17]. The vaginal transducer should be inserted into the anterior fornix of the vagina. A sagittal, long-axis image of the entire cervix should be obtained [18]. The cervix should occupy two-thirds of the screen, ensuring that the internal and external os are seen clearly. The cervical length should be measured between the internal and external os, along the endocervical canal [18]. At least three measurements should be taken. The shortest, best image should be used. See ◘ Fig. 6.1 for a transvaginal ultrasound image and schematic illustrating a cervical length measurement.

6.5.2 When to Perform Cervical Length Measurement

If transvaginal cervical screening is performed, the cervix should be assessed between 16 and 24 weeks of gestation [19]. It should not be routinely measured prior to 16 weeks

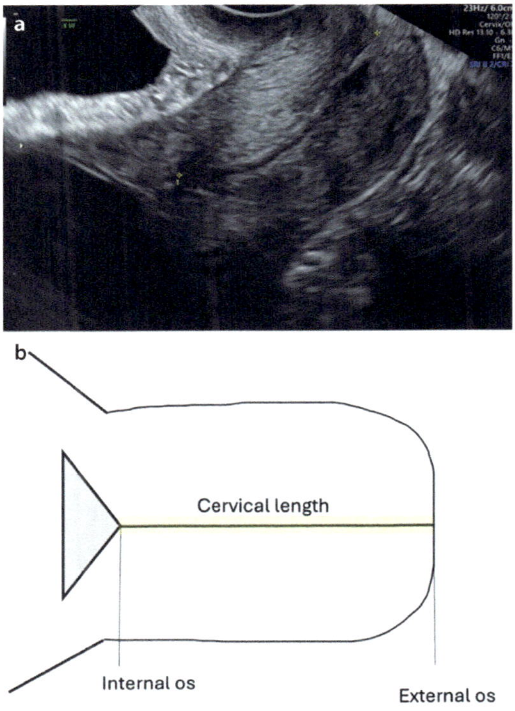

◘ **Fig. 6.1** **a** Transvaginal ultrasound scan image and **b** schematic diagram of cervical length measurement. The cervical length should be measured between the internal and external os, along the endocervical canal

of gestation, as evidence suggests that first- and early-second-trimester cervical lengths are not predictive for preterm birth [20, 21]. This is likely because at early gestations, the lower uterine segment is less developed, making it difficult to delineate clearly from the endocervical canal.

Routine cervical length screening is not recommended beyond 24 weeks of gestation in asymptomatic women. Studies investigating interventions for preterm birth, such as cerclage and progesterone, have used this gestation as the upper limit for the initiation of treatment [22–24]. Therefore, scanning after this threshold in asymptomatic populations, confers limited benefit.

6.5.3 Cervical Length Threshold for Prediction

Most major guidelines suggest using a mid-trimester cervical length threshold of 25 mm for risk assessment [25–28]. See ◘ Fig. 6.2 for a transvaginal ultrasound image of cervical lengths <25 mm and >25 mm.

This is based on the hallmark study by Iams et al. in 1996, where the cervical lengths of 2915 women with singleton pregnancies were assessed at 24 and 28 weeks, with the associated risks of preterm birth [5]. They found that at 24 weeks' gestation, only 10% of women had a cervical length of <26 mm, and the risk of preterm birth was inversely related to the cervical length. A cervical length <26 mm at 24 weeks had a better predictive value compared to a cervical length <26 mm at 28 weeks for predicting preterm birth <35 weeks [5].

This was reproduced in another study where the cervical length and the risk of preterm birth were assessed at 16–22 weeks [29]. The mean cervical length in this study was 38.5 mm, with an increasing relative risk of preterm birth <37 weeks with shortening cervical length [29].

6.6 Singleton Pregnancies

The approach to cervical length screening varies based on patient characteristics and risk factors. Guidelines vary; see ◘ Table 6.2 for a summary of international guidelines.

6.6.1 Previous Preterm Birth and Mid-trimester Loss

There is a consensus that women with a singleton pregnancy and a history of previous preterm birth or mid-trimester loss should be offered cervical length screening [25–28]. This is because a history of preterm birth and/or mid-trimester loss is the strongest predictor of preterm birth [30].

Several studies have been conducted where serial cervical length screening was performed in women with a history of preterm birth and/or mid-trimester loss. In these studies, 40–70% of women maintained a cervical length >25 mm before 24 weeks of gestation [31–34].

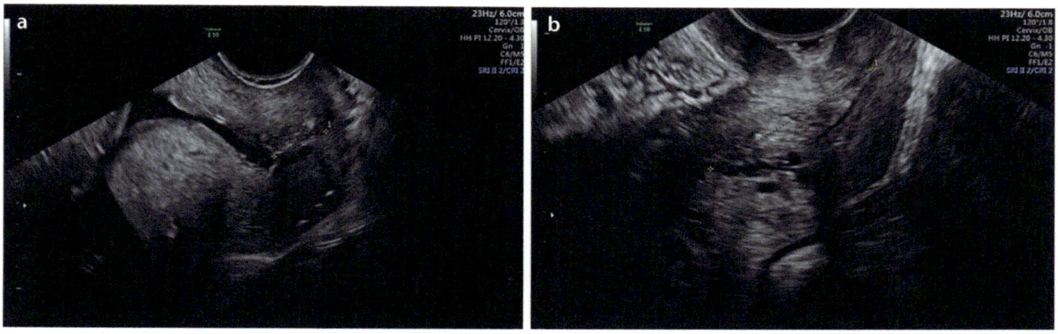

◘ **Fig. 6.2** **a** Transvaginal ultrasound scan image of cervix measuring 13 mm and **b** transvaginal ultrasound scan image of cervix measuring 31 mm

Table 6.2 Summary of current international guidelines

	NICE [30]	FIGO [31, 32]	IUSOG [33]	ACOG [34]	RANZCOG [25]	SMFM [35]	RCOG [36]
Title (year)	Preterm labour and birth (2022)	Best Practice in Maternal-Fetal Medicine (2015); FIGO good practice recommen-dations for reducing preterm birth and improving child outcomes (2021)	ISUOG practice guidelines: Role of ultrasound in the prediction of spontaneous preterm birth (2022)	Prediction and prevention of spontaneous preterm birth ACOG practice bulletin, number 234 (2021)	Measurement of cervical length for prediction of preterm birth (C-Obs 27) (2021)	The role of routine cervical length screening in selected high- and low-risk women for preterm birth prevention (2016)	Cervical Cerclage green-top guideline no. 75 (2022)
Gestational range	16 + 0–24 + 0 weeks	Not mentioned	14–16–24 + 0 weeks	16 + 0–24 + 0 weeks	Not mentioned	16 + 0–24 + 0 weeks	Not mentioned
Method of assessment	Transvaginal ultrasound	Transvaginal ultrasound	Transvaginal ultrasound	Transabdominal and transvaginal ultrasound	Transabdominal or transvaginal if poor views or <35 mm	Transvaginal ultrasound	Transvaginal ultrasound
Cervical length cut-off	<25 mm; <15 mm if >30/40	<25 mm	<25 mm	<25 mm	<35 mm on transabdominal ultrasound <25 mm	<25 mm	<25 mm
Previous preterm birth/mid-trimester loss	Recommended	Recommended	Recommended	Recommended	Recommended	Recommended	Recommended
Other risk factors (uterine anomaly or LLETZ)	Recommended for 'cervical trauma'	Individualised surveillance	Assess as with universal screening	Assess as with universal screening	May be useful	Not recommended	>10 mm or more than one cervical surgery, recommended for uterine anomaly
Multiple pregnancy	Not mentioned	Not recommended	Recommended	Assess as with universal screening	May be useful	Not recommended	Recommended
Symptomatic assessment	>30 + 0 weeks	Not mentioned	Recommended 22 + 0–34 + 0 weeks	Not mentioned	May be useful 24 + 0–34 + 0 weeks	Recommended	Not mentioned
Universal screening	Not mentioned	19–24 weeks recommended, progesterone as intervention	18 + 0–24 + 0 weeks	18 + 0–22 + 6 weeks	Transabdominal at mid-trimester ultrasound scan	If implemented, to adhere to struct guidelines	Not mentioned

Moreover, a meta-analysis was performed comparing pregnancy outcomes in singleton pregnancies with prior preterm birth, which were managed either by ultrasound-indicated cerclage for surveillance-detected cervical shortening or history-indicated cerclage. This study found that only 42% of women receiving cervical length surveillance needed a cerclage for a short cervix [14]. Outcomes, including preterm birth before 37 weeks, preterm birth before 34 weeks, and perinatal mortality, were similar between the groups [14].

These findings support the guidance that women with previous preterm birth and/or mid-trimester loss can be safely monitored by cervical length screening.

6.6.2 Cervical Surgery

Cervical dysplasia managed surgically by excisional treatment, such as large loop excision of the transformation zone (LLETZ) or cone biopsy, is associated with preterm birth. The risk increases with the increasing volume of tissue removed and following multiple procedures [35]. Studies have demonstrated that women with a previous cervical surgery and a mid-trimester cervical length less than 25 or 30 mm have a greater risk of preterm birth [36, 37]. Therefore, cervical length may be a useful predictive tool in those with previous cervical surgery.

6.6.3 Uterine Anomaly

Cervical surveillance may have a role in uterine anomalies, a recognised risk factor for preterm birth. Evidence suggests that women with a unicornuate and a bicornuate uterus tend to have a shorter cervical length and that shortening occurs earlier in the uterus didelphys or uterine septum compared to low-risk controls [38]. A cervical length of >30 mm was demonstrated to have a strong negative predictive value of 100%; however, the positive predictive value was only 37.5% [38]. Another study demonstrated that a cervical length <25 mm did not predict preterm birth <37 or <34 weeks in women with uterine anomalies overall. However, in subgroup analysis, it was predictive in women with resorption defects and not fusion defects [39]. Therefore, the role of cervical length in uterine anomalies remains to be fully elucidated.

6.6.4 Full-Dilatation Caesarean Section

There has been an increasing recognition of an association between delivery by in-labour caesarean section and an increased risk of subsequent mid-trimester loss and preterm birth [40–42]. The risks appear to be greater with increasing dilatation and are highest when the cervix is fully dilated [40]. In women who have a subsequent preterm birth following an in-labour caesarean section, this is more likely to recur in a future pregnancy [43]. In the UK, Saving Babies Lives Care Bundle Version 3 recommends that all women with a previous full-dilatation caesarean section should be referred for cervical length scanning between 18 and 22 weeks [11].

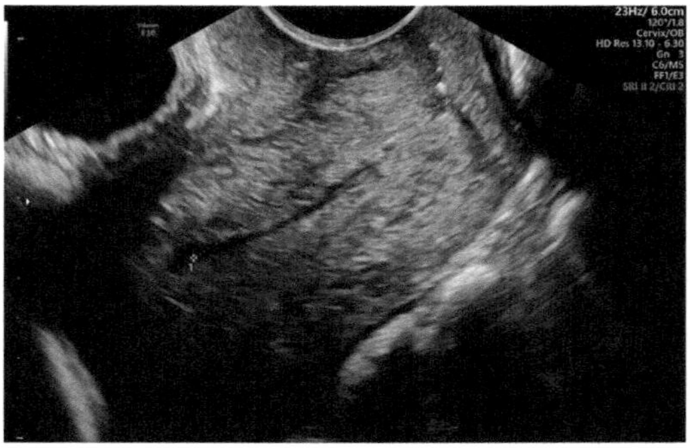

6.7 Multiple Pregnancies

There is an increased risk of preterm birth in multiple pregnancies. Women with multiple pregnancies have a shorter cervical length than those with singleton pregnancies [44, 45]. In a study that followed 1163 women with twin pregnancies until delivery, the median cervical length at 22–24 weeks was 35 mm, and the rates of cervical length ≤25 mm, ≤20 mm, and ≤15 mm were 16%, 8%, and 5%, respectively [46].

Cervical length has a predictive value in multiple pregnancies. For example, one meta-analysis demonstrated that among asymptomatic women, a cervical length <20 mm was the most accurate threshold for predicting preterm birth <32 and <34 weeks' gestation (pooled sensitivities: 39% and 29%; specificities: 96% and 97%) [47].

However, the limitation for its use is the paucity of evidence regarding therapeutic intervention for those with a short cervix. At present, it is suggested that progesterone may be considered at <25 mm and that, for consideration of cerclage, a threshold of <15 mm should be met [48–51].

As with singleton pregnancies, there may be some additional benefit in recognising multiple pregnancies at increased risk of preterm delivery, so that appropriate arrangements can be made to optimise outcomes should early birth occur..

Overall, international guidelines for the prediction and prevention of preterm birth in multiple pregnancies vary across different countries, as summarised in ◘ Table 6.2.

6.8 Symptomatic Women

Transvaginal ultrasound cervical length measurement may be used in addition to clinical history and examination in the assessment of women presenting with symptoms of threatened preterm labour [52]. This can facilitate admission, in utero transfer to a tertiary centre, and the initiation of preterm optimisation with antenatal corticosteroids. The cervical length threshold recommended in the UK by national institute for health and care excellence (NICE) for symptomatic women is 15 mm; however, the use of the quantitative innovation in predicting preterm birth (QUIPP) application and adjunct biomarkers can facilitate making individualised management plans [27, 53, 54].

6.8.1 International Guidelines

While guidelines have a crucial role in ensuring standards of care and patient safety, by optimising evidence-based medicine while aiming to reduce variation in practice, often, international guidelines are conflicting in some of the nuances relating to preterm birth surveillance. In September 2024, Ramachandran et al. published a quality assessment and systematic review of practice in international journal of obstetrics and gynaecology (*IJOG*) using the appraisal of guidelines for research & evaluation II (AGREE II) framework [61], examining practices across 37 clinical guidelines from 20 different organisations.

Differences in preconception care, management of modifiable risk factors, indications for surveillance, and interventions were all interrogated with few consistencies. These inter-organisational differences reflect the work that is still required and is ongoing in optimising management of those at risk of preterm birth.

Interestingly, when we examine international guidelines on cervical length surveillance from obstetric colleges, foetal medicine institutions, and ultrasound societies, similar inconsistencies were identified. While mid-trimester surveillance is recommended for women with a history of previous preterm birth in almost all of these and via transvaginal ultrasound in all but two, variations in practice in situations such as multiple pregnancies, women with previous cervical surgery, and women who require assessment for symptoms of threatened preterm labour are apparent.

Interestingly, both americal college of obstetricians and gynaecologists (ACOG) [34] and royal australian and new zealand college of obstetricians and gynaecologists (RANZCOG) [25] suggest the option of transabdominal cervical length assessment and progressing to transvaginal scan if needed. Universal assessment of the cervix in the late mid-trimester is also discussed in the Australian and North American guidelines but not in the British guidelines [30, 36]. This is summarised in ◘ Table 6.2.

6.9 Challenges of Cervical Length Measurements

6.9.1 Inter- and Intra-user Variability

While transvaginal ultrasound remains one of the key assessments in pregnancy for the prediction of preterm birth, a major limitation includes concerns about user reliability and both inter- and intra-operator dependence. While it is generally accepted that a cut-off of <25 mm is short, concerns regarding both under- and overtreatment if scans are not accurate must be considered [62].

When taking measurements, often while the image quality can be acceptable, consistent placement of the callipers consistently at both the internal and external os can be challenging, especially in settings where strong isthmic contraction or placenta praevia may obstruct a clear view of the internal os. Generally, it is accepted that an inter-observer ratio of 5 mm is acceptable [62], and Health et al., in 1998, reported an intra-observer variability of <3.5 mm as acceptable in 100 patients [63]. It is accepted clinically and in research that the lowest obtained measurement is used in decision-making.

Concern regarding ensuring reproducibility is valid and has been examined in multiple populations [62, 64–66]. Robust training pathways and frequent revalidation of clinicians performing cervical length assessments are imperative to ensure that those who require further teaching or support are identified early.

6.9.2 Access to Care

Ensuring equal access to care is vital to reducing maternal morbidity and mortality. Disparities among ethnicities remain present in the UK obstetric care, with higher rates of morbidity and mortality among Black and Asian women [67]. Late booking [68] and differences in key factors in major obstetric incidents have also been noted to be inequalities in maternity services. The so-called postcode lottery for access to specialist care has led women to travel long distances for many years to seek assistance that their local units may not have the expertise to provide.

To counteract this, the UK government released the 'Saving Babies Lives' Care Bundle. Version 2 [69] recommended a preterm birth pathway for all identified as being at risk at booking. This focused on prediction, prevention, and preparation for imminent preterm birth. As part of this, a pathway to access a transvaginal cervical length scan, either with a clinician with an interest locally or a referral pathway, should be present in every obstetric unit. Version 3 [70] additionally supported the introduction of a local multidisciplinary team and a preterm birth prevention clinic and access to tertiary level care for those with complex medical or obstetric history and needs. If implemented correctly, these care pathways could ensure that all intermediate- and high-risk women have equal access to cervical length surveillance and appropriate interventions. Where appropriately trained clinicians are not available, care pathways to another unit should be in place to ensure smooth transitions to other clinics, avoiding delays and unnecessary parental stress.

Improvements in training and exposure are also necessary to ensure that those taking on these roles have adequate training and experience to be able to support this at-risk population safely.

It should be noted that, in low- and middle-income settings, access to an ultrasound machine with a transvaginal ultrasound probe and a trained professional can be difficult, especially in rural or non-tertiary-level settings; women at high risk in these settings may not ever receive access to specialty care or ultrasound.

6.9.3 Variation in Care

As we saw above, international guidelines have some significant differences in the recommended care pathways. Notably, there are often differences between units, often even within the same hospital groups, on some of the more nuanced steps in preterm birth care.

Guidelines on frequency of surveillance are not defined, although most clinics offer routine appointments every 2–4 weeks, dependent on clinical picture, in combination with obstetric history. Additionally, the interpretation of high risk may be different within certain settings (multiple pregnancies, uterine anomalies, or cervical surgery), which may lead to less consistent monitoring.

Access to resources and staff trained in preterm birth prevention may impact the ability to provide more frequent appointments for patients. Urban areas with established foetal medicine units and advanced neonatal care can change the approach of the care providers more used to involvement in high-risk pregnancies and their ability to offer interventions.

Additionally, a clinician may have a particular preference for what intervention they feel is best, and this may guide management. Follow-up following the intervention is also variable. While evidence to support monitoring of cervical length following the insertion of a cerclage has been examined, often, individual departments do not offer follow-up, as it is felt that if the intervention has already been offered, what benefit is there in surveillance. When considering this, the goal should not be focused on a preventative intervention but rather on anticipating a need for proactive optimisation if that intervention is not successful [71]. See ◘ Fig. 6.3 for a post-cerclage cervical length.

Likewise, the administration of perinatal optimisation such as antenatal corticosteroids to enhance foetal lung maturity in the event of anticipated preterm birth is not always standardised. The timing and dosage of steroids can differ based on regional guidelines, available facilities, and individual clinical judgement.

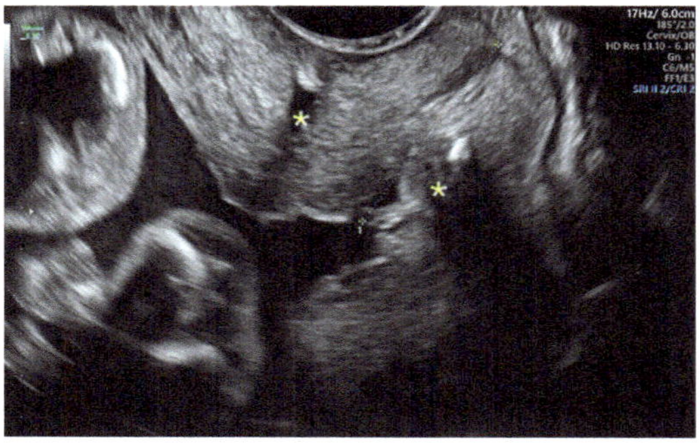

◘ **Fig. 6.3** Transvaginal ultrasound scan image of cervix following cerclage: the cerclage can be visualised as two small hyperechoic circles (*)

6.10 Other Ultrasound Markers

While transvaginal cervical length is the most used and most researched ultrasound marker for preterm birth prediction, there are many others that help to create a more complete clinical picture. Variation in practices means that, often, these may not be consistently included in imaging, and some more novel investigations are still being investigated for more robust supporting evidence; however, it is important to be aware of them and their implications for risk.

6.10.1 Sludge

During transvaginal ultrasound, 'sludge' appears as free-floating hyperechogenic, often particulate, material, close to the cervix [72] The presence of amniotic fluid sludge, while not diagnostic, is associated with an increased risk of mid-trimester loss, chorioamnionitis, and preterm delivery [73, 74] and can be used as a poor prognostic marker and prompt close observation and review.

6.10.2 Funnelling

The occurrence of opening of the internal cervical os, or funnelling, is also a marker noted during ultrasound assessment of the cervix. The internal os develops a V- or U-shaped appearance, and membranes push down into the cervical canal, often before women report significant associated symptoms. The occurrence of funnelling appears to be associated with an increased risk of PPROM and earlier gestation at delivery [75, 76]. Length and width measurements of the funnel can be taken, in addition to routine measurements; however, evidence does not appear to suggest the size of the funnel or use it as a single measurement independent of the cervical length that improves prediction in addition to the cervical length [77].

Case Study 2

A 26-year-old patient is referred to a preterm surveillance clinic from booking. It is her fourth pregnancy. She has a history of a previous 16 18-week and 15 mid-trimester losses. She has a history of indicated cerclage placed at 14 weeks. She has ongoing follow-up in the preterm surveillance clinic, and at her 18-week review, she is found to have a cervical length of 15 mm, with a funnel measuring 17 × 17 mm; see image below.

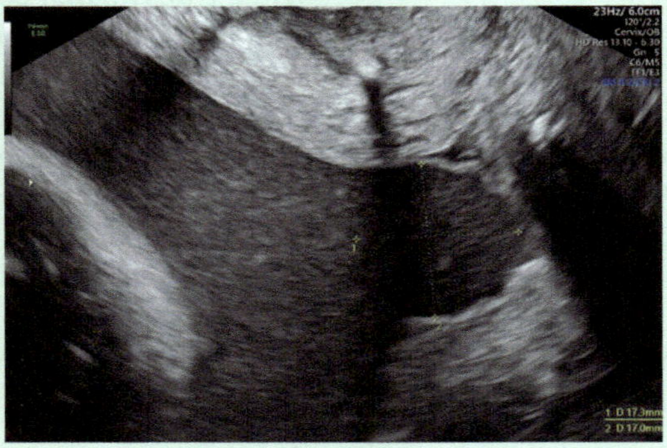

She is asymptomatic, and her QUIPP risk score of delivery in <1 week is 0.5%; see image below. Therefore, she is not admitted to the hospital and is not given steroids. Follow-up in clinic is arranged, and safety netting advice is provided.

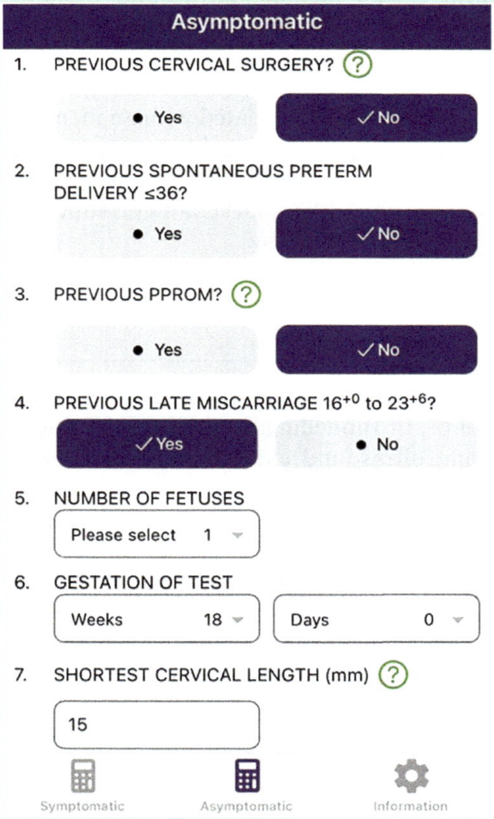

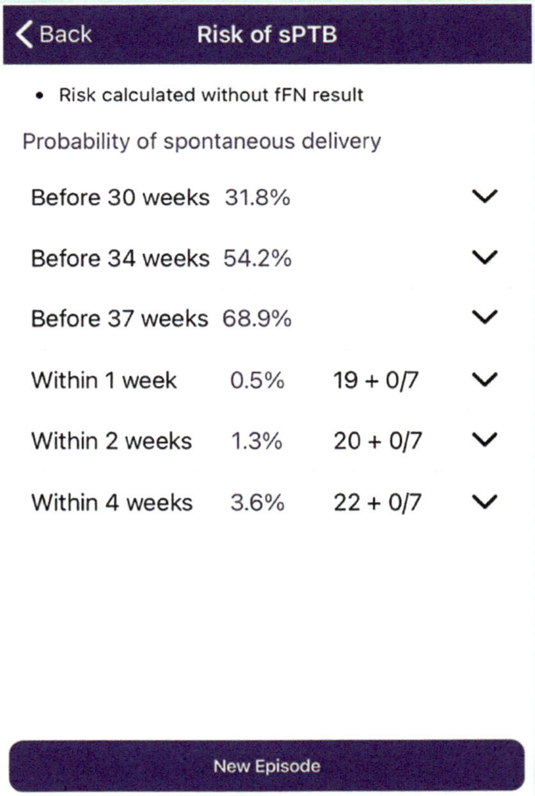

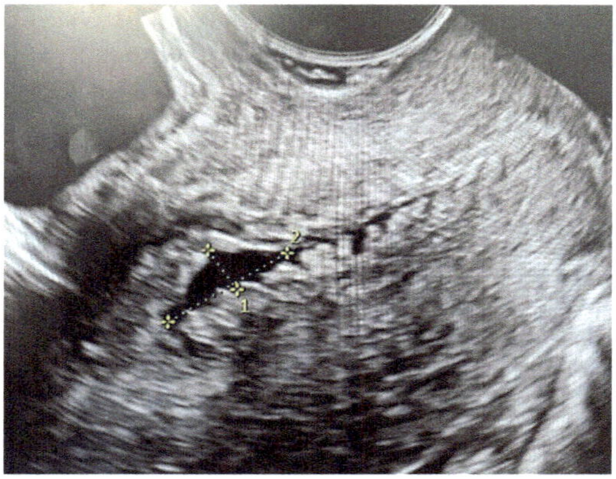

Fig. 6.4 Transvaginal ultrasound scan image of the cervix, illustrating a caesarean section niche

6.10.3 Caesarean Scar Niche

As knowledge of the impact of a full-dilatation caesarean section on subsequent preterm birth risk evolves, approaches to try and identify additional risk markers grow with it. Transvaginal cervical length has not been validated as an accurate predictive marker in this cohort [78]. Multiple studies have shown that the identification of a caesarean scar niche is a reproducible marker [79–81], and a recent single-centre prospective cohort study showed that the distance of a caesarean scar niche from the internal os may identify women at risk of spontaneous preterm birth [82]; see Fig. 6.4.

6.11 Novel Ultrasound Markers

6.11.1 Cervical Consistency Index

Cervical consistency index (CCI) has been investigated as a sonographic marker to assess cervical softness as a predictor of spontaneous preterm birth. The rationale for this test is that the cervix progressively softens and then shortens prior to birth; therefore, it may be possible to identify cervical softening before shortening occurs. With pressure applied to the anterior lip of the cervix, it is compressed, with the anterior–posterior diameter measured before and after pressure is applied and then calculated as a ratio [83]. A limitation of this method is the inability to objectively compare the force applied to the cervix by different operators.

6.11.2 Uterocervical Angle

Uterocervical angle (UCA) is a novel sonographic marker defined as the triangular segment measured between the lower uterine segment and the cervical canal. It is measured using a line that starts from the internal cervical os and a second line that tracks the internal segment of the anterior uterine wall. Two systematic reviews looking at this marker have examined this marker. Daskalakis et al. [83] suggested that a wider uterocervical angle *may* be a marker for preterm birth prediction, but Goldstein et al. looked at the uterocervical angle compared to the cervical length, and while an increased uterocervical angle was associated with an increased risk of preterm birth and was a reproducible measurement, they found that UCA had a significantly greater sensitivity than cervical length but demonstrated a significantly lower specificity and did not show improvement in prediction compared to or in combination with the cervical length 84].

6.11.3 Cervical Elastography

Ultrasound elastography is an imaging technique that can visualise the change in the stiffness of an examined region. Previously, it was used to identify lesions and tumours on other organs, but it has shown promise in assessing cervical consistency. Different approaches, such as strain elastography (SE) and shear wave elastography (SWE), have been examined. In the prediction of preterm birth, SE has a sensitivity and specificity of 84% (95% CI: 68–100%) and 80% (95% CI: 60–100%), respectively. A recent systematic review reported that it had a better diagnostic performance than cervical length alone [85]. As yet, research into this subject has not translated to routine practise.

6.12 Additional Predictive Tools and Cervical Length Integration

Predictive tools and decision-making algorithms are playing an increasingly important role in clinical medicine. They help provide more targeted and accurate planning for individuals and for optimising resource allocation.

6.12.1 Saving Babies' Lives

This care bundle, previously discussed, works to reduce the rates of preterm birth and improve neonatal outcomes by identifying those at risk earlier and ensuring that they are appropriately referred for cervical length screening, ideally by 12 weeks [70. The emphasis on early screening in high-risk patients aims to allow for earlier intervention where needed [70]. Patients are risk-stratified into low-, intermediate-, or high-risk pathways and managed accordingly. Additionally, the bundle has proactive discussions around modifiable risk factors such as smoking cessation.

6.12.2 Tommy's Clinical Decision Tool

This decision-making tool is a web-based (Conformité Européene (European Conformity), standards ensuring goods meet EU standards of safety, health and environmental standards) CE-marked medical device where women input their history directly, in conjunction with test results. It uses this information to more accurately and automatically assess a woman's risk of preterm birth and pregnancy complications, thus allowing her to be streamed into an appropriate antenatal care pathway, undergoing cervical length assessment, if and when it is deemed appropriate [80] .

While risk stratification is key in decision-making for the allocation of appropriate resources, it is important to be able to interpret the results of these tests in the context of past obstetric history and current pregnancy complications. Several algorithms have been developed with the aim of integration into clinical care to support both clinician and shared decision-making.

6.12.3 Fetal Medicine Foundation

The foetal medicine foundation's (FMF) second-trimester screening group carried out a prospective observational study using risk factors for preterm birth, in combination with transvaginal cervical length assessment [81]. This showed a higher detection rate of preterm birth risk than either alone, advocating for combined screening in this population to provide a percentage risk for the clinician and woman to use for further care planning.

6.12.4 QUIPP

The QUIPP app was developed at King's College London, in conjunction with Guy's and St. Thomas' Charity, Tommy's Charity, and the National Institute for Health and Care Research, as a clinical decision-making tool for medical professionals caring for women at risk of preterm birth [82]. It has been designed for use in both asymptomatic women at a high risk of preterm birth and for the management of women with symptoms suggestive of threatened preterm labour. By inputting relevant clinical history and test results available (transvaginal cervical length, quantitative foetal fibronectin, or both), the algorithm provides an individual percentage risk based on the assessment of the imminent risk of preterm birth, as well as the risk of delivery before 30, 34, and 37 weeks of gestation. For women presenting with symptoms of threatened preterm labour, it is a safe alternative to the NICE guidelines' 'treat all' approach, potentially reducing the risk of unnecessary admission or antenatal corticosteroids [83]. The app has also been externally validated outside of the UK [84] .

6.12.5 QUIDS

The quantitative fibronectin to help decision-making in women with symptoms of preterm labour (QUIDS) study used risk factors, in combination with foetal fibronectin (fFN), to create a predictive model for spontaneous preterm birth [85]. While the results showed promise, the loss of quantitative fFN from current clinical use has highlighted the limitations of relying on one single commercially available biomarker to predict this multimodal issue.

6.13 Summary

- Shortening of the cervix can be measured by transvaginal cervical length scanning.
- The assessment of risk factors for the prediction of preterm birth can allow appropriate surveillance of at-risk cohorts.
- Performing a cervical length should be undertaken with a standardised technique by someone with formal training in obtaining these measurements.
- The threshold for ultrasound-indicated interventions for the prevention of preterm birth is <25 mm before 24 + 0 weeks of gestation.
- In multiple pregnancies, there is a paucity of evidence regarding interventions, and it is suggested that different thresholds should be used if offering interventions.
- Transvaginal ultrasound cervical length measurement may be used in the assessment of symptomatic women.
- Guidelines on transvaginal ultrasound cervical length are not consistent internationally.
- Access to standard and high-level care is imperative to reduce preterm birth rates.
- Additional predictive algorithms and tests may be useful in care planning.
- Novel ultrasound markers in the prediction of preterm birth risk show promise for the future.

Chapter Key Points

- Role of cervical length as a screening tool for prediction of preterm birth.
- Principles and the technique of transvaginal cervical length measurement.
- Clinical application in singleton and multiple pregnancies.
- Assessment and relevance of risk factors, including cervical surgery, uterine anomalies, and prior obstetric history.
- Use of cervical length in symptomatic women and integration with predictive tools (QUIPP and (Fetal medicine foundation) FMF algorithms).
- Limitations, variability, and access considerations in cervical length screening.

Pearls and Pitfalls

Pearls

- Risk stratification at booking will help identify those who will most benefit from cervical length scanning for preterm prediction.
- Transvaginal cervical length scanning is a useful tool in asymptomatic and symptomatic pregnancies.
- A consistent and systematic approach is needed to be able to provide a reproducible assessment and accurate results.
- Cervical length measurements can be used with other biomarkers.

Pitfalls

- Cervical length scanning requires appropriate training and access to an ultrasound machine.
- There is intra-operator variability in cervical length scanning, which may lead to inconsistencies and implications for clinical care.
- Further work is needed to establish the use of cervical length in certain clinical situations, such as multiple pregnancies and universal screening.

References

1. Saigal S, Doyle LW. An overview of mortality and sequelae of preterm birth from infancy to adulthood. The Lancet [Internet]. 2008;371(9608):261–9. [cited 2023 Nov 14]; Available from: http://www.thelancet.com/article/S0140673608601361/fulltext
2. World Health Organisation. Born too soon: decade of action on preterm birth. 2023.
3. Blencowe H, Cousens S, Oestergaard MZ, Chou D, Moller AB, Narwal R, Adler A, Vera Garcia C,

Rohde S, Say L, Lawn JE. National, regional, and worldwide estimates of preterm birth rates in the year 2010 with time trends since 1990 for selected countries: a systematic analysis and implications. Lancet. 2012;379(9832):2162–72.

4. Romero R, Dey SK, Fisher SJ. Preterm labor: one syndrome, many causes. Science [Internet]. 2014;345(6198):760–5. [cited 2024 May 28]; Available from: https://pubmed.ncbi.nlm.nih.gov/25124429/
5. Iams JD, Goldenberg RL, Meis PJ, Mercer BM, Moawad A, Das A, Thom E, McNellis D, Copper RL, Johnson F, Roberts JM. The length of the cervix and the risk of spontaneous premature delivery. National Institute of Child Health and Human Development Maternal Fetal Medicine Unit Network. N Engl J Med [Internet]. 1996;334(9):567–72. [cited 2025 Feb 25]; Available from: https://pubmed.ncbi.nlm.nih.gov/8569824/
6. Naim A, Haberman S, Burgess T, Navizedeh N, Minkoff H. Changes in cervical length and the risk of preterm labor. Am J Obstet Gynecol [Internet]. 2002;186(5):887–9. [cited 2025 Feb 25]; Available from: https://pubmed.ncbi.nlm.nih.gov/12015503/
7. Principles and practice of screening for disease [Internet]. [cited 2025 Feb 25]. Available from: https://iris.who.int/handle/10665/37650
8. Iams JD, Goldenberg RL, Mercer BM, Moawad A, Thom E, Meis PJ, McNellis D, Caritis SN, Miodovnik M, Menard MK, Thurnau GR, Bottoms SF, Roberts JM. The Preterm Prediction Study: recurrence risk of spontaneous preterm birth. National Institute of Child Health and Human Development Maternal-Fetal Medicine Units Network. Am J Obstet Gynecol [Internet]. 1998;178(5):1035–40. [cited 2025 Feb 25]; Available from: https://pubmed.ncbi.nlm.nih.gov/9609580/
9. Nageotte MP, Casal D, Senyei AE. Fetal fibronectin in patients at increased risk for premature birth. Am J Obstet Gynecol [Internet]. 1994;170(1 Pt 1):20–5. [cited 2025 Feb 25]; Available from: https://pubmed.ncbi.nlm.nih.gov/8296822/
10. Phillips C, Velji Z, Hanly C, Metcalfe A. Risk of recurrent spontaneous preterm birth: a systematic review and meta-analysis. BMJ Open [Internet]. 2017;7(6) [cited 2025 Feb 25]; Available from: https://pubmed.ncbi.nlm.nih.gov/28679674/
11. NHS England. Saving babies' lives version three a care bundle for reducing perinatal mortality [Internet]. 2023 [cited 2023 Dec 14]. Available from: https://www.england.nhs.uk/long-read/saving-babies-lives-version-3/
12. Berghella V, Saccone G. Cervical assessment by ultrasound for preventing preterm delivery. Cochrane Database Syst Rev [Internet]. 2019;2019(9):CD007235. [cited 2025 Feb 25]; Available from: https://pmc.ncbi.nlm.nih.gov/articles/PMC6953418/
13. Melamed N, Hiersch L, Domniz N, Maresky A, Bardin R, Yogev Y. Predictive value of cervical length in women with threatened preterm labor. Obstet Gynecol [Internet]. 2013;122(6):1279–87. [cited 2025 Feb 25]; Available from: https://journals.lww.com/greenjournal/fulltext/2013/12000/predictive_value_of_cervical_length_in_women_with.19.aspx
14. Berghella V, Palacio M, Ness A, Alfirevic Z, Nicolaides KH, Saccone G. Cervical length screening for prevention of preterm birth in singleton pregnancy with threatened preterm labor: systematic review and meta-analysis of randomized controlled trials using individual patient-level data. Ultrasound Obstet Gynecol [Internet]. 2017;49(3):322–9. [cited 2025 Feb 25]; Available from: https://onlinelibrary.wiley.com/doi/full/10.1002/uog.17388
15. Doyle NM, Monga M. Role of ultrasound in screening patients at risk for preterm delivery. Obstet Gynecol Clin N Am. 2004;31(1):125–39.
16. França C, Carraca T, Monteiro SB, Rodrigues T, Montenegro N, Severo M, Matias A. Inter- and intra-observer variability in cervical measurement by ultrasound in the first and second trimesters of pregnancy: does it matter? J Perinat Med [Internet]. 2015;43(1):67–73. [cited 2025 Feb 25]; Available from: https://pubmed.ncbi.nlm.nih.gov/24846957/
17. Farràs A, Catalán S, Casellas A, Higueras T, Calero I, Goya M, Maiz N, Brik M, Carreras E. Real-time ultrasound demonstration of uterine isthmus contractions during pregnancy. Am J Obstet Gynecol [Internet]. 2024;230(1):89.e1–89.e12. [cited 2025 Feb 25]; Available from: https://pubmed.ncbi.nlm.nih.gov/37481152/
18. Kagan KO, Sonek J. How to measure cervical length. Ultrasound Obstet Gynecol [Internet]. 2015;45(3):358–62. [cited 2025 Feb 25]; Available from: https://pubmed.ncbi.nlm.nih.gov/25632014/
19. McIntosh J, Feltovich H, Berghella V, Manuck T. The role of routine cervical length screening in selected high- and low-risk women for preterm birth prevention. Am J Obstet Gynecol [Internet]. 2016;215(3):B2–7. [cited 2025 Feb 25]; Available from: https://www.ajog.org/action/showFullText?pii=S0002937816301120
20. Berghella V, Talucci M, Desai A. Does transvaginal sonographic measurement of cervical length before 14 weeks predict preterm delivery in high-risk pregnancies? Ultrasound Obstet Gynecol [Internet]. 2003;21(2):140–4. [cited 2025 Feb 25]; Available from: https://onlinelibrary.wiley.com/doi/full/10.1002/uog.28
21. Greco E, Gupta R, Syngelaki A, Poon LCY, Nicolaides KH. First-trimester screening for spontaneous preterm delivery with maternal characteristics and cervical length. Fetal Diagn Ther [Internet]. 2012;31(3):154–61. [cited 2025 Feb 25]; Available from: https://doi.org/10.1159/000335686
22. Goya M, Pratcorona L, Merced C, Rodó C, Valle L, Romero A, Juan M, Rodríguez A, Muñoz B, Santacruz B, Bello-Muñoz JC, Llurba E, Higueras

T, Cabero L, Carreras E. Cervical pessary in pregnant women with a short cervix (PECEP): an open-label randomised controlled trial. The Lancet [Internet]. 2012;379(9828):1800–6. [cited 2025 Feb 25]; Available from: https://www.thelancet.com/action/showFullText?pii=S0140673612600300
23. Fonseca EB, Celik E, Parra M, Singh M, Nicolaides KH. Progesterone and the risk of preterm birth among women with a short cervix. N Engl J Med [Internet]. 2007;357(5):462–9. [cited 2025 Feb 25]; Available from: https://www.nejm.org/doi/full/10.1056/NEJMoa067815
24. Shennan A, Story L, Jacobsson B, Grobman WA, Simpson JL, Norman J, Bianchi A, Munjanja S, González CMV, Mol BW. FIGO good practice recommendations on cervical cerclage for prevention of preterm birth. Int J Gynaecol Obstet [Internet]. 2021;155(1):19–22. [cited 2024 May 31]; Available from: https://pubmed.ncbi.nlm.nih.gov/34520055/
25. Ranzcog. Measurement of cervical length for prediction of preterm birth (C-Obs 27).
26. Salomon LJ, Alfirevic Z, Berghella V, Bilardo C, Hernandez-Andrade E, Johnsen SL, Kalache K, Leung KY, Malinger G, Munoz H, Prefumo F, Toi A, Lee W. Practice guidelines for performance of the routine mid-trimester fetal ultrasound scan. Ultrasound Obstet Gynecol [Internet]. 2011;37(1):116–26. [cited 2025 Feb 25]; Available from: https://onlinelibrary.wiley.com/doi/full/10.1002/uog.8831
27. Overview | Preterm labour and birth | Guidance | NICE.
28. Committee on Practice Bulletins-Obstetrics, The American College of, Obstetricians. Practice bulletin no. 130: prediction and prevention of preterm birth. Obstet Gynecol [Internet]. 2012;120(4):964–73. [cited 2025 Feb 25]; Available from: https://journals.lww.com/greenjournal/fulltext/2012/10000/practice_bulletin_no__130__prediction_and.42.aspx
29. Hibbard JU, Tart M, Moawad AH. Cervical length at 16-22 weeks' gestation and risk for preterm delivery. Obstet Gynecol [Internet]. 2000;96(6):972–8. [cited 2025 Feb 25]; Available from: https://pubmed.ncbi.nlm.nih.gov/11084188/
30. Laughon SK, Albert PS, Leishear K, Mendola P. The NICHD consecutive pregnancies study: recurrent preterm delivery by subtype. Am J Obstet Gynecol [Internet]. 2014;210(2):131.e1–8. [cited 2025 Feb 25]; Available from: https://www.ajog.org/action/showFullText?pii=S0002937813009551
31. To MS, Skentou C, Liao AW, Cacho A, Nicolaides KH. Cervical length and funneling at 23 weeks of gestation in the prediction of spontaneous early preterm delivery. Ultrasound Obstet Gynecol [Internet]. 2001;18(3):200–3. [cited 2025 Feb 25]; Available from: https://pubmed.ncbi.nlm.nih.gov/11555446/
32. Berghella V, Haas S, Chervoneva I, Hyslop T. Patients with prior second-trimester loss: prophylactic cerclage or serial transvaginal sonograms? Am J Obstet Gynecol [Internet]. 2002;187(3):747–51. [cited 2025 Feb 25]; Available from: https://pubmed.ncbi.nlm.nih.gov/12237658/
33. Althuisius SM, Dekker GA, Van Geijn HP, Bekedam DJ, Hummel P. Cervical incompetence prevention randomized cerclage trial (CIPRACT): study design and preliminary results. Am J Obstet Gynecol [Internet]. 2000;183(4):823–9. [cited 2025 Feb 25]; Available from: https://pubmed.ncbi.nlm.nih.gov/11035320/
34. To MS, Palaniappan V, Skentou C, Gibb D, Nicolaides KH. Elective cerclage vs. ultrasound-indicated cerclage in high-risk pregnancies. Ultrasound Obstet Gynecol [Internet]. 2002;19(5):475–7. [cited 2025 Feb 25]; Available from: https://pubmed.ncbi.nlm.nih.gov/11982981/
35. Kyrgiou M, Athanasiou A, Paraskevaidi M, Mitra A, Kalliala I, Martin-Hirsch P, Arbyn M, Bennett P, Paraskevaidis E. Adverse obstetric outcomes after local treatment for cervical preinvasive and early invasive disease according to cone depth: systematic review and meta-analysis. BMJ [Internet]. 2016;354. [cited 2025 Feb 25]; Available from: https://pubmed.ncbi.nlm.nih.gov/27469988/
36. Berghella V, Pereira L, Gariepy A, Simonazzi G. Prior cone biopsy: prediction of preterm birth by cervical ultrasound. Am J Obstet Gynecol [Internet]. 2004;191(4):1393–7. [cited 2025 Feb 25]; Available from: https://pubmed.ncbi.nlm.nih.gov/15507971/
37. Crane JMG, Delaney T, Hutchens D. Transvaginal ultrasonography in the prediction of preterm birth after treatment for cervical intraepithelial neoplasia. Obstet Gynecol [Internet]. 2006;107(1):37–44. [cited 2025 Feb 25]; Available from: https://journals.lww.com/greenjournal/fulltext/2006/01000/transvaginal_ultrasonography_in_the_prediction_of.8.aspx
38. Crane J, Scott H, Stewart A, Chandra S, Whittle W, Hutchens D. Transvaginal ultrasonography to predict preterm birth in women with bicornuate or didelphus uterus. J Matern Fetal Neonatal Med [Internet]. 2012;25(10):1960–4. [cited 2025 Feb 25]; Available from: https://www.tandfonline.com/doi/abs/10.3109/14767058.2012.675372
39. Ridout AE, Ibeto LA, Ross GN, Cook JR, Sykes L, David AL, Seed PT, Tribe RM, Bennett PR, Terzidou V, Shennan AH, Chandiramani M, Brown RG, Chatfield S, Sadeh D. Cervical length and quantitative fetal fibronectin in the prediction of spontaneous preterm birth in asymptomatic women with congenital uterine anomaly. Am J Obstet Gynecol [Internet]. 2019;221(4):341.e1–9. [cited 2025 Feb 25]; Available from: https://www.ajog.org/action/showFullText?pii=S0002937819307045
40. Levine LD, Sammel MD, Hirshberg A, Elovitz MA, Srinivas SK. Does stage of labor at time of

6

cesarean delivery affect risk of subsequent preterm birth? Am J Obstet Gynecol. 2015;212(3):360.e1–7.
41. Cong A, de Vries B, Ludlow J. Does previous caesarean section at full dilatation increase the likelihood of subsequent spontaneous preterm birth? Aust NZ J Obstet Gynaecol [Internet]. 2018;58(3):267–73. [cited 2023 Dec 19]; Available from: https://onlinelibrary.wiley.com/doi/full/10.1111/ajo.12713
42. Ewington LJ, Quenby S. Full dilatation caesarean section and the risk of preterm delivery in a subsequent pregnancy: a historical cohort study. J Clin Med. 2020;9(12):1–10.
43. Suff N, Xu VX, Glazewska-Hallin A, Carter J, Brennecke S, Shennan A. Previous term emergency caesarean section is a risk factor for recurrent spontaneous preterm birth; a retrospective cohort study. Eur J Obstet Gynecol. 2022;271:108–11.
44. Gordon MC, McKenna DS, Stewart TL, Howard BC, Foster KF, Higby K, Cypher RL, Barth WH. Transvaginal cervical length scans to prevent prematurity in twins: a randomized controlled trial presented in abstract form at the 27th Annual Clinic Meeting of the Society for Maternal-Fetal Medicine, San Francisco, CA, Feb 5–10, 2007. Am J Obstet Gynecol [Internet]. 2016;214(2):277.e1–7. [cited 2025 Feb 25]; Available from: https://www.ajog.org/action/showFullText?pii=S0002937815010133
45. Pagani G, Stagnati V, Fichera A, Prefumo F. Cervical length at mid-gestation in screening for preterm birth in twin pregnancy. Ultrasound Obstet Gynecol [Internet]. 2016;48(1):56–60. [cited 2025 Feb 25]; Available from: https://onlinelibrary.wiley.com/doi/full/10.1002/uog.15668
46. To MS, Fonseca EB, Molina FS, Cacho AM, Nicolaides KH. Maternal characteristics and cervical length in the prediction of spontaneous early preterm delivery in twins. Am J Obstet Gynecol [Internet]. 2006;194(5):1360–5. [cited 2025 Feb 25]; Available from: https://www.ajog.org/action/showFullText?pii=S0002937805024464
47. Lim AC, Hegeman MA, Huis In 'T Veld MA, Opmeer BC, Bruinse HW, Mol BWJ. Cervical length measurement for the prediction of preterm birth in multiple pregnancies: a systematic review and bivariate meta-analysis. Ultrasound Obstet Gynecol [Internet]. 2011;38(1):10–7. [cited 2025 Feb 25]; Available from: https://onlinelibrary.wiley.com/doi/full/10.1002/uog.9013
48. Conde-Agudelo A, Romero R, Rehal A, Brizot ML, Serra V, Da Fonseca E, Cetingoz E, Syngelaki A, Perales A, Hassan SS, Nicolaides KH. Vaginal progesterone for preventing preterm birth and adverse perinatal outcomes in twin gestations: a systematic review and meta-analysis. Am J Obstet Gynecol. 2023;229(6):599–616.e3.
49. D'Antonio F, Berghella V, Di Mascio D, Saccone G, Sileo F, Flacco ME, Odibo AO, Liberati M, Manzoli L, Khalil A. Role of progesterone, cerclage and pessary in preventing preterm birth in twin pregnancies: a systematic review and network meta-analysis. Eur J Obstet Gynecol Reprod Biol [Internet]. 2021;261:166–77. [cited 2025 Jan 3]; Available from: http://www.ejog.org/article/S0301211521001949/fulltext
50. Shennan AH, Story L. Cervical Cerclage: green-top guideline no. 75. BJOG. 2022;129(7):1178–210.
51. Khalil A, Rodgers M, Baschat A, Bhide A, Gratacos E, Hecher K, Kilby MD, Lewi L, Nicolaides KH, Oepkes D, Raine-Fenning N, Reed K, Salomon LJ, Sotiriadis A, Thilaganathan B, Ville Y. ISUOG practice guidelines: role of ultrasound in twin pregnancy. Ultrasound Obstet Gynecol [Internet]. 2016;47(2):247–63. [cited 2025 Feb 25]; Available from: https://onlinelibrary.wiley.com/doi/full/10.1002/uog.15821
52. Sotiriadis A, Papatheodorou S, Kavvadias A, Makrydimas G. Transvaginal cervical length measurement for prediction of preterm birth in women with threatened preterm labor: a meta-analysis. Ultrasound Obstet Gynecol [Internet]. 2010;35(1):54–64. [cited 2025 Feb 25]; Available from: https://onlinelibrary.wiley.com/doi/full/10.1002/uog.7457
53. Watson HA, Carlisle N, Seed PT, Carter J, Kuhrt K, Tribe RM, Shennan AH. Evaluating the use of the QUiPP app and its impact on the management of threatened preterm labour: a cluster randomised trial. PLoS Med [Internet]. 2021;18(7) [cited 2025 Feb 25]; Available from: https://pubmed.ncbi.nlm.nih.gov/34228735/
54. Berghella V, Saccone G. Fetal fibronectin testing for prevention of preterm birth in singleton pregnancies with threatened preterm labor: a systematic review and metaanalysis of randomized controlled trials. Am J Obstet Gynecol. 2016;215(4):431–8.
55. Ramachandran A, Clottey KD, Gordon A, Hyett JA. Prediction and prevention of preterm birth: Quality assessment and systematic review of clinical practice guidelines using the AGREE II framework. Int J Gynaecol Obstet. 2024;166(3):932–42. https://doi.org/10.1002/IJGO.15514. PubMed PMID: 38619379.
56. Kuusela P, Wennerholm UB, Fadl H, Wesström J, Lindgren P, Hagberg H, et al. Second trimester cervical length measurements with transvaginal ultrasound: a prospective observational agreement and reliability study. Acta Obstet Gynecol Scand. 2020;99(11):1476–85. https://doi.org/10.1111/AOGS.13895. PubMed PMID: 32392356.
57. Heath VCF, Southall TR, Souka AP, Novakov A, Nicolaides KH. Cervical length at 23 weeks of gestation: relation to demographic characteristics and previous obstetric history. Ultrasound Obstetr Gynecol. 1998;12(5):304–11. https://doi.org/10.1046/j.1469-0705.1998.12050304.x. PubMed PMID: 9819867.
58. Stein W, Hellmeyer L, Schmidt S, Tekesin I. Intraobserver and interobserver reliability of transvagi-

nal cervical length measurements and quantitative ultrasound tissue characterization of the cervix in the second and third trimester of pregnancy. Ultraschall Med. 2011;32 Suppl 2(SUPPL. 2) https://doi.org/10.1055/S-0031-1273409. PubMed PMID: 21630183./pp9.
59. França C, Carraca T, Monteiro SB, Rodrigues T, Montenegro N, Severo M, et al. Inter- and intra-observer variability in cervical measurement by ultrasound in the first and second trimesters of pregnancy: does it matter? J Perinat Med. 2015;43(1):67–73. https://doi.org/10.1515/JPM-2014-0123/MACHINEREADABLECITATION/RIS. PubMed PMID: 24846957./pp10.
60. Baños N, Burgos-Artizzu XP, Valenzuela-Alcaraz B, Coronado-Gutiérrez D, Perez-Moreno Á, Ponce J, et al. Intra- and interobserver reproducibility of second trimester ultrasound cervical length measurement in a general population. J Matern Fetal Neonatal Med. 2022;35(5):999–1002. https://doi.org/10.1080/14767058.2020.1733516. PubMed PMID: 32164477./p
61. Farrant K, Faluyi D, Watson K, Vause S, Birds H, Rowbotham S, et al. Role of ethnicity in high-level obstetric clinical incidents: a review of cases from a large UK NHS maternity unit. BMJ Open Qual. 2022;11(4):e001862. https://doi.org/10.1136/BMJOQ-2022-001862. PubMed PMID: 36379618.
62. Puthussery S, Tseng PC, Sharma E, Harden A, Griffiths M, Bamfo J, et al. Disparities in the timing of antenatal care initiation and associated factors in an ethnically dense maternal cohort with high levels of area deprivation. BMC Pregn Childbirth. 2022;22(1) https://doi.org/10.1186/S12884-022-04984-6. PubMed PMID: 36123628.
63. NHS England. https://www.england.nhs.uk/publication/saving-babies-livesversiontwo-a-care-bundle-for-reducing-perinatal-mortality/. 2019. Saving Babies Lives Care Bundle Version 2.
64. Saving Babies' Lives Version Three A care bundle for reducing perinatal mortality
65. Story L, Shennan A. Cervical cerclage: an evolving evidence base. BJOG. 2024;131(12):1579–86. https://doi.org/10.1111/1471-0528.17905.
66. Romero R, Kusanovic JP, Espinoza J, Gotsch F, Nhan-Chang CL, Erez O, et al. What is amniotic fluid 'sludge'? Ultrasound Obstet Gynecol. 2007;30(5):793. https://doi.org/10.1002/UOG.5173. PubMed PMID: 17899615.
67. Pannain GD, Pereira AMG, Da RMLTLF, Lopes RGC. Amniotic sludge and prematurity: systematic review and meta-analysis. Rev Bras Ginecol Obstet. 2023;45(8):E489–98. https://doi.org/10.1055/S-0043-1772189. PubMed PMID: 37683661./pp24.
68. Suff N, Webley E, Hall M, Tribe RM, Shennan AH. Amniotic fluid sludge is associated with earlier preterm delivery and raised cervicovaginal interleukin 8 concentrations. Am J Obstet Gynecol MFM. 2023;5(11) https://doi.org/10.1016/J.AJOGMF.2023.101161. PubMed PMID: 37709051./p
69. Rust OA, Atlas RO, Kimmel S, Roberts WE, Hess LW. Does the presence of a funnel increase the risk of adverse perinatal outcome in a patient with a short cervix? Am J Obstet Gynecol. 2005;192(4):1060–6. https://doi.org/10.1016/j.ajog.2005.01.076. PubMed PMID: 15846180./pp26.
70. Berghella V, Owen J, MacPherson C, Yost N, Swain M, Dildy GA, et al. Natural history of cervical funneling in women at high risk for spontaneous preterm birth. Obstetr Gynecol. 2007;109(4):863–9. https://doi.org/10.1097/01.AOG.0000258276.64005.CE. PubMed PMID: 17400847./p
71. To MS, Skentou C, Liao AW, Cacho A, Nicolaides KH. Cervical length and funneling at 23 weeks of gestation in the prediction of spontaneous early preterm delivery. Ultrasound Obstet Gynecol. 2001;18(3):200–3. https://doi.org/10.1046/J.1469-0705.2001.00437.X. PubMed PMID: 11555446.
72. Carlisle N, Glazewska-Hallin A, Story L, Carter J, Seed PT, Suff N, et al. CRAFT (Cerclage after full dilatation caesarean section): protocol of a mixed methods study investigating the role of previous in-labour caesarean section in preterm birth risk. BMC Pregn Childbirth. 2020;20(1) https://doi.org/10.1186/S12884-020-03375-Z. PubMed PMID: 33198663.
73. Naji O, Daemen A, Smith A, Abdallah Y, Saso S, Stalder C, et al. Visibility and measurement of cesarean section scars in pregnancy: a reproducibility study. Ultrasound Obstet Gynecol. 2012;40(5):549–56. https://doi.org/10.1002/UOG.11132. PubMed PMID: 22323065./pp30.
74. Savukyne E, Machtejeviene E, Paskauskas S, Ramoniene G, Nadisauskiene RJ. Transvaginal sonographic evaluation of Cesarean section Scar Niche in pregnancy: a prospective longitudinal study. Medicina (Kaunas). 2021;57(10) https://doi.org/10.3390/MEDICINA57101091. PubMed PMID: 34684128./pp31.
75. Banerjee A, Al-Dabbach Z, Bredaki FE, Casagrandi D, Tetteh A, Greenwold N, et al. Reproducibility of assessment of full-dilatation Cesarean section scar in women undergoing second-trimester screening for preterm birth. Ultrasound Obstetr Gynecol. 2022;60(3):396–403. https://doi.org/10.1002/UOG.26027. PubMed PMID: 35809243./p
76. Banerjee A, Ivan M, Nazarenko T, Solda R, Bredaki EF, Casagrandi D, et al. Prediction of spontaneous preterm birth in women with previous full dilatation cesarean delivery. Am J Obstet Gynecol MFM. 2024;6(3) https://doi.org/10.1016/J.AJOGMF.2024.101298. PubMed PMID: 38278178.
77. Parra-Saavedra M, Gómez L, Barrero A, Parra G, Vergara F, Navarro E. Prediction of preterm birth

using the cervical consistency index. Ultrasound Obstet Gynecol. 2011;38(1):44–51. https://doi.org/10.1002/UOG.9010. PubMed PMID: 21465603.

78. Goldstein MJ, Bailer JM, Gonzalez-Brown VM. Uterocervical angle in predicting spontaneous preterm birth: a systematic review and meta-analysis. AJOG Glob Rep. 2023;3(3) https://doi.org/10.1016/J.XAGR.2023.100240. PubMed PMID: 37396342.
79. Wang B, Zhang Y, Chen S, Xiang X, Wen J, Yi M, et al. Diagnostic accuracy of cervical elastography in predicting preterm delivery: a systematic review and meta-analysis. Medicine. 2019;98(29):e16449. https://doi.org/10.1097/MD.0000000000016449. PubMed PMID: 31335700.
80. Carter J, Anumba D, Brigante L, Burden C, Draycott T, Gillespie S, et al. The Tommy's Clinical Decision Tool, a device for reducing the clinical impact of placental dysfunction and preterm birth: protocol for a mixed-methods early implementation evaluation study. BMC Pregn Childbirth. 2022;22(1):639. https://doi.org/10.1186/S12884-022-04867-W. PubMed PMID: 35971107.
81. Celik E, To M, Gajewska K, Smith GCS, Nicolaides KH. Cervical length and obstetric history predict spontaneous preterm birth: development and validation of a model to provide individualized risk assessment. Ultrasound Obstetr Gynecol. 2008;31(5):549–54. https://doi.org/10.1002/uog.5333.
82. Carter J, Seed PT, Watson HA, David AL, Sandall J, Shennan AH, et al. Development and validation of predictive models for QUiPP App v.2: tool for predicting preterm birth in women with symptoms of threatened preterm labor. Ultrasound Obstetr Gynecol. 2020;55(3):357–67. https://doi.org/10.1002/uog.20422.
83. Watson HA, Carter J, Seed PT, Tribe RM, Shennan AH. The QUiPP App: a safe alternative to a treat-all strategy for threatened preterm labor. Ultrasound Obstetr Gynecol. 2017;50(3):342–6. https://doi.org/10.1002/uog.17499.
84. Creswell L, Rolnik DL, Burke B, Daly S, O'Gorman N. Performance of QUiPP App v.2 tool for prediction of preterm birth in asymptomatic high-risk women attending preterm specialist clinic: external validation study. Ultrasound Obstet Gynecol. 2024;64(1):71–8. https://doi.org/10.1002/UOG.27619. PubMed PMID: 38379428.
85. Stock SJE, Horne M, Bruijn M, White H, Boyd KA, Heggie R, et al. Development and validation of a risk prediction model of preterm birth for women with preterm labour symptoms (the QUIDS study): a prospective cohort study and individual participant data meta-analysis. PLoS Med. 2021;18(7) https://doi.org/10.1371/JOURNAL.PMED.1003686. PubMed PMID: 34228732.

The Role of Cerclage in Singleton and Twins

Anastasia Martin and Andrew Shennan

Contents

Y. Yogev, A. Khalil (eds.), *Prevention of Complications in Obstetrics*,
https://doi.org/10.1007/978-3-032-23479-7_7

Learning Objectives

- Recognise the significance of preterm birth and its implications.
- Identify the key indications and contra-indications for cervical cerclage.
- Differentiate between the types of cervical cerclage.
- Understand the current evidence surrounding cerclage and its limitations.
- Understand the role of cerclage in different subgroups of women.

Chapter Introduction

Preterm birth <37 weeks is the leading cause of neonatal death. While the majority of cases are of unknown causes, women with known risk factors can be appropriately monitored and managed to reduce risk. Interventions such as cervical cerclage have been used since the 1950s to reduce the risk of preterm birth. In this chapter, you will gain a basic understanding of the use of cervical cerclage, its indications, and its evidence base in different subgroups.

7.1 Introduction

Cervical cerclage is a surgical procedure that involves placing a stitch around the cervix. It is used as a way of preventing spontaneous preterm birth and has become established as an intervention in women with a risk of second-trimester foetal loss or early preterm birth.

Initial descriptions of this technique were in the 1950s, followed by widespread uptake in view of the apparent success following the use of cerclage. Controlled trials into the effectiveness of the procedure were not conducted until the 1980s, and they established that its efficacy was somewhat limited and that there was uncertainty around its value in different subgroups. Currently, approximately 1–2% of all pregnancies receive a cerclage in high-income settings [1]. Accurate data is unavailable for its uptake in large parts of the world, although it is common practice in India. Given the poor evidence base for cerclage, there is a need for contemporary, well-controlled clinical trials to elucidate those populations who are likely to benefit from it.

There is uncertainty regarding the optimal technique, and many details surrounding cerclage indications and management are yet to be determined. However, evidence is evolving, and this chapter will elucidate some of this.

7.1.1 The Impact of Preterm Birth and the Concept of Cervical Insufficiency

Preterm birth is a major health problem in the world and contributes more to lost health capital than any other health issue [2]. Approximately 15 million babies are born before 37 weeks of gestation each year, and around one million will die, with rates varying widely across countries, ranging from about 4% to 16% [3]. Consequences of preterm birth are well-described, and it is a significant cause of neonatal morbidity and mortality, as well as long-term health outcomes to women and society [4, 5]. There are multiple reasons why women deliver early, but for many, there is no identifiable factor.

The use of cerclage has been directed primarily to women with prior adverse events, usually second-trimester loss or early preterm birth, although occasionally, when there is a very deficient cervix, cerclage can be used to target the cervix as the primary cause of a potential problem. Given the complex nature of preterm birth and our poor understanding of the mechanism, along with the multiple aetiologies, the use of cerclage has not been sufficiently researched in most subgroups. There are plausible reasons why its action could vary depending on aetiology. In those women with underlying risk factors, such as smoking, low BMI, or other socio-demographic features linked to preterm birth, the use of cerclage is unclear, and no adequate research has been done targeting women specifically in these subgroups unless they have been related to a prior event. In situations where there is likely to be cervical deficiency, for example, Large loop excision of the transformation zone (LLETZ) or cone biopsy, cerclage is a more logical procedure, as it will provide structural support to a likely physical deficiency; however, very few trials have evaluated its efficacy in these subgroups. More recently, women with previous caesarean sections in labour are known to have cervical trauma that results in subsequent preterm birth, and this is also likely to be related to cervical trauma [6, 7]. This is a good example of where aetiology may be critical in determining efficacy: vaginal cerclage in these women is known to have a much higher failure rate (×10), and abdominal cerclage may be required to prevent loss [8, 9].

The cervix is not only required to provide mechanical strength but also acts as a barrier to avoid ascending infection. This final common pathway for many preterm births can still be prevented with cervical cerclage, so it may be therapeutic as well as prophylactic in many cases, which may explain why abdominal cerclage has such high success rates in spite of these multiple aetiologies. However, direct evidence of this as a mechanism is lacking, although the success of abdominal and other cerclages is directly linked to maintaining a long cervical canal [10, 11].

Therefore, the ability of the cerclage to maintain cervical length may assist in ensuring that an endocervical mucus plug remains intact with its antimicrobial properties.

Cerclage remains an under-researched but commonly used technique, with multiple variations. The interaction between cervical integrity, the risk of preterm birth, and how it is modified needs to be elucidated.

7.2 Classification of Cerclage

There are a number of classifications used over the years, but these are often related to either the indication or the level of placement. An indication can be due to prior poor obstetric history, in which case, a history-indicated cerclage can be performed. Alternatively, an ultrasound-indicated cerclage can be used when the cervix shortens, often in a woman with a prior poor history. An examination-indicated cerclage, sometimes known as an emergency or rescue cerclage, is used when the cervix is open and membranes are visible, a high-risk situation in view of the exposure to the vaginal microbiome.

A history-indicated cerclage is usually performed only when there is significant concern of preterm birth, and in practice, this would be done in a woman who has had multiple prior events. In modern practice, where women and clinicians feel more comfortable with action, cerclage is often placed in women for whom there has been little evidence of benefit. However, this must be a joint decision between the patient and her doctor, although if we are to progress in our knowledge of efficacy in this intervention, clinicians should be clear about the uncertainty of benefit and encourage participation in research when available.

An alternative to surgery is to rely on ultrasound and only insert a cerclage if the cervix shortens [12]. This is known as an ultrasound-indicated cerclage, and the conventional threshold is 25 mm or less for action (usually between 16 and 24 weeks of gestation). This is a very reasonable strategy, particularly in women without a clear evidence base for insertion, such as those with only one or two prior events. In practice, even those with multiple events or those with a prior cerclage can rely on ultrasound to inform the need for cerclage if they prefer, as a long cervix is a reliable indication that cerclage would not be indicated.

When the cerclage is defined by its placement, it can be classified as low when inserted vaginally without additional surgery to move the bladder. This is sometimes referred to as a low-vaginal cerclage, a purse-string cerclage, or a McDonald cerclage (◘ Fig. 7.1). In fact, the anatomical variation in women means that the height may not be related to bladder mobilisation, i.e. a higher suture can be placed without mobilisation, and each case needs to be individualised. When there has been extensive cervical surgery, for example, with large loop excisions, bladder mobilisation may be necessary to be able to insert the suture, but it need not necessarily be high. A high cerclage is referred in cases where bladder mobilisation allows for higher placement but where there is little evidence that routinely placing it with bladder mobilisation is beneficial (◘ Fig. 7.1) [13]. Transabdominal cerclage is performed by the abdominal route, which allows higher placement of the cerclage (◘ Fig. 7.2).

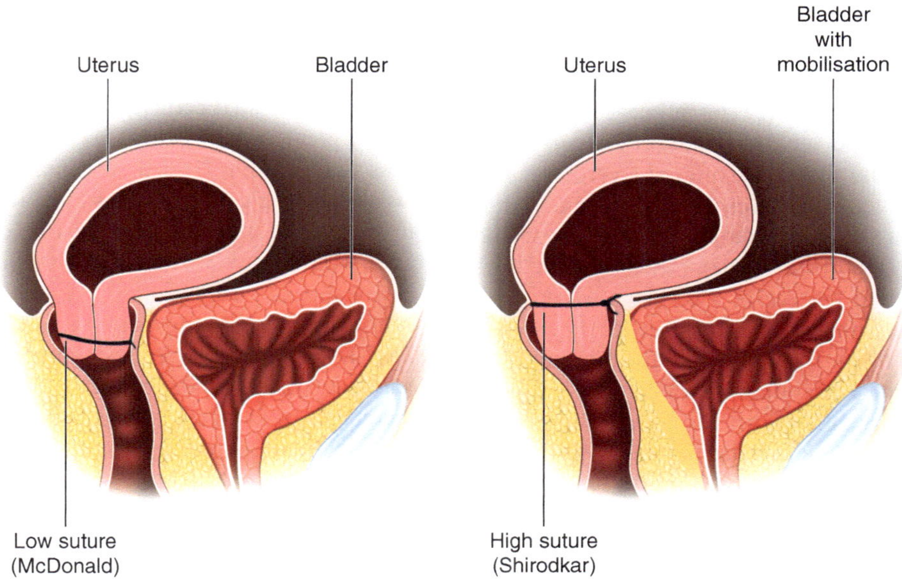

Fig. 7.1 Low (McDonald) suture (left) and high (Shirodkar) suture with bladder mobilisation (right)

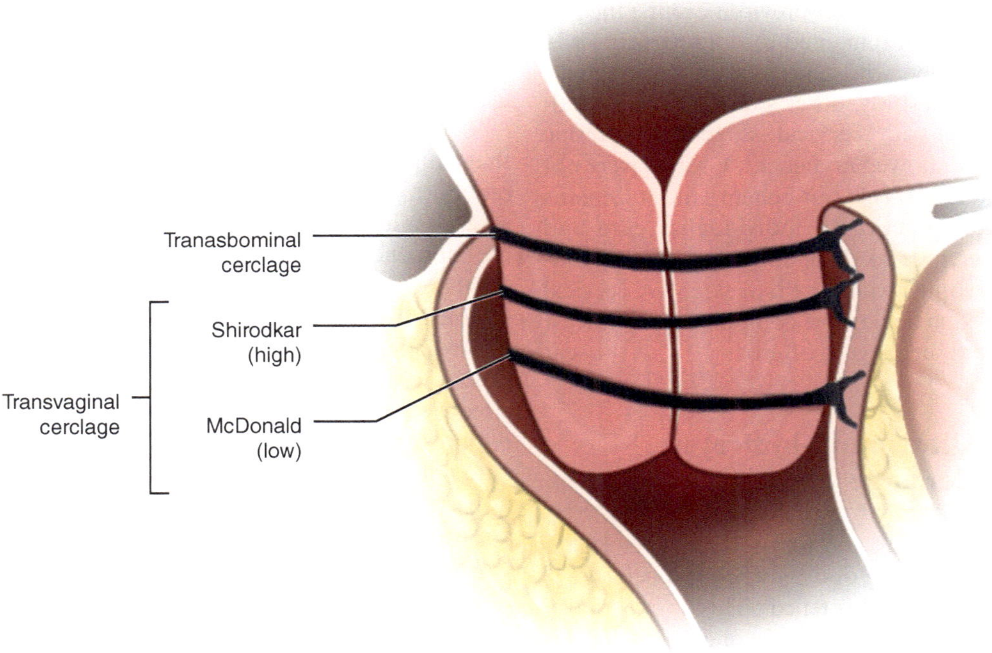

Fig. 7.2 Types of sutures, including both transvaginal and transabdominal

7.2.1 History-Indicated Cerclage

Currently, women with a singleton pregnancy who have had three or more prior events (either in the second trimester or early preterm births) should be offered a cerclage. The evidence base for this is not strong and is based on subgroup analysis on the largest trial to date (from the 1980s), when women were randomised to receive a cerclage when clinicians were uncertain as to whether they would benefit from it or not. This international multi-centre trial demonstrated that in a subgroup of women with three or more events, the chance of delivering before 30 weeks was halved from 32% to 15% [14]. This implies that only 1 in 25 women receiving a cerclage would benefit from its insertion, and it is important that women are counselled that the procedure does not often change the outcome. However, most women (>80%) will achieve a successful pregnancy, unrelated to the cerclage. In this trial, no effect was seen on those who had two or fewer previous events; the recommendation remained to only perform it in those women who had at least three events. Within this study, other sub-analyses, including those with cervical surgery or uterine anomaly, showed no benefit. Groups were not big enough to rule out benefit, and it remains common practice to individualise care and offer cerclage to these subgroups. For example, in women who have had extensive cervical surgery, particularly if combined with at least one event, cerclage is offered.

7.2.2 Ultrasound-Indicated Cerclage

An alternative to a history-indicated cerclage is to scan a woman and only insert a cerclage if the cervix has shortened. This is a strategy often used for those with one or two prior spontaneous preterm births, where the evidence does not indicate a benefit for history-indicated cerclage. Current evidence suggests cervical scanning every 2–4 weeks from 16 to 24 weeks and inserting a cerclage if the cervical length is less than 25 mm. One randomised control trial has demonstrated that in women with prior preterm birth, the risk of delivery before 35 weeks was approximately halved when an ultrasound-indicated cerclage is used, and this benefit is greatest in those with a cervical length of less than 15 mm [15]. If a woman reaches 24 weeks and the cervix remains long, there is a high chance of passing 34 weeks, and most women would not have continued surveillance.

Care should always be individualised, and it is not unreasonable to perform a scan in a high-risk woman at her request, given the lack of clinical trial evidence regarding the benefit of cerclage. In low-risk women, the value of routine cervical scanning has not been established, and this tends to be reserved for women with risk factors.

The meta-analysis of vaginal cerclage use demonstrates benefit, with a modest relative risk reduction of around 20–25% for preterm delivery (before 35 weeks) for all cerclage types [16]. Of note, vaginal cerclage has not been linked to a reduction in mortality, but this is probably related to a lack of evidence rather than evidence of no effect. It supports the need for more research for a commonly used and established intervention.

There is often a perception from women that a higher suture is beneficial, and they may request a procedure that is not indicated (e.g. an abdominal cerclage). This can be driven by the nomenclature and the perception that "higher" is better. Clinicians should not be tempted to offer more complex procedures to lower-risk cases, as the potential complications likely outweigh any benefits. In practice, effective counseling for suture procedures requires experienced clinicians who are up-to-date with the latest evidence. In cases where non-evidence-based practices are used, it is essential to document the agreement and the reasons for the chosen approach.

7.3 Multiple and Higher-Order Pregnancies

Currently, the use of history- or ultrasound-indicated cerclage is not routinely recommended in twin pregnancies [17, 18]. Clinical trials are often performed on twins without additional risk factors, and this evidence should not be extrapolated to twins with other risk factors, such as a prior event or cervical surgery. The benefit of cerclage in twins is not strong, and there are few randomised controlled trials. Women with other risk factors that would normally have ultrasound surveillance can still be managed on an individualised basis. However, there is increasing evidence that there may be a benefit in observational studies where cerclage appears to reduce risks, particularly in cervixes that are less than 15 mm [19].

7.4 When Not to Use a Cerclage

Contraindications are related to situations where continuing the pregnancy may be dangerous, if a woman is in active preterm labour, has evidence of infection, has ruptured membranes, or is actively bleeding. If a foetus is compromised through foetal distress or has a lethal defect, a cerclage should not be performed. It is important that women who have a cerclage have access to appropriate care after the procedure, and if this is not guaranteed, then the need for cerclage should be reconsidered. The importance of appropriate counselling and informed consent cannot be overstated.

7.5 Other Prophylactic Therapies and Interactions with Cerclage

Progesterone as a vaginal pessary or intramuscular 17-hydroxyprogesterone caproate has been extensively investigated, and it is currently recommended that a woman with a prior history of preterm birth or second-trimester loss should receive prophylactic therapy, usually from 16 to 34 weeks [20, 21]. If the cervix is short, this can also be an indication. Conversely, a long cervix may allow this to be withheld.

There have been a few studies looking at the interaction between progesterone and cerclage when given together. Some of these have been criticised and have not yet substantively informed clinical practice.

It seems pragmatic, as the evidence evolves, to recommend giving progesterone to all women who have had a prior preterm event, but the criteria for using cerclage can still be valid in this group of women. Further studies are needed to assess whether this interaction should influence this practice. Based on the innocuous nature of natural progesterone and its simplicity in treatment, it would be appropriate to continue to use it in women with cerclage.

Alternative therapies, such as the Arabin pessary, have been less extensively evaluated, and there have been more negative trials [22]. Most clinicians would not prescribe an Arabin pessary together with a cerclage, as they are mechanistically very similar, and this would appear less logical.

One recent trial, the Stitch, Pessary, or Progesterone Randomised Trial (SuPPoRT) trial, is the first study to compare, in a three-way randomised design, cerclage with pessary or progesterone. In this study, there was considerable crossover, but there was no clear indication that there was one indication superior to another [23].

7.6 Practical Consideration to Cerclage Insertion

Transvaginal cerclage is generally inserted once the first-trimester ultrasound is complete to ensure that aneuploidy is unlikely. This will also ensure viability and prevent unnecessary sutures from being put in. The number of pregnancies can be confirmed, along with possible lethal or major foetal anomalies. It is important to ensure that women understand that in the case of miscarriage (which is possible with a cerclage) or an incidental complication that requires the termination of pregnancy, the suture will need to be removed. As with all surgical procedures, appropriate informed consent should be obtained, both with verbal and written information, with clear indications of the benefits and risks. Direct risks are hard to elucidate, as these are high-risk pregnancies, but there is little evidence to suggest that the cerclage itself will increase the risk of pregnancy loss, and women can be reassured that the purpose of the suture is to reduce these risks. There is a theoretical concern that there may be surgical trauma (i.e. damage to the bladder or cervix) or possible lacerations; however, in practice, these are rare and not prevalent in large series of cerclage use. At the time of the procedure, it is also a theoretical concern that membranes could be inadvertently ruptured, but again, this is an extremely rare event. More of a concern is that if there is an intrauterine infection, cerclage may delay a miscarriage, which itself may increase risks of sepsis to the mother. Serious sepsis is rare but occasionally can be severe and life-threatening, and women should be counselled considering this. In practice, women can be assured that the cerclage is not likely to increase risks to the baby.

7.6.1 Need for Anaesthesia

When inserting a cerclage, it is necessary to give adequate analgesia generally, with a regional block or a general anaesthetic. There is no operative advantage in performing a general anaesthesia. In modern practice, these anaesthetic techniques are very safe, and therefore, both are reasonable if requested, but regional anaesthesia is believed to be safer. Most procedures are now performed with regional anaesthesia.

7.6.2 Operative Technique

There is little research evaluating the operative technique and its relative merits. In practice, the choice of cerclage technique is largely related to the experience and discretion of the surgeon. However, it is established that a cerclage placed high is likely to be better, as it maintains the integrity of the internal os and is related to improved outcomes [11]. Mobilisation of the bladder may be required to achieve a high cervical cerclage, although routine mobilisation does not appear to be advantageous. In practice, therefore, a deficient cervix may require bladder mobilisation in order to insert the suture high enough for benefit. Assessment prior to the procedure can be performed with a vaginal examination in the clinic.

The material used should be non-absorbable and, again, is largely related to the discretion of the surgeon. The two commonly used materials are monofilament or braided. The recent C-Stitch trial randomised women to receive either monofilament or braided sutures to compare their efficacy. The primary outcome was pregnancy loss; however, the study found no significant difference between the two, with both groups experiencing a loss rate of approximately 8%. However, in the study, there was no difference, with both groups having around 8% loss [24]. Monofilament may be associated with less disruption of the vaginal microbiome [25]. However, this does not translate into differences in pregnancy success. One outcome in this study, which was the reporting of maternal sepsis and clinical chorioamnionitis, appeared to be less in monofilament but, again, with no influence on outcomes. Therefore, it remains reasonable for surgeons to use either based on their preference. One notable finding was that it was significantly more difficult to remove the monofilament suture in this study, requiring more anaesthesia.

7.6.3 Details of Low-Vaginal Cerclage Insertion

Following normal practice, using standard surgical preparation and safety procedures, it is common to place the patient in lithotomy position and then to clean the surrounding skin and vagina with antiseptic, often chlorhexidine- or iodine-based. Standard retractors such as the Simms speculum and lateral wall retractors can allow the cervix to be visualised, and generally, one or two assistants will facilitate this (◘ Fig. 7.3). Usually, between four and six bites are taken of the cervix in a purse-string fashion, circumferentially around the cervix (◘ Fig. 7.4). Often, the cervix can be held using appropriate atraumatic clamps or sponge-holding forceps (Fig. 7.3). Most surgeons tend to tie the knot anteriorly. Posterior knot placement is also practised and may reduce effects on the bladder (not evidenced), although it is harder to identify for retrieval. Blood loss is minimal, but if present, once the knot is tied, haemostasis is generally good, and it is rare to need additional sutures to stop bleeding. A catheter is usually inserted after the procedure to ensure that the urine is clear and that there is no bladder trauma. Depending on the surgeon's preference, the bladder can also be emptied at the beginning of the procedure, although this is not necessary and may, in fact, aid identification.

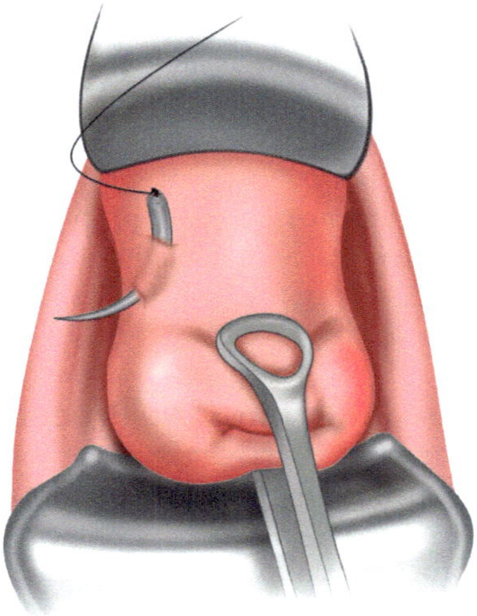

Fig. 7.3 Suture placement through the vaginal route

The technique of the high-vaginal cerclage is variable but generally follows the same principles but following bladder mobilisation. This is usually achieved by a small transverse incision (about 4 cm) below the bladder and blunt dissection used to mobilise the bladder. This can be facilitated by using fluid dissection (e.g. 20 ml of normal saline in the space prior to incision). The suture can be buried, or a tail can be left through the skin incision to allow retrieval. The skin should be sutured to ensure haemostasis.

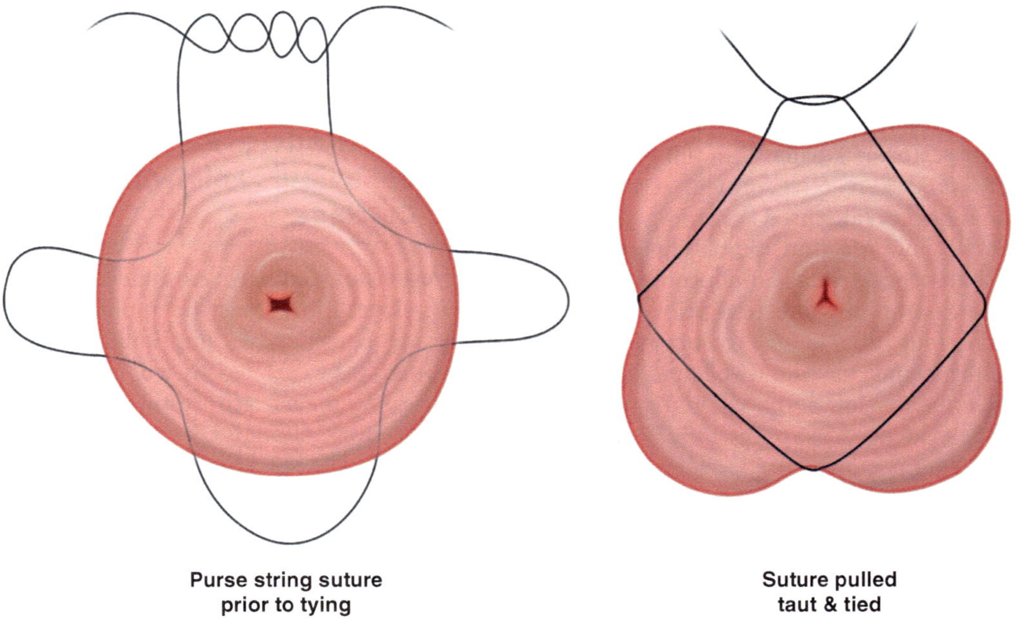

Fig. 7.4 Purse-string suture

7.7 Exam-Indicated Cerclage (Cerclage with Exposed Membranes)

When membranes are exposed to the vaginal microbiome, it creates a high-risk situation that can lead to sepsis [20]. The purpose of the procedure is to reform the barrier between the intrauterine environment and the vagina and allow recovery before sepsis takes hold. Appropriate counselling is required, and the woman should understand that this is a high-risk situation and that these types of cerclages would often fail. However, on average, pregnancy tends to be prolonged, often by about 6 weeks [26]. There are ongoing large clinical trials to evaluate the risks and benefits of this approach. One study has demonstrated an average latency of 34 days [27]. Certain factors can indicate a higher risk of failure; these include advanced dilatation at the time of diagnosis, the presence of sludge in the amniotic fluid, or if foetal parts have descended through the cervix [28]. However, none of these are absolute contraindications to performing the stitch. There are anecdotal successes of women going to term in many of these difficult cases, usually because these sutures had been inserted before there had been any intrauterine sepsis. Because of the concern for sepsis, standard infection screens can be performed, usually an full blood count (FBC) and C-reactive protein (CRP). Care should be individualised according to the possible risk of infection. Some clinicians have advocated performing amniocentesis to rule out intra-amniotic infection prior to the procedure, but this is not common practice. Equally, people have removed fluid in order to reduce the tension in the sac, but again, there is little evidence to support this. Preoperative interventions can be used, such as screening for genital tract infections and urine cultures. Other adjuvant therapies that have been used include tocolysis and other agents, such as non-steroidal anti-inflammatories, which may also achieve some uterine quiescence. Biomarkers have been used to ascertain the risk; for example, quantitative foetal fibronectin, even with exposed membranes, is related to the success of the procedure [29]. Given the difficulties of performing this procedure and replacing the membranes and the proximity of the needle to the sac, this should only be performed by experienced surgeons. The use of antibiotics can be prescribed at the time of the procedure, but their role in longer-term use in this situation is not established. As antibiotics in intact membranes in women at risk of preterm delivery are associated with longer-term poor outcomes, prolonged antibiotics should not be used prophylactically until further research elucidates their risk/benefit [30].

7.8 Care Following the Procedure

Most women having a history- or ultrasound-indicated cerclage can be sent home on the day of the procedure, although occasionally, problems with urinary retention or discomfort may warrant an overnight stay and appropriate management. Following emergency cerclage, the risk of sepsis is far higher; the gestational age and the circumstance will dictate the need for inpatient management, particularly if the cerclage is performed around viability.

7.9 Other Advice Regarding Behaviours Following Cerclage

Bed rest is not routinely recommended following cerclage. But it must be appreciated that there are considerable emotional, financial, and other issues related to women requiring cerclage, and the need for resting at home and avoiding work should be supported on an individual basis as is appropriate. Equally, there is no evidence to suggest the need to abstain from sexual intercourse, but in the case of a short cervix or an exam-indicated cerclage, the possibility of introducing infection must be considered. Following the procedure, measuring cervical length is a reliable way to assess the risk, i.e. a short cervix is associated with a much higher chance of delivery in spite of the cerclage, and a long cervix indicates a higher chance of success [10]. Again, these can be used on an individual basis to ascertain management. Biomarkers such as foetal fibronectin are also reliable in women with a cerclage, although slightly more false positives have been reported [31]. Other biomarkers are available, and cerclage is not a contraindication to their use, although there is little evidence to support it in common management.

7.10 Delivery Following Cerclage

An elective cerclage can be removed at or before 37 weeks to minimise labour, resulting in trauma to the cervix. If an elective caesarean section is being planned, then the need for removal can be delayed until this point for convenience's sake. Most sutures can be removed without a regional or general anaesthetic unless they were buried during a high-vaginal procedure. If labour does occur or if there are signs of chorioamnionitis, active vaginal bleeding, or other indications for delivery, then the transvaginal cerclage can be removed at any time. Should rupture of membranes occur, then again, there should be individualised care depending on gestation; however, in earlier gestations, as long as there were no signs of chorioamnionitis, sutures can be left in situ if there is benefit in management, such as the need for antenatal steroids for foetal lung maturity [32].

7.11 Transabdominal Cerclage

In women who have had a previous unsuccessful transcervical cerclage or in women who have a very deficient cervix, where a vaginal cerclage would be extremely difficult, a transabdominal cerclage can be considered. They are performed either periconceptually or in the first trimester of pregnancy. Preconception sutures allow the surgeon to place the sutures higher without concern for the pregnancy, and it has also been proven that it is not associated with any fertility issues [33]. One randomised controlled trial has demonstrated that transabdominal cerclage, when used in women with a prior failed cerclage, significantly reduces the risk of delivery before 32 weeks, as well as foetal loss; the number needed to treat is very modest at less than one in five. This is a much stronger evidence base than for vaginal sutures but in a much rarer group. Following this trial, most women with two failed cerclages achieved a successful outcome, even when managed by the team with the failed cerclage, suggesting that the technique alone explains the success. Given the complexity of performing a laparotomy and the need for subsequent caesarean section, this should not be a first-line procedure and should only be reserved for those with a failed cerclage or a very deficient cervix, where a vaginal cerclage would be challenging [34]. Transabdominal cerclage can be performed either laparoscopically or through a small transverse scar by laparotomy. Both appear to be efficacious, although laparotomy is currently a more common procedure (83% in the UK) [35]. Women receiving a laparoscopic approach have a small conversion rate to an open procedure of around 5% and, because they require a caesarean section, will end up with more abdominal scarring overall; these factors should be discussed with the woman. Although more surgery is required, overall significant morbidity is probably reduced with transabdominal cerclage in view of the fact that it has more success (i.e. women with mid-trimester losses can have serious complications). Women should be counselled as to the normal risks of a laparotomy but reassured that the success overall will not significantly increase serious morbidity.

The procedure involves dissecting the uterovesical fold to expose the lower part of the uterus and the upper cervix; the suture is sited above the uterosacral and cardinal ligaments; both monofilament and braided sutures are described, and variable practice is common; some people will use one, others two. There is little evidence to support one technique over others, but overall, large series of abdominal sutures have been remarkably successful. A recent publication provides free access to a video of both laparoscopic and open techniques [36]. Following viewing of this video, there have been reports of remarkable success in Africa [37].

Generally, knots are tied posteriorly to avoid bladder irritation. And this has not been associated with issues with the bowel. Removing the suture via colpotomy has been described. Prolonged hospital stay is generally not required in women with transabdominal cerclage, and early mobilisation is encouraged.

In the event that there is early miscarriage or foetal death with a transabdominal cerclage, generally, if this is early, for example, in the first trimester, this can be managed as in a woman without the cerclage. In slightly later mid-trimester miscarriages or intrauterine demise, dilatation and evacuation have been described up to 18 weeks. Beyond 18 weeks, the cerclage can be cut either through colpotomy or laparoscopy to facilitate a vaginal delivery. Failing this, a hysterotomy is performed. Given the high success of a transabdominal cerclage, the need for these procedures related to failure is rare. If an abdominal cerclage is successful, then a caesarean section should be booked; the timing of this should be as per any elective caesarean and planned for 39 weeks or later. If labour occurs earlier, then surgery can be performed at this time. Threatened preterm labour can occur in these women and should be managed in the normal way and will often settle down; it is rare for a serious complication to ensue.

Case Study

A woman presents at 13 weeks of gestation with a history of a large loop excision of her cervix (of unknown dimensions) performed under local anaesthesia 10 years ago. She had a subsequent 20-week mid-trimester loss associated with chorioamnionitis. She has a sufficient vaginal cervix to perform a cerclage.

Management: A plan is made to perform serial vaginal cervical scans every 2 weeks from 16 weeks of gestation and commence progesterone vaginally.

Rationale: There is little evidence that a routine history-indicated cerclage would benefit this woman, as she has only had one prior loss, even taking into account the large loop excision. Cervical surveillance is a reasonable option.

Cervical measurements were 32 mm at 16 weeks of gestation and 28 mm at 18 weeks of gestation. At 20 weeks, following a normal anomaly scan, the cervix is 24 mm.

Management: An ultrasound-indicated cerclage is performed using a braided suture the following day.

Rationale: A cerclage performed in women with additional risk factors (such as a prior mid-trimester loss) is known to reduce the risk of early birth in a cervix under 25 mm.

Following cerclage, the cervix is noted to be shorter at 11 mm at 24 weeks. She is admitted and subsequently delivers at 25 weeks following treatment with antenatal steroids and magnesium sulphate. The baby is admitted to the neonatal intensive care unit but is discharged without significant morbidity.

Management: She is seen postnatally, and a transabdominal cerclage is recommended prior to her next pregnancy.

Rationale: As a delivery has occurred before 28 weeks, an abdominal cerclage is known to significantly improve outcomes in future pregnancies and should be offered.

7.12 Cervical Cerclage Simulator

More recently, a simulator to perform vaginal cervical cerclage has been developed, given the surgical challenges of operating in a confined space. Simulators offer the opportunity to mimic real-life situations, which is particularly useful when inserting stitches and tying knots, particularly in a confined space [38]. Research on the simulator has demonstrated a wide variety of techniques performed even by experienced clinicians, including variable height, depth, and tension of the suture, and there is a need for consensus regarding the optimal technique [39]. However, it is generally agreed that a high suture is desirable without inserting the needle too deeply and with reasonable tension. A loose suture may allow prolapse of membranes through the canal if cervical changes occur. If sutures are too tight or too deep, there is a risk of migrating to the cervical os, and the suture would be ineffective. Of concern, during these in vitro simulator studies, 15% of sutures were actually placed through the cervical os, probably rendering them ineffective. As most cerclages make little difference to the outcome, these ineffective techniques could go unnoticed. There is a pressing need to evaluate and standardise techniques, both in clinical trials and in clinical practice.

7.13 Conclusion

Cerclage is a common practice in the world. Very few women have been evaluated in clinical trials in spite of this, and the evidence base is from randomised trials some decades ago. Our increasing knowledge of the complex nature of preterm birth and the lack of understanding of the mechanism mean that the role of cerclage requires further evaluation. Some subgroups (e.g. cervical caesarean damage) have much higher failure rates. The technique is variable and needs standardisation. The role of adjuvant therapies with cerclage, both perioperatively and with other prophylactic measures, is not clear. There are ongoing trials in twins, examination-indicated cerclage, and subgroups such as women with cervical caesarean damage, which will improve the evidence base. In the meantime, there is evidence that it has value and can reduce preterm delivery in women with a poor obstetric history. Ultrasound can be used to target the need. Some techniques in certain subgroups (e.g. abdominal cerclage) have strong evidence of efficacy and can reduce mortality.

Chapter Key Points

- Epidemiology and burden of preterm birth and rationale for cerclage
- Definition, indications, and contraindications of cervical cerclage
- Differences between history-, ultrasound-, and exam-indicated cerclage
- Role and evidence for cerclage in twins and other high-risk subgroups
- Comparison of transvaginal and transabdominal techniques and indications
- Interaction of cerclage with progesterone, pessary, and adjunct therapies
- Key procedural considerations, including anaesthesia, technique, and post-operative care

Chapter-End Summary

This chapter outlines the role of cervical cerclage as a preventive intervention for preterm birth, reviewing its indications, mechanisms, and limitations. It describes the major types of cerclages—history-indicated, ultrasound-indicated, and exam-indicated—and highlights the importance of aetiology, as efficacy differs depending on whether cervical weakness, surgical trauma, or other risk factors are present. Evidence for benefit is strongest in women with multiple prior losses or a very short cervix, while its role in twins remains uncertain. The chapter also reviews technical aspects of insertion, compares transvaginal and abdominal approaches, and discusses adjunct therapies, such as progesterone. Despite widespread use, cerclage remains under-researched, and ongoing trials will refine its role in diverse subgroups. Clinicians should individualise care, balancing risks and benefits while ensuring informed shared decision-making.

Bibliography

1. Shennan A, Story L. Cervical cerclage: green-top guideline no. 75. BJOG. 2022;129(7):1178–210.
2. World Health Organization. Born too soon: decade of action on preterm birth. Geneva: World Health Organization; 2023.
3. World Health Organization. https://www.who.int/news-room/fact-sheets/detail/preterm-birth. Preterm Birth.
4. Vos T, Lim SS, Abbafati C, Abbas KM, Abbasi M, Abbasifard M, et al. Global burden of 369 diseases and injuries in 204 countries and territories, 1990–2019: a systematic analysis for the Global Burden of Disease Study 2019. Lancet. 2020;396(10258):1204–22.
5. Saigal S, Doyle LW. An overview of mortality and sequelae of preterm birth from infancy to adulthood. Lancet. 2008;371(9608):261–9.
6. van der Krogt L, Shennan A. Cervical cesarean damage as a growing clinical problem: the association between in-labour cesarean section and recurrent preterm birth in subsequent pregnancies. PLoS Med. 2024;21(12):e1004497.
7. Banerjee A, Ivan M, Nazarenko T, Solda R, Bredaki EF, Casagrandi D, et al. Prediction of spontaneous preterm birth in women with previous full dilatation cesarean delivery. Am J Obstet Gynecol MFM. 2024;6(3):101298.
8. Hickland MM, Story L, Glazewska-Hallin A, Suff N, Cauldwell M, Watson HA, et al. Efficacy of transvaginal cervical cerclage in women at risk of preterm birth following previous emergency cesarean section. Acta Obstet Gynecol Scand. 2020;99(11):1486–91.
9. Rosen O'Sullivan H, Glazewska-Hallin A, Suff N, Seed P, Shennan A. The role of transabdominal cerclage in preventing recurrent preterm delivery in women with a history of term full dilatation cesarean section followed by a spontaneous preterm birth or late miscarriage and a subsequent pregnancy with cerclage: a retrospective cohort study. Am J Obstet Gynecol MFM. 2023;5(11):101144.
10. Ridout AE, Carter J, Seed PT, Chandiramani M, David AL, Tribe RM, et al. Longitudinal change in cervical length following vaginal or abdominal cervical cerclage: a randomized comparison. Am J Obstet Gynecol MFM. 2023;5(7):100987.
11. Cook JR, Chatfield S, Chandiramani M, Kindinger L, Cacciatore S, Sykes L, et al. Cerclage position, cervical length and preterm delivery in women undergoing ultrasound indicated cervical cerclage: a retrospective cohort study. PLoS One. 2017;12(6):e0178072.
12. Coutinho CM, Sotiriadis A, Odibo A, Khalil A, D'Antonio F, Feltovich H, et al. ISUOG Practice Guidelines: role of ultrasound in the prediction of spontaneous preterm birth. Ultrasound Obstet Gynecol. 2022;60(3):435–56.
13. Shennan A, Chandiramani M, Bennett P, David AL, Girling J, Ridout A, et al. MAVRIC: a multicenter randomized controlled trial of transabdominal vs transvaginal cervical cerclage. Am J Obstet Gynecol. 2020;222(3):261.e1–9.
14. McNaughton MC, Chalmers IG, Dubowitz V, Dunn PM, Grant AM, McPherson K, et al. Final report of the Medical Research Council/Royal College of Obstetricians and Gynaecologists Multicentre randomised trial of cervical cerclage. BJOG. 1993;100(6):516–23.
15. Owen J, Hankins G, Iams JD, Berghella V, Sheffield JS, Perez-Delboy A, et al. Multicenter randomized trial of cerclage for preterm birth prevention in high-risk women with shortened midtrimester cervical length. Am J Obstet Gynecol. 2009;201(4):375.e1–8.
16. Alfirevic Z, Stampalija T, Medley N. Cervical stitch (cerclage) for preventing preterm birth in singleton pregnancy. Cochrane Database Syst Rev. 2017;2017(6):CD008991.
17. Rafael TJ, Berghella V, Alfirevic Z. Cervical stitch (cerclage) for preventing preterm birth in multiple pregnancy. Cochrane Database Syst Rev. 2014;2014(9):CD009166.
18. Jarde A, Lutsiv O, Park C, Barrett J, Beyene J, Saito S, et al. Preterm birth prevention in twin pregnancies with progesterone, pessary, or cerclage: a systematic review and meta-analysis. BJOG. 2017;124(8):1163–73.
19. Roman A, Rochelson B, Fox NS, Hoffman M, Berghella V, Patel V, et al. Efficacy of ultrasound-indicated cerclage in twin pregnancies. Am J Obstet Gynecol. 2015;212(6):788.e1–6.
20. Shennan A, Suff N, Leigh Simpson J, Jacobsson B, Mol BW, Grobman WA. FIGO good practice recommendations on progestogens for prevention of preterm delivery. Int J Gynecol Obstet. 2021;155(1):16–8.
21. Grobman WA, Norman J, Jacobsson B. FIGO good practice recommendations on the use of pessary for reducing the frequency and improving outcomes of preterm birth. Int J Gynecol Obstet. 2021;155(1):23–5.
22. Norman JE, Norrie J, MacLennan G, Cooper D, Whyte S, Chowdhry S, et al. Evaluation of the

Arabin cervical pessary for prevention of preterm birth in women with a twin pregnancy and short cervix (STOPPIT-2): an open-label randomised trial and updated meta-analysis. PLoS Med. 2021;18(3):e1003506.
23. Hezelgrave NL, Suff N, Seed P, Robinson V, Carter J, Watson H, et al. Comparing cervical cerclage, pessary and vaginal progesterone for prevention of preterm birth in women with a short cervix (SuPPoRT): a multicentre randomised controlled trial. PLoS Med. 2024;21(7):e1004427.
24. Hodgetts Morton V, Moakes CA, Daniels J, Middleton L, Shennan A, Brocklehurst P, et al. Cerclage suture type to prevent pregnancy loss in women requiring a vaginal cervical cerclage: the C-STICH RCT. Health Technol Assess. 2024;28(40):1–44.
25. Kindinger LM, MacIntyre DA, Lee YS, Marchesi JR, Smith A, McDonald JAK, et al. Relationship between vaginal microbial dysbiosis, inflammation, and pregnancy outcomes in cervical cerclage. Sci Transl Med. 2016;8(350):350ra102.
26. Hulshoff CC, Bosgraaf RP, Spaanderman MEA, Inthout J, Scholten RR, Van Drongelen J. The efficacy of emergency cervical cerclage in singleton and twin pregnancies: a systematic review with meta-analysis. Am J Obstet Gynecol MFM. 2023;5(7):100971.
27. Ehsanipoor RM, Seligman NS, Saccone G, Szymanski LM, Wissinger C, Werner EF, et al. Physical examination–indicated cerclage. Obstet Gynecol. 2015;126(1):125–35.
28. Lee SE, Romero R, Park CW, Jun JK, Yoon BH. The frequency and significance of intraamniotic inflammation in patients with cervical insufficiency. Am J Obstet Gynecol. 2008;198(6):633.e1–8.
29. Suff N, Hall M, Shennan A, Chandiramani M. The use of quantitative fetal fibronectin for the prediction of preterm birth in women with exposed fetal membranes undergoing emergency cervical cerclage. Eur J Obstet Gynecol Reprod Biol. 2020;246:19–22.
30. Kenyon S, Taylor D, Tarnow-Mordi W. Broad-spectrum antibiotics for spontaneous preterm labour: the ORACLE II randomised trial. Lancet. 2001;357(9261):989–94.
31. Duhig K, Chandiramani M, Seed P, Briley A, Kenyon A, Shennan A. Fetal fibronectin as a predictor of spontaneous preterm labour in asymptomatic women with a cervical cerclage. BJOG. 2009;116(6):799–803.
32. Suff N, Kunitsyna M, Shennan A, Chandiramani M. Optimal timing of cervical cerclage removal following preterm premature rupture of membranes; a retrospective analysis. Eur J Obstet Gynecol Reprod Biol. 2021;259:75–80.
33. Vousden NJ, Carter J, Seed PT, Shennan AH. What is the impact of preconception abdominal cerclage on fertility: evidence from a randomized controlled trial. Acta Obstet Gynecol Scand. 2017;96(5):543–6.
34. Suff N, Carter J, Chandiramani M, Shennan A. Pregnancy outcomes following transabdominal cerclage after recurrent failed vaginal cerclage. Eur J Obstet Gynecol Reprod Biol. 2021;258:469–70.
35. Carter J, Deery J, Chandiramani M, Shennan A. "I had given up on being a mother": a survey of 183 women's experience of transabdominal cerclage (TAC). BMC Pregnancy Childbirth. 2023;23(1):751.
36. Suff N, Kuhrt K, Chandiramani M, Saridogan E, David A, Shennan AH. Development of a video to teach clinicians how to perform a transabdominal cerclage. Am J Obstet Gynecol MFM. 2020;2(4):100238.
37. Kuhrt K, Martin A, Mwaikasu LP, Shennan A. "A stitch in time saves nine": the impact of video-based training for surgical procedures in low-resource settings. Am J Obstet Gynecol MFM. 2023;5(6):100967.
38. Hall M, Suff N, Stirrat L, Coary C, Abernethy J, Debray R, et al. Cervical cerclage training: development and assessment of a simulator. Am J Obstet Gynecol MFM. 2023;5(3):100853.
39. Stirrat LI, Tydeman F, Suff N, Hall M, English WJ, Shennan AH, et al. Cervical cerclage technique: what do experts actually achieve? Am J Obstet Gynecol MFM. 2023;5(7):100961.

Effectiveness of Cervical Pessaries for Preventing Preterm Birth in Singleton and Twin Pregnancies: Current Evidence and Clinical Insights

Chen Ben David, Naphtali Justman, and Ido Solt

Contents

Y. Yogev, A. Khalil (eds.), *Prevention of Complications in Obstetrics*,
https://doi.org/10.1007/978-3-032-23479-7_8

Learning Objectives

- Explain the rationale for pessary use in preventing preterm birth.
- Summarize key evidence from RCTs evaluating pessary effectiveness.
- Compare pessary outcomes with progesterone and other interventions.
- Identify limitations and controversies in pessary research.
- Discuss future directions and potential subgroups for targeted pessary use.

8.1 Background

8

Preterm birth (PTB) remains one of the most significant challenges in obstetrics, accounting for a large proportion of neonatal morbidity and mortality globally. Cervical insufficiency, diagnosed as a short cervical length (CL) measured on ultrasound, is a well-established risk factor [1]. Over the past two decades, vaginal pessaries have emerged as a noninvasive intervention aimed at preventing PTB. However, despite widespread clinical interest, evidence supporting their effectiveness has evolved inconsistently [2].

The use of pessaries in medicine dates back thousands of years, primarily for the treatment of pelvic organ prolapse. Early examples of pessary use can be found in ancient Egypt, where materials such as linen, wool, or honey-soaked cotton were employed to create rudimentary devices. As medical knowledge evolved, so did the materials and designs of pessaries. Modern pessaries are now constructed from medical-grade silicone and come in various forms, such as the ring, cube, and dish pessaries, each tailored to address different types of pelvic organ prolapse and other gynecological conditions [3].

Pessaries are available in a variety of designs and materials, each tailored for specific indications. These devices are typically made from silicone, rubber, or plastic and are inserted into the vagina to offer support or address specific conditions [4].

While pessaries have been used in general gynecology for centuries, their application in obstetrics is relatively recent. Cervical pessaries were first systematically studied for their role in preventing preterm birth in the early twentieth century, but it was not until the development of the Arabin pessary in the 1980s that their use in obstetrics became more widespread. The Arabin pessary was specifically shaped to prevent premature dilation of the cervix in pregnant women at risk of preterm labor. Its design allows for the redistribution of uterine pressure, effectively reducing stress on the cervix and helping prevent preterm birth [5].

The early interest in pessaries as a preventive measure for PTB stems from their mechanical design. This device alters the orientation of the cervix, reducing the risk of premature cervical dilation by redistributing pressure from the growing uterus [6]. The initial theoretical basis for this intervention was supported by smaller observational studies suggesting that pessaries might prevent cervical shortening and thereby delay delivery. Some studies also suggest that pessaries might reduce inflammatory processes, which are often associated with preterm labor [7] (Fig. 8.1).

This chapter describes the evolving studies and current evidence on the use of cervical pessaries for the prevention of PTB in singleton and twin gestations.

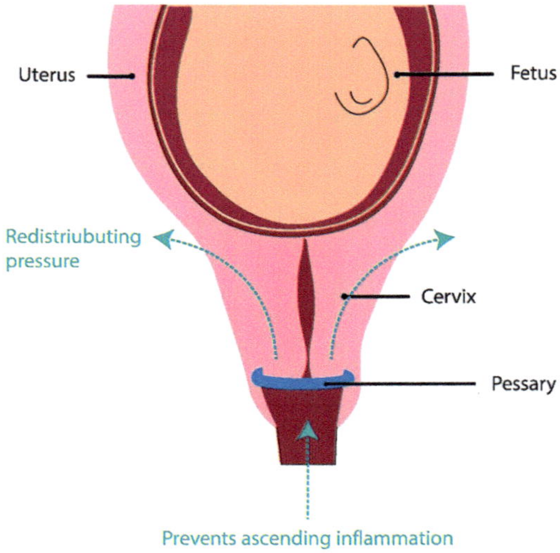

Fig. 8.1 Pessary positioning and its mechanism in preventing preterm birth

8.2 Early Evidence and Initial Studies

The early study by Arabin et al. [8] assessed the use of vaginal pessary to reduce the risk of spontaneous preterm birth (sPTB) in 258 singleton and 282 twin pregnancies in women with short cervical length (CL), defined as a CL < 10th percentile. The study found that for singleton pregnancies, the mean gestational age at delivery was significantly prolonged in the pessary group (38 weeks) compared to the control group (33 + 4 weeks). In twin pregnancies also, the pessary significantly extended the pregnancy, with an average gestational age at delivery of 35 + 6 weeks compared to 33 + 2 weeks in the control group.

An additional study further supported the efficacy of the pessary in prolonging pregnancy in patients with cervical incompetence [9]. These authors concluded that the Arabin cervical pessary is a safe and effective intervention for reducing the rate of preterm birth in high-risk women with cervical insufficiency.

Despite these encouraging findings, early studies, while promising, were limited by sample size and lacked long-term follow-up data. Nonetheless, the results laid the foundation for further research and clinical trials to evaluate the role of cervical pessary in preterm birth prevention more conclusively.

8.3 The Cervical Pessary in Pregnant Women with a Short Cervix (PECEP) Trial: A Breakthrough or a Limited Victory?

The PECEP trial, conducted by Goya et al. [5] in 2012, was one of the first large randomized controlled trials (RCTs) designed to evaluate the effectiveness of vaginal pessaries in preventing PTB in women with singleton pregnancies and a short cervix. The trial included 385 women and reported a significant reduction in PTB before 34 weeks, with rates dropping from 27% in the control group to 6% in the pessary group.

The PECEP trial marked a turning point in clinical interest regarding pessaries. It was one of the first studies to offer statistically significant evidence in favor of pessary use, and as a result, the pessary gained traction as a noninvasive alternative to treatments such as cervical cerclage or vaginal progesterone. However, the trial had limitations, including a relatively small sample size and its focus on a highly specific population (women with a cervical length ≤25 mm). Subsequent RCTs and meta-analyses attempted to validate these findings.

8.4 Expanding the Research: RCTs

Building on the momentum of the PECEP trial, Nicolaides et al. [10] conducted another large-scale multicenter RCT in 2016. This study focused on twin pregnancies with a short cervix (≤25 mm) and randomized women to pessary insertion or expectant management. The researchers found no significant differences between the pessary and control groups in the rates of PTB <34 weeks (13.6% vs. 12.9%; relative risk 1.054, 95% confidence interval (CI) 0.787-1.413; p=0.722). Also, rates of adverse perinatal outcomes did not differ between the intervention and control groups.

Following that, two additional RCTs published in 2017 evaluated the effectiveness of cervical pessary in reducing sPTB among asymptomatic women with a short cervical length in singleton [11] and twin gestations [12]. The former, which was performed in Italy, randomized patients to either receive a cervical pessary or undergo standard care. The primary outcome was sPTB <34 weeks of gestation. Results showed that the pessary group had a significantly lower rate of sPTB <34 weeks compared to the control group (7.3% vs. 15.3%; RR: 0.48; 95% CI: 0.24–0.95). Additionally, the pessary group had a longer gestational age at delivery, higher birth weight, and lower neonatal intensive care unit admissions and adverse perinatal outcomes [11]. The latter trial, in twin pregnancies, showed no significant difference in PTB rates before

34 weeks between the pessary group (39%) and the control group (35%) (RR: 1.13; 95% CI: 0.53–2.40). Secondary outcomes, including PTB before 37, 32, and 28 weeks, gestational age at delivery, birth weight, and neonatal outcomes, also showed no significant differences between the groups [12].

In an attempt to solve these inconsistent results, the randomized Trial of Pessary in Singleton Pregnancies With a Short Cervix (TOPS) RCT [13], published in 2023, evaluated whether cervical pessary placement could reduce the risk of PTB or fetal death in nonlaboring individuals with singleton pregnancies and a CL of ≤20 mm. The primary outcome, defined as PTB fetal death <37 weeks, occurred in 45.5% of the pessary group and 45.6% of the usual care group (RR: 1.00; 95% CI: 0.83–1.20), showing no significant difference between the groups. Despite that, the rate of fetal or neonatal/infant death was notably higher in the pessary group (13.3% vs. 6.8%; RR: 1.94; 95% CI: 1.13–3.32). The trial was terminated early due to concerns regarding the increased risk of fetal and neonatal death in the pessary group, as well as the lack of efficacy in reducing PTB.

These trials highlighted a recurring issue in the literature—while many studies suggested some benefit from pessary use, the magnitude of this benefit was often inconsistent, with the last RCT raising concerns regarding increased perinatal mortality.

8.5 Emerging Skepticism: Comparing Pessaries with Progesterone

As the use of pessaries expanded, researchers began to compare their efficacy with that of other interventions, particularly vaginal progesterone.

An RCT by Cruz-Melguizo et al. [14] randomized 246 women with singleton pregnancies and a short cervix to receive either a cervical pessary or vaginal progesterone. The study found no significant difference in sPTB rates <34 weeks of gestation between the pessary (14%) and progesterone (14%) groups. Increased vaginal discharge and discomfort were more common in the pessary group.

Additionally, in another RCT by van Dijk et al. [15], the researchers compared the effectiveness of cervical pessary with vaginal progesterone for the prevention of adverse perinatal outcomes in singletons with a short CL. A total of 612 were included in the final analysis. The authors detected no difference in the rates of adverse perinatal outcomes when comparing women with cervical pessary as compared to vaginal progesterone. Furthermore, in a subgroup of women with a CL ≤25 mm, the rates of PTB <28 weeks of gestation were higher in the cervical pessary group (16% vs. 4%; relative risk: 3.7; 95% CI: 1.1–12.9).

These studies cast doubt on whether pessaries provided any additional benefit over progesterone, a well-established therapy [16]. In fact, some clinicians began to question the role of pessaries, given that they offered no clear advantage over progesterone and were associated with patient discomfort and early withdrawal in some cases. Additionally, these trials failed to detect any significant difference in neonatal outcomes between the two groups, further undermining the case for pessaries.

8.6 Systematic Reviews and Meta-Analyses: A Mixed Picture

Over the past decade, several systematic reviews and meta-analyses have attempted to consolidate the available evidence on pessaries. In a systematic review and meta-analysis by Conde-Agudelo et al. [17], the efficacy of cervical pessaries in preventing PTB in asymptomatic women at high risk was evaluated. The results indicated that there were no significant differences in the risk of sPTB <34 weeks between women who received a cervical pessary and those who did not, across both singleton and twin gestations, even in women with a short CL. Moreover, no improvements in perinatal outcomes were observed.

A Cochrane review in 2022 [18] evaluated the role of cervical pessary for preventing PTB in women with singleton pregnancies and risk factors for cervical insufficiency. The eight studies that were included compared cervical pessary to no treatment, vaginal progesterone, or cervical cerclage. The review found that in women with singleton pregnancy, cervical pessary compared to no treatment may reduce the risk of delivery <34 weeks (risk ratio (RR): 0.72; 95% CI: 0.33–1.55) and <37 weeks (RR: 0.68; 95% CI: 0.44–1.05), although the certainty of this evidence was low due to inconsistency and imprecision. In comparison to vaginal progesterone, cervical pessary reduced the risk of delivery before 34 weeks (RR: 0.72; 95% CI: 0.52–1.02; moderate-certainty evidence) and before 37 weeks (RR: 0.89; 95% CI: 0.73–1.09; moderate-certainty evidence), although the evidence is uncertain [18].

Furthermore, in a meta-analysis by Saccone et al. [19], the effectiveness of cervical Arabin pessaries in preventing sPTB in singleton pregnancies with a short CL was assessed. A review of three randomized clinical trials, involving 1420 participants, found that the use of the Arabin pessary did not significantly reduce the incidence of sPTB at various gestational ages (<37, <34, <32, and <28 weeks) compared to expectant management. No improvements were noted in perinatal outcomes or delivery timing. However, the pessary was linked to an increased risk of vaginal discharge.

In a recently published meta-analysis by Norooznezhad et al. [20], the data from six RCTs was analyzed regarding the use of cervical pessaries for the prevention of PTB in twin gestations with asymptomatic, short CL. The authors noted that the cervical pessary did not significantly increase the gestational age at delivery or reduce the incidence of PTB before 28, 32, or 37 weeks. Additionally, no significant reductions in neonatal morbidity or composite adverse neonatal outcomes were observed.

These reviews further question the effectiveness of cervical pessaries both in singleton and twin gestations.

8.7 Long-Term Neonatal Outcomes

Long-term follow-up studies have provided additional insights into the safety of pessaries but have not strengthened the case for their routine use. The ProTWIN study [21] and its follow-up analysis [22] examined the neurodevelopmental outcomes of children born to mothers who used pessaries. At 3 years of age, no significant differences in neurodevelopment were observed between children whose mothers used a pessary and those who did not.

These findings suggest that while pessaries may not pose significant long-term risks, they also do not confer notable long-term benefits, at least in terms of neurodevelopment. This neutral outcome has contributed to the ongoing debate about whether the modest short-term benefits of pessary use justify its widespread adoption in clinical practice.

8.8 Long-Term Maternal Effect

In another follow-up study, conducted 4 years after the ProTWIN trial, van Limburg Stirum et al. [23] examined the effects of cervical pessary use on subsequent pregnancy outcomes and maternal quality of life. Of 408 participants, 68.4% had a live birth, with no significant difference between the pessary group (35 births) and the control group (32 births) (RR: 0.93; 95% CI: 0.8–1.07). Preterm birth (<37 weeks) occurred in three pessary group cases vs. one in the control group. No differences were found in maternal quality of life or in women with a short cervix, though the sample size was limited. The study concluded that pessary use had no long-term impact on pregnancy outcomes or maternal quality of life.

8.9 Prediction Model

The most recent studies, such as those by Merced et al. [24], have attempted to refine the understanding of which populations benefit most from pessary use. The authors developed a risk prediction model that included cervical length, maternal age, and smoking status as factors influencing pessary effectiveness. Their findings suggested that pessaries may be more effective in women with cervical lengths ≤25 mm, but even in these cases, the benefit was modest and heavily dependent on other risk factors.

Furthermore, this study noted that in some populations, pessary use was associated with a higher rate of PTB, particularly among women who smoked during pregnancy. These findings underscored the need for more personalized approaches to PTB prevention.

8

8.10 Conclusion

PTB remains a significant obstetric challenge, with evidence on the effectiveness of cervical pessaries for its prevention in both singleton and twin pregnancies remaining inconclusive. While early studies suggested potential benefits in specific subgroups, such as women with a short CL, more recent large-scale trials and meta-analyses have yielded mixed results. There has been no consistent evidence that pessary use significantly reduces PTB rates, particularly when compared to other interventions like vaginal progesterone.

Despite the inconsistent evidence regarding the effectiveness of cervical pessaries in preventing PTB, they remain a safe and noninvasive intervention. Thus, we believe that future research should focus on identifying specific subpopulations who may benefit from this intervention.

Chapter Key Points

- Preterm birth remains a major global cause of neonatal morbidity and mortality.
- Role and historical evolution of the cervical pessary as a noninvasive intervention.
- Evidence from RCTs shows inconsistent benefits of pessaries in singleton and twin pregnancies.
- Comparisons with progesterone show no clear advantage for pessaries and possible harms in subgroups.
- Findings from systematic reviews and meta-analyses do not support routine pessary use.
- Long-term neonatal and maternal outcomes show no significant benefit.
- Cervical pessary effectiveness may depend on specific high-risk subgroups.

Chapter-End Summary

This chapter reviews the development, rationale, and clinical evidence concerning the use of cervical pessaries for preventing preterm birth in singleton and twin pregnancies. Early observational studies and small trials suggested potential benefit, particularly in women with a short cervix. However, results from large randomized controlled trials and recent meta-analyses have been inconsistent, with some studies showing no benefit and others raising concerns about increased perinatal morbidity. Comparisons with vaginal progesterone—a well-established intervention—have not demonstrated clear superiority of pessaries. Long-term maternal and neonatal outcomes also suggest limited impact. While pessaries remain a safe, noninvasive option, current evidence does not support their routine use, highlighting the need for future research to identify specific subgroups that may benefit.

References

1. Goldenberg RL, Culhane JF, Iams JD, Romero R. Epidemiology and causes of preterm birth. Lancet. 2008;371(9606):75–84.
2. Piccioni MG, Del Negro V, Bruno Vecchio RC, Faralli I, Savastano G, Galoppi P, Perrone G. Is the Arabin Pessary really useful in preventing preterm birth? A review of literature. J Gynecol Obstet Hum Reprod. 2021;50(4):101824.
3. Oliver R, Thakar R, Sultan AH. The history and usage of the vaginal pessary: a review. Eur J Obstet Gynecol Reprod Biol. 2011;156(2):125–30.
4. Arabin B, Alfirevic Z. Cervical pessaries for prevention of spontaneous preterm birth: past, present and future. Ultrasound Obstet Gynecol. 2013;42(4):390–9.
5. Goya M, Pratcorona L, Merced C, Rodó C, Valle L, Romero A, et al. Cervical pessary in pregnant women with a short cervix (PECEP): an open-label randomised controlled trial. Lancet. 2012;379(9828):1800–6.
6. Grobman WA, Norman J, Jacobsson B, FIGO Working Group for Preterm Birth. FIGO good practice recommendations on the use of pessary for reducing the frequency and improving outcomes of preterm birth. Int J Gynaecol Obstet. 2021;155(1):23–5.
7. van Limburg Stirum EVJ, Zegveld SJ, Simons NE, de Boer MA, Pajkrt E, Mol BWJ, et al. Consequences of cervical pessary for subsequent pregnancy: follow-up of randomized clinical trial (ProTWIN). Ultrasound Obstet Gynecol. 2022;59(6):771–7.
8. Arabin B, Halbesma JR, Vork F, Hübener M, van Eyck J. Is treatment with vaginal pessaries an option in patients with a sonographically detected short cervix? J Perinat Med. 2003;31(2):122–33.
9. Sieroszewski P, Jasiński A, Perenc M, Banach R, Oszukowski P. The Arabin pessary for the treatment of threatened mid-trimester miscarriage or premature labour and miscarriage: a case series. J Matern Fetal Neonatal Med. 2009;22(6):469–72.
10. Nicolaides KH, Syngelaki A, Poon LC, De Paco Matallana C, Plasencia W, Molina FS, et al. Cervical pessary placement for prevention of preterm birth in unselected twin pregnancies: a randomized controlled trial. Am J Obstet Gynecol. 2016;214(1):3.e1–9.
11. Saccone G, Maruotti GM, Giudicepietro A, Martinelli P, Mazzarelli L, Visentin S, et al. Effect of cervical pessary on spontaneous preterm birth in women with singleton pregnancies and short cervical length a randomized clinical trial. JAMA. 2017;318(23):2317–24.
12. Berghella V, Dugoff L, Ludmir J. Prevention of preterm birth with pessary in twins (PoPPT): a randomized controlled trial. Ultrasound Obstet Gynecol. 2017;49(5):567–72.
13. Hoffman MK, Clifton RG, Biggio JR, Saade GR, Ugwu LG, Longo M, et al. Cervical pessary for prevention of preterm birth in individuals with a short cervix: the TOPS randomized clinical trial. JAMA. 2023;330(4):340–8.
14. Cruz-Melguizo S, San-Frutos L, Martínez-Payo C, Ruiz-Antorán B, Adiego-Burgos B, Campillos-Maza JM, et al. Cervical pessary compared with vaginal progesterone for preventing early preterm birth: a randomized controlled trial. Obstet Gynecol. 2018;132(4):907–15.
15. van Dijk CE, van Gils AL, van Zijl MD, Koullali B, van der Weide MC, van den Akker ES, et al. Cervical pessary versus vaginal progesterone in women with a singleton pregnancy, a short cervix, and no history of spontaneous preterm birth at less than 34 weeks' gestation: open label, multicentre, randomised, controlled trial. BMJ. 2024;384:e077033.
16. Berghella V, Gulersen M, Roman A, Boelig RC. Vaginal progesterone for the prevention of recurrent spontaneous preterm birth. Am J Obstet Gynecol MFM. 2023;5(10):101116.
17. Conde-Agudelo A, Romero R, Nicolaides KH. Cervical pessary to prevent preterm birth in asymptomatic high-risk women: a systematic review and meta-analysis. Am J Obstet Gynecol. 2020;223(1):42–65.e2.
18. Abdel-Aleem H, Shaaban OM, Abdel-Aleem MA, Aboelfadle Mohamed A. Cervical pessary for preventing preterm birth in singleton pregnancies. Cochrane Database Syst Rev. 2022;12(12):CD014508.
19. Saccone G, Ciardulli A, Xodo S, Dugoff L, Ludmir J, Pagani G, et al. Cervical pessary for preventing preterm birth in singleton pregnancies with short cervical length: a systematic review and meta-analysis. J Ultrasound Med. 2017;36(8):1535–43.
20. Norooznezhad AH, Zargarzadeh N, Javinani A, Nabavian SM, Qaderi S, Mostafaei S, Berghella V, et al. The effect of cervical pessary on increasing gestational age at delivery in twin pregnancies with asymptomatic short cervix: a systematic review and meta-analysis of randomized controlled trials. AJOG Glob Rep. 2024;4(2):100347.
21. Liem S, Schuit E, Hegeman M, Bais J, de Boer K, Bloemenkamp K, Brons J, et al. Cervical pessaries for prevention of preterm birth in women with a multiple pregnancy (ProTWIN): a multicentre, open-label randomised controlled trial. Lancet. 2013;382(9901):1341–9.

22. van 't Hooft J, van der Lee JH, Opmeer BC, van Wassenaer-Leemhuis AG, van Baar AL, et al. Pessary for prevention of preterm birth in twin pregnancy with short cervix: 3-year follow-up study. Ultrasound Obstet Gynecol. 2018;51(5):621–8.
23. van Limburg Stirum EVJ, van der Windt LI, van Dijk CE, van Baar AL, Leemhuis AG, van Wely M, et al. Pessary or progesterone to prevent preterm birth in women with short cervical length: protocol of the 4-6 year follow-up of a randomised controlled trial (Quadruple-P). BMJ Open. 2022;12(8):e064049.
24. Merced C, Pratcorona L, Higueras T, Vargas M, Del Barco E, Solà J, et al. Risk factors of early spontaneous preterm birth despite carrying a cervical pessary in singleton pregnancies with a short cervix: development of a risk prediction model. Eur J Obstet Gynecol Reprod Biol X. 2024;22:100305.

The Role of Progesterone in Singleton and Twin Pregnancies: Prevention of Preterm Birth

Rinat Gabbay-Benziv, Esther Maor-Sagie, and Amir Naeh

Contents

Y. Yogev, A. Khalil (eds.), *Prevention of Complications in Obstetrics*,
https://doi.org/10.1007/978-3-032-23479-7_9

Learning Objectives

- Explain biological mechanisms underpinning progesterone's role in preterm birth prevention.
- Summarize evidence for progesterone use in singleton and twin pregnancies.
- Distinguish between indications with proven benefit and those with uncertain efficacy.
- Compare progesterone to alternative interventions, including cerclage and pessary.
- Identify gaps in evidence and areas requiring further research.

9.1 Mechanism of Action

Progesterone plays a key role in extending pregnancy and preventing preterm labor through several mechanisms, though these are not fully elucidated. In the myometrium, it promotes smooth muscle relaxation, counteracts the stimulating effects of oxytocin, and inhibits the formation of gap junctions that facilitate coordinated uterine contractions, [1, 2] thus maintaining the uterine quiescence. Research on animals such as sheep and goats has shown that labor onset follows a decline in plasma progesterone levels and a rise in estrogen. [3] While this pattern does not occur in primates, including humans, localized changes in progesterone levels or in the progesterone-to-estrogen ratio in the placenta, decidua, or fetal membranes may play a role in labor initiation. [4] Supporting this, studies have found that administering progesterone antagonists at term can expedite labor onset, indicating a relationship between progesterone and maintaining uterine inactivity. [5]

The rationale for exogenous progesterone supplementation to prevent preterm birth stems from the various biological functions of endogenous progesterone. Progesterone from the corpus luteum during early pregnancy is critical for maintaining gestation until the placenta takes over at around 7–9 weeks. Disruption of corpus luteum activity or blocking of progesterone receptors before this transition readily induces abortion [6, 7], highlighting its importance in pregnancy maintenance. Progesterone also appears to suppress uterine contractility by sustaining a state of functional withdrawal at the uterine level, evident in both term and preterm labor. [8–15] Additionally, progesterone exerts immune-modulating effects that mitigate pro-inflammatory pathways involved in preterm labor, which underscores its role in preventing early delivery. [16–19] In vitro studies further demonstrate that progesterone can prevent apoptosis in fetal membrane tissues, potentially lowering the risk of preterm pre-labor rupture of membranes and subsequent preterm birth. [20–22] Last, progesterone slows down cervical remodeling, thus delaying cervical shortening, a known precursor to labor. [23–25]

Despite these mechanisms, the biological justification for exogenous progesterone supplementation is complex, especially as endogenous progesterone levels are already elevated in late pregnancy. These high levels are believed to saturate progesterone receptors, which do not decrease before labor nor respond significantly to additional supplementation. Furthermore, both term and preterm labor are linked to increased activity of progesterone-metabolizing enzymes and reduced progesterone receptor functionality, implying that local rises in progesterone may have limited effects. This understanding has fueled ongoing discussions regarding the precise mechanisms by which exogenous progesterone prevents spontaneous preterm birth.

9.2 Progesterone Preparations

Progesterone can be administered in the form of natural or micronized progesterone, either vaginally or orally. The intramuscular form, 17-hydroxyprogesterone caproate (17-OHPC), which has been withdrawn from the market, will be discussed in the following section.

The strongest evidence for efficacy lies with vaginally administered progesterone. This route is highly effective, likely due to its superior uterine bioavailability, as it reaches the uterus directly before undergoing first-pass metabolism in the liver. Vaginal progesterone has minimal systemic side effects; however, it may cause local irritation, and daily administration is required. Dosages typically range from 90 to 400 mg, starting as early as 16 weeks of gestation, and are available in gel, tablet, or capsule forms.

Oral progesterone—A micronized oral preparation of natural progesterone is also available. Despite its convenience, the evidence for oral progesterone is insufficient to inform clinical guidelines. The evaluating progestogens for preventing preterm birth international collaborative (EPPPIC) [26] individual patient data meta-analysis reported a 40 percent reduction in preterm birth before 34 weeks (relative risk (RR): 0.60, 95% confidence interval (CI): 0.41–0.90) with oral progesterone, but these findings were based on limited data from only two trials involving 181 patients. [26]

9.3 The Rise and Fall of 17-Alpha-Hydroxyprogesterone Caproate: From Promising Hope to FDA Withdrawal

The use of 17-OHPC in preterm birth prevention has had a complex history, starting with early support in the 2000s and culminating in its recent FDA withdrawal. Early studies in the 1950s explored synthetic progesterone for preventing preterm birth and found controversial results on efficacy. [27–29] The Meis trial in 2003 brought significant attention to 17-OHPC after demonstrating a 34% reduction in recurrent preterm birth among women with a history of preterm delivery. [30] Meis and coinvestigators randomly assigned 459 patients with a documented history of spontaneous singleton preterm birth <37 completed weeks to weekly intramuscular injections of 17-OHPC or placebo beginning at 16–20 weeks of gestation and continuing until 36 weeks. Based on these promising findings, the FDA granted accelerated approval to the drug in 2011 under the trade name Makena, subject to further confirmatory trials. The approval was temporary, and sponsors were mandated to conduct post-market follow-up studies to confirm the anticipated clinical benefit and safety, suggested by the surrogate end point.

However, subsequent evidence raised questions about its efficacy. The FDA-mandated randomized placebo-controlled multicenter international trial, the prevent recurrent preterm birth in singleton gestations (PROLONG) trial, a large international study published in 2020, failed to replicate the initial benefits, finding no significant difference in preterm birth rates or neonatal outcomes between the treatment and placebo groups. [31] The trial assessed the safety and efficacy of 17-OHPC in over 1700 patients with a singleton gestation and a history of preterm birth. It did not include US sites since the drug was already widely used and was considered a "standard of care." Although no safety concerns were identified, the trial found that the intervention did not significantly reduce preterm birth <35 weeks or fetal/early infant death. This discrepancy, coupled with the high-profile trial outcomes, led to widespread reevaluation of the drug's role in obstetric practice. The FDA, reviewing the body of evidence—including the PROLONG trial [31] and additional meta-analyses—ultimately determined that 17-OHPC did not provide a clinically meaningful benefit for preterm birth prevention. In April 2023, the FDA [32] withdrew its approval, citing a lack of efficacy rather than safety concerns, a decision endorsed by major organizations such as the American College of Obstetricians and Gynecologists (ACOG) and the Society for Maternal-Fetal Medicine (SMFM). [33] This withdrawal marks a critical moment in the treatment landscape for preterm birth, highlighting the need for rigorous, large-scale trials to substantiate therapies in high-risk pregnancies.

9.4 Progesterone's Role in Singleton Pregnancies

The recommendations for progesterone supplementation to reduce the risk of spontaneous preterm birth have evolved significantly in recent years, as discussed in this section. The effectiveness of progesterone in preventing preterm birth hinges on selecting the appropriate patient population, a topic that remains a subject of ongoing debate.

9.4.1 Patients with a Previous Preterm Delivery

The history of preterm birth is a powerful predictor of subsequent preterm deliveries. [34, 35] The recurrence risk is significantly influenced by both the number of prior preterm births and the gestational age at delivery in those cases. McManemy et al. demonstrated that the risk of preterm delivery was 5% in patients with two prior term deliveries; however, it increased markedly to 21% and 42% in patients with one and two previous preterm births, respectively. [36]

As previously discussed, 17-OHPC was initially proposed as an effective treatment for preventing preterm delivery; however, the FDA later withdrew its approval. [32]

Vaginal progesterone has long been studied for its effectiveness in patients with a history of prior preterm birth. The first landmark study to evaluate vaginal progesterone efficacy for the prevention of recurrent preterm birth was published by Fonseca in 2003. [37] This randomized, double-blind, placebo-controlled study of 142 high-risk singleton pregnancies found that daily prophylactic vaginal progesterone (100 mg) significantly reduced both uterine contraction frequency (23.6% vs. 54.3%, $p < 0.05$) and the rate of preterm birth (13.8% vs. 28.5%, $p < 0.05$). Additionally, fewer women in the progesterone group delivered before 34 weeks (2.7% vs. 18.5%, $p < 0.05$), demonstrating its efficacy in decreasing preterm birth rates. High-risk women included women with a history of preterm birth. [37]

Following this and with 17-OHPC as an alternative treatment, two meta-analyses evaluated vaginal progesterone vs. 17-OHPC for the prevention of preterm birth among high-risk women. The first meta-analysis was published in 2017 by Saccone et al. [38] and included three randomized trials comparing 17-OHPC with vaginal progesterone, demonstrating that vaginal progesterone was associated with a lower risk of preterm birth before 34 weeks of gestation. The rate of preterm birth was 17.5% among those receiving vaginal progesterone, compared to 25% in those treated with 17-OHPC. [38] However, the studies included different doses of vaginal progesterone, and the quality level of the summary estimates was low. The second systematic review and network meta-analysis was published in 2019 and assessed 40 studies comparing the relative effects of different types and routes of administration of progesterone, cerclage, and pessary at preventing preterm birth and concluded that vaginal progesterone was the only intervention with consistent effectiveness for preventing preterm birth in singleton at-risk pregnancies overall and in those with a previous preterm birth. [39]

In parallel to these studies, three randomized controlled double-blind studies evaluated the efficacy of vaginal progesterone vs. placebo for preventing recurrent preterm birth, including the OPTIMMUM study [40] and the progesterone to prevent neonatal respiratory distress syndrome (PROGRESS) study [41], as well as O'Brien's earlier trial. [42] All three studies failed to demonstrate any benefit of progesterone supplementation in reducing recurrent preterm birth. The OPTIMMUM study, [40] published in 2016, included women with previous preterm deliveries at or before 34 gestational weeks, and the PROGRESS study [41] included women with a previous preterm delivery at or before 37 gestational weeks. In the OPTIMMUM study, [40] 78–80% of the women enrolled had a previous preterm birth. The study failed to show not only the benefit of vaginal progesterone in terms of prolonging pregnancy but also improved composite neonatal adverse outcomes and showed that it had no significant long-term benefit or harm on outcomes in children at 2 years of age [40]. A fourth recent prospective, observational cohort study further supported the lack of benefit of vaginal progesterone for women with a history of preterm birth. [43]

The most recent systematic review and meta-analysis assessing ten randomized controlled trials (RCTs) comparing vaginal progesterone to placebo or no treatment in asymptomatic women with a singleton gestation and a history of spontaneous preterm birth [44] found that vaginal progesterone reduced the risk of preterm birth <37 weeks (32% vs. 37.8%, RR: 0.64, 95% CI: 0.50–0.81) and <34 weeks (13.5% vs. 17%, RR: 0.62, 95% CI: 0.42–0.92). Nevertheless, none of the reductions in preterm birth remained statistically significant after restriction to trials at low risk of bias and adjustment for small-study effects. The authors concluded that there was no convincing evidence to support the use of vaginal progesterone to prevent recurrent preterm birth in singleton gestations with a history of spontaneous preterm birth. [44]

Concluding all the evidence, in 2023, the ACOG published an updated clinical guidance recommending against the use of vaginal progesterone to prevent recurrent preterm birth in patients who do not have a short cervix. [45] The SMFM recommends a shared decision-making process regarding the use of vaginal progesterone for the prevention of recurrent preterm birth in patients who do not have a short cervix (Table 9.1). [33]

Table 9.1 Guidelines for administration of progeterone in different clinical settings

	ACOG, 2024	SMFM, 2024	NICE, 2022	SOGC, 2019	FIGO, 2021
Singleton pregnancy					
Previous PTD	Should not be offered	Discuss VP	Consider	Recommend VP	Should be offered
Mid-trimester cervical length ≤25 mm	Recommend VP	Consider VP if Cx 21–25 mm Administer VP if Cx ≤20 mm	Consider	Recommend VP	Should be offered
Previous PTD and mid-trimester cervical length ≤25 mm	Consider VP		Offer		
Timing			Start between 16 + 0 and 24 + 0 weeks. Continue until at least 34 weeks	Initiate between 16 and 24 weeks of gestation; continue to 34–36 weeks	
Preparation			Vaginal 200 mg capsules	Vaginal micronized progesterone, daily dose of 200 mg	Daily vaginal progesterone or weekly 17-OHPC treatment

(continued)

Table 9.1 (continued)

	ACOG, 2024	SMFM, 2024	NICE, 2022	SOGC, 2019	FIGO, 2021
Twin pregnancy					
Previous PTD	Insufficient data				
Mid-trimester cervical length ≤25 mm	Insufficient data		Offer VP	Recommend VP	
Previous PTD and mid- trimester cervical length ≤25 mm	Insufficient data				
Timing			Start between 16 + 0 and 20 + 0 weeks. Continue until at least 34 weeks	Initiate between 16 and 24 weeks of gestation; continue to 34–36 weeks	
Preparation			Vaginal 200 mg capsules	Vaginal micronized progesterone, daily dose of 400 mg	Daily vaginal progesterone or weekly 17-OHPC treatment

ACOG: American College of Obstetrics and Gynecology [45], SMFM: Society for Fetal Maternal Medicine [70], NICE: National Institute for Health and Care Excellence [71], SOGC: Society of Obstetricians and Gynaecologists of Canada [72], FIGO: International Federation of Gynecology and Obstetrics [73], *PTD* preterm delivery, *VP* vaginal progesterone

9.4.2 Mid-trimester Short Cervix

Assessment of cervical length in the second trimester has proven valuable in identifying women at an increased risk of preterm birth. [46] Moreover, there is an inverse correlation between cervical length and the risk of early delivery: The shorter the cervix, the higher the risk. [47]

In a landmark study in 2007, Fonseca et al. [48] randomized 250 asymptomatic women with a measured cervical length <15 mm to receive vaginal progesterone or placebo from 24 to 34 weeks of gestation. Vaginal progesterone treatment significantly reduced the risk of spontaneous preterm delivery before 34 weeks compared to the placebo group (19.2% vs. 34.4%, RR: 0.56, 95% CI: 0.36–0.86). [48] This pivotal study spurred further research, and in the following PREGNANT trial, [49] conducted in 2011, treatment with vaginal progesterone at 19–24 gestational weeks for women with a cervical length of 10–20 mm resulted in a significant reduction in the rate of preterm birth before 28, 33, and 35 weeks (RR: 0.50, 95% CI: 0.25–0.97; RR: 0.55, 95% CI: 0.33–0.92; and RR: 0.62, 95% CI: 0.42–0.92). Moreover, the study demonstrated a neonatal benefit with a significant reduction in respiratory distress syndrome. Only 16% of the study population had a history of previous preterm birth, and even after excluding these participants, progesterone continued to show a significant benefit in managing an isolated short cervix. [49] Existing data culminated in a 2018 meta-analysis of individual patient data. [50] The meta-analysis published by Romero et al. demonstrated that vaginal progesterone treatment in women with a cervical length of <25 mm significantly reduced the risk of preterm birth before 33 weeks of gestation. Additionally, it was associated with lower rates of preterm deliveries before 28, 30, 34, and 36 gestational weeks. Last, neonatal respiratory distress syndrome, neonatal intensive care unit admissions, composite neonatal adverse outcomes, and birth weight below 1500 and 2500 grams were also reduced. Unexpectedly, the authors did not find any difference in neonatal neurodevelopment scores at 2 years between the study and control groups. The authors concluded that vaginal progesterone reduces the risk of preterm birth and improves perinatal outcomes in singleton pregnancies with a mid-trimester sonographic short cervix, without any detectable adverse effects on childhood neurodevelopment. [50]

Based on the evidence, there is a well-established Level A recommendation to administer vaginal progesterone to asymptomatic individuals with a singleton pregnancy and a mid-trimester short cervix. [51]

9.4.3 Comparison with Other Treatments

The main alternative for vaginal progesterone in the context of preterm delivery prevention is cerclage—a cervical stitch.

In general, cervical cerclage is of uncertain effectiveness in patients with a short cervix and no history of preterm birth. A systematic review and meta-analysis of five randomized controlled trials using individual patient-level data showed that in women without prior spontaneous preterm birth and a cervical length <25 mm, placement of cerclage did not prevent preterm delivery or improve the neonatal outcome [52], thus making vaginal progesterone the treatment of choice. However, in a planned subgroup analysis of 126 patients with a cervical length of less than 10 mm, those who received cerclage had a lower risk of delivery before 35 weeks, suggesting that in this specific group, cerclage may be comparable to vaginal progesterone.

Special consideration is warranted for patients with a history of preterm delivery and a short cervix in the current pregnancy, as both are significant risk factors for early delivery, and their effects are additive. [53] A meta-analysis demonstrated that in patients with a previous spontaneous preterm birth and a cervical length of <25 mm before 24 weeks of gestation, cerclage reduced the rate of preterm birth before 35 weeks (28% vs. 41%, RR: 0.70, 95% CI: 0.55–0.89). [54]

While no adequately powered trials have directly compared cerclage to vaginal progesterone in patients with a prior spontaneous preterm birth and a short cervix, existing data suggest that both treatments yield similar benefits. An indirect comparison meta-analysis of five randomized trials of vaginal progesterone vs. placebo and five trials of cerclage vs. no cerclage in this population reported comparable outcomes. The relative risk of preterm birth before 35 weeks was 0.68 (95% CI: 0.50–0.93) with vaginal progesterone and 0.70 (95% CI: 0.55–0.89) with cerclage. Composite neonatal morbidity and mortality outcomes were also similar. Indirect comparison analysis found no significant difference between the two treatments. [55]

Consequently, the ACOG recommends that in cases of prior preterm delivery and a short cervix, both treatment options should be discussed with the patient. If the patient is already receiving progesterone supplementation, cerclage may be offered in addition to continuing progesterone therapy. [51]

9.4.4 Arrested Preterm Labor/Progesterone After 24 Gestational Weeks

Another clinical scenario in which the role of progesterone supplementation is controversial is arrested preterm labor or if an asymptomatic short cervix is identified after 24 gestational weeks.

Several RCTs have shown no clear benefit of progesterone treatment in this setting. [56, 57] A recent systematic review and meta-analysis of 13 RCTs found that progestogen maintenance therapy was associated with a modestly longer latency period, extending it by an average of 4.3 days compared to controls, and slightly higher neonatal birth weight. However, no significant differences were observed in other perinatal outcomes. The authors concluded that while progestogen maintenance therapy after arrested preterm labor may have a modest effect on prolonging latency, its overall impact on perinatal outcomes remains limited and that validation through further research is highly recommended. [58]

9.5 Progesterone's Role in Multifetal Pregnancies

The risk of preterm delivery is substantially higher in twin pregnancies compared to singleton pregnancies, with twin gestations having a sevenfold increased risk of delivery before 37 weeks (62.1% vs. 8.8%) and a ninefold increased risk of delivery before 34 weeks (20.3% vs. 2.2%). [59] This heightened risk of prematurity contributes to significant adverse outcomes in twin pregnancies, including increased rates of fetal and neonatal mortality, cerebral palsy, and long-term neurodevelopmental impairment. The impact of these complications extends beyond individual families, affecting both quality of life and healthcare resource utilization, underscoring the importance of preventive strategies in twin gestations. While twin pregnancy itself carries inherent risks of preterm birth, the presence of additional risk factors can substantially modify this baseline risk and influence therapeutic decisions. Understanding these additive risk factors and their interplay has become crucial in developing optimal preventive strategies in contemporary obstetric practice. In unselected twin pregnancies, there is no convincing evidence that vaginal progesterone reduces the rate of preterm deliveries or improves outcomes. [26, 60, 61] Moreover, a recent comprehensive meta-analysis encompassing 11 studies with 3401 women and 6802 fetuses/infants found no significant difference in the risk of preterm birth before 34 or 37 weeks between those receiving vaginal progesterone and those given a placebo or no treatment. [62]

9.5.1 Patients with a Previous Preterm Delivery

For twin pregnancies with a history of preterm delivery, the evidence regarding the role of vaginal progesterone in preventing recurrent preterm birth remains limited. Among the three randomized controlled trials evaluating progesterone vs. placebo for this indication, only the PROGRESS trial [41] included twin pregnancies. In this study, just 12 out of 787 participants had twin gestations. As previously noted, the trial did not demonstrate any benefit of vaginal progesterone in reducing the risk of preterm birth or improving neonatal outcomes in women with prior preterm deliveries. A meta-analysis conducted in 2021 by the EPPPIC group further assessed the use of vaginal progesterone for preterm birth prevention, including data from 61 twin pregnancies with prior preterm deliveries. This analysis also found no reduction in early preterm birth for women with multifetal pregnancies receiving vaginal progesterone (RR: 1.01, 95% CI: 0.84–1.20). [26]

For singleton pregnancies, current guidelines from ACOG [45] do not support the routine use of vaginal progesterone for preterm birth prevention, reflecting broader uncertainties about its efficacy. While these recommendations specifically address singletons, they highlight the ongoing lack of robust evidence to guide clinical decisions in twin pregnancies. Given this uncertainty, healthcare providers should carefully assess individual patient risk factors and engage in shared decision-making when discussing strategies to prevent preterm birth in twin pregnancies.

9.5.2 Mid-trimester Short Cervix

As in singleton pregnancies, mid-trimester cervical length is a strong predictor of preterm delivery risk. [63, 64] In 2012, the SMFM stated that there was no evidence supporting the use of progesterone to prevent preterm birth in multifetal pregnancies. However, this position was challenged in 2015 by Schuit et al., who conducted an individual patient data meta-analysis on the efficacy of progesterone in twin pregnancies. [65] Their analysis revealed that progesterone did not reduce adverse perinatal outcomes in an unselected twin population and may even increase certain risks. However, in a subgroup analysis of women with a cervical length ≤25 mm, progesterone use was associated with a 44% reduction in composite perinatal outcomes.

Building on this, Romero et al. conducted an individual patient data meta-analysis in 2017, providing further insights. [66] Their analysis included 303 women with twin pregnancies and a short mid-trimester cervical length (≤25 mm), showing that vaginal progesterone significantly reduced the risk of preterm birth before 33 weeks. Additionally, vaginal progesterone was associated with decreased risks of preterm birth at <35, <34, <32, and <30 weeks; neonatal death; respiratory distress syndrome; composite neonatal morbidity and mortality; mechanical ventilation; and low birth weight (<1500 g). Neurodevelopmental outcomes at 4–5 years were similar between the progesterone and placebo groups. A subsequent update of this meta-analysis in 2022, incorporating new data and excluding a study lacking ethical committee approval, confirmed these findings, demonstrating consistent reductions in preterm birth and neonatal complications across various gestational age thresholds in twin pregnancies with a mid-trimester short cervix. [67]

Additionally, in a 2023 meta-analysis by Conde-Agudelo et al., vaginal progesterone was evaluated for twin gestations with a cervical length <30 mm. [62] The analysis (six studies, 306 women, and 612 fetuses) showed significant reductions in preterm birth before 28–32 weeks (RR 0.48–0.65), neonatal death, and low birth weight <1500 g. For twin pregnancies with a cervical length ≤25 mm, the authors demonstrated that vaginal progesterone also reduced preterm birth at <28–34 weeks (RR: 0.41–0.68), composite neonatal morbidity and mortality, and low birth weight <1500 g, with moderate-quality evidence supporting these outcomes.

In conclusion, existing evidence indicates that vaginal progesterone might lower the risk of early preterm birth and neonatal complications in twin pregnancies with a mid-trimester short cervix. The recommended dosage and timing, as outlined by professional society guidelines, are summarized in ◘ Table 9.1. However, further robust, high-quality research is required to definitively determine progesterone's effectiveness in twin gestations, as well as the appropriate dosage. Upcoming studies, such as the pessary and progesterone for preterm prevention in twin (PROSPECT) trial, are anticipated to shed more light on the role of progesterone in twin pregnancies with a mid-trimester short cervix.

9.5.3 Comparison with Other Treatments

Data comparing progesterone to other interventions for the prevention of preterm birth in twin pregnancies remain limited and yield conflicting results.

In 2019, Dang et al. [68] conducted a randomized controlled trial involving 300 women with twin gestations and a cervical length shorter than 38 mm, comparing the efficacy of vaginal progesterone (400 mg daily) to the Arabin pessary. The primary outcome was delivery before 34 weeks, with subgroup analysis based on cervical length. The study found no overall difference in the primary outcome between the groups. However, in women with a cervical length <28 mm, the pessary significantly reduced the preterm birth rate at less than 34 weeks from 46% (16/35) to 21% (10/47) (RR: 0.47, 95% CI: 0.24–0.90) and significantly improved composite poor perinatal outcomes. [68]

A 2021 meta-analysis by D'Antonioi et al. [61] evaluated the role of vaginal progesterone, intramuscular 17-OHPC, cervical cerclage, and pessary in preventing preterm birth in twin pregnancies. Including 26 studies, the analysis revealed that in an unselected twin population, none of these interventions significantly reduced the risk of preterm birth before 34 weeks (all $p > 0.05$). Similarly, when focusing on spontaneous preterm birth, no intervention demonstrated a significant risk reduction. In twin pregnancies with a short cervical length (≤25 mm), there was no evidence that any of these interventions, including cerclage, pessary, or progesterone (vaginal or intramuscular), significantly reduced preterm birth before 34 weeks. [61]

An Israeli study further explored this issue by comparing vaginal progesterone alone to a combination of vaginal progesterone and an Arabin pessary in twin pregnancies with a cervical length <25 mm between 16 and 28 weeks of gestation. The study included 68 women in the treatment group and 78 in the control group. Despite shorter cervical length at intervention and later initiation of treatment in the study group, the rate of spontaneous preterm delivery <34 weeks was similar between the two groups (36.8% vs. 37.2%, $p > 0.05$). [69]

In conclusion, the current literature highlights the lack of strong evidence supporting the use of progesterone, cerclage, or pessary for the prevention of preterm birth in twin pregnancies, especially in those without a short cervix. The data underscore the need for continued research to identify effective preventive strategies for preterm birth in twin pregnancies.

9.5.4 Arrested Preterm Labor/ Progesterone After 24 Gestational Weeks

Women with arrested preterm labor represent a high-risk population for spontaneous preterm delivery, which remains the primary cause of neonatal mortality and morbidity. Despite this critical clinical challenge, no maintenance therapy has been definitively established as effective for pregnancy prolongation. Literature addressing this issue is limited, with particularly scant research on twin gestations. In a recent multicenter Israeli study, [56] the authors examined 200 mg of vaginal progesterone administered twice daily after arrested preterm labor at 24–34 weeks in singleton and twin pregnancies. Comparing 12 women with twin pregnancies to 15 without treatment, the findings revealed that while 400 mg of vaginal progesterone was ineffective in prolonging pregnancy for singleton pregnancies, it demonstrated potentially beneficial effects in twin pregnancies, suggesting the need for further investigative research.

9.6 Conclusion

Progesterone therapy has been extensively studied in the context of preventing preterm birth, with varying outcomes depending on the clinical scenario and method of administration:

1. **17-Alpha-Hydroxyprogesterone Caproate (17-OHPC):** Current evidence does not support its effectiveness in preventing preterm birth.
2. **Vaginal Progesterone in Singleton Pregnancies:**
   I. Short Cervix (<25 mm in the Mid-trimester): Studies demonstrate a clear benefit in reducing the risk of preterm birth, supporting its use in this population.
   II. History of Preterm Birth with Normal Mid-trimester Cervix: There is no consistent evidence of benefit in this group. In these cases, shared decision-making with the patient is recommended.
3. **Vaginal Progesterone in Twin Pregnancies:**
   I. Although fewer studies are available, the data suggest a benefit for twin pregnancies with a short cervix (<25 mm in the mid-trimester), supporting its use in this population.
   II. For women with a history of preterm birth and a normal mid-trimester cervix, the evidence does not clearly show

a benefit, and shared decision-making with the patient is advised.

4. **Timing and Dosage Considerations:** The optimal timing and dosage of vaginal progesterone remain unclear, with significant variation across studies.

Conclusion: Vaginal progesterone shows promise in reducing preterm birth in singleton pregnancies and possibly in twin pregnancies with a short cervix. However, its role in cases with a normal mid-trimester cervix, regardless of the history of preterm birth, is less clear. Further research is needed to establish definitive guidelines, particularly for twin pregnancies.

Chapter Key Points

- Progesterone mechanisms, including uterine quiescence and anti-inflammatory and cervical stabilization effects.
- Evidence for vaginal progesterone efficacy in singleton pregnancies with mid-trimester short cervix.
- Limited or absent benefit for progesterone in recurrent preterm birth without a short cervix.
- Evolving evidence and mixed results regarding progesterone use in twin pregnancies.
- Comparison with other interventions, such as cerclage and pessary.
- Uncertain role of progesterone after 24 weeks or in arrested preterm labor.

Chapter-End Summary

This chapter outlines progesterone's role in preventing spontaneous preterm birth across different clinical contexts. Strong evidence supports vaginal progesterone in singleton pregnancies with a mid-trimester short cervix, demonstrating reductions in preterm birth and improved neonatal outcomes. In contrast, progesterone has not shown consistent benefit for women with prior preterm birth who have a normal cervical length, leading to updated guidelines advising against routine use. Evidence in twin pregnancies is mixed: While unselected twins do not appear to benefit, those with a short cervix may experience reduced risk of early preterm birth and neonatal complications. Progesterone shows limited effectiveness after 24 weeks or following arrested preterm labor. Comparison with cerclage suggests a similar benefit in certain high-risk groups, though optimal selection criteria, timing, and dosing require further investigation.

References

1. Siiteri PK, Serón-Ferré M. Some new thoughts on the feto-placental unit and parturition in primates. In: Novy MJ, Res¬ko JA, editors. Fetal endocrinology. New York: Academic; 1981. p. 1–34.
2. Garfield RE, Kannan MS, Daniel EE. Gap junction formation in myometrium: control by estrogens, progesterone, and prostaglandins. Am J Phys. 1980;238(3):C81–9. https://doi.org/10.1152/ajpcell.1980.238.3.C81.
3. Challis JR. Sharp increase in free circulating oestrogens immediately before parturition in sheep. Nature. 1971;229(5281):208. https://doi.org/10.1038/229208a0.
4. Mitchell B, Cruickshank B, McLean D, Challis J. Local modulation of progesterone production in human fetal membranes. J Clin Endocrinol Metab. 1982;55(6):1237–9. https://doi.org/10.1210/jcem-55-6-1237.
5. Frydman R, Lelaidier C, Baton-Saint-Mleux C, Fernandez H, Vial M, Bourget P. Labor induction in women at term with mifepristone (RU 486): a double-blind, randomized, placebo-controlled study. Obstet Gynecol. 1992;80(6):972–5.
6. Csapo AI, Pulkkinen M. Indispensability of the human corpus luteum in the maintenance of early pregnancy. Luteectomy evidence. Obstetrical & gynecological survey. 1978;33(2):69–81. https://doi.org/10.1097/00006254-197802000-00001.
7. Peyron R, Aubény E, Targosz V, Silvestre L, Renault M, Elkik F, Leclerc P, Ulmann A, Baulieu EE. Early termination of pregnancy with mifepristone (RU 486) and the orally active prostaglandin misoprostol. N Engl J Med. 1993;328(21):1509–13. https://doi.org/10.1056/NEJM199305273282101.

8. Norwitz ER, Robinson JN, Challis JR. The control of labor. N Engl J Med. 1999;341(9):660–6. https://doi.org/10.1056/NEJM199908263410906.
9. Challis JRG, Matthews SG, Gibb W, Lye SJ. Endocrine and paracrine regulation of birth at term and preterm. Endocr Rev. 2000;21(5):514–50. https://doi.org/10.1210/edrv.21.5.0407.
10. Norwitz ER, Lye SJ. Biology of parturition. In: Creasy RK, Resnick R, Iams JD, et al., editors. Creasy & Resnick's maternal-fetal medicine. 6th ed. Philadelphia: Elsevier; 2009. p. 69.
11. Condon JC, Jeyasuria P, Faust JM, Wilson JW, Mendelson CR. A decline in the levels of progesterone receptor coactivators in the pregnant uterus at term may antagonize progesterone receptor function and contribute to the initiation of parturition. Proc Natl Acad Sci USA. 2003;100(16):9518–23. https://doi.org/10.1073/pnas.1633616100.
12. Oh SY, Kim CJ, Park I, Romero R, Sohn YK, Moon KC, Yoon BH. Progesterone receptor isoform (A/B) ratio of human fetal membranes increases during term parturition. Am J Obstet Gynecol. 2005;193(3 Pt 2):1156–60. https://doi.org/10.1016/j.ajog.2005.05.071.
13. Renthal NE, Chen CC, Williams KC, Gerard RD, Prange-Kiel J, Mendelson CR. miR-200 family and targets, ZEB1 and ZEB2, modulate uterine quiescence and contractility during pregnancy and labor. Proc Natl Acad Sci USA. 2010;107(48):20828–33. https://doi.org/10.1073/pnas.1008301107.
14. Mesiano S, Wang Y, Norwitz ER. Progesterone receptors in the human pregnancy uterus: do they hold the key to birth timing? Reprod Sci. 2011;18(1):6–19. https://doi.org/10.1177/1933719110382922.
15. Lockwood CJ, Stocco C, Murk W, Kayisli UA, Funai EF, Schatz F. Human labor is associated with reduced decidual cell expression of progesterone, but not glucocorticoid, receptors. J Clin Endocrinol Metab. 2010;95(5):2271–5. https://doi.org/10.1210/jc.2009-2136.
16. Shah NM, Lai PF, Imami N, Johnson MR. Progesterone-related immune modulation of pregnancy and labor. Front Endocrinol. 2019;10:198. https://doi.org/10.3389/fendo.2019.00198.
17. Berghella V, Gulersen M, Roman A, Boelig RC. Vaginal progesterone for the prevention of recurrent spontaneous preterm birth. Am J Obstet Gynecol MFM. 2023;5(10):101116. https://doi.org/10.1016/j.ajogmf.2023.101116.
18. Garry DJ, Baker DA, Persad MD, Peresleni T, Kocis C, Demishev M. Progesterone effects on vaginal cytokines in women with a history of preterm birth. PLoS One. 2018;13(12):e0209346. https://doi.org/10.1371/journal.pone.0209346.
19. Hung TH, Chen SF, Wu CP, Li MJ, Yeh YL, Hsieh TT. Micronized progesterone pretreatment affects the inflammatory response of human gestational tissues and the cervix to lipopolysaccharide stimulation. Placenta. 2017;57:1–8. https://doi.org/10.1016/j.placenta.2017.05.013.
20. Luo G, Abrahams VM, Tadesse S, Funai EF, Hodgson EJ, Gao J, Norwitz ER. Progesterone inhibits basal and TNF-alpha-induced apoptosis in fetal membranes: a novel mechanism to explain progesterone-mediated prevention of preterm birth. Reprod Sci. 2010;17(6):532–9. https://doi.org/10.1177/1933719110363618.
21. Kumar D, Springel E, Moore RM, Mercer BM, Philipson E, Mansour JM, Mesiano S, Schatz F, Lockwood CJ, Moore JJ. Progesterone inhibits in vitro fetal membrane weakening. Am J Obstet Gynecol. 2015;213(4):520.e1–520.e5209. https://doi.org/10.1016/j.ajog.2015.06.014.
22. Wang Y, Abrahams VM, Luo G, Norwitz NG, Snegovskikh VV, Ng SW, Norwitz ER. Progesterone inhibits apoptosis in fetal membranes by altering expression of both pro- and antiapoptotic proteins. Reprod Sci. 2018;25(8):1161–7. https://doi.org/10.1177/1933719118759440.
23. O'Brien JM, Defranco EA, Adair CD, Lewis DF, Hall DR, How H, Bsharat M, Creasy GW, Progesterone Vaginal Gel Study Group. Effect of progesterone on cervical shortening in women at risk for preterm birth: secondary analysis from a multinational, randomized, double-blind, placebo-controlled trial. Ultrasound Obstet Gynecol. 2009;34(6):653–9. https://doi.org/10.1002/uog.7338.
24. House M, Kelly J, Klebanov N, Yoshida K, Myers K, Kaplan DL. Mechanical and biochemical effects of progesterone on engineered cervical tissue. Tissue Eng Part A. 2018;24(23–24):1765–74. https://doi.org/10.1089/ten.TEA.2018.0036.
25. Nallasamy S, Yoshida K, Akins M, Myers K, Iozzo R, Mahendroo M. Steroid hormones are key modulators of tissue mechanical function via regulation of collagen and elastic fibers. Endocrinology. 2017;158(4):950–62. https://doi.org/10.1210/en.2016-1930.
26. EPPPIC Group. Evaluating Progestogens for Preventing Preterm birth International Collaborative (EPPPIC): meta-analysis of individual participant data from randomised controlled trials. Lancet (London, England). 2021;397(10280):1183–94. https://doi.org/10.1016/S0140-6736(21)00217-8.
27. Papiernik E. Double blind study of an agent to prevent pre-term delivery among women at increased risk. Schering ed Serie. 1970;4:65–8.
28. Yemini M, Borenstein R, Dreazen E, Apelman Z, Mogilner BM, Kessler I, Lancet M. Prevention of premature labor by 17 alpha-hydroxyprogesterone caproate. Am J Obstet Gynecol. 1985;151(5):574–7. https://doi.org/10.1016/0002-9378(85)90141-3.
29. Johnson JW, Austin KL, Jones GS, Davis GH, King TM. Efficacy of 17alpha-hydroxyprogesterone caproate in the prevention

of premature labor. N Engl J Med. 1975;293(14):675–80. https://doi.org/10.1056/NEJM197510022931401.
30. Meis PJ, Klebanoff M, Thom E, Dombrowski MP, Sibai B, Moawad AH, Spong CY, Hauth JC, Miodovnik M, Varner MW, Leveno KJ, Caritis SN, Iams JD, Wapner RJ, Conway D, O'Sullivan MJ, Carpenter M, Mercer B, Ramin SM, Thorp JM, et al. Prevention of recurrent preterm delivery by 17 alpha-hydroxyprogesterone caproate. N Engl J Med. 2003;348(24):2379–85. https://doi.org/10.1056/NEJMoa035140.
31. Blackwell SC, Gyamfi-Bannerman C, Biggio JR Jr, Chauhan SP, Hughes BL, Louis JM, Manuck TA, Miller HS, Das AF, Saade GR, Nielsen P, Baker J, Yuzko OM, Reznichenko GI, Reznichenko NY, Pekarev O, Tatarova N, Gudeman J, Birch R, Jozwiakowski MJ, et al. 17-OHPC to Prevent Recurrent Preterm Birth in Singleton Gestations (PROLONG study): a multicenter, international, randomized double-blind Trial. Am J Perinatol. 2020;37(2):127–36. https://doi.org/10.1055/s-0039-3400227.
32. Final Decision on Withdrawal of MAKENA (Hydroxyprogesterone Caproate) and Eight Abbreviated New Drug Applications Following Public Hearing; Availability of Final Decision. Federal Register: The Daily Journal of the United States Government [Internet]. 2023 May 15 [cited 2024 Jun 12]. Available from: https://www.federalregister.gov/d/2023-10264
33. Society for Maternal-Fetal Medicine (SMFM). Electronic address: pubs@smfm.org, & SMFM Publications Committee. Society for maternal-fetal medicine statement: response to the food and drug administration's withdrawal of 17-alpha hydroxyprogesterone caproate. Am J Obstet Gynecol. 2023;229(1):B2–6. https://doi.org/10.1016/j.ajog.2023.04.012.
34. Spong CY. Prediction and prevention of recurrent spontaneous preterm birth. Obstet Gynecol. 2007;110(2 Pt 1):405–15. https://doi.org/10.1097/01.AOG.0000275287.08520.4a.
35. Yang J, Baer RJ, Berghella V, Chambers C, Chung P, Coker T, Currier RJ, Druzin ML, Kuppermann M, Muglia LJ, Norton ME, Rand L, Ryckman K, Shaw GM, Stevenson D, Jelliffe-Pawlowski LL. Recurrence of preterm birth and early term birth. Obstet Gynecol. 2016;128(2):364–72. https://doi.org/10.1097/AOG.0000000000001506.
36. McManemy J, Cooke E, Amon E, Leet T. Recurrence risk for preterm delivery. Am J Obstet Gynecol. 2007;196(6):576.e1-6. https://doi.org/10.1016/j.ajog.2007.01.039.
37. da Fonseca EB, Bittar RE, Carvalho MH, Zugaib M. Prophylactic administration of progesterone by vaginal suppository to reduce the incidence of spontaneous preterm birth in women at increased risk: a randomized placebo-controlled double-blind study. Am J Obstet Gynecol. 2003;188(2):419–24. https://doi.org/10.1067/mob.2003.41.
38. Saccone G, Khalifeh A, Elimian A, Bahrami E, Chaman-Ara K, Bahrami MA, Berghella V. Vaginal progesterone vs intramuscular 17α-hydroxyprogesterone caproate for prevention of recurrent spontaneous preterm birth in singleton gestations: systematic review and meta-analysis of randomized controlled trials. Ultrasound Obstet Gynecol. 2017;49(3):315–21. https://doi.org/10.1002/uog.17245.
39. Jarde A, Lutsiv O, Beyene J, McDonald SD. Vaginal progesterone, oral progesterone, 17-OHPC, cerclage, and pessary for preventing preterm birth in at-risk singleton pregnancies: an updated systematic review and network meta-analysis. BJOG. 2019;126(5):556–67. https://doi.org/10.1111/1471-0528.15566.
40. Norman JE, Marlow N, Messow CM, Shennan A, Bennett PR, Thornton S, Robson SC, McConnachie A, Petrou S, Sebire NJ, Lavender T, Whyte S, Norrie J, OPPTIMUM study group. Vaginal progesterone prophylaxis for preterm birth (the OPPTIMUM study): a multicentre, randomised, double-blind trial. Lancet (London, England). 2016;387(10033):2106–16. https://doi.org/10.1016/S0140-6736(16)00350-0.
41. Crowther CA, Ashwood P, McPhee AJ, Flenady V, Tran T, Dodd JM, Robinson JS, PROGRESS Study Group. Vaginal progesterone pessaries for pregnant women with a previous preterm birth to prevent neonatal respiratory distress syndrome (the PROGRESS study): a multicentre, randomised, placebo-controlled trial. PLoS Med. 2017;14(9):e1002390. https://doi.org/10.1371/journal.pmed.1002390.
42. O'Brien JM, Adair CD, Lewis DF, Hall DR, Defranco EA, Fusey S, Soma-Pillay P, Porter K, How H, Schackis R, Eller D, Trivedi Y, Vanburen G, Khandelwal M, Trofatter K, Vidyadhari D, Vijayaraghavan J, Weeks J, Dattel B, Newton E, et al. Progesterone vaginal gel for the reduction of recurrent preterm birth: primary results from a randomized, double-blind, placebo-controlled trial. Ultrasound Obstet Gynecol. 2007;30(5):687–96. https://doi.org/10.1002/uog.5158.
43. Nelson DB, Lafferty A, Venkatraman C, McDonald JG, Eckert KM, McIntire DD, Spong CY. Association of vaginal progesterone treatment with prevention of recurrent preterm birth. JAMA Netw Open. 2022;5(10):e2237600. https://doi.org/10.1001/jamanetworkopen.2022.37600.
44. Conde-Agudelo A, Romero R. Does vaginal progesterone prevent recurrent preterm birth in women with a singleton gestation and a history of spontaneous preterm birth? Evidence from a systematic review and meta-analysis. Am J Obstet Gynecol. 2022;227(3):440–461.e2. https://doi.org/10.1016/j.ajog.2022.04.023.

45. Updated Clinical Guidance for the Use of Progesterone Supplementation for the Prevention of Recurrent Preterm Birth [Internet]. [cited 2024 Nov 16]. Available from: https://www.acog.org/clinical/clinical-guidance/practice-advisory/articles/2023/04/updated-guidance-use-of-progesterone-supplementation-for-prevention-of-recurrent-preterm-birth
46. Crane JM, Hutchens D. Transvaginal sonographic measurement of cervical length to predict preterm birth in asymptomatic women at increased risk: a systematic review. Ultrasound Obstet Gynecol. 2008;31(5):579–87. https://doi.org/10.1002/uog.5323.
47. Iams JD, Goldenberg RL, Meis PJ, Mercer BM, Moawad A, Das A, Thom E, McNellis D, Copper RL, Johnson F, Roberts JM. The length of the cervix and the risk of spontaneous premature delivery. National Institute of Child Health and Human Development maternal fetal medicine unit network. N Engl J Med. 1996;334(9):567–72. https://doi.org/10.1056/NEJM199602293340904.
48. Fonseca EB, Celik E, Parra M, Singh M, Nicolaides KH, Fetal Medicine Foundation Second Trimester Screening Group. Progesterone and the risk of preterm birth among women with a short cervix. N Engl J Med. 2007;357(5):462–9. https://doi.org/10.1056/NEJMoa067815.
49. Hassan SS, Romero R, Vidyadhari D, Fusey S, Baxter JK, Khandelwal M, Vijayaraghavan J, Trivedi Y, Soma-Pillay P, Sambarey P, Dayal A, Potapov V, O'Brien J, Astakhov V, Yuzko O, Kinzler W, Dattel B, Sehdev H, Mazheika L, Manchulenko D, et al. Vaginal progesterone reduces the rate of preterm birth in women with a sonographic short cervix: a multicenter, randomized, double-blind, placebo-controlled trial. Ultrasound Obstet Gynecol. 2011;38(1):18–31. https://doi.org/10.1002/uog.9017.
50. Romero R, Conde-Agudelo A, Da Fonseca E, O'Brien JM, Cetingoz E, Creasy GW, Hassan SS, Nicolaides KH. Vaginal progesterone for preventing preterm birth and adverse perinatal outcomes in singleton gestations with a short cervix: a meta-analysis of individual patient data. Am J Obstet Gynecol. 2018;218(2):161–80. https://doi.org/10.1016/j.ajog.2017.11.576.
51. Prediction and Prevention of Spontaneous Preterm Birth. ACOG practice bulletin, number 234. Obstet Gynecol. 2021;138(2):e65–90. https://doi.org/10.1097/AOG.0000000000004479.
52. Berghella V, Ciardulli A, Rust OA, To M, Otsuki K, Althuisius S, Nicolaides KH, Roman A, Saccone G. Cerclage for sonographic short cervix in singleton gestations without prior spontaneous preterm birth: systematic review and meta-analysis of randomized controlled trials using individual patient-level data. Ultrasound Obstet Gynecol. 2017;50(5):569–77. https://doi.org/10.1002/uog.17457.
53. To MS, Skentou CA, Royston P, Yu CK, Nicolaides KH. Prediction of patient-specific risk of early preterm delivery using maternal history and sonographic measurement of cervical length: a population-based prospective study. Ultrasound Obstet Gynecol. 2006;27(4):362–7. https://doi.org/10.1002/uog.2773.
54. Berghella V, Rafael TJ, Szychowski JM, Rust OA, Owen J. Cerclage for short cervix on ultrasonography in women with singleton gestations and previous preterm birth: a meta-analysis. Obstet Gynecol. 2011;117(3):663–71.
55. Conde-Agudelo A, Romero R, Da Fonseca E, O'Brien JM, Cetingoz E, Creasy GW, Hassan SS, Erez O, Pacora P, Nicolaides KH. Vaginal progesterone is as effective as cervical cerclage to prevent preterm birth in women with a singleton gestation, previous spontaneous preterm birth, and a short cervix: updated indirect comparison meta-analysis. Am J Obstet Gynecol. 2018;219(1):10–25. https://doi.org/10.1016/j.ajog.2018.03.028.
56. Nachum Z, Ganor Paz Y, Massalha M, Wated M, Harel N, Yefet E. Vaginal progesterone for pregnancy prolongation after arrested preterm labor: a randomized clinical Trial. JAMA Netw Open. 2024;7(7):e2419894. https://doi.org/10.1001/jamanetworkopen.2024.19894.
57. Martinez de Tejada B, Karolinski A, Ocampo MC, Laterra C, Hösli I, Fernández D, Surbek D, Huespe M, Drack G, Bunader A, Rouillier S, López de Degani G, Seidenstein E, Prentl E, Antón J, Krähenmann F, Nowacki D, Poncelas M, Nassif JC, Papera R, et al. Prevention of preterm delivery with vaginal progesterone in women with preterm labour (4P): randomised double-blind placebo-controlled trial. BJOG. 2015;122(1):80–91. https://doi.org/10.1111/1471-0528.13061.
58. Breuking SH, De Ruigh AA, Hermans FJR, Schuit E, Combs CA, de Tejada BM, Oudijk MA, Mol BW, Pajkrt E. Progestogen maintenance therapy for prolongation of pregnancy after an episode of preterm labour: a systematic review and meta-analysis. BJOG. 2023;130(11):1306–16. https://doi.org/10.1111/1471-0528.17499.
59. Osterman MJK, Hamilton BE, Martin JA, Driscoll AK, Valenzuela CP. Births: final data for 2021. Natl Vital Stat Rep. 2023;72(1):1–53.
60. Dodd JM, Grivell RM, OBrien CM, Dowswell T, Deussen AR. Prenatal administration of progestogens for preventing spontaneous preterm birth in women with a multiple pregnancy. Cochrane Database Syst Rev. 2019;2019(11):CD012024. https://doi.org/10.1002/14651858.CD012024.pub3.
61. D'Antonio F, Berghella V, Di Mascio D, Saccone G, Sileo F, Flacco ME, Odibo AO, Liberati M, Manzoli L, Khalil A. Role of progesterone, cerclage and pessary in preventing preterm birth in twin pregnancies: a systematic review and network meta-analysis. Eur J Obstet Gynecol Reprod Biol. 2021;261:166–77. https://doi.org/10.1016/j.ejogrb.2021.04.023.

62. Conde-Agudelo A, Romero R, Rehal A, Brizot ML, Serra V, Da Fonseca E, Cetingoz E, Syngelaki A, Perales A, Hassan SS, Nicolaides KH. Vaginal progesterone for preventing preterm birth and adverse perinatal outcomes in twin gestations: a systematic review and meta-analysis. Am J Obstet Gynecol. 2023;229(6):599–616.e3. https://doi.org/10.1016/j.ajog.2023.05.010.
63. Lim AC, Hegeman MA, Huis In 'T Veld MA, Opmeer BC, Bruinse HW, Mol BW. Cervical length measurement for the prediction of preterm birth in multiple pregnancies: a systematic review and bivariate meta-analysis. Ultrasound Obstet Gynecol. 2011;38(1):10–7. https://doi.org/10.1002/uog.9013.
64. Conde-Agudelo A, Romero R, Hassan SS, Yeo L. Transvaginal sonographic cervical length for the prediction of spontaneous preterm birth in twin pregnancies: a systematic review and metaanalysis. Am J Obstet Gynecol. 2010;203(2):128.e1–12. https://doi.org/10.1016/j.ajog.2010.02.064.
65. Schuit E, Stock S, Rode L, Rouse DJ, Lim AC, Norman JE, Nassar AH, Serra V, Combs CA, Vayssiere C, Aboulghar MM, Wood S, Çetingöz E, Briery CM, Fonseca EB, Worda K, Tabor A, Thom EA, Caritis SN, Awwad J, et al. Effectiveness of progestogens to improve perinatal outcome in twin pregnancies: an individual participant data meta-analysis. BJOG. 2015;122(1):27–37. https://doi.org/10.1111/1471-0528.13032.
66. Romero R, Conde-Agudelo A, El-Refaie W, Rode L, Brizot ML, Cetingoz E, Serra V, Da Fonseca E, Abdelhafez MS, Tabor A, Perales A, Hassan SS, Nicolaides KH. Vaginal progesterone decreases preterm birth and neonatal morbidity and mortality in women with a twin gestation and a short cervix: an updated meta-analysis of individual patient data. Ultrasound Obstet Gynecol. 2017;49(3):303–14. https://doi.org/10.1002/uog.17397.
67. Romero R, Conde-Agudelo A, Rehal A, Da Fonseca E, Brizot ML, Rode L, Serra V, Cetingoz E, Syngelaki A, Tabor A, Perales A, Hassan SS, Nicolaides KH. Vaginal progesterone for the prevention of preterm birth and adverse perinatal outcomes in twin gestations with a short cervix: an updated individual patient data meta-analysis. Ultrasound Obstet Gynecol. 2022;59(2):263–6. https://doi.org/10.1002/uog.24839.
68. Dang VQ, Nguyen LK, Pham TD, He YTN, Vu KN, Phan MTN, Le TQ, Le CH, Vuong LN, Mol BW. Pessary compared with vaginal progesterone for the prevention of preterm birth in women with twin pregnancies and cervical length less than 38 mm: a randomized controlled Trial. Obstet Gynecol. 2019;133(3):459–67. https://doi.org/10.1097/AOG.0000000000003136.
69. Yaniv-Nachmani H, Melcer Y, Weiner I, Bar K, Kovo M, Hershko C, Frank Wolf M, Zimerman A, Maymon R. Harefuah. 2021;160(1):13–8.
70. SMFM Consult Series #70: Management of short cervix in individuals without a history of spontaneous preterm birth. Am J Obstet Gynecol. 2024;231(2):B2–B13.
71. NICE, https://www.nice.org.uk/guidance/NG25 ; https://www.nice.org.uk/guidance/ng137
72. SOGC, Jain V, McDonald SD, Mundle WR, Farine D. Guideline No. 398: progesterone for prevention of spontaneous preterm birth. J Obstet Gynaecol Can. 202042(6):806–12.
73. FIGO, Shennan A, Suff N, Leigh Simpson J, Jacobsson B, Mol BW, Grobman WA, FIGO Working Group for Preterm Birth. FIGO good practice recommendations on progestogens for prevention of preterm delivery. Int J Gynaecol Obstet. 2021;155(1):16–8.

The Role of Biomarkers

Daniel Gabbai and Yariv Yogev

Contents

Y. Yogev, A. Khalil (eds.), *Prevention of Complications in Obstetrics*,
https://doi.org/10.1007/978-3-032-23479-7_10

Learning Objectives

- Explain the biological and clinical rationale for biomarker use in predicting preterm birth.
- Describe the major biomarker categories (fFN, inflammatory markers, placental proteins, and genetic biomarkers).
- Summarize the strength of evidence supporting each biomarker in predicting PTB.
- Identify limitations of biomarker-based prediction and the challenge of applying results clinically.
- Understand emerging molecular biomarkers such as plasma cell-free RNA and their potential role in future screening.

10.1 Introduction

Maternal biomarkers have been implicated in the prediction of preterm birth (PTB), with various studies underscoring their potential significance. Systematic reviews are indispensable to evidence-based healthcare, offering the highest tier of evidence to inform clinical decision-making [1]. However, the limited sample sizes, variability in inclusion criteria, discrepancies in gestational age at assessment, and inconsistencies in outcome definitions have obstructed a comprehensive quantification of the predictive capabilities of these biomarkers in relation to PTB. This chapter endeavors to synthesize evidence from multiple investigations, thereby providing a concise overview of the current understanding regarding the role of maternal biomarkers in predicting preterm birth.

10.2 Fibronectin

Fetal fibronectin (fFN), a glycoprotein, was initially identified within the extracellular matrix of the normal human implantation site, specifically connecting extravillous trophoblasts and trophoblastic cell columns to the uterine decidua [2]. By 1991, evidence had accumulated regarding its potential role in preventing PTB [3]. fFN is present in the amniotic fluid and on the decidual chorionic surface; thus, any mechanical disruption or inflammatory damage to the amniotic membrane can result in the release of fFN into the cervical–vaginal secretions.

Numerous studies have investigated the role of fFN in predicting PTB. These studies have explored its utility both as a stand-alone marker and in combination with other clinical parameters, assessing its effectiveness in symptomatic vs. asymptomatic patients, using it qualitatively or quantitatively, sampling from cervical secretions and blood, and evaluating its application in specific populations such as those with multiple gestations.

Some studies have explored the role of fFN as a stand-alone predictor of PTB. A meta-analysis by Berghella V. in 2019 included six randomized controlled trials (RCTs) involving 546 symptomatic women with singleton pregnancies between 23 + 0 and 34 + 6 weeks of gestation. These women were randomized based on whether the attending physician was aware of the fFN results. The analysis did not find sufficient evidence to support fFN as a reliable predictor of PTB on its own [4]. Additionally, no significant advantage was found in management strategies based on fFN results for various outcomes, including preterm birth before 28 weeks, gestational age at delivery, birth weight less than 2500 g, perinatal death, use of tocolysis, administration of steroids for fetal lung maturity, time to evaluation, respiratory distress syndrome, neonatal intensive care unit (NICU) admission, or the duration of NICU stay. Moreover, the use of fFN was associated with higher costs and increased hospitalization charges [5].

Several studies have sought to enhance the prediction of PTB by combining fFN with other clinical parameters. A systematic review and meta-analysis by Boot et al. [6] investigated the diagnostic accuracy of fFN, fetal breathing movements (FBM), and cervical length (CL) for the short-term prediction of PTB. The pooled analysis, which included 72 studies, revealed significant associations: Positive fFN was linked to PTB within 24 h (odds ratio (OR): 7, 95% CI: 3–17) and 7 days

(OR: 12, 95% CI: 8–16), CL <15 mm was associated with PTB within 24 h (OR: 24, 95% CI: 9–65) and 7 days (OR: 23, 95% CI: 12–46), and FBM emerged as the best predictor of PTB within 24 h (OR: 37.8, 95% CI: 9–164) and 7 days (OR: 93, 95% CI: 15–592). Similar findings were reported in another meta-analysis of 32 studies involving symptomatic women, which found positive cervicovaginal fFN to be an independent risk factor for PTB, with an overall OR of 14.4 (95% CI: 9.7–21.3) and a sensitivity and specificity of 0.76 and 0.82, respectively [7].

As a commercially available tool, the qualitative measurement of fFN (greater than or equal to 50 ng/mL) is commonly used in practice. However, false-negative results can occur, often due to factors such as recent intercourse, a grossly bloody specimen, or a recent digital cervical examination [8–10].

Abbott et al. explored the dose-dependent relationship between quantitative cervicovaginal fFN and PTB, aiming to improve predictive accuracy [11]. In symptomatic women, the positive predictive value for PTB before 34 weeks increased progressively with higher fFN thresholds: 19% at 10 ng/mL, 32% at 50 ng/mL, 61% at 200 ng/mL, and 75% at 500 ng/mL. The predictive value of quantitative fFN, when combined with CL, improved both the negative and positive predictive values [12]. Combining quantitative fFN with other parameters, such as CL, demographic information, and obstetric history, has been used to develop algorithms that predict the risk of PTB [13, 14]. This approach has shown high accuracy in asymptomatic high-risk women for predicting spontaneous PTB at <30, <34, and <37 weeks' gestation and within 1, 2, and 4 weeks of testing, with AUCs ranging from 0.75 to 0.90 for fFN and CL combined, from 0.68 to 0.90 for fFN alone, and from 0.71 to 0.87 for CL alone [15]. In symptomatic women, the predictive value varies by gestational age, with areas under the curve (AUCs) of 0.96 at <30 weeks, 0.85 at <34 weeks, 0.77 at <37 weeks, 0.91 at <1 week from testing, and 0.92 at <2 weeks from testing [16].

Regarding multiple gestations, particularly twin pregnancies, studies have shown minimal-to-moderate predictive accuracy using fFN [17]. Compared to singleton pregnancies, Singer et al. demonstrated that fFN predicted delivery within 14 days of testing with sensitivity, specificity, and positive and negative predictive values of 71%, 74%, 19%, and 97%, respectively, in twin gestations and 82%, 90%, 17%, and 99%, respectively, in singleton gestations [18]. A systematic review and meta-analysis by Conde-Agudelo and Romero emphasized the accuracy of fFN, particularly its negative predictive value, in women with twin pregnancies and threatened preterm labor for predicting spontaneous preterm birth within 7 days [19].

10.3 Alpha-Fetoprotein (AFP)

AFP is a glycoprotein synthesized primarily by the yolk sac early in pregnancy, with the fetal liver taking over as the main site of production as gestation progresses. Fetal AFP levels peak around 13 weeks of gestation before gradually declining until birth. AFP is believed to enter maternal circulation primarily through the placenta from the fetal bloodstream and, to a lesser extent, from the amniotic fluid via the fetal membranes and decidua [20]. While the exact physiological role of AFP in maternal circulation remains unclear, its association with adverse obstetric outcomes has led to its use as part of second-trimester screening, alongside other biomarkers [21].

Since 1992, several studies have explored the association between AFP and PTB, consistently finding a potential link between the two [22–25]. Xu Wang et al. investigated 13,828 pregnant women with available second-trimester serum biomarker data and found that AFP levels greater than 1.8 MoM were associated with an increased risk of PTB, even after controlling for potential confounders such as gestational age, maternal age, infant gender, and delivery method. The adjusted odds ratio (aOR) was 1.387 (95% CI: 1.140–1.689), with a p-value of 0.001 [26]. Additionally, "The Preterm Prediction Study" identified AFP measurement at 24 weeks of gestation as an independent predictive factor for PTB, with an aOR of 3.95 (95% CI: 1.77–8.85) and a p-value of 0.001 [27].

However, it remains unclear whether this association is influenced by other confounding factors or by PTB-related biomarkers included in these studies, such as human chorionic gonadotropin (hCG). For instance, isolated elevated AFP, where other biomarkers are within normal ranges, was not found to be associated with PTB [28].

Wei Yuan conducted a meta-analysis on the role of AFP in predicting PTB, reviewing 24 studies and including data from 207,135 women. The analysis concluded that AFP demonstrated high specificity but low sensitivity in predicting PTB. However, the overall predictive value remains inconclusive due to the influence of other biomarker confounders. In cases of isolated elevated AFP levels, the predictive value for PTB was not statistically significant, with an OR of 1.80 (95% CI: 0.92–2.68). Although using a cutoff of 2.5 MoM instead of 2 MoM could improve prediction accuracy, it does not enhance the positive or negative predictive value [29].

10.4 C-Reactive Protein (CRP)

CRP is an inflammatory marker that can be detected in blood and other bodily fluids, with levels increasing in response to inflammatory or infectious conditions. Its role in predicting PTB has been investigated in several studies [30].

A systematic review and meta-analysis demonstrated an association between elevated CRP levels and PTB in asymptomatic women, suggesting that CRP may play a role in the sequence of events leading to spontaneous PTB. This review analyzed eight studies, encompassing a total of 4190 women. The overall crude OR was 1.53 (95% CI: 1.22–1.90) for elevated CRP levels in blood samples and 7.85 (95% CI: 3.88–15.87) for elevated CRP levels in the amniotic fluid [31]. Another meta-analysis investigated elevated CRP levels in the amniotic fluid of patients in the second or third trimester, comparing two groups: those who experienced PTB and a control group. The analysis revealed a mean difference of 21.34 (95% CI: 11.69–30.89, $p < 0.01$), suggesting a significant association between elevated CRP in the amniotic fluid and PTB [32].

Vogel et al. demonstrated an association between elevated CRP and PTB in asymptomatic women, with a positive likelihood ratio (LR+) of 1.8, sensitivity of 26%, and a false-positive (FP) rate of 15%. In symptomatic women, the association was stronger, with an LR+ of 6.3, sensitivity of 38%, and FP of 6% [33].

10.5 Other Biomarkers

10.5.1 Cytokines

Several studies have explored the relationship between maternal cytokines and PTB. Interleukin-6 (IL-6), a pro-inflammatory cytokine, plays a key role in the body's inflammatory response and is thought to contribute to the mechanism of PTB. A systematic review of 17 studies found that PTB was strongly associated with increased IL-6 levels in mid-trimester cervicovaginal fluid (OR: 3.05, 95% CI: 2.00–4.67, number needed to treat = 7) and amniotic fluid (OR: 4.52, 95% CI: 2.67–7.65, number needed to treat = 7). However, there was no association between IL-6 levels in plasma specimens and PTB (OR: 1.5, 95% CI: 0.7–3.0) [31]. Additionally, a meta-analysis, which included nine studies and 1904 patients, demonstrated a significant association between elevated IL-6 levels in the amniotic fluid and cervicovaginal samples with PTB. The standardized mean difference (SMD) was 1.87 (95% CI: 0.82–2.93, $p < 0.001$) for amniotic fluid, and 0.46 (95% CI: 0.09–0.84, $p = 0.022$) for cervicovaginal samples. However, no significant association was found between IL-6 levels in maternal blood and PTB (SMD: -0.11, 95% CI: −0.57–0.34, $p = 0.623$) [34].

Interleukin-1 (IL-1), produced by the decidua, stimulates prostaglandin production by the human amnion and is elevated in cases of PTB with infection, as well as in spontaneous labor at term [35]. Research examining the relationship between IL-1 and its receptor antagonist, which can modulate the inflammatory response and varies by specific genetic variants, has found an association between this cytokine and PTB. An analysis of maternal genotypes revealed that IL-1 is a risk factor for PTB, with an OR of 2.02 (95% CI: 1.44–2.85) in the subgroup including preterm prelabour rupture of membranes (PPROM) and an OR of 1.55 (95% CI: 0.82–2.94) in the subgroup excluding PPROM. In the fetal genotype analysis, the risk was OR = 1.42 (95% CI: 1.02–1.99) in the subgroup with PPROM and OR = 1.05 (95% CI: 0.56–1.97) in the subgroup without PPROM [36].

Other genetic variants have been investigated for their role in modulating inflammation through cytokine activity, such as tumor necrosis factor-alpha (TNF-α). In 2006, a meta-analysis by Menon found no significant correlation between TNF-α and PTB [37]. Similar results were observed in another meta-analysis, which reported that TNF-α was not associated with PTB (OR = 0.84, 95% CI: 0.65–1.07, $p = 0.167$) [38]. However, a separate study reported a positive likelihood ratio (LR) of 3.9 (95% CI: 2.6–5.9) and a negative LR of 0.2 (95% CI: 0.1–0.4) when TNF-α was detected in amniotic fluid samples of women with PTB [39]. Furthermore, it was revealed that the presence of TNF-α in amniotic fluid increases the positive LR for PTB to +10 and the negative LR to −6 in asymptomatic women. For symptomatic women, the positive LR was +8, while the negative LR was −0.4 [40].

10.5.2 Thyroid Antibodies (TPO and TG-Ab)

Several studies have investigated the association between thyroid antibodies and PTB. A meta-analysis [41] of 11 prospective cohort studies, involving 35,467 women, revealed that the presence of thyroid antibodies is associated with an increased risk of PTB, with an Relative Risk (RR) of 1.41 (95% CI: 1.08–1.84, $p = 0.011$). In subgroup analyses, thyroid peroxidase (TPO) antibodies were identified as the primary risk factor for PTB, with an RR of 1.69 (95% CI: 1.19–2.41, $p = 0.003$), whereas thyroglobulin antibodies (TG-Ab) showed no significant association with PTB.

Another meta-analysis of 19 studies [42], involving 47,045 pregnant women without overt thyroid disease, found that subclinical hypothyroidism, isolated hypothyroxinemia, and TPO antibody positivity were significantly associated with an increased risk of PTB. TPO antibody–positive women had a higher risk of PTB compared to TPO antibody–negative women (6.6% vs. 4.9%, respectively; absolute risk difference: 1.6% [95% CI: 0.7%–2.8%], OR: 1.33 [95% CI: 1.15–1.56]). The American Thyroid Association's 2017 guidelines also support this association, stating that TPO antibody positivity is linked to an increased risk of PTB [43].

Moreover, the Generation R study reported that TPO antibody positivity was associated with a 1.7-fold increased risk of PTB, independent of thyroid function [44]. Another study, which developed a nomogram for predicting PTB based on multivariate logistic regression analysis [45], identified a combination of previous PTB (OR: 5.25, 95% CI: 2.13–12.90, $p < 0.01$), TPO antibody positivity (OR: 1.01, 95% CI: 1.01–1.02), and T4 levels (OR: 0.90, 95% CI: 0.83–0.97, $p = 0.04$) as independent risk factors that most accurately predicted preterm birth. The area under the curve (AUC) for the model was 0.66 (95% CI: 0.61–0.72).

10.5.3 Matrix Metalloproteins

Based on strong evidence suggesting that subclinical intra-amniotic inflammation or infection may be causally linked to early PTB, several studies have demonstrated the predictive value of matrix metalloproteinases (MMPs), particularly MMP-8 and MMP-9, in identifying the risk of PTB. MMPs are released by inflammatory cells in response to microbial products or inflammatory signals. A case-control study by Kim et al. [46] investigated amniotic fluid from asymptomatic singleton pregnant women who underwent mid-trimester genetic amniocentesis and found that elevated levels of MMP-8 in amniotic fluid, measured by a rapid bedside test, identified 42% of patients at risk of early spontaneous PTB (<30 weeks).

Additionally, Davis et al. recruited patients at both low and high risk of PTB and reported that elevated vaginal MMP-9 levels were significantly higher in patients who experienced PTB compared to those who delivered at term (85.46% ± 19.79 vs. 53.20% ± 31.47, $p = 0.01$), suggesting its potential as an early predictor of PTB [47]. Similarly, Duran-Chávez et al. found that the adjusted odds ratios were 1.42 (95% CI: 0.80–2.53) for MMP-2 and 2.71 (95% CI: 1.52–4.83) for MMP-9, indicating an increased risk of PTB, along with other associated covariates [48].

10.5.4 Placental Proteins

10

Placental proteins, such as human chorionic gonadotropin, prolactin, relaxin, angiogenin, and proteomics-related biomarkers (desmoplakin isoform-1, stratifin, and thrombospondin-1 precursor), have all demonstrated good predictive accuracy for PTB.

Low levels of pregnancy-associated plasma protein-A (PAPP-A) in the first trimester (11–13 + 6 weeks) are associated with an increased risk of PTB. Swiercz et al. found that diminished PAPP-A levels significantly contributed to the risk of preterm deliveries before 35 and 37 weeks, as well as PPROM. The greatest discriminatory potential was observed for PAPP-A levels below 0.688, providing an OR of 2.66 (95% CI: 1.51–4.66) [49].

Chiu et al., in a study of 9298 singleton pregnancies, reported that low PAPP-A levels and serum placental growth factor (PlGF) were associated with increased risks of PTB and PPROM. Screening using a combination of maternal risk factors, PAPP-A, and PlGF achieved better performance in predicting PTB before 37 weeks (AUC: 0.630 vs. 0.555, detection rate (DR): 24.8% vs. 16.6% at an FP rate of 10%, $p \leq 0.0001$) and PPROM before 37 weeks (AUC: 0.643 vs. 0.558, DR: 28.1% vs. 17.0% at an FP rate of 10%, $p \leq 0.0001$) compared to using maternal risk factors alone [50].

Reduced first-trimester concentrations of free beta-human chorionic gonadotropin (beta-hCG) have been identified as a risk factor for deliveries before 37 weeks, PPROM, and PTB before 35 weeks of gestation. Additionally, cervicovaginal hCG levels have been shown to predict preterm delivery in symptomatic patients. A positive rapid qualitative assay from cervicovaginal secretions between 24 and 34 weeks' gestation was associated with a significant increase in the incidence of preterm delivery (RR: 2.62, 95% CI: 1.38–4.98) [51, 52].

Moreover, elevated cervicovaginal prolactin levels have been found to be significantly higher in women with PTB compared to those who delivered at term [53]. High serum relaxin levels have also been associated with an increased risk of PTB in symptomatic women [54]. Pantelis et al. demonstrated that a combination of serum relaxin and cervical length increased the predictive accuracy for PTB. Another protein, mid-trimester amniotic fluid angiogenin, has been investigated in several studies, with findings showing that higher angiogenin levels were significantly correlated with PTB [55].

Proteomic analyses have identified several novel biomarkers associated with PTB [56]. Three proteins—desmoplakin isoform-1, stratifin, and thrombospondin-1 precursor—were significantly elevated in cervicovaginal fluid collected at 24–28 weeks of gestation in women who delivered between 28 and 32 weeks, compared with controls who delivered after 37 weeks [39].

10.5.5 Genetic Biomarkers

The IFN-γ A874T polymorphism has been associated with an increased risk of PTB. A meta-analysis by Liu et al. demonstrated that the A allele of the IFN-γ A874T polymorphism is linked to a heightened risk of PTB (OR = 1.14, 95% CI: 1.11–1.73, $p = 0.004$) [38]. Similarly, the GSTT1 polymorphism has also been linked to PTB. Mustafa et al. found that the GSTT1 null genotype was significantly more frequent in PTB cases compared to those with full-term labor (p = 0.028, OR = 3.4) [57]. Additionally, Tsai et al. reported significant associations between GSTT1–smoking interactions in individuals of African ancestry and PTB (22% in the GSTT1 null group compared to 31% in the non-null group, OR = 1.11, 95% CI: 1.02–1.20) and very preterm birth (gestational age less than 34 weeks: 23% compared to 33%, OR = 1.17, 95% CI: 1.03–1.33) [58].

10.5.6 Miscellaneous Biomarkers

Other biomarkers found to be related to PTB include vascular endothelial growth factor (VEGF), adrenocorticotropic hormone (ACTH), lactate dehydrogenase (LDH), ferritin, and placental protein 13 (PP-13). Elevated levels of VEGF in amniotic fluid during the second trimester have been associated with an increased risk of PTB, particularly in cases of placenta previa and other placental complications [59, 60]. Elevated maternal serum levels of ACTH have also been found to be predictive of PTB; women with higher ACTH levels were more likely to deliver preterm compared to those with lower levels [61]. Higher concentrations of LDH in mid-trimester amniotic fluid (above 120 IU/L) have shown a sensitivity of 59% and a specificity of 81% for predicting PTB [62, 63]. Additionally, elevated cervical and serum ferritin levels have been linked to an increased risk of PTB and are thought to reflect an acute-phase reaction to subclinical infections, which are closely associated with PTB [64, 65]. Decreased levels of PP-13 in the first trimester, along with other markers like PAPP-A and uterine artery Doppler indices, have also been associated with an increased risk of PTB [66, 67].

10.6 Under Investigation

As mentioned above, PTB is a leading cause of maternal and neonatal morbidity and mortality. The development of predictive tools for identifying the risk of PTB in the antenatal population is of clinical relevance. Several studies aim to find more accurate ways to predict PTB, with one of the most investigated fields being plasma cell-free (PCF) RNA.

PCF RNAs include both coding and non-coding RNAs that can modulate angiogenesis, cell proliferation and death, tumor cell invasion, and cell-to-cell communication. A recently published study provides a comprehensive assessment of alterations in the placental transcriptome correlated with spontaneous PTB, offering novel insights into the mechanisms of PTB by highlighting molecular differences in the placenta. Measuring RNA levels in maternal plasma may serve as a useful and convenient approach to reflect placental gene expression profiles. Thus, PCF RNA profiles in maternal blood can function as predictive biomarkers for PTB.

A study by Camunas-Soler et al. identified 25 transcripts associated with an increased risk of PTB, developing a logistic regression model with an AUC of 0.80, indicating good predictive accuracy [68]. This study also highlighted the enrichment of genes related to collagen and extracellular matrix pathways, which may be involved in premature cervical remodeling. Jin et al. identified 15 genes with consistent regulatory trends in both the placenta and plasma of PTB cases [69]. They validated seven PCF RNAs, with ARHGEF28 showing excellent predictive performance for PTB, achieving an AUC of 0.990. Weiner et al. discovered 297 differentially expressed RNAs in women who delivered preterm before 32 weeks [70]. They validated a panel of four RNAs that were significantly higher in PTB cases, demonstrating the potential for early prediction by 16 weeks of gestation.

10.7 Conclusion

As previously described, numerous biomarkers have been investigated to predict PTB. Among these, cervical fibronectin, AFP, CRP, and cytokines, particularly IL-6, exhibit the strongest associations with the occurrence of PTB. In contrast, other identified biomarkers demonstrate only mild-to-moderate associations in predicting PTB. Consequently, large-scale prospective studies are warranted to elucidate the roles of these biomarkers, both individually and in combination, in predicting spontaneous PTB.

Chapter Key Points

- Biomarkers aim to improve the prediction of spontaneous preterm birth (PTB) but vary greatly in accuracy and clinical utility.
- Fetal fibronectin (fFN) shows the strongest negative predictive value, with enhanced accuracy when combined with cervical length.
- AFP and CRP show associations with PTB but limited predictive precision due to low sensitivity or confounding factors.
- Cytokines, particularly IL-6, correlate strongly with PTB when measured in cervicovaginal or amniotic fluid.
- Placental biomarkers (PAPP-A, PlGF, and beta-hCG) and proteomic signatures contribute moderate predictive value.
- Emerging biomarkers, such as plasma cell-free RNA profiles, show high potential but require validation in large cohorts.

Chapter-End Summary

This chapter reviews the current evidence on biochemical, inflammatory, placental, and genetic biomarkers used to predict spontaneous preterm birth. Fetal fibronectin remains the most clinically validated tool, particularly as a strong negative predictor, with improved accuracy when integrated with cervical length or incorporated into risk prediction algorithms. Inflammatory biomarkers such as CRP, IL-6, and matrix metalloproteinases demonstrate strong associations with PTB, especially when measured in cervicovaginal or amniotic samples, though their predictive value varies by patient population. Placental biomarkers, including PAPP-A, PlGF, and beta-hCG, show moderate predictive performance, while genetic and proteomic markers offer emerging promise. Novel approaches such as plasma cell-free RNA profiling demonstrate high accuracy in early gestation but require further validation. Overall, while multiple biomarkers correlate with the PTB risk, few are ready for widespread clinical application, underscoring the need for large-scale, prospective studies evaluating combined biomarker strategies.

References

1. Lucaroni F, Morciano L, Rizzo G, D'Antonio F, Buonuomo E, Palombi L, et al. Biomarkers for predicting spontaneous preterm birth: an umbrella systematic review. J Matern Fetal Neonatal Med. 2018;31(6):726–34.
2. Feinberg RF, Kliman HJ, Lockwood CJ. Is oncofetal fibronectin a trophoblast glue for human implantation? Am J Pathol. 1991;138(3):537–43.
3. Lockwood CJ, Senyei AE, Dische MR, Casal D, Shah KD, Thung SN, et al. Fetal fibronectin in cervical and vaginal secretions as a predictor of preterm delivery. N Engl J Med. 1991;325(10):669–74.
4. Berghella V, Saccone G. Fetal fibronectin testing for reducing the risk of preterm birth. Cochrane Database Syst Rev. 2019;7(7):CD006843.
5. Berghella V, Saccone G. Fetal fibronectin testing for prevention of preterm birth in singleton pregnancies with threatened preterm labor: a systematic review and metaanalysis of randomized controlled trials. Am J Obstet Gynecol. 2016;215(4):431–8.
6. Boots AB, Sanchez-Ramos L, Bowers DM, Kaunitz AM, Zamora J, Schlattmann P. The short-term prediction of preterm birth: a systematic review and diagnostic metaanalysis. Am J Obstet Gynecol. 2014;210(1):54.e1–54.e10.
7. Sanchez-Ramos L, Delke I, Zamora J, Kaunitz AM. Fetal fibronectin as a short-term predictor of preterm birth in symptomatic patients: a meta-analysis. Obstet Gynecol. 2009;114(3):631–40.
8. Shimoya K, Hashimoto K, Shimizu T, Koyama M, Azuma C, Murata Y. Cervical fluid oncofetal fibronectin as a predictor of early ectopic pregnancy. Is it affected by blood contamination? J Reprod Med. 2002;47(8):640–4.
9. McLaren JS, Hezelgrave NL, Ayubi H, Seed PT, Shennan AH. Prediction of spontaneous preterm birth using quantitative fetal fibronectin after

recent sexual intercourse. Am J Obstet Gynecol. 2015;212(1):89.e1–5.
10. McKenna DS, Chung K, Iams JD. Effect of digital cervical examination on the expression of fetal fibronectin. J Reprod Med. 1999;44(9):796–800.
11. Abbott DS, Radford SK, Seed PT, Tribe RM, Shennan AH. Evaluation of a quantitative fetal fibronectin test for spontaneous preterm birth in symptomatic women. Am J Obstet Gynecol. 2013;208(2):122.e1–6.
12. Bruijn MMC, Kamphuis EI, Hoesli IM, Martinez de Tejada B, Loccufier AR, Kühnert M, et al. The predictive value of quantitative fibronectin testing in combination with cervical length measurement in symptomatic women. Am J Obstet Gynecol. 2016;215(6):793.e1–8.
13. Kuhrt K, Smout E, Hezelgrave N, Seed PT, Carter J, Shennan AH. Development and validation of a tool incorporating cervical length and quantitative fetal fibronectin to predict spontaneous preterm birth in asymptomatic high-risk women. Ultrasound Obstet Gynecol. 2016;47(1):104–9.
14. Watson HA, Carter J, Seed PT, Tribe RM, Shennan AH. The QUiPP App: a safe alternative to a treat-all strategy for threatened preterm labor. Ultrasound Obstet Gynecol. 2017;50(3):342–6.
15. Watson HA, Seed PT, Carter J, Hezelgrave NL, Kuhrt K, Tribe RM, et al. Development and validation of predictive models for QUiPP App v.2: tool for predicting preterm birth in asymptomatic high-risk women. Ultrasound Obstet Gynecol. 2020;55(3):348–56.
16. Carter J, Seed PT, Watson HA, David AL, Sandall J, Shennan AH, et al. Development and validation of predictive models for QUiPP App v.2: tool for predicting preterm birth in women with symptoms of threatened preterm labor. Ultrasound Obstet Gynecol. 2020;55(3):357–67.
17. Conde-Agudelo A, Romero R. Prediction of preterm birth in twin gestations using biophysical and biochemical tests. Am J Obstet Gynecol. 2014;211(6):583–95.
18. Singer E, Pilpel S, Bsat F, Plevyak M, Healy A, Markenson G. Accuracy of fetal fibronectin to predict preterm birth in twin gestations with symptoms of labor. Obstet Gynecol. 2007;109(5):1083–7.
19. Conde-Agudelo A, Romero R. Cervicovaginal fetal fibronectin for the prediction of spontaneous preterm birth in multiple pregnancies: a systematic review and meta-analysis. J Matern Fetal Neonatal Med. 2010;23(12):1365–76.
20. Newby D, Dalgliesh G, Lyall F, Aitken DA. Alphafetoprotein and alphafetoprotein receptor expression in the normal human placenta at term. Placenta. 2005;26(2–3):190–200.
21. Canick JA, MacRae AR. Second trimester serum markers. Semin Perinatol. 2005;29(4):203–8.
22. Cho S, Durfee KK, Keel BA, Parks LH. Perinatal outcomes in a prospective matched pair study of pregnancy and unexplained elevated or low AFP screening. J Perinat Med. 1997;25(6):476–83.
23. Chitayat D, Farrell SA, Huang T, Meier C, Wyatt PR, Summers AM. Double-positive maternal serum screening results for down syndrome and open neural tube defects: an indicator for fetal structural or chromosomal abnormalities and adverse obstetric outcomes. Am J Obstet Gynecol. 2002;187(3):758–63.
24. Williams MA, Hickok DE, Zingheim RW, Luthy DA, Kimelman J, Nyberg DA, et al. Elevated maternal serum alpha-fetoprotein levels and midtrimester placental abnormalities in relation to subsequent adverse pregnancy outcomes. Am J Obstet Gynecol. 1992;167(4 Pt 1):1032–7.
25. Bernstein IM, Barth RA, Miller R, Capeless EL. Elevated maternal serum alpha-fetoprotein: association with placental sonolucencies, fetomaternal hemorrhage, vaginal bleeding, and pregnancy outcome in the absence of fetal anomalies. Obstet Gynecol. 1992;79(1):71–4.
26. Wang X, Chen Y, Kuang H, Yang R, Chen D, Chen A, et al. Associations between maternal AFP and β-HCG and preterm birth. Am J Perinatol. 2019;36(14):1459–63.
27. Moawad AH, Goldenberg RL, Mercer B, Meis PJ, Iams JD, Das A, et al. The Preterm Prediction Study: the value of serum alkaline phosphatase, alpha-fetoprotein, plasma corticotropin-releasing hormone, and other serum markers for the prediction of spontaneous preterm birth. Am J Obstet Gynecol. 2002;186(5):990–6.
28. Duric K, Skrablin S, Lesin J, Kalafatic D, Kuvacic I, Suchanek E. Second trimester total human chorionic gonadotropin, alpha-fetoprotein and unconjugated estriol in predicting pregnancy complications other than fetal aneuploidy. Eur J Obstet Gynecol Reprod Biol. 2003;110(1):12–5.
29. Yuan W, Chen L, Bernal AL. Is elevated maternal serum alpha-fetoprotein in the second trimester of pregnancy associated with increased preterm birth risk? A systematic review and meta-analysis. Eur J Obstet Gynecol Reprod Biol. 2009;145(1):57–64.
30. Shahshahan Z, Rasouli O. The use of maternal C-reactive protein in the predicting of preterm labor and tocolytic therapy in preterm labor women. Adv Biomed Res. 2014;3:154.
31. Wei SQ, Fraser W, Luo ZC. Inflammatory cytokines and spontaneous preterm birth in asymptomatic women: a systematic review. Obstet Gynecol. 2010;116(2 Pt 1):393–401.
32. Wang C, Chen Q, Wang Y. Correlation of amniotic fluid inflammatory markers with preterm birth: a meta-analysis. J Obstet Gynaecol. 2024;44(1):2368764.
33. Vogel I, Thorsen P, Curry A, Sandager P, Uldbjerg N. Biomarkers for the prediction of preterm delivery. Acta Obstet Gynecol Scand. 2005;84(6):516–25.
34. Chang Y, Li W, Shen Y, Li S, Chen X. Association between interleukin-6 and preterm birth: a meta-analysis. Ann Med. 2023;55(2):2284384.

35. Mitchell MD, Edwin S, Romero RJ. Prostaglandin biosynthesis by human decidual cells: effects of inflammatory mediators. Prostaglandins Leukot Essent Fat Acids. 1990;41(1):35–8.
36. Cui J, Wang F, Zhang X, Liu L. Maternal and fetal IL1RN polymorphisms and the risk of preterm delivery: a meta-analysis. J Matern Fetal Neonatal Med. 2015;28(1):100–5.
37. Menon R, Merialdi M, Betrán AP, Dolan S, Jiang L, Fortunato SJ, et al. Analysis of association between maternal tumor necrosis factor-alpha promoter polymorphism (−308), tumor necrosis factor concentration, and preterm birth. Am J Obstet Gynecol. 2006;195(5):1240–8.
38. Liu Y, Yao CJ, Tao FB, Luo CM, Cao Y, Su-Juan Z, et al. Association between maternal tumor necrosis factor-α G308A polymorphism and interferon-γ A874T polymorphism and risk of preterm birth: a meta-analysis. Eur J Obstet Gynecol Reprod Biol. 2015;190:11–9.
39. Conde-Agudelo A, Papageorghiou AT, Kennedy SH, Villar J. Novel biomarkers for the prediction of the spontaneous preterm birth phenotype: a systematic review and meta-analysis. BJOG. 2011;118(9):1042–54.
40. Hee L. Likelihood ratios for the prediction of preterm delivery with biomarkers. Acta Obstet Gynecol Scand. 2011;90(11):1189–99.
41. He X, Wang P, Wang Z, He X, Xu D, Wang B. Thyroid antibodies and risk of preterm delivery: a meta-analysis of prospective cohort studies. Eur J Endocrinol. 2012;167(4):455–64.
42. Consortium on Thyroid and Pregnancy—Study Group on Preterm Birth, Korevaar TIM, Derakhshan A, Taylor PN, Meima M, Chen L, et al. Association of thyroid function test abnormalities and thyroid autoimmunity with preterm birth: a systematic review and meta-analysis. JAMA. 2019;322(7):632–41.
43. Alexander EK, Pearce EN, Brent GA, Brown RS, Chen H, Dosiou C, et al. 2017 guidelines of the American Thyroid Association for the diagnosis and management of thyroid disease during pregnancy and the postpartum. Thyroid. 2017;27(3):315–89.
44. Korevaar TIM, Schalekamp-Timmermans S, de Rijke YB, Visser WE, Visser W, de Muinck Keizer-Schrama SMPF, et al. Hypothyroxinemia and TPO-antibody positivity are risk factors for premature delivery: the generation R study. J Clin Endocrinol Metab. 2013;98(11):4382–90.
45. Nazarpour S, Ramezani Tehrani F, Rahmati M, Azizi F. Prediction of preterm delivery based on thyroid peroxidase antibody levels and other identified risk factors. Eur J Obstet Gynecol Reprod Biol. 2023;284:125–30.
46. Kim SM, Romero R, Lee J, Chaemsaithong P, Lee MW, Chaiyasit N, et al. About one-half of early spontaneous preterm deliveries can be identified by a rapid matrix metalloproteinase-8 (MMP-8) bedside test at the time of mid-trimester genetic amniocentesis. J Matern Fetal Neonatal Med. 2016;29(15):2414–22.
47. Davis JA, Baker D, Peresleni T, Heiselman C, Kocis C, Demishev M, et al. Vaginal matrix metalloproteinase-9 (MMP-9) as a potential early predictor of preterm birth. J Perinat Med. 2024;52(6):591–6.
48. Duran-Chávez J, Grandi C, Dos S Rodrigues L, de Freitas SF, Cardoso VC, Carvalho Cavalli R. Relationship between metalloproteinase-2 and -9 levels in plasma and vaginal secretion with preterm birth. Eur J Obstet Gynecol Reprod Biol. 2021;261:217–21.
49. Swiercz G, Zmelonek-Znamirowska A, Szwabowicz K, Armanska J, Detka K, Mlodawska M, et al. Evaluating the predictive efficacy of first trimester biochemical markers (PAPP-A, fβ-hCG) in forecasting preterm delivery incidences. Sci Rep. 2024;14(1):16206.
50. Chiu CPH, Feng Q, Chaemsaithong P, Sahota DS, Lau YY, Yeung YK, et al. Prediction of spontaneous preterm birth and preterm prelabor rupture of membranes using maternal factors, obstetric history and biomarkers of placental function at 11-13 weeks. Ultrasound Obstet Gynecol. 2022;60(2):192–9.
51. Gurbuz A, Karateke A, Ozturkmen M, Kabaca C. Human chorionic gonadotropin assay in cervical secretions for accurate diagnosis of preterm labor. Int J Gynaecol Obstet. 2004;85(2):132–8.
52. Sanchez-Ramos L, Mentel C, Bertholf R, Kaunitz AM, Delke I, Loge C. Human chorionic gonadotropin in cervicovaginal secretions as a predictor of preterm delivery. Int J Gynaecol Obstet. 2003;83(2):151–7.
53. Guvenal T, Kantas E, Erselcan T, Culhaoglu Y, Cetin A. Beta-human chorionic gonadotropin and prolactin assays in cervicovaginal secretions as a predictor of preterm delivery. Int J Gynaecol Obstet. 2001;75(3):229–34.
54. Pantelis A, Sotiriadis A, Chatzistamatiou K, Pratilas G, Dinas K. Serum relaxin and cervical length for prediction of spontaneous preterm birth in second-trimester symptomatic women. Ultrasound Obstet Gynecol. 2018;52(6):763–8.
55. Spong CY, Ghidini A, Sherer DM, Pezzullo JC, Ossandon M, Eglinton GS. Angiogenin: a marker for preterm delivery in midtrimester amniotic fluid. Am J Obstet Gynecol. 1997;176(2):415–8.
56. Marić I, Stevenson DK, Aghaeepour N, Gaudillière B, Wong RJ, Angst MS. Predicting preterm birth using proteomics. Clin Perinatol. 2024;51(2):391–409.
57. Mustafa MD, Pathak R, Ahmed T, Ahmed RS, Tripathi AK, Guleria K, et al. Association of glutathione S-transferase M1 and T1 gene polymor-

phisms and oxidative stress markers in preterm labor. Clin Biochem. 2010;43(13–14):1124–8.
58. Tsai HJ, Hong X, Chen J, Liu X, Pearson C, Ortiz K, et al. Role of African ancestry and gene-environment interactions in predicting preterm birth. Obstet Gynecol. 2011;118(5):1081–9.
59. Hong SN, Joo BS, Chun S, Kim A, Kim HY. Prediction of preterm delivery using levels of vascular endothelial growth factor and leptin in amniotic fluid from the second trimester. Arch Gynecol Obstet. 2015;291(2):265–71.
60. Kim A, Lee ES, Shin JC, Kim HY. Identification of biomarkers for preterm delivery in mid-trimester amniotic fluid. Placenta. 2013;34(10):873–8.
61. Makrigiannakis A, Semmler M, Briese V, Eckerle H, Minas V, Mylonas I, et al. Maternal serum corticotropin-releasing hormone and ACTH levels as predictive markers of premature labor. Int J Gynaecol Obstet. 2007;97(2):115–9.
62. Borna S, Mirzaie F, Abdollahi A. Mid-trimester amniotic fluid C-reactive protein, ferritin and lactate dehydrogenase concentrations and subsequent risk of spontaneous preterm labour. Aust N Z J Obstet Gynaecol. 2009;49(4):400–3.
63. Madazli R, Atiş A, Uzun H, Aksu F. Mid-trimester amniotic fluid angiogenin, lactate dehydrogenase and fibronectin in the prediction of preterm delivery. Eur J Obstet Gynecol Reprod Biol. 2003;106(2):160–4.
64. Ramsey PS, Tamura T, Goldenberg RL, Mercer BM, Iams JD, Meis PJ, et al. The preterm prediction study: elevated cervical ferritin levels at 22 to 24 weeks of gestation are associated with spontaneous preterm delivery in asymptomatic women. Am J Obstet Gynecol. 2002;186(3):458–63.
65. Tamura T, Goldenberg RL, Johnston KE, Cliver SP, Hickey CA. Serum ferritin: a predictor of early spontaneous preterm delivery. Obstet Gynecol. 1996;87(3):360–5.
66. Stout MJ, Goetzinger KR, Tuuli MG, Cahill AG, Macones GA, Odibo AO. First trimester serum analytes, maternal characteristics and ultrasound markers to predict pregnancies at risk for preterm birth. Placenta. 2013;34(1):14–9.
67. Kazatsker MM, Sharabi-Nov A, Meiri H, Sammour R, Sammar M. Augmented placental protein 13 in placental-associated extracellular vesicles in term and preterm preeclampsia is further elevated by corticosteroids. Int J Mol Sci. 2023;24(15)
68. Camunas-Soler J, Gee EPS, Reddy M, Mi JD, Thao M, Brundage T, et al. Predictive RNA profiles for early and very early spontaneous preterm birth. Am J Obstet Gynecol. 2022;227(1):72.e1–72.e16.
69. Jin H, Zhang Y, Fan Z, Wang X, Rui C, Xing S, et al. Identification of novel cell-free RNAs in maternal plasma as preterm biomarkers in combination with placental RNA profiles. J Transl Med. 2023;21(1):256.
70. Weiner CP, Dong Y, Zhou H, Cuckle H, Ramsey R, Egerman R, et al. Early pregnancy prediction of spontaneous preterm birth before 32 completed weeks of pregnancy using plasma RNA: transcriptome discovery and initial validation of an RNA panel of markers. BJOG. 2021;128(11):1870–80.

Prevention of Gestational Diabetes Mellitus

Roy Bitan, Tomer Avnon, and Yariv Yogev

Contents

Y. Yogev, A. Khalil (eds.), *Prevention of Complications in Obstetrics*,
https://doi.org/10.1007/978-3-032-23479-7_11

Learning Objectives

- Understand the epidemiology and pathophysiology of GDM.
- Identify evidence-based lifestyle and dietary and physical activity interventions for prevention.
- Evaluate the role of probiotics, metformin, and myo-inositol in GDM prevention.
- Differentiate between effective interventions and those with insufficient evidence.
- Apply current evidence to counsel women before and during pregnancy.

11.1 Introduction

11

Gestational diabetes mellitus (GDM) is a condition characterized by glucose intolerance of varying degrees that first manifests or is diagnosed during pregnancy. It typically resolves after delivery but has significant implications for both maternal and fetal health [1, 2]. GDM is one of the most common complications of pregnancy, affecting about 6–14% of pregnancies worldwide, with varying prevalence depending on the population, the prevalence of type 2 diabetes, and the diagnostic criteria used [2–7].

The pathophysiology of GDM primarily involves insulin resistance, which is physiologically heightened during pregnancy due to hormonal changes. Mild insulin resistance is a normal adaptation to pregnancy, which is thought to ensure adequate glucose supply to the fetus. Some women experience an exaggerated insulin resistance, have a limited ability to increase insulin secretion, or a mixture of both, which will later lead to hyperglycemia. This imbalance underlies the development of GDM in susceptible individuals [6, 8].

GDM is commonly diagnosed after 24 weeks of gestation when the physiological insulin resistance of pregnancy becomes more pronounced. The primary diagnostic method is the oral glucose tolerance test (OGTT) by a one-step or two-step approach [1, 2, 9, 10].

GDM is associated with several maternal and fetal complications. For the mother, these include an increased risk of hypertensive disorders such as preeclampsia, obstetric complications such as operative assisted delivery, postpartum hemorrhage, vaginal lacerations, and the need for cesarean delivery and a lifetime risk of developing future type 2 diabetes mellitus. For the fetus, GDM increases the likelihood of macrosomia, labor trauma such as clavicle fracture and Erb's palsy, neonatal hypoglycemia, jaundice, and later-life metabolic syndrome. Despite advances in screening and management, these complications emphasize the importance of addressing GDM proactively [1, 2, 4].

The management of GDM requires ongoing glucose monitoring and individualized care to achieve optimal outcomes. Treatment usually begins with lifestyle modifications. Dietary changes and regular physical activity (PA) form the cornerstone of treatment, aiming to control glucose levels and reduce pregnancy-associated risks. If glycemic control cannot be achieved through lifestyle measures, pharmacological treatments, such as insulin or oral hypoglycemic agents, may be required [2, 11–13].

Primary prevention is thought to produce a better outcome than treating an ongoing GDM. Pregnancy and, possibly, the preconception period represent unique opportunities for intervention in women's health. Pregnant women are typically in frequent contact with healthcare providers and are highly motivated to adopt healthier lifestyle choices, especially when these changes are framed as beneficial for their babies [14–16].

The question of whether GDM can be effectively prevented remains a critical and complex issue. The current body of literature on GDM prevention highlights considerable variability in findings. This chapter aims to provide a comprehensive review of the existing evidence, examining strategies both before and during pregnancy for preventing the appearance of GDM and exploring the challenges and gaps in current knowledge.

11.2 Lifestyle Interventions for Preventing GDM

11.2.1 Dietary Approaches to Preventing GDM

One of the most extensively studied approaches to preventing GDM is lifestyle intervention. Proper nutrition plays a crucial role in managing maternal weight, improving glucose metabolism, and reducing insulin resistance, all of which are key factors in GDM prevention, though the effectiveness remains controversial [17]. Studies have shown that factors like a high intake of sugar-sweetened beverages, heme iron, and fried foods increase GDM risk, while a prudent diet rich in fruits, vegetables, fiber, and fish can be beneficial [17–19]. Additionally, research has shown that a Mediterranean diet may be particularly effective in preventing GDM [18]. Moreover, there is some evidence suggesting that insufficient vitamin D in early pregnancy may increase the risk of GDM, but its overall impact remains unclear, with conflicting study results [18].

Since in many cases maternity care starts only after a significant portion of pregnancy has already passed, preventing GDM and obesity during pregnancy could be more challenging [16]. Lifestyle and dietary changes require time to show meaningful effects. In contrast to long-term lifestyle modifications that have been shown to prevent progress to diabetes among women with a history of impaired fasting glucose (IFG) outside of pregnancy [16, 20], the prevention of GDM is not fully proven. Most studies on the prevention of GDM have shown better outcomes when lifestyle interventions, particularly those combining diet and physical activity, are implemented earlier in pregnancy or even before pregnancy [17, 21]. The effectiveness of lifestyle interventions in preventing GDM varies among studies and depends on factors such as the criteria used to define GDM and the composition of the study population, including whether it focuses on low-risk individuals or high-risk groups, such as women with obesity, a prior history of GDM, or polycystic ovary syndrome (PCOS) [17, 21].

Several studies have failed to demonstrate a clear benefit for successful GDM prevention with dietary change. A network meta-analysis of 46 randomized controlled trials (RCTs) with 16,545 participants found that dietary interventions compared to placebo did not significantly reduce the risk of GDM (odds ratio (OR): 0.76, 95% confidence interval (CI): 0.55–1.05) [22]. Similarly, combined interventions involving both physical activity and dietary modifications showed no significant reduction in GDM risk (OR: 0.74, 95% CI: 0.54–1.01) [22]. In addition, a Cochrane review that included 11 trials with 3744 women reported that combined diet and exercise interventions during pregnancy did not significantly reduce GDM risk (relative risk (RR): 0.92, 95% CI: 0.68–1.23) [23]. A systematic review and network meta-analysis including 23 studies with 8877 participants concluded that physical activity, dietary interventions, and their combination did not significantly reduce the risk of GDM in overweight or obese women, though to be mentioned, this study still demonstrated that physical activity combined with dietary intervention was more effective and showed a trend in lowering GDM risk compared to no intervention at all [24].

On the positive side, a growing body of evidence supports the effectiveness of lifestyle interventions, particularly when implemented during prepregnancy time or in the early stages of pregnancy [17, 21]. For example, the Finnish Gestational Diabetes Prevention Study (RADIEL) demonstrated that individualized lifestyle interventions, encompassing dietary counseling, physical activity, and weight management, significantly reduced the incidence of GDM by 39% (13.9% vs. 21.6%, P-value = 0.044) in high-risk women, such as those with a prepregnancy body mass index (BMI) ≥30 kg/m^2 or a history of GDM [25]. Additionally, a systematic review and meta-analysis of 257,876 pregnancies showed that women who were physically active before pregnancy, followed a low carbohydrate/low sugar diet, or had higher quality diet scores were 29% (OR: 0.71, 95% CI: 0.57–0.88), 14% (OR: 0.86, 95% CI: 0.68–1.09), and 28% (OR: 0.72, 95% CI: 0.60–0.87), respectively, less likely to develop GDM [19].

Despite some conflicting findings, most studies indicate that lifestyle and dietary interventions, especially those started early, hold promise for reducing GDM risk and improving maternal and fetal outcomes.

11.2.2 Physical Activity and Its Role in Preventing GDM

Several studies have highlighted the potential benefits of physical activity (PA) in reducing the risk of GDM. These studies suggest that engaging in regular exercise can improve insulin sensitivity, promote better glucose metabolism, and prevent excessive weight gain, all of which contribute to lowering GDM incidence [16]. A meta-analysis of 13 RCTs (2873 pregnant women) demonstrated that structured moderate-intensity physical exercise during pregnancy significantly reduced the risk of GDM by 31%, with an even greater reduction of 36% when the exercise program was performed throughout pregnancy. Combined exercise programs, including both aerobic and strength training, were most effective in reducing the risk of GDM [26]. A meta-analysis by Song et al. showed that lifestyle interventions, including diet and PA, reduced the risk of GDM by 18% (95% CI: 5–30%). The effect was most significant when interventions started before the 15th gestational week (RR: 0.80, 95% CI: 0.66–0.97) [27]. A systematic review and meta-analysis found that greater PA, particularly before pregnancy, was significantly associated with a reduced risk of GDM, with prepregnancy activity linked to a 55% risk reduction and early pregnancy activity to a 25% reduction. This comprehensive review included data from 12 studies with over 34,000 participants for prepregnancy activity and over 4400 participants for early pregnancy activity, showing pooled ORs of 0.45 and 0.76, respectively, for the highest vs. the lowest activity levels [28]. A network meta-analysis by Tang et al. demonstrated that PA significantly reduced the risk of GDM compared to placebo (OR: 0.64, 95% CI: 0.46–0.88), further emphasizing its role as an effective preventive strategy [22].

In contrast, other studies have failed to show a significant effect of PA on reducing the risk of GDM. A meta-analysis of six RCTs found no significant difference in the risk of developing GDM between the intervention and control groups, with an RR of 0.91 and 95% CI of 0.57–1.44 [29]. A study by Stafne et al. found no significant effect of a 12-week exercise program on preventing gestational diabetes or improving insulin resistance. The prevalence of GDM was 7% in the exercise group vs. 6% in the control group (P-value = 0.52), and only 55% of women adhered to the program [30]. A Cochrane review of five trials, including 1115 women, found no significant differences in the incidence of GDM (RR: 1.10, 95% CI: 0.66–1.84) between women receiving exercise interventions and routine care [31]. Similarly, a recent review of combined diet and exercise interventions also found no clear difference in GDM risk [24]. Such evidence challenges the assumption that PA alone is sufficient for GDM prevention and raises questions about its practical implementation and efficacy.

To conclude, the evidence of PA alone for the prevention of GDM is not completely certain, though there is some good evidence for a positive effect, especially during prepregnancy time.

11.3 Probiotics and Gut Health in GDM Prevention

The role of probiotics for preventing GDM has garnered increasing attention in recent years, as gut microbiota (GM) is believed to influence metabolic pathways, including glucose metabolism and insulin sensitivity. Zeevi et al. demonstrated GM's position in glucose regulation. In this study, high variability was observed in postprandial glucose responses to identical meals among 800 people, highlighting the limitations of universal dietary recommendations. Using a machine learning algorithm that incorporated microbiome data, the researchers accurately predicted personalized glycemic responses. Dietary interventions based on these predictions significantly lowered glucose levels and altered GM, suggesting that personalized strategies targeting the microbiome could aid in GDM prevention [32].

Several studies have examined the potential of probiotic supplementation during pregnancy to reduce the risk of GDM, though with mixed results [33–36]. Research supporting the efficacy of probiotics includes a New Zealand study by Barthow and Wickens et al., which found that supplementation with *Lactobacillus rhamnosus* HN001 beginning at 14–16 weeks of pregnancy reduced the prevalence of GDM by 40%, particularly among women aged 35 or older and among women with a previous GDM history [37]. Tang et al.'s analysis also highlighted the effectiveness of probiotic interventions compared to placebo, with a significant reduction in GDM incidence (OR: 0.57, 95% CI: 0.34–0.96) [22]. Another promising study by Luoto et al. reported a reduced risk of GDM (13% in the probiotic group vs. 36% in the placebo group, P-value = 0.003) when dietary counseling was combined with *Lactobacillus rhamnosus* GG and *Bifidobacterium lactis* Bb12 [38].

In contrast, other studies have failed to show a clear benefit of probiotics in preventing GDM. For instance, a double-blind randomized trial by Callaway et al. in overweight and obese Australian women found no significant difference in GDM incidence between the probiotic group (18.4%) and the placebo group (12.3%, P-value = 0.10) [39]. Additionally, a systematic review and meta-analysis by Alexander Jarde et al. reported no significant impact of probiotics on GDM risk (RR: 1.25, 95% CI: 0.61–2.56) [40]. Similarly, Pellonperä et al. evaluated probiotics combined with fish oil supplementation in overweight women and found no significant differences in GDM rates between intervention groups [41]. Furthermore, a Cochrane review of six trials with 1440 participants concluded that probiotics did not significantly lower the risk of GDM (RR: 0.80, 95% CI: 0.54–1.20) [42]. Likewise, a recent meta-analysis by Zhang et al., including six RCTs, confirmed no significant benefits of probiotic supplementation for preventing GDM (OR: 0.68, 95% CI: 0.39–1.20, *P*-value = 0.18) [43].

While some studies suggest that probiotics may play a role in reducing the risk of GDM, particularly in high-risk populations, the evidence remains inconclusive. Variability in probiotic strains, dosages, study designs, and patient populations is likely to contribute to these conflicting results. There is no consistent and reliable data to support their routine use in clinical practice for preventing GDM. Further clinical trials should continue to conclude of probiotics efficacy for this use..

11.4 Metformin as a Preventive Strategy for Gestational Diabetes Mellitus

Metformin, a well-established treatment for type 2 diabetes, has been explored for its potential role in preventing GDM. By improving insulin sensitivity and reducing hepatic glucose production, metformin may help regulate glucose levels during pregnancy [44]. While its role in preventing and delaying the occurrence of type 2 diabetes mellitus in women with or without a history of GDM is well-documented in the literature [45, 46], its efficacy in preventing GDM specifically remains less clear.

A meta-analysis by Yu et al. focused on high-risk populations, including women with PCOS, obesity, or pregestational insulin resistance. This study, which included 20 trials with 3911 participants, found that prophylactic metformin significantly reduced the incidence of GDM compared to control treatments (RR: 0.59, 95% CI: 0.43–0.80). Subgroup analyses demonstrated even greater reductions in Asian populations, women with PCOS, and those receiving higher doses of metformin (>1000 mg). However, among women with obesity, the analysis did not show a statistically significant reduction in GDM incidence with metformin treatment (RR: 0.73, 95% CI: 0.49–1.07, P-value = 0.105) [47]. Additionally, Zhao et al. analyzed six studies, including three RCTs and three observational studies with 643 women. They showed a significant reduction in GDM development among women with PCOS receiving metformin (log OR: -1.27, 95% CI: −2.24—0.30) [48]. In contrast, Zhuo et al. conducted a meta-analysis of 13 studies (five RCTs and eight non-RCTs) on women with PCOS, which showed conflicting results: While the RCTs found no significant effect of metformin on GDM prevention (OR: 1.07, 95% CI: 0.60–1.92), the non-RCTs indicated a significant reduction in GDM incidence (OR: 0.19, 95% CI: 0.13–0.27) [49]. These discrepancies may reflect differences in study design, population characteristics, and methodology.

While the evidence for metformin's role in preventing GDM is promising, it remains inconclusive, with variability in results across studies. The data suggest that metformin is most effective in high-risk groups. Furthermore, metformin's proven long-term efficacy in preventing type 2 diabetes highlights its potential for broader applications. Unlike type 2 diabetes, where intervention typically spans extended periods, the relatively short duration of treatment during pregnancy may limit metformin's preventive effects for GDM. Initiating treatment earlier, potentially even in the preconception period, may enhance its effectiveness in preventing GDM and improving pregnancy outcomes.

11.5 Myo-inositol and Its Potential in GDM Prevention

Myo-inositol, a naturally occurring carbohydrate, has gained significant attention for its potential role in improving insulin sensitivity and regulating glucose metabolism, making it a promising candidate for preventing GDM [18, 50]. A meta-analysis by Motuhifonua et al. involving seven RCTs and 1319 women reported a 47% reduction in the risk of GDM among women who received myo-inositol supplementation (RR: 0.53, 95% CI: 0.31–0.90) [51]. Similarly, Wei et al. reviewed seven RCTs and found a 70% reduction in GDM risk (RR: 0.30, 95% CI: 0.18–0.49) among women who took 4 grams of myo-inositol daily, alongside significant improvements in fasting glucose levels and glucose tolerance during pregnancy [52]. A review by Crawford et al., which included four RCTs with 567 women who were less than 24 weeks pregnant, also found that myo-inositol supplementation reduced the incidence of GDM compared to controls (RR: 0.43, 95% CI: 0.29–0.64) [53]. A collection of meta-analyses highlights the potential of myo-inositol supplementation in reducing GDM risk. Guo et al. (586 participants) reported a 56% reduction in GDM risk (RR: 0.44, 95% CI: 0.32–0.62) with a number needed to treat of seven, alongside improvements in fasting glucose and OGTT results [54]. Similarly, Vitagliano et al. (965 participants) and Liu et al. (involving data from eight RCTs) demonstrated reductions in GDM incidence ranging from 51% to 60% (OR: 0.49, 95% CI: 0.24–1.03, and OR: 0.40, 95% CI: 0.19–0.84, respectively), underscoring the potential of myo-inositol to significantly lower GDM rates [55, 56].

While myo-inositol supplementation has shown promise in some studies, a comprehensive network meta-analysis, which included 46 RCTs involving 16,545 patients, found that it did not significantly reduce the risk of GDM compared to placebo (OR: 0.82, 95% CI: 0.43–1.56) [22].

In conclusion, there is still not enough data to support myo-inositol use to reduce the incidence of GDM, and further research is required.

11.6 Conclusion

Prevention of GDM has been explored by numerous studies and different methods. Lifestyle change, dietary and physical activity, probiotics, medical intervention, and supplementation were all evaluated. So far, no method has shown consistent effectiveness. PA remains the most supported strategy with the best results, with/without diet intervention. Early intervention, starting in the preconception period and sustained over time, is crucial for improving metabolic health and reducing GDM risk. Further research is needed to refine prevention strategies for this condition, which significantly affects maternal and future child health and carries a major economic burden.

Chapter Key Points

- Gestational diabetes mellitus (GDM) is common and linked to adverse maternal and fetal outcomes.
- Lifestyle interventions (diet and physical activity) show mixed evidence, but early/prepregnancy initiation is most beneficial.
- Physical activity demonstrates the strongest preventive effect, especially before and early in pregnancy.
- Probiotics show inconsistent results and are not recommended routinely.
- Metformin shows preventive benefit, mainly in high-risk groups such as PCOS.
- Myo-inositol demonstrates promising results, but evidence remains insufficient for routine use.

Chapter-End Summary

This chapter reviews strategies for preventing gestational diabetes mellitus, including lifestyle and dietary and physical activity interventions, as well as probiotics, metformin, and myo-inositol. While lifestyle and exercise interventions show the strongest evidence—particularly when initiated before or early in pregnancy—other approaches such as probiotics and inositol supplementation yield inconsistent results. Metformin demonstrates preventive benefit, mainly in high-risk populations such as women with PCOS. Overall, early intervention, risk stratification, and long-term metabolic health optimization are the cornerstones of GDM prevention, though further research is needed to clarify the effectiveness of several emerging strategies.

References

1. HAPO Study Cooperative Research Group, Metzger BE, Lowe LP, Dyer AR, Trimble ER, Chaovarindr U, Coustan DR, et al. Hyperglycemia and adverse pregnancy outcomes. N Engl J Med. 2008;358(19):1991–2002.
2. ACOG. Practice bulletin no. 190: gestational diabetes mellitus. Obstet Gynecol. 2018;131(2):e49–64.
3. Sacks DA, Hadden DR, Maresh M, Deerochanawong C, Dyer AR, Metzger BE, HAPO Study Cooperative Research Group, et al. Frequency of gestational diabetes mellitus at collaborating centers based on IADPSG consensus panel-recommended criteria: the Hyperglycemia and Adverse Pregnancy Outcome (HAPO) study. Diabetes Care. 2012;35(3):526–8.
4. Zhu Y, Zhang C. Prevalence of gestational diabetes and risk of progression to type 2 diabetes: a global perspective. Curr Diab Rep. 2016;16(1):7.
5. Casagrande SS, Linder B, Cowie CC. Prevalence of gestational diabetes and subsequent type 2 diabetes among U.S. women. Diabetes Res Clin Pract. 2018;141:200–8.
6. Modzelewski R, Stefanowicz-Rutkowska MM, Matuszewski W, Bandurska-Stankiewicz EM. Gestational diabetes mellitus-recent literature review. J Clin Med. 2022;11(19):5736.
7. Wang H, Li N, Chivese T, Werfalli M, Sun H, Yuen L, IDF Diabetes Atlas Committee Hyperglycaemia in Pregnancy Special Interest Group, et al. IDF diabetes atlas: estimation of global and regional gestational diabetes mellitus prevalence for 2021 by International Association of Diabetes in Pregnancy Study Group's Criteria. Diabetes Res Clin Pract. 2022;183:109050.
8. Sacks DB, Arnold M, Bakris GL, Bruns DE, Horvath AR, Lernmark Å, et al. Guidelines and recommendations for laboratory analysis in the diagnosis and management of diabetes mellitus. Diabetes Care. 2023;46(10):e151–99.
9. American Diabetes Association Professional Practice Committee. 2. Diagnosis and classification of diabetes: standards of Care in Diabetes-2024. Diabetes Care. 2024;47(Suppl 1):S20–42.
10. US Preventive Services Task Force, Davidson KW, Barry MJ, Mangione CM, Cabana M, Caughey AB, Davis EM, et al. Screening for gestational diabetes: US Preventive Services Task Force recommendation statement. JAMA. 2021;326(6):531–8.
11. Crowther CA, Hiller JE, Moss JR, McPhee AJ, Jeffries WS, Robinson JS, Australian Carbohydrate Intolerance Study in Pregnant Women (ACHOIS) Trial Group. Effect of treatment of gestational diabetes mellitus on pregnancy outcomes. N Engl J Med. 2005;352(24):2477–86.
12. Langer O, Yogev Y, Most O, Xenakis EM. Gestational diabetes: the consequences of not treating. Am J Obstet Gynecol. 2005;192(4):989–97.
13. Landon MB, Spong CY, Thom E, Carpenter MW, Ramin SM, Casey B, Eunice Kennedy Shriver National Institute of Child Health and Human Development Maternal-Fetal Medicine Units Network, et al. A multicenter, randomized trial of treatment for mild gestational diabetes. N Engl J Med. 2009;361(14):1339–48.

14. Hoover EA, Louis JM. Optimizing health: weight, exercise, and nutrition in pregnancy and beyond. Obstet Gynecol Clin N Am. 2019;46(3):431–40.
15. Phelan S. Pregnancy: a "teachable moment" for weight control and obesity prevention. Am J Obstet Gynecol. 2010;202(2):135.e1–8.
16. Langer O. Prevention of obesity and diabetes in pregnancy: is it an impossible dream? Am J Obstet Gynecol. 2018;218(6):581–9.
17. Zhang C, Rawal S, Chong YS. Risk factors for gestational diabetes: is prevention possible? Diabetologia. 2016;59(7):1385–90.
18. Mierzyński R, Poniedziałek-Czajkowska E, Sotowski M, Szydełko-Gorzkowicz M. Nutrition as prevention factor of gestational diabetes mellitus: a narrative review. Nutrients. 2021;13(11):3787.
19. Sampathkumar S, Parkhi D, Ghebremichael-Weldeselassie Y, Sukumar N, Saravanan P. Effectiveness of pre-pregnancy lifestyle in preventing gestational diabetes mellitus-a systematic review and meta-analysis of 257,876 pregnancies. Nutr Diabetes. 2023;13(1):22.
20. Tuomilehto J, Lindström J, Eriksson JG, Valle TT, Hämäläinen H, Ilanne-Parikka P, Finnish Diabetes Prevention Study Group, et al. Prevention of type 2 diabetes mellitus by changes in lifestyle among subjects with impaired glucose tolerance. N Engl J Med. 2001;344(18):1343–50.
21. Zito G, Della Corte L, Giampaolino P, Terzic M, Terzic S, Di Guardo F, et al. Gestational diabetes mellitus: prevention, diagnosis and treatment. A fresh look to a busy corner. J Neonatal Perinatal Med. 2020;13(4):529–41.
22. Tang Q, Zhong Y, Xu C, Li W, Wang H, Hou Y. Effectiveness of five interventions used for prevention of gestational diabetes: a network meta-analysis. Medicine (Baltimore). 2022;101(15):e29126.
23. Bain E, Crane M, Tieu J, Han S, Crowther CA, Middleton P. Diet and exercise interventions for preventing gestational diabetes mellitus. Cochrane Database Syst Rev. 2015;4:CD010443.
24. Wu S, Jin J, Hu KL, Wu Y, Zhang D. Prevention of gestational diabetes mellitus and gestational weight gain restriction in overweight/obese pregnant women: a systematic review and network meta-analysis. Nutrients. 2022;14(12):2383.
25. Koivusalo SB, Rönö K, Klemetti MM, Roine RP, Lindström J, Erkkola M, et al. Gestational diabetes mellitus can be prevented by lifestyle intervention: the Finnish gestational diabetes prevention study (RADIEL): a randomized controlled trial. Diabetes Care. 2016;39(1):24–30.
26. Sanabria-Martínez G, García-Hermoso A, Poyatos-León R, Álvarez-Bueno C, Sánchez-López M, Martínez-Vizcaíno V. Effectiveness of physical activity interventions on preventing gestational diabetes mellitus and excessive maternal weight gain: a meta-analysis. BJOG. 2015;122(9):1167–74.
27. Song C, Li J, Leng J, Ma RC, Yang X. Lifestyle intervention can reduce the risk of gestational diabetes: a meta-analysis of randomized controlled trials. Obes Rev. 2016;17(10):960–9.
28. Tobias DK, Zhang C, van Dam RM, Bowers K, Hu FB. Physical activity before and during pregnancy and risk of gestational diabetes mellitus: a meta-analysis. Diabetes Care. 2011;34(1):223–9.
29. Yin YN, Li XL, Tao TJ, Luo BR, Liao SJ. Physical activity during pregnancy and the risk of gestational diabetes mellitus: a systematic review and meta-analysis of randomised controlled trials. Br J Sports Med. 2014;48(4):290–5.
30. Stafne SN, Salvesen KÅ, Romundstad PR, Eggebø TM, Carlsen SM, Mørkved S. Regular exercise during pregnancy to prevent gestational diabetes: a randomized controlled trial. Obstet Gynecol. 2012;119(1):29–36.
31. Han S, Middleton P, Crowther CA. Exercise for pregnant women for preventing gestational diabetes mellitus. Cochrane Database Syst Rev. 2012;2012(7):CD009021.
32. Zeevi D, Korem T, Zmora N, Israeli D, Rothschild D, Weinberger A, et al. Personalized nutrition by prediction of glycemic responses. Cell. 2015;163(5):1079–94.
33. Kamińska K, Stenclik D, Błażejewska W, Bogdański P, Moszak M. Probiotics in the prevention and treatment of gestational diabetes mellitus (GDM): a review. Nutrients. 2022;14(20):4303.
34. Plows JF, Reynolds CM, Vickers MH, Baker PN, Stanley JL. Nutritional supplementation for the prevention and/or treatment of gestational diabetes mellitus. Curr Diab Rep. 2019;19(9):73.
35. Tsarna E, Christopoulos P. The role of gut microbiome in prevention, diagnosis and treatment of gestational diabetes mellitus. J Obstet Gynaecol. 2022;42(5):719–25.
36. Homayouni A, Bagheri N, Mohammad-Alizadeh-Charandabi S, Kashani N, Mobaraki-Asl N, Mirghafurvand M, et al. Prevention of gestational diabetes mellitus (GDM) and probiotics: mechanism of action: a review. Curr Diabetes Rev. 2020;16(6):538–45.
37. Wickens KL, Barthow CA, Murphy R, Abels PR, Maude RM, Stone PR, et al. Early pregnancy probiotic supplementation with Lactobacillus rhamnosus HN001 may reduce the prevalence of gestational diabetes mellitus: a randomised controlled trial. Br J Nutr. 2017;117(6):804–13.
38. Luoto R, Laitinen K, Nermes M, Isolauri E. Impact of maternal probiotic-supplemented dietary counselling on pregnancy outcome and prenatal and postnatal growth: a double-blind, placebo-controlled study. Br J Nutr. 2010;103(12):1792–9.
39. Callaway LK, McIntyre HD, Barrett HL, Foxcroft K, Tremellen A, Lingwood BE, et al. Probiotics for the prevention of gestational diabetes mellitus in overweight and obese women: findings from the

SPRING double-blind randomized controlled trial. Diabetes Care. 2019;42(3):364–71.
40. Jarde A, Lewis-Mikhael AM, Moayyedi P, Stearns JC, Collins SM, Beyene J. Pregnancy outcomes in women taking probiotics or prebiotics: a systematic review and meta-analysis. BMC Pregnancy Childbirth. 2018;18(1):14.
41. Pellonperä O, Mokkala K, Houttu N, Vahlberg T, Koivuniemi E, Tertti K, et al. Efficacy of fish oil and/or probiotic intervention on the incidence of gestational diabetes mellitus in an at-risk group of overweight and obese women: a randomized, placebo-controlled, double-blind clinical trial. Diabetes Care. 2019;42(6):1009–17.
42. Davidson SJ, Barrett HL, Price SA, Callaway LK, Dekker Nitert M. Probiotics for preventing gestational diabetes. Cochrane Database Syst Rev. 2021;4(4):CD009951.
43. Zhang Z, Niu R, Zhang H, Ma T, Chen X, Pan L. Probiotic supplement for the prevention of gestational diabetes: a meta-analysis of randomized controlled trials. Z Geburtshilfe Neonatol. 2023;227(1):24–30.
44. Romero R, Erez O, Hüttemann M, Maymon E, Panaitescu B, Conde-Agudelo A, et al. Metformin, the aspirin of the 21st century: its role in gestational diabetes mellitus, prevention of preeclampsia and cancer, and the promotion of longevity. Am J Obstet Gynecol. 2017;217(3):282–302.
45. Aroda VR, Christophi CA, Edelstein SL, Zhang P, Herman WH, Barrett-Connor E, Diabetes Prevention Program Research Group, et al. The effect of lifestyle intervention and metformin on preventing or delaying diabetes among women with and without gestational diabetes: the diabetes prevention program outcomes study 10-year follow-up. J Clin Endocrinol Metab. 2015;100(4):1646–53.
46. Ratner RE, Christophi CA, Metzger BE, Dabelea D, Bennett PH, Pi-Sunyer X, Diabetes Prevention Program Research Group, et al. Prevention of diabetes in women with a history of gestational diabetes: effects of metformin and lifestyle interventions. J Clin Endocrinol Metab. 2008;93(12):4774–9.
47. Yu H, Sun J, Hu H. Prophylactic administration of metformin reduces gestational diabetes mellitus incidence in the high-risk populations: a meta-analysis: metformin for gestational diabetes prevention. Ir J Med Sci. 2024;193(1):199–209.
48. Zhao J, Liu X, Zhang W. The effect of metformin therapy for preventing gestational diabetes mellitus in women with polycystic ovary syndrome: a meta-analysis. Exp Clin Endocrinol Diabetes. 2020;128(3):199–205.
49. Zhuo Z, Wang A, Yu H. Effect of metformin intervention during pregnancy on the gestational diabetes mellitus in women with polycystic ovary syndrome: a systematic review and meta-analysis. J Diabetes Res. 2014;2014:381231.
50. Noventa M, Vitagliano A, Quaranta M, Borgato S, Abdulrahim B, Gizzo S. Preventive and therapeutic role of dietary inositol supplementation in periconceptional period and during pregnancy: a summary of evidences and future applications. Reprod Sci. 2016;23(3):278–88.
51. Motuhifonua SK, Lin L, Alsweiler J, Crawford TJ, Crowther CA. Antenatal dietary supplementation with myo-inositol for preventing gestational diabetes. Cochrane Database Syst Rev. 2023;2(2):CD011507.
52. Wei J, Yan J, Yang H. Inositol nutritional supplementation for the prevention of gestational diabetes mellitus: a systematic review and meta-analysis of randomized controlled trials. Nutrients. 2022;14(14):2831.
53. Crawford TJ, Crowther CA, Alsweiler J, Brown J. Antenatal dietary supplementation with myo-inositol in women during pregnancy for preventing gestational diabetes. Cochrane Database Syst Rev. 2015;2015(12):CD011507.
54. Guo X, Guo S, Miao Z, Li Z, Zhang H. Myo-inositol lowers the risk of developing gestational diabetic mellitus in pregnancies: a systematic review and meta-analysis of randomized controlled trials with trial sequential analysis. J Diabetes Complicat. 2018;32(3):342–8.
55. Vitagliano A, Saccone G, Cosmi E, Visentin S, Dessole F, Ambrosini G, et al. Inositol for the prevention of gestational diabetes: a systematic review and meta-analysis of randomized controlled trials. Arch Gynecol Obstet. 2019;299(1):55–68.
56. Liu Q, Liu Z. The efficacy of myo-inositol supplementation to reduce the incidence of gestational diabetes: a meta-analysis. Gynecol Endocrinol. 2022;38(6):450–4.

Antenatal Corticosteroids for the Prevention of Mortality and Morbidity in Preterm Infants

Nir Melamed and Elizabeth Asztalos

Contents

Y. Yogev, A. Khalil (eds.), *Prevention of Complications in Obstetrics*,
https://doi.org/10.1007/978-3-032-23479-7_12

What You Will Learn in This Chapter

Preterm birth is the leading cause of neonatal mortality and morbidity. Antenatal corticosteroids (ACS) for fetal lung maturation are the single most effective intervention for the prevention of mortality and morbidity in preterm infants. In the current chapter, we will review the rationale, mechanism of action, optimal use, and current recommendations of professional societies regarding ACS.

Learning Objectives

- Explain the ACS mechanism and rationale
- Describe evidence of benefits across gestational ages
- Identify potential short- and long-term risks
- Compare ACS use in specific subgroups
- Discuss dosing regimens and emerging alternatives
- Understand optimal timing and strategies to improve appropriate use
- Evaluate evidence on repeat and rescue courses

Learning Objectives

- Understand the rationale behind using ACS for fetal lung maturation.
- Describe how ACS promotes fetal lung development and enhances lung function.
- Identify the effects of ACS on both respiratory and non-respiratory neonatal short- and long-term morbidities.
- Discuss the benefits of ACS across different gestational age periods.
- Recognize the potential short- and long-term risks to infants exposed to ACS in utero.
- Understand the benefits and risks of ACS in specific subgroups.
- Identify the different types of ACS used in antenatal care and understand the efficacy and safety of different ACS regimens.
- Understand the optimal timing for ACS administration and discuss strategies to optimize ACS timing.

12.1 Introduction

12.1.1 Prevalence and Impact of Preterm Birth

Preterm birth (PTB), defined as any infant born alive before 37 weeks of pregnancy, is the leading cause of neonatal mortality and morbidity [67]. Preterm births are further categorized based on the gestational age at the time of birth as extremely PTB (<28 weeks), very PTB (28 weeks to <32 weeks), moderate PTB (32 weeks to <34 weeks), and late PTB (34 weeks to <37 weeks) [125]. It is estimated that 13.4 million babies were born too early in 2020. This is more than 1 in 10 babies. Approximately 900,000 children died in 2019 of complications related to a PTB [125]. Many survivors face a lifetime of disability, including learning disabilities and visual and hearing problems.

The majority of preterm births occur in southern Asia and sub-Saharan Africa, but PTB is truly a global problem. There is a dramatic difference in the survival of preterm babies depending on where they are born. Inequalities in survival rates around the world are striking. In low-income settings, half of the babies born at ≤32 weeks die due to a lack of feasible, cost-effective care such as warmth, breastfeeding support, and basic care for infections and breathing difficulties, yet less than 10% of extremely preterm babies die in high-income settings. Consequently, the approaches to this global problem may vary by region.

Globally, prematurity is the leading cause of death in children under the age of 5 years [127]. Yet, in high-income countries, almost all these babies survive. In addition, suboptimal use of technology in middle-income settings is causing an increased burden of disability among preterm babies who survive the neonatal period.

While research is underway to identify factors contributing to PTB, treatments are available to help protect the preterm infant from common neonatal complications, which include breathing difficulties and infections. These include the provision of positive pressure support and medicines like caffeine to assist in breathing, as well as kangaroo care and the provision of breast milk. However, from the obstetrical side, the single most effective intervention available to reduce the risk of mortality and morbidity of preterm infants is the administration of antenatal corticosteroids (ACS) to improve fetal lung maturation.

12.1.2 Antenatal Corticosteroids: Historical Perspective and Rationale

In 1972, the first trial evaluating ACS was published by Liggins and Howie, demonstrating the use of ACS to reduce respiratory distress syndrome (RDS) in preterm infants. In this study, which randomized 1142 women to ACS vs. placebo, RDS was reduced from 26% to 9%, and mortality was reduced from 11% to 6% in the ACS group [89]. Over the next 20 years, a number of trials took place to confirm and validate the findings of this historic trial. By the early 1990s, a consensus statement was issued in many countries that ACS should be considered standard treatment for any pregnant patients between 24 and 34 weeks of gestation who were considered to be at risk of PTB (1994).

12

The initial Liggins and Howie trial used betamethasone as a 1:1 mixture of betamethasone phosphate and betamethasone acetate (currently available as Celestone), as did most of the subsequent trials [89]. The regimen, consisting of two doses of 12 mg given at a 24-hour interval, was empirically chosen by Liggins and Howie [89]. Despite clear evidence of the effectiveness of this therapy, this regimen has never been rigorously tested in clinical studies but has become the standard practice. Trials to evaluate different aspects of ACS treatment, including the dose or frequency, are only now slowly being considered. In addition, the analysis from this initial trial indicated that the effectiveness of ACS peaked from 2 to 7 days after the first dose, suggesting that patients receiving ACS would be considered to have completed a course of ACS after 48 hours and that the optimal timing of administration is within 7 days before birth.

12.2 Mechanism of Action of Antenatal Corticosteroids

12.2.1 Impact on Fetal Lung Development

As pregnancy progresses toward term, the fetal hypothalamic-pituitary axis (HPA) becomes activated. This critical developmental process results in a fetal adrenal glucocorticoid surge, which is an essential component of lung maturation in the developing fetus. The glucocorticoid surge acts on the type 2 pneumocytes, resulting in a transient increase in surfactant production. In addition, this endogenous glucocorticoid surge enhances lung compliance and volume by promoting persistent structural maturation of the lung parenchyma, reducing vascular permeability, and increasing clearance of lung water, all to facilitate adequate transition in respiration upon birth at term gestation [19, 63, 69, 81, 189]. Fetal 11β-hydroxysteroid dehydrogenase-2 is an enzyme that is heavily concentrated in the placenta and the fetal brain and has the capacity to metabolize cortisol into inactive metabolites. It is a natural fetal protective buffer to any surges in maternal glucocorticoids and only allows fetal glucocorticoids to drive fetal maturation [148].

It is these principles that helped to understand how ACS functions in the fetal environment. ACS therapy is known to be resistant to the fetal 11β-hydroxysteroid dehydrogenase-2 buffer and effectively reach its target organ, the fetal lung. ACS have the same action as seen with endogenous fetal cortisol of increasing the production of surfactant and promoting structural changes in the lungs, which in turn reduces the incidence of life-threatening respiratory conditions in the event of a PTB.

Repeated meta-analyses and systematic reviews have supported this finding that ACS administration before an anticipated PTB is associated with a reduction in perinatal death, neonatal death, acute respiratory distress, and, indirectly, severe intraventricular hemorrhage (IVH) [94].

12.2.2 Non-pulmonary Effects

During predetermined periods of fetal development, the fetal HPA axis is responsible for glucocorticoid surges to facilitate normal organ maturation in preparation for a term birth. However, precocious activation of the glucocorticoid receptors can be induced by endogenous cortisol release in response to an adverse intrauterine environment, yielding a stress response in the fetus that promotes early release of glucocorticoids. If a stressor results in a significant period of elevated fetal glucocorticoid concentrations, this can lead to permanent maladaptive changes after birth and predispose the infant to an increased risk of physical and mental disease and form the basis of the process referred to as "developmental programming."[24, 60, 135].

A similar scenario can take place when synthetic glucocorticoids such as ACS are administered to mothers at risk of PTB. This results in the activation of a number of fetal glucocorticoid receptors on a wide variety of fetal organs, most importantly, the fetal brain. Glucocorticoids are central to all aspects of brain and neuronal development and maturation. Abnormal glucocorticoid elevations, such as in the case of ACS administration, can lead to abnormal processes/programming in fetal brain development and maturation, particularly in the hippocampus, hypothalamus, and pituitary gland. The precise pathways are unclear but are felt to be related to abnormal DNA methylation in response to elevated glucocorticoids presented to the developing fetus [24]. Prolonged or unnecessary fetal exposure to ACS may contribute to a negative "programming" signal to the fetus and set the stage for long-term effects in the child [80].

12.3 Evidence on the Benefits of Antenatal Corticosteroids

12.3.1 Neonatal Mortality and Morbidity

RDS is a serious complication of PTB and remains the primary cause of early neonatal death and childhood disability in many countries worldwide. It can affect up to 50% of infants born before 28 weeks of gestation and up to 30% of those infants born under 32 weeks of gestation. Of note, up to 42% of infants under 1500 grams will have RDS [74]. RDS is secondary to a qualitative and quantitative surfactant deficiency. In the 20 years following the initial trial by Liggins and Howie, repeated reviews showed that ACS given before a PTB was effective in preventing significant RDS and reducing perinatal and neonatal mortality [48, 139]. Corticosteroids appear to exert major vasoconstrictive effects on fetal cerebral blood flow, protecting the fetus against IVH at rest and when challenged by conditions causing vasodilation, such as hypercapnia. This contributes to a reduction of IVH in the first few days after birth. In the most recently published meta-analysis, ACS were associated with a significant reduction in neonatal death (RR 0.78 [95% CI 0.70–0.87]), RDS (RR 0.71 [95% CI 0.65–0.78]), and IVH (RR 0.58 [95% CI 0.45–0.75]) [94]. ACS do not affect evolving chronic lung disease. These beneficial effects of ACS on the risk of neonatal mortality and severe neurological injury among extremely preterm infants have been shown to remain stable over the past decades despite the ongoing improvements in neonatal care of preterm infants [103].

12.3.2 Neurodevelopmental Outcomes in Early Childhood

In a review that evaluated studies comparing a single course of ACS to either no treatment or a placebo, a single course of ACS was found to increase the rates of intact survival and reduce the rates of severe disability, cerebral palsy, and a psychomotor developmental index less than 70 [163]. No difference was found in the rate of minor disability or the full, verbal, or performance IQ on the Wechsler Intelligence Scale in early childhood. These findings are consistent with the biological concept that improved respiratory performance of preterm neonates facilitates the use of ventilation techniques that are associated with a lower rate of IVH and motor impairment in infancy. The comparable scores in the Wechsler Intelligence Scale suggest that ACS do not have a measurable negative effect on the maturation of higher brain functions. However, few studies have evaluated children consistently to allow for clearer comparisons. In summary, data from randomized as well as non-randomized studies suggest that a single course of ACS administered in pregnancies where the fetus is born preterm is associated with improved rates of intact survival and severe disability compared with no ACS.

12.3.3 Benefits by Gestational Period

Overall, exposure to ACS is associated with lower rates of mortality and serious neonatal morbidities and is recommended by all professional societies between $24^{0/7}$ and $33^{6/7}$ weeks (◘ Table 12.1). However, the benefits of ACS on specific outcomes vary by gestational age. A large prospective cohort study from the United States examined the association of ACS with a range of outcomes by gestational age at birth in a cohort of 117,941 infants born between $23^{0/7}$ and $34^{6/7}$ weeks [171]. Exposure to ACS was associated with a reduction in neonatal mortality at nearly all gestational weeks (23–29, 31, 33, and 34 weeks), but the number needed to treat increased sharply from 6 at 23–24 weeks to 798 at 34 weeks. ACS were also associated with a reduction in the risk of severe intracranial hemorrhage or death at 23–31 weeks, the risk of stage ≥2 necrotizing enterocolitis or death at 23–30 weeks, and the risk of retinopathy of prematurity or death at 23–29 weeks. Finally, ACS were associated with survival without major hospital morbidity only among infants born at 23, 24, 26, and 27 weeks [171].

12.3.3.1 Periviable Period (22–25 Weeks)

In the trials that followed the initial trial by Liggins and Howie, only a small proportion of them included infants born at or before 28 weeks. However, with the improvement of not only perinatal but also neonatal management, fetuses at risk of PTB between 24 and 27 completed weeks are now routinely exposed to current obstetrical and neonatal care. Large data sets from research and clinical care groups provide information to evaluate ACS treatment for extremely preterm infants. Unlike clinical trials, these data sets use death and neurodevelopmental outcomes to evaluate ACS treatment for very preterm pregnancies. In all, infants exposed to ACS treatment were found to have decreased rates of mortality and IVH and improved neurodevelopmental outcomes by 24 months corrected age. Because of effective but limited evidence of action, decisions on utilizing ACS are based on the biological plausibility that ACS treatment will be effective in the extreme gestation period. The use of ACS treatment for these extreme preterm pregnancies at risk is, in general, 80–90% of pregnancies presenting at 24–25 weeks of gestation and almost 60% at 23 weeks of gestation. An advantage to ACS treatment is less certain at 22 weeks of gestation [38, 73, 111, 171, 174]. Several professional societies recommend consideration of ACS for pregnancies at risk of PTB at 22 and 23 weeks of gestation (◘ Table 12.1). Thus, discussion at the early gestation of 22–23 weeks should include the utilization of ACS should active neonatal care be considered in the event of a PTB.

12.3.3.2 Later Preterm Period ($34^{0/7}$–$36^{6/7}$ Weeks)

Late preterm infants ($34^{0/7}$–$36^{6/7}$ weeks) have an increased risk of respiratory and neurodevelopmental complications compared to term infants, but the absolute risk is low (11–12%). However, the burden presented by this group of preterm infants is high because the majority (>70%) of preterm births worldwide are in this group of infants. The most notable clinical trial to evaluate the benefits of ACS in this group of preterm infants was the Antenatal Late Preterm Steroids trial (ALPS), which included patients with a singleton pregnancy at risk for a PTB between $34^{0/7}$ and $36^{5/7}$ weeks [70]. Patients were randomized to receive a course of ACS (beta-

Table 12.1 Recommendations of professional societies regarding the administration of antenatal corticosteroids

Society	Gestational age				Subpopulations			Repeated courses	Regimen
	Periviable period	24 + 0 to 33 + 6 weeks	Late preterm period	Planned CS at term	PPROM	Fetal growth restriction	Twins		
United States									
ACOG 2020, 2021 [6, 47]	Consider at 22 + 0 to 23 + 6 weeks	Yes	Yes (34 + 0 to 36 + 6 weeks) Not if chorioamnionitis		No change	No change	No change	A single repeat course until 34 + 0 weeks If >7–14 days from prior course	**Betamethasone** 12 mg IM 2 doses q24h **Dexamethasone** 6 mg IM 4 doses q12h
SMFM 2021 [160]			Yes (34 + 0 to 36 + 6 weeks), if: Singleton pregnancies Dilation ≥3 cm or effacement ≥75% No pregestational diabetes Avoid tocolysis to delay delivery						**Betamethasone** 12 mg IM 2 doses q24h
Canada									
SOGC 2018, 2023 [88, 156]	Consider at 22 + 0 to 23 + 6 weeks	Yes	Consider based on absolute harms and benefits specific to the gestational week. Not if pregestational diabetes	No	No change	No change	No change	Not recommended routinely	**Betamethasone** 12 mg IM 2 doses q24h **Dexamethasone** 6 mg IM 4 doses q12h

(continued)

■ **Table 12.1** (continued)

Society	Gestational age				Subpopulations			Repeated courses	Regimen
United Kingdom									
RCOG 2022 [165]	Consider at <24 + 0 weeks	Yes	Offer up to 34 + 6 weeks. Consider 35 + 0 to 36 + 6 weeks	Consider at 37 + 0 to 38 + 6 weeks	No change	No change	No change	Should be discussed if >7 days from prior course. No more than three courses	**Dexametha-sone** <u>12 mg IM 2 dose q24h</u> OR 6 mg IM 4 doses q12h **Betametha-sone** 12 mg IM 2 doses q24h
NICE 2022 [7]	Consider at 22 + 0 to 23 + 6 weeks	Yes	Consider 34 + 0 to 35 + 6 weeks		No change	No change	No change	A single repeat course Until 34 + 0 weeks If >7 days from prior course If <30w or FGR, consider the potential impact on fetal growth	
Australia and New Zealand									
RAN-ZCOG 2015 [5]		Yes	Up to 34 + 6 weeks		No change	No change	No change	A single repeat dose or course Until 32 + 6 weeks If >7 days from prior course	**Betametha-sone** 12 mg IM 2 doses q24h **Dexametha-sone** 6 mg IM 4 doses q12h

Society	Gestational age				Subpopulations			Repeated courses	Regimen
Interna-tional									
FIGO 2021 [122]	Consider	Yes (up to 34 + 0 weeks)	No	No	No change	Insuf-ficient evidence	No change	A single repeat course Until 34 + 0 weeks If >7 days from prior course If delivery is anticipated within the next 72 h	**Betametha-sone** 12 mg IM 2 doses q24h **Dexametha-sone** 12 mg IM 2 doses q24h
WHO 2022 [8, 182]		Yes (up to 34 + 0 weeks)	No	No	No change (unless chorio-amnionitis)	No change	No change	A single repeat course if >7 days from prior course	**Betamethasone** 12 mg IM 2 doses q24h **Dexametha-sone** 6 mg IM 4 doses q12h

CS cesarean section, *PPROM* preterm pre-labor rupture of membranes, *ACOG* American College of Obstetricians and Gynecologists, *SMFM* Society for Maternal-Fetal Medicine, *SOGC* Society of Obstetricians and Gynecologists of Canada, *RCOG* Royal College of Obstetricians and Gynecologists; National Institute for Health and Care Excellence, *RANZCOG* Royal Australian and New Zealand College of Obstetricians and Gynecologists, *FIGO* The International Federation of Gynecology and Obstetrics, *WHO* Word Health Organization methasone) or a placebo. The primary outcome was a composite of treatment in the first 72 hours (the use of continuous positive airway pressure or high-flow nasal cannula for at least 2 h, supplemental oxygen with a fraction of inspired oxygen of at least 0.30 for at least 4 h, extracorporeal membrane oxygenation, or mechanical ventilation) or stillbirth or neonatal death within 72 h after delivery. The risk of the primary outcome was significantly lower in the ACS group (11.6% vs. 14.4%, RR 0.80 [95%-CI 0.66–0.97]). This finding was mainly driven by a reduction in the need for continuous positive airway pressure or supplemental oxygen due to transient tachypnea of the newborn (TTN), which is viewed in neonatal care as a mild, self-limited condition. There were no differences between the groups in the risk of neonatal mortality, RDS, neonatal intensive care unit admission, pneumothorax, or mechanical ventilation. Of note, ACS was associated with an increased risk of neonatal hypoglycemia (24.0% vs. 15.0%; RR 1.60 [95%-CI 1.37–1.87]). The findings of the trial and similar ones have been somewhat controversial since the incidence of significant RDS was not different between groups.

A recent secondary analysis of this trial quantified the risk reduction by gestational age at presentation and planned mode of delivery [43]. The benefit of ACS was greater for patients planned for cesarean compared with vaginal birth and decreased with gestational age at presentation. The absolute risk reduction was highest for those presenting at 34 weeks and planned for cesarean delivery (32.0% vs. 39.4%, risk difference – 7.3% [95%-CI -14.1% to –0.6%]) and lowest among those presenting at 36 weeks and planned for vaginal birth (5.6% vs. 6.9%, risk difference – 1.3% [95%-CI -2.5% to –0.1%]). This study suggests that the decision regarding the administration of ACS during the late preterm period may be adjusted by mode of delivery and gestational age.

We identified considerable variation in the recommendations of professional societies (◘ Table 12.1). In the United States, ACS is recommended throughout the late preterm period. In the United Kingdom, it is recommended that ACS be offered up to $34^{6/7}$ weeks and be considered up to $35^{6/7}$ or $36^{6/7}$ weeks. The Canadian guidelines recommend that the decision be discussed based on absolute harms and benefits specific to the gestational week, as described in the secondary analysis of the APLS study. In contrast, international societies do not support the administration of ACS during the late preterm period, in part due to the potential increased risk of neonatal hypoglycemia. Further information and, most notably, neurodevelopmental outcomes in childhood and beyond will help determine this approach to care in the future.

12.3.3.3 Early-Term Period ($37^{0/7}$–$38^{6/7}$ Weeks)

Early-term neonates ($37^{0/7}$–$38^{6/7}$ weeks) also have a slightly higher risk of RDS, primarily if born without labor in place. There have been a series of trials evaluating the role of ACS for a planned cesarean section at term gestation [162, 166]. Although some benefits were observed, consideration should be given to the difference between statistical significance and clinical significance, particularly in view of the very low event rates of significant respiratory morbidity in the early-term population [166]. At present, this approach has not been adopted by most obstetrical societies worldwide (◘ Table 12.1).

12.4 Emerging Concerns of Antenatal Corticosteroids

12.4.1 Maternal Risks

In general, ACS are safe for pregnant patients in high-income countries. Most reports have not identified an association with maternal complications, including death, endometritis, or chorioamnionitis [139]. However, evidence from low-income settings suggests that harm in the form of infectious complications may be increased. Further studies in low-income settings are needed to guide optimal administration [13].

12.4.2 Short-Term Risks for the Infant

ACS may have potential negative effects on the fetus/infant. There has been an association between ACS exposure and reduced infant anthropometry at birth. ACS exposure has been associated with a reduced head circumference by at least 0.6 cm at birth [36, 117, 142]. These can have consequences for the child later on. In addition, in late preterm pregnancies, ACS was associated with an increased risk of neonatal hypoglycemia, which, in itself, is associated with poor cognitive and motor function in early childhood [70, 95].

12.4.3 Long-Term Risks for the Child

Due to the limited precision in identifying patients "at risk for preterm birth," many patients may inappropriately receive ACS. Up to a third or even half of patients treated with ACS are noted to carry the pregnancy to term or near term, leading to many children being unnecessarily exposed to in-utero ACS without any benefit [119, 134]. The exposure to ACS in utero, coupled with the natural cortisol surge in late gestation, can potentially contribute to negative programming within the developing brain, HPA axis, and cardiometabolic functions, as previously described [135]. There is a growing body of information to suggest that term-born infants who have been exposed to ACS during pregnancy may be at increased risk of poor emotional and neurodevelopmental outcomes not only in infancy but also in early childhood. Clinical trials evaluating ACS have been difficult to interpret due to the need to separate preterm from term children; this holds true for the short-term benefits but, more importantly, long-term benefits or risks. However, a body of knowledge has been emerging. A long-term study evaluating the 5-year outcome of children born to the patients who participated in the Multiple Courses of Antenatal Corticosteroids for Preterm Birth Study (MACS-5 and MCAS, respectively) [20, 116] highlighted concerns regarding prolonged in-utero exposure to ACS [20]. Overall, MACS-5 showed no long-term benefits or risks between single or multiple courses of ACS. However, in both single and multiple ACS-exposed children, over 13% demonstrated abnormalities in neurobehavioral function, which is higher than reported for the general population. This increase was seen irrespective of the gestational age at birth, but most importantly, it was seen in term-born children. Furthermore, children born at term who received multiple courses of ACS exhibited negative effects with an increase in vision and hearing difficulties [16]. This increase in neurosensory difficulties may reflect the impaired myelination that has been identified in animal studies (sheep and rat), which evaluated optic and auditory nerve function following ACS exposure [41, 130]. The lack of a control group of infants unexposed to ACS, though, limited the interpretation of these findings. Still, these findings led to a signal of potential harm.

The Antenatal Steroids for Term Elective Cesarean Section (ASTECS) trial demonstrated that ACS given before an elective cesarean delivery at term reduced short-term respiratory morbidity. In the follow-up assessment for this trial, there were no differences in behavior and health for the subjects at 8–15 years of age [167]. However, though not statistically significant, there was an increased incidence of being in the lowest quarter of academic ability in the ACS group compared to the controls. Although there are limitations to the interpretation of these results, again, the signal for concern for potential difficulties is there.

More recently, population-based studies have explored the association between ACS exposure in term and also near-term-born children and neurodevelopmental challenges. Two important Canadian-based population studies evaluated over half a million term and over 25,000 near-term pregnancies. They revealed that these children, but more specifically those born at term gestation, were more likely to experience neurosensory and neurocognitive concerns by the age of 5 years [21, 101]. There has been a question as to whether familial confounders may play a role in explaining the associations. A study from Finland explored this relationship and found that ACS exposure was still significantly associated with a higher risk of mental and behavioral challenges than nonexposed sibling pairs [132]. A more recent study from the same group found that exposure to ACS was also associated with an increased hazard of disorders of speech and language, disorders of scholastic skills, disorders of motor function, pervasive developmental disorder, epilepsy, and cerebral palsy [133].

Finally, animal studies have shown that elevated levels of glucocorticoids, both endogenous and exogenous, can lead to altered programming of functions involving epigenetic processes in the limbic system, hypothalamus, and pituitary gland. This altered programming can contribute to the neurobehavioral dysfunction alluded to in the aforementioned studies but also affect HPA function on a long-term basis [108, 109].

Further studies are required to ascertain when ACS should be given and to whom in order to ensure the maximum benefit of the intervention with the minimum amount of harm to the fetus to minimize long-term concerns. The concerns about the long-term harm to the ACS-exposed fetus who is born beyond the period of greatest benefit from ACS, namely, the term-born fetus, are important signals that should not be ignored nor put aside.

12.5 Role of Antenatal Corticosteroids in Specific Groups

As described before, ACS reduces neonatal morbidity and mortality when administered to patients at risk of PTB between 24 and 34 weeks. However, certain subgroups of high-risk pregnancies have been traditionally excluded or underrepresented in most ACS trials. These include pregnancies complicated by fetal growth restriction (FGR), multifetal pregnancies, and pregnancies with preterm pre-labor rupture of membranes (PPROM). In addition to the limited evidence, the unique physiological and clinical characteristics of these pregnancies raise theoretical concerns that the balance between the benefits and risks of ACS in these subgroups may be different than observed in uncomplicated singleton preterm pregnancies.

12.5.1 Fetal Growth Restriction

The benefit of ACS in cases of FGR has been questioned based on reports showing already higher endogenous cortisol levels within this population compared with pregnancies of normally grown fetuses [56, 98, 112, 151]. In addition, the unique cardiovascular, hormonal, and metabolic characteristics of growth-restricted fetuses raised concerns that exposure to exogenous steroids may produce potentially harmful cardiovascular and metabolic effects in these already compromised fetuses [25, 30, 75, 138, 172, 180]. Indeed, ACS exposure has been shown to affect Doppler changes in growth-restricted fetuses, such as a transient increase in diastolic flow in the umbilical artery [141, 150, 154, 183] and the middle cerebral artery, [113, 128, 190], which have been attributed to peripheral vasodilatation and an increase in cardiac output and circulatory stress [97, 128].

Data from randomized trials on the benefits and risks of ACS in this population are limited, as most randomized controlled trials excluded pregnancies complicated by FGR due to the association between ACS and increased mortality within this subgroup originally reported by Liggins and Howie in the first randomized controlled trial on ACS [89]. Data from observational studies provided conflicting results [31, 58, 78, 87, 91, 107, 137, 144, 164, 170, 176]. However, many of these studies were small, did not account for potential confounding factors, and did not include a positive control group of normally grown fetuses that would allow for a direct comparison of the benefit of ACS between FGR and non-FGR fetuses. In a large population-based study from the Canadian Neonatal Network, we compared the association of ACS with neonatal outcomes when administered within the optimal interval of 1–7 days before birth, between small for gestational age (SGA) and appropriate for gestational age (AGA) fetuses. Exposure to ACS in SGA and AGA pregnancies was associated with a similar reduction in neonatal death (adjusted odds ratio [aOR] 0.27 [95%-CI 0.14–0.52] vs. 0.40 [95%-CI 0.29–0.54], $p = 0.29$), mechanical ventilation (aOR 0.56 [95%-CI 0.38–0.85] vs. 0.54 [95%-CI 0.46–0.64], p = 0.87), and severe brain injury (aOR 0.43 [95%-CI 0.22–0.84] vs. 0.39 [95%-CI 0.30–0.51], $p = 0.77$) [104, 106]. Similar findings were reported by others [137]. In a large study from the Vermont Oxford Network of very low birth weight SGA neonates born at 25–30 weeks, Bernstein et al. found no interaction between the effects of ACS and SGA and concluded that the benefits of ACS for growth-restricted newborns are similar to those among normally grown infants [31]. These findings are further supported by two recent meta-analyses that reported that exposure to ACS in pregnancies complicated by FGR was associated with a significant reduction in neonatal mortality and morbidity [32, 143]. Most available guidelines recommend that the administration of ACS in FGR pregnancies should follow the same protocol used in pregnancies not affected by FGR (◘ Table 12.1), although close monitoring has been advised when ACS is administered in fetuses with severe FGR with late Doppler changes [102].

12.5.2 Multifetal Pregnancies

The question of whether ACS has similar effects in multifetal pregnancies is based on physiologic and metabolic differences between twin and singleton pregnancies, such as a higher volume of distribution and a shorter half-life of betamethasone in twin pregnancies [22]. Data on the benefit of ACS in this population are limited, given that multifetal pregnancies were either excluded [14, 86, 105, 110, 118, 129, 136, 149, 177, 185] or constituted a small proportion of subjects in prior trials on ACS [55, 59, 62, 66, 83, 89, 126, 147, 153, 168, 169]. Data from observational studies are limited and conflicting [2, 15, 27, 33, 34, 37, 40, 72, 84, 115, 131, 173] in part due to limitations of available studies, including small sample size [27, 114, 164] and the lack of a positive control group of singleton pregnancies. In a recent large population-based study from Canada, we compared the association of exposure to ACS within the optimal interval of 1–7 days before birth with neonatal outcomes between twin and singleton pregnancies. We found that exposure to ACS in twin and singleton pregnancies was associated with a similar reduction in neonatal death (aOR 0.42 [95%CI 0.24–0.76] vs. 0.38 [95%CI 0.28–0.50]; $p = 0.7$), mechanical ventilation (aOR 0.47 [95%CI 0.35–0.63] vs. 0.47 [95%CI 0.41–0.55]; $p = 0.9$), RDS (aOR 0.53 [95%CI 0.40–0.69] vs. 0.54 [95%CI 0.47–0.62]; $p = 0.9$), and severe neurologic injury (aOR 0.50 [95%CI 0.30–0.83] vs. 0.45 [95%CI 0.34–0.59]; $p = 0.7$) [104, 106]. Another large study from the National Institute of Child Health and Human Development Neonatal Research Network center of twin infants born at 22–28 weeks found that exposure to ACS was associated with a lower risk of mortality, with no significant differences in the composite of neurodevelopmental impairment or death at 18–22 months [35]. A recent meta-analysis of observational studies reported that exposure to ACS was associated with a reduction in the risk of neonatal mortality (aOR 0.59 [95%-CI 0.43–0.80]) and RDS (aOR 0.70 [95%-CI 0.57–0.86]) [159]. Most professional societies recommend that the administration of ACS in multifetal pregnancies follow the same protocols used in singleton pregnancies (◘ Table 12.1) [99, 188].

12.5.3 Preterm Pre-labor Rupture of Membranes

The main concern with regard to the use of ACS in cases of PPROM is the potential for an increased risk of infectious morbidity in the mother (chorioamnionitis and endometritis) and newborn (early neonatal sepsis) [26, 64, 76, 77]. Based on these concerns, the initial National Institute of Health (NIH) Consensus panel recommended that ACS be used only up to 30–32 weeks of gestation in patients with PPROM (1995). However, subsequent studies demonstrated that ACS reduces neonatal morbidity and mortality without increasing the risk of maternal or neonatal infectious morbidity [29, 71, 91, 139, 152]. In the most recent meta-analysis on ACS, there were no differences in the effect of ACS on perinatal mortality and morbidity, RDS, chorioamnionitis, or endometritis between patients with PPROM and those with intact membranes [94]. Accordingly, current guidelines recommend that the administration of ACS in patients with PPROM should follow the same protocols used in cases with intact membranes (◘ Table 12.1).

12.6 Types and Regimens of Antenatal Corticosteroids

12.6.1 Commonly Used Antenatal Corticosteroid Regimens

12

The two most widely used types of ACS are betamethasone and dexamethasone. These drugs are less extensively metabolized by the placenta than other steroids, such as hydrocortisone, which is cleared by the enzyme 11β-hydroxysteroid dehydrogenase type 2 [94, 191].

Betamethasone is administered intramuscularly in two doses of 12 mg 24 hours apart. It consists of a 1:1 mixture of betamethasone sodium phosphate (which is rapidly absorbed) and betamethasone acetate (which is less soluble and is slowly hydrolyzed, resulting in a longer duration of action) [82]. As a result, this formulation of betamethasone provides both immediate and sustained release properties and results in detectable plasma levels up to 14 days after administration.

For dexamethasone, the most common regimen consists of four doses of 6 mg intramuscularly 12 hours apart. It consists of dexamethasone sodium phosphate, which has a more rapid onset and shorter duration of action than betamethasone, explaining the shorter dosing interval. However, a recent trial used an alternative regimen of dexamethasone (two doses of 12 mg 24 hours apart, similar to betamethasone), which was found to be equivalent to that of betamethasone [50, 52] and is currently recommended by some professional societies [122, 165] (◘ Table 12.1).

Whether one of these drugs should be preferred over the other remains unclear. Dexamethasone is approximately 3% of the cost of betamethasone and is more readily available [50, 52]. However, the choice of drug is often affected by other factors, such as local practices and data on the relative efficacy and safety of the two drugs. Overall, both drugs are associated with similar reductions in RDS and neonatal death. Some providers tend to prefer betamethasone based on data demonstrating a clearer reduction in IVH compared with dexamethasone (RR 0.48 [95% CI 0.34–0.68] for betamethasone vs. placebo, and RR 0.78 [95% CI 0.54–1.13] for dexamethasone vs. placebo) [94]. However, studies directly comparing betamethasone with dexamethasone did not find a difference between the two drugs in the reduction of IVH and other neonatal outcomes [42, 191]. A recent large trial comparing betamethasone with a modified regimen of dexamethasone (2 doses of 12 mg 24 h apart) found no difference in the rate of death or neurosensory disability at age 2 years of age [50, 52]. With respect to maternal outcomes, two recent systematic reviews found that dexamethasone may be associated with a lower risk of chorioamnionitis and maternal adverse effects, although the results were inconclusive [42, 191]. Most professional societies support using either of these drugs (◘ Table 12.1).

12.6.2 Alternative Regimens

The optimal regimen with respect to the dose, frequency, and duration of treatment remains unclear. This information is important given the potential long-term risks associated with fetal ACS exposure [19]. Preliminary studies in animal models suggest that the dose required for lung maturation may be much lower than the standard dosing regimens described above [145]. Such lower doses may potentially reduce the risk of adverse effects while maintaining the same efficacy [175]. The WHO ACTION-III study is an ongoing multicenter trial investigating the efficacy and safety of a reduced betamethasone regimen (betamethasone phosphate, four doses of 2 mg 12 h apart) compared to the standard dexamethasone regimen and placebo in the late preterm period [45].

Another approach to reducing fetal ACS exposure is to provide a single, as opposed to a double, dose of betamethasone. A recent trial (BETADOSE study) tested the hypothesis that a single dose of betamethasone is non-inferior to the standard double-dose regimen among singleton pregnancies at risk of delivery before 32 weeks [100, 146]. The rate of the primary outcome, the need for exogenous intratracheal surfactant within 48 hours after birth, was 20.0% in the half-dose group compared to 17.5% in the full-dose group. The study failed to demonstrate non-inferiority of the half-dose regimen, as the upper limit of the 95% CI exceeded the predefined non-inferiority margin of 4%. However, no significant differences were observed between the groups in secondary outcomes such as neonatal death, severe IVH, necrotizing enterocolitis, or survival without severe neonatal morbidity [28]. A similar trial (SNACS study, NCT05114096) currently ongoing in Canada and Australia may provide additional data regarding the efficacy of a single dose of betamethasone.

Some care providers have used "accelerated" dosing regimens with a shorter interval between doses when delivery appears to be imminent. However, there is currently no evidence to suggest that this approach is beneficial [47].

12.7 Timing of Administration

12.7.1 Optimal Timing of Administration

ACS is the single most effective intervention for reducing mortality and morbidity of preterm infants [48], 1994, 1995, [49, 94, 103, 139, 156]. Therefore, it is imperative that this intervention be utilized in a manner that maximizes its benefits. The initial studies of Liggins and Howie indicated that the effect of ACS starts to decline after 7 days [89]. This observation was subsequently supported by meta-analyses of randomized controlled trials [93, 96, 140] and in vitro studies showing that the effects of ACS on surfactant production by type-2 pneumocytes are transient [23, 79, 178]. For example, in a large population-based study from Canada, the odds of neonatal mortality and severe morbidity were higher among infants exposed to ACS <24 hours (aOR 1.48 [95%-CI 1.22–1.80]) or >7 days (aOR 1.46 [95%-CI 1.20–1.77]) before birth compared to infants exposed to ACS within 1–7 days before birth [105]. As a result, most professional societies recommend that ACS be administered when PTB is anticipated within the next 7 days.

However, the interpretation of available data regarding the optimal ACS-to-birth interval is limited by the fact that most studies considered the ACS-to-birth interval as a categorical variable using a wide range of arbitrary, predetermined categories. A recent systematic review identified 65 different intervals, concluding that this variation is one of the leading reasons for the failure to synthesize data and refine our understanding of the relationship between the timing of ACS in relation to birth and its effect [93]. As a result, it remains unclear how soon within the first 24 hours ACS start to take effect, when their maximal effect is achieved, and how long after the first 7 days their effect persists. These questions, which define the *beneficial interval of ACS* (the period through which they exert any benefit) as well as the *optimal interval of ACS* (the period through which they exert their maximal benefit), are of major importance as they may determine whether ACS should be administered in cases where PTB is imminent, determine the optimal timing of ACS, and guide the timing of a repeat ('rescue') course of ACS [47, 53]. Therefore, it was recommended that advanced statistical modeling, where the interval is expressed as a continuous variable rather than an arbitrary predetermined range, is essential to improve our understanding of this relationship.

Data on the association of the ACS-to-birth interval as a continuous variable with neonatal outcomes are scarce. In an observational study of 4594 singleton infants born between 24 and 31 weeks, Norman et al. reported that the association of ACS with a reduction in neonatal mortality was noticed as early as the first few hours following administration, increased rapidly over the first 12 hours, and remained significant for up to 3–4 weeks following administration [123]. With regard to the optimal interval, they found a gradual decrease in the benefit of ACS starting at 5–7 days post-administration. Thus, the optimal interval according to their study was between 12 hours and 5–7 days. In a recent secondary analysis of data from a multicenter randomized controlled trial in low-resource countries that included 2904 infants exposed to dexamethasone vs. placebo between $26^{0/7}$ and $33^{6/7}$ weeks (WHO ACTION-I trial), the authors found that the benefit of dexamethasone increased gradually over time, reaching a peak at approximately 14 days and then diminished as the interval approached 28 days [44]. The authors concluded that the neonatal benefits of dexamethasone appear to increase with longer administration-to-birth intervals than previously thought.

12.7.2 Strategies to Optimize the Timing of Antenatal Corticosteroids

Despite the evidence described above regarding an optimal time window for the administration of ACS, only 15–40% of pregnant patients treated with ACS received it within 1–7 days before birth [9, 61, 85, 105, 119, 121, 123, 134, 146, 157, 158, 181]. In addition, up to 40% of patients who receive ACS ultimately give birth at term (≥37 weeks), in which case the fetus was unnecessarily exposed to ACS [116, 119, 146, 161, 184]. This finding is concerning, given the recent observational data suggesting that ACS given inappropriately may be harmful to newborns due to long-term neurodevelopmental, neurosensory, cardiovascular, metabolic, and hormonal effects [10, 11, 16–18, 54, 57, 80, 101, 120, 124, 132, 166].

Several factors may contribute to the suboptimal timing of ACS. First, care providers may be unfamiliar with the most up-to-date evidence regarding the likelihood of PTB in various clinical scenarios and may thus administer ACS in cases where the risk of PTB within the next 1–2 weeks is relatively low. Second, the decision to administer ACS is most commonly based on the clinical judgment of the attending physician rather than on quantitative decision tools. In the absence of clear guidance, care providers often choose to administer ACS even when they are aware that the risk of PTB is small, in part for medico-legal reasons. Third, some professional organizations implemented performance metrics that are focused solely on the administration of ACS irrespective of the timing of ACS administration in relation to birth, thereby encouraging an aggressive approach to ACS administration, even when the likelihood of PTB is low [46, 161].

Strategies to improve the timing of ACS should address the factors described above. Educational interventions can promote knowledge of care providers regarding the indications for ACS, the likelihood of PTB in different clinical scenarios, and the potential long-term risks of inappropriately administered ACS. The implementation of decision support tools that quantify the risk of PTB based on patient-specific factors and the most up-to-date evidence can contribute to an objective, standardized, and personalized decision regarding the administration of ACS. Several studies attempted to quantify the risk of PTB within the next 1–2 weeks in cases of preterm labor [39, 68, 186, 187], bleeding placenta previa [12], and other conditions associated with PTB [90, 92, 155, 158, 179, 193]. Finally, quality indicators and performance metrics should focus on the appropriate administration of ACS (including administration within 1–7 days before birth and administration to patients who gave birth prematurely) rather than the overall administration of ACS [46, 161].

12.7.3 Role of Multiple Courses and Rescue Dose

As mentioned earlier, the maximal effect of ACS lasts approximately 7 days, after which its effect seems to be reduced by approximately 50% [105]. However, the fact that a large proportion of patients remain pregnant more than 7–14 days after an initial course of ACS [116] led to the question of continuing ACS weekly or biweekly to maintain the benefits of ACS for the fetus or providing an extra dose or course in the form of a rescue approach. Several trials evaluated repeated courses, and their pooled results showed that infants had reduced risks of early respiratory morbidities [51]. However, no benefit was seen for chronic lung disease, IVH, or perinatal mortality. In addition, there was a negative effect on neonatal head circumference at birth. The trials' varying approaches questioned the generalizability of the findings for clinical management, and there still remains a lack of consensus on whether this approach should be used in practice [50, 52, 192].

In addition to the consideration of repeated courses of ACS, should women remain pregnant 14 days after the initial course, a modified rescue approach to the repeat dosing concept has also been considered. In 2009, a trial enrolled over 400 patients who had received an initial course of ACS and had remained pregnant 14 days later [65]. These women were randomized to receive a repeat single course of ACS vs. placebo. A rescue course was associated with a significant reduction in the primary outcome of composite neonatal morbidity <34 weeks and significantly decreased RDS, ventilator support, and surfactant use. Perinatal mortality and other morbidities were similar in both groups. Including all neonates in the analysis (regardless of gestational age at birth) still demonstrated a significant reduction in composite morbidity in the rescue course group and an improvement in respiratory morbidities. These findings supported a move to endorse a rescue approach in a patient who had received a single course of ACS and was actively at risk of a PTB <34 weeks of gestation more than 14 days after the initial administration of ACS [192]. However, questions arise whether multiple "rescue" courses of ACS are beneficial or only one such course would be needed, independent of delivery not taking place. Further evaluation is needed before it may be fully endorsed for general care. With the exception of the Canadian guidelines [88, 156], most professional societies support considering a single rescue course (◘ Table 12.1).

12.8 Future Directions and Research

ACS is the single most effective intervention for reducing the risk of mortality and morbidity of preterm infants. While the benefits of ACS are well established, several questions remain regarding how this intervention can be optimized, including the choice of drug, dose, frequency, and timing of administration. In addition, recent data from observational studies raise concerns that fetal exposure to ACS may be associated with adverse long-term neurodevelopmental, neurosensory, and endocrine effects, especially among infants born at term. These concerns have triggered efforts to identify the lowest dose of ACS that provides the same benefits while minimizing potential risks. Future studies should focus on identifying the optimal regimen and timing of ACS with regard to their efficacy and safety, investigating the benefit of ACS in specific subgroups of pregnancies, and developing decision tools to optimize the timing and the decision to administer ACS.

12.9 Summary Points

- Antenatal corticosteroids (ACS) are the single most effective intervention to improve the outcomes of preterm infants, including a reduction in neonatal death, respiratory morbidity, severe intraventricular hemorrhage, and long-term disability.
- The benefits of ACS are achieved through a combination of transient biochemical

effects (e.g., increase in surfactant production) and persistent structural effects (e.g., promoting structural maturation of the lung parenchyma).

- Most professional societies recommend routine administration of ACS between $24^{0/7}$ and $33^{6/7}$ weeks. Recommendations are less consistent with regard to the administration of ACS in the periviable period ($22^{0/7}$–$23^{6/7}$ weeks), the late preterm period ($34^{0/7}$–$36^{6/7}$ weeks), and before planned cesarean deliveries at term.
- Despite limited direct evidence, most professional societies recommend that the administration of ACS in specific subgroups of pregnancies (e.g., pregnancies affected by fetal growth restriction, multifetal pregnancies, and cases of preterm pre-labor rupture of membranes) follow the same protocols used in uncomplicated singleton preterm births.
- ACS may be associated with potential short-term neonatal risks, primarily neonatal hypoglycemia. In addition, repeated courses of ACS have been associated with reduced weight and smaller head circumference at birth.
- Data from animal models and observational studies suggest that ACS may be associated with long-term neurodevelopmental, neurosensory, cardiometabolic, endocrine, and mental adverse effects, especially among infants born at term following exposure to ACS.
- The two most widely used ACS regimens are betamethasone (2 doses of 12 mg IM injections 24 hours apart) and dexamethasone (4 doses of 6 mg IM injections 12 hours apart). Whether one of these regimens should be preferred over the other remains unclear.
- Data from animal studies suggest that the dose required for lung maturation may be much lower than the current standard dosing regimens. There are ongoing efforts to determine whether modified regimens (reduced dosing or a single as opposed to double dose of betamethasone) can maintain the same efficacy while reducing the potential short- and long-term adverse effects of ACS.
- Most studies suggest the optimal timing for ACS administration is approximately 1–7 days before birth. However, recent evidence suggests that the effect of ACS is observed as early as the first few hours following administration.
- Only 15–40% of pregnant patients treated with ACS received it within the optimal window of 1–7 days before birth, and up to 40% of patients who receive ACS ultimately give birth at term. The implementation of educational interventions, decision support tools, and performance metrics that consider the timing of ACS are possible strategies to optimize the timing of ACS.
- Most professional societies support considering a single rescue course of ACS in patients remaining at risk of PTB >7–14 days following the first course of ACS.

12

Chapter Key Points

- ACS reduces neonatal mortality, respiratory morbidity, IVH, and long-term disability
- Mechanism includes surfactant induction and structural lung maturation
- Benefit varies by gestational age; strongest 24–34 weeks
- Use in periviable, late preterm, and early-term periods remains debated
- ACS efficacy similar across subgroups (FGR, twins, PPROM)
- Betamethasone and dexamethasone are standard regimens
- Optimal timing is 1–7 days before birth; only a minority receive ACS in this window
- Potential risks include neonatal hypoglycemia and long-term neurodevelopmental concerns when given unnecessarily
- Role of repeated or rescue courses remains controversial

Chapter-End Summary

This chapter reviews evidence supporting antenatal corticosteroids as the most effective intervention to reduce mortality and morbidity in preterm infants. It explains mechanisms of action, benefits by gestational age, and considerations for periviable, late preterm, and early-term periods. Data in subgroups such as FGR, twins, and PPROM support use similar to singletons, while concerns remain about unnecessary exposure, neonatal hypoglycemia, and potential long-term neurodevelopmental effects. The chapter describes standard ACS regimens, alternative dosing strategies, and the importance of timing within 1–7 days before birth. Emerging models and decision tools aim to optimize timing and reduce inappropriate use. Evidence for repeat or rescue courses is mixed, with most societies supporting a single rescue course in select cases

References

1. Single dose of antenatal corticosteroids for pregnancies at risk of preterm delivery (SNACS) (SNACS). https://clinicaltrials.gov/study/NCT05114096.
2. Effect of antenatal dexamethasone administration on the prevention of respiratory distress syndrome. Am J Obstet Gynecol. 1981;141(3):276–87. PMID: 70256s38.
3. Effect of corticosteroids for fetal maturation on perinatal outcomes. NIH Consens Statement. 1994;12(2):1–24.
4. NIH Consensus Development Panel on the Effect of Corticosteroids for Fetal Maturation on Perinatal Outcomes. Effect of corticosteroids for fetal maturation on perinatal outcomes. JAMA. 1995;273(5):413–8.
5. New Zealand and Australian Clinical Practice Guidelines Antenatal Corticosteroids Given To Women Prior To Birth To Improve Fetal, Infant, Child and Adult Health. 2015. https://ranzcog.edu.au/wp-content/uploads/2022/05/Antenatal-Corticosteroids-Given-to-Women-Prior-to-Birth-to-Improve-Fetal-Infant-Child-and-Adult-Health.pdf.
6. Use of Antenatal Corticosteroids at 22 Weeks of Gestation. ACOG practice advisory. 2021. https://www.acog.org/clinical/clinical-guidance/practice-advisory/articles/2021/09/use-of-antenatal-corticosteroids-at-22-weeks-of-gestation.
7. NICE Guideline Preterm labour and birth (NG25). 2022. https://www.nice.org.uk/guidance/ng25.
8. WHO. WHO recommendations on antenatal corticosteroids for improving preterm birth outcomes. 2022. https://www.who.int/publications/i/item/9789240057296.
9. Adams TM, Kinzler WL, Chavez MR, Fazzari MJ, Vintzileos AM. Practice patterns in the timing of antenatal corticosteroids for fetal lung maturity. J Matern Fetal Neonatal Med. 2015;28(13):1598–601.
10. Aiken CE, Fowden AL, Smith GC. Antenatal glucocorticoids prior to cesarean delivery at term. JAMA Pediatr. 2014;168(6):507–8.
11. Alexander N, Rosenlocher F, Stalder T, Linke J, Distler W, Morgner J, Kirschbaum C. Impact of antenatal synthetic glucocorticoid exposure on endocrine stress reactivity in term-born children. J Clin Endocrinol Metab. 2012;97(10):3538–44.
12. Alsayegh E, Barrett J, Melamed N. Optimal timing of antenatal corticosteroids in women with bleeding placenta previa or low-lying placent. J Matern Fetal Neonatal Med. 2018;32(12):1971–7.
13. Althabe F, Belizán JM, McClure EM, Hemingway-Foday J, Berrueta M, Mazzoni A, Ciganda A, Goudar SS, Kodkany BS, Mahantshetti NS, Dhaded SM, Katageri GM, Metgud MC, Joshi AM, Bellad MB, Honnungar NV, Derman RJ, Saleem S, Pasha O, Ali S, Hasnain F, Goldenberg RL, Esamai F, Nyongesa P, Ayunga S, Liechty EA, Garces AL, Figueroa L, Hambidge KM, Krebs NF, Patel A, Bhandarkar A, Waikar M, Hibberd PL, Chomba E, Carlo WA, Mwiche A, Chiwila M, Manasyan A, Pineda S, Meleth S, Thorsten V, Stolka K, Wallace D.D., Koso-Thomas M, Jobe AH, Buekens PM. A population-based, multifaceted strategy to implement antenatal corticosteroid treatment versus standard care for the reduction of neonatal mortality due to preterm birth in low-income and middle-income countries: the ACT cluster-randomised trial. Lancet. 2014;385(9968):629–39.
14. Amorim MM, Santos LC, Faundes A. Corticosteroid therapy for prevention of respiratory distress syndrome in severe preeclampsia. Am J Obstet Gynecol. 1999;180(5):1283–8.
15. Ardila J, Le Guennec JC, Papageorgiou A. Influence of antenatal betamethasone and gender cohabitation on outcome of twin pregnancies 24 to 34 weeks of gestation. Semin Perinatol. 1994;18(1):15–8.
16. Asztalos E, Willan A, Murphy K, Matthews S, Ohlsson A, Saigal S, Armson A, Kelly E, Delisle MF, Gafni A, Lee S, Sananes R, Rovet J, Guselle P, Amankwah K, MACS-5 Collaborative Group. Association between gestational age at birth, antenatal corticosteroids, and outcomes at 5 years: multiple courses of antenatal corticosteroids for preterm birth study at 5 years of age

(MACS-5). BMC Pregnancy Childbirth. 2014;14:272.
17. Asztalos EV. Antenatal corticosteroids are currently used excessively and more stringent controls on their use should be established: FOR: the use of antenatal corticosteroids should be restricted if we are to avoid causing harm. BJOG. 2016;123(11):1787.
18. Asztalos EV, Murphy KE, Matthews SG. A growing dilemma: antenatal corticosteroids and long-term consequences. Am J Perinatol. 2020;39:592.
19. Asztalos EV, Murphy KE, Matthews SG. A growing dilemma: antenatal corticosteroids and long-term consequences. Am J Perinatol. 2022;39(6):592–600.
20. Asztalos EV, Murphy KE, Willan AR, Matthews SG, Ohlsson A, Saigal S, Armson BA, Kelly EN, Delisle MF, Gafni A, Lee SK, Sananes R, Rovet J, Guselle P, Amankwah K, Saleem M, Sanchez J, MACS-5 Collaborative Group. Multiple courses of antenatal corticosteroids for preterm birth study: outcomes in children at 5 years of age (MACS-5). JAMA Pediatr. 2013;167(12):1102–10.
21. Aviram A, Murphy K, McDonald S, Asztalos E, Zaltz A, Redelmeier D, Shah B, Barrett J, Melamed N. Antenatal corticosteroids and neurodevelopmental outcomes in late preterm births. Arch Dis Child Fetal Neonatal Ed. 2022;107(3):250–5.
22. Ballabh P, Lo ES, Kumari J, Cooper TB, Zervoudakis I, Auld PA, Krauss AN. Pharmacokinetics of betamethasone in twin and singleton pregnancy. Clin Pharmacol Ther. 2002;71(1):39–45.
23. Ballard PL, Ballard RA. Scientific basis and therapeutic regimens for use of antenatal glucocorticoids. Am J Obstet Gynecol. 1995;173(1):254–62.
24. Barker DJ. In utero programming of chronic disease. Clin Sci (Lond). 1998;95(2):115–28.
25. Baschat AA. Pathophysiology of fetal growth restriction: implications for diagnosis and surveillance. Obstet Gynecol Surv. 2004;59(8):617–27.
26. Battarbee AN. Use of antenatal corticosteroids in preterm Prelabor rupture of membranes. Obstet Gynecol Clin N Am. 2020;47(4):587–94.
27. Battista L, Winovitch KC, Rumney PJ, Davis E, Hagemann C, Wing DA. A case-control comparison of the effectiveness of betamethasone to prevent neonatal morbidity and mortality in preterm twin and singleton pregnancies. Am J Perinatol. 2008;25(7):449–53.
28. Baud O, Sentilhes L, Ursino M, Doret-Dion M, Alberti C, Aupiais C, Schmitz T, BETADOSE trial study group and the GROG. Survival without severe neonatal morbidity after antenatal betamethasone dose reduction: a post hoc analysis of a randomized non-inferiority trial. Am J Obstet Gynecol. 2024;231(4):458 e451–16.
29. Been JV, Degraeuwe PL, Kramer BW, Zimmermann LJ. Antenatal steroids and neonatal outcome after chorioamnionitis: a meta-analysis. BJOG. 2011;118(2):113–22.
30. Beltrand J, Verkauskiene R, Nicolescu R, Sibony O, Gaucherand P, Chevenne D, Claris O, Levy-Marchal C. Adaptive changes in neonatal hormonal and metabolic profiles induced by fetal growth restriction. J Clin Endocrinol Metab. 2008;93(10):4027–32.
31. Bernstein IM, Horbar JD, Badger GJ, Ohlsson A, Golan A. Morbidity and mortality among very-low-birth-weight neonates with intrauterine growth restriction. The Vermont Oxford Network. Am J Obstet Gynecol. 2000;182(1 Pt 1):198–206.
32. Blankenship SA, Brown KE, Simon LE, Stout MJ, Tuuli MG. Antenatal corticosteroids in preterm small-for-gestational age infants: a systematic review and meta-analysis. Am J Obstet Gynecol MFM. 2020;2(4):100215.
33. Blickstein I, Reichman B, Lusky A, Shinwell ES, Israel Neonatal Network. Plurality-dependent risk of severe intraventricular hemorrhage among very low birth weight infants and antepartum corticosteroid treatment. Am J Obstet Gynecol. 2006;194(5):1329–33.
34. Blickstein I, Shinwell ES, Lusky A, Reichman B, Israel Neonatal N. Plurality-dependent risk of respiratory distress syndrome among very-low-birth-weight infants and antepartum corticosteroid treatment. Am J Obstet Gynecol. 2005;192(2):360–4.
35. Boghossian NS, McDonald SA, Bell EF, Carlo WA, Brumbaugh JE, Stoll BJ, Laptook AR, Shankaran S, Walsh MC, Das A, Higgins RD, H. Eunice Kennedy Shriver National Institute of Child and N. Human Development Neonatal Research. Association of antenatal corticosteroids with mortality, morbidity, and neurodevelopmental outcomes in extremely preterm multiple gestation infants. JAMA Pediatr. 2016;170(6):593–601.
36. Braun T, Husar A, Challis JR, Dudenhausen JW, Henrich W, Plagemann A, Sloboda DM. Growth restricting effects of a single course of antenatal betamethasone treatment and the role of human placental lactogen. Placenta. 2013;34(5):407–15.
37. Burkett G, Bauer CR, Morrison J, Curet LB. Effect of prenatal dexamethasone administration on prevention of respiratory distress syndrome in twin pregnancies. J Perinatol. 1986;6:304–8.
38. Carlo WA, McDonald SA, Fanaroff AA, Vohr BR, Stoll BJ, Ehrenkranz RA, Andrews WW, Wallace D, Das A, Bell EF, Walsh MC, Laptook AR, Shankaran S, Poindexter BB, Hale EC, Newman NS, Davis AS, Schibler K, Kennedy KA, Sanchez PJ, Van Meurs KP, Goldberg RN, Watterberg KL, Faix RG, Frantz ID 3rd, Higgins RD, H. Eunice Kennedy Shriver National Institute of Child and N. Human Development Neonatal Research. Association of antenatal cor-

ticosteroids with mortality and neurodevelopmental outcomes among infants born at 22 to 25 weeks' gestation. JAMA. 2011;306(21):2348–58.
39. Carter J, Seed PT, Watson HA, David AL, Sandall J, Shennan AH, Tribe RM. Development and validation of predictive models for QUiPP App v.2: tool for predicting preterm birth in women with symptoms of threatened preterm labor. Ultrasound Obstet Gynecol. 2020;55(3):357–67.
40. Choi SJ, Song SE, Seo ES, Oh SY, Kim JH, Roh CR. The effect of single or multiple courses of antenatal corticosteroid therapy on neonatal respiratory distress syndrome in singleton versus twin pregnancies. Aust N Z J Obstet Gynaecol. 2009;49(2):173–9.
41. Church MW, Adams BR, Anumba JI, Jackson DA, Kruger ML, Jen KL. Repeated antenatal corticosteroid treatments adversely affect neural transmission time and auditory thresholds in laboratory rats. Neurotoxicol Teratol. 2012;34(1):196–205.
42. Ciapponi A, Klein K, Colaci D, Althabe F, Belizan JM, Deegan A, Veroniki AA, Florez ID. Dexamethasone versus betamethasone for preterm birth: a systematic review and network meta-analysis. Am J Obstet Gynecol MFM. 2021;3(3):100312.
43. Clapp MA, Li S, Cohen JL, Gyamfi-Bannerman C, Knudsen AB, Lorch SA, Thaweethai T, Wright JD, Kaimal AJ, Melamed A. Betamethasone exposure and Neonatal respiratory morbidity among late preterm births by planned mode of delivery and gestational age. Obstet Gynecol. 2024;144:747.
44. WHO ACTION Trials Collaborators. Effect of dexamethasone on newborn survival at different administration-to-birth intervals: a secondary analysis of the WHO ACTION (Antenatal CorticosTeroids for Improving Outcomes in Preterm Newborn)-I trial. EClinicalMedicine. 2022;53:101744.
45. Collaborators WAT. The World Health Organization Antenatal CorTicosteroids for Improving Outcomes in Preterm Newborns (ACTION-III) trial: study protocol for a multicountry, multi-centre, double-blind, three-arm, placebo-controlled, individually randomized trial of antenatal corticosteroids for women at high probability of late preterm birth in hospitals in low- resource countries. Trials. 2024;25(1):258.
46. Combs CA, Handler DL, Clark RH. Antenatal corticosteroids before early preterm birth: interval from administration to birth in contemporary practice and association with neonatal mortality. Am J Obstet Gynecol MFM. 2023;5(10):101130.
47. Committee on Obstetric Practice. Committee opinion no. 713: antenatal corticosteroid therapy for fetal maturation. Obstet Gynecol. 2017;130(2):e102–9.
48. Crowley P, Chalmers I, Keirse MJ. The effects of corticosteroid administration before preterm delivery: an overview of the evidence from controlled trials. Br J Obstet Gynaecol. 1990;97(1):11–25.
49. Crowley PA. Antenatal corticosteroid therapy: a meta-analysis of the randomized trials, 1972 to 1994. Am J Obstet Gynecol. 1995;173(1):322–35.
50. Crowther CA, Ashwood P, Andersen CC, Middleton PF, Tran T, Doyle LW, Robinson JS, Harding JE, ASTEROID Study Group. Maternal intramuscular dexamethasone versus betamethasone before preterm birth (ASTEROID): a multicentre, double-blind, randomised controlled trial. Lancet Child Adolesc Health. 2019a;3(11):769–80.
51. Crowther CA, McKinlay CJ, Middleton P, Harding JE. Repeat doses of prenatal corticosteroids for women at risk of preterm birth for improving neonatal health outcomes. Cochrane Database Syst Rev. 2015;7:CD003935.
52. Crowther CA, Middleton PF, Voysey M, Askie L, Zhang S, Martlow TK, Aghajafari F, Asztalos EV, Brocklehurst P, Dutta S, Garite TJ, Guinn DA, Hallman M, Hardy P, Lee MJ, Maurel K, Mazumder P, McEvoy C, Murphy KE, Peltoniemi OM, Thom EA, Wapner RJ, Doyle LW, PRECISE Group. Effects of repeat prenatal corticosteroids given to women at risk of preterm birth: an individual participant data meta-analysis. PLoS Med. 2019b;16(4):e1002771.
53. Datkhaeva I, Dray D, Has P, Stifani B, Hughes BL, Rouse DJ. Uptake of a guideline for the administration of a rescue course of antenatal corticosteroids. Obstet Gynecol. 2017;129(4):720–6.
54. Davis EP, Sandman CA, Buss C, Wing DA, Head K. Fetal glucocorticoid exposure is associated with preadolescent brain development. Biol Psychiatry. 2013;74(9):647–55.
55. Doran TA, Swyer P, MacMurray B, Mahon W, Enhorning G, Bernstein A, Falk M, Wood MM. Results of a double-blind controlled study on the use of betamethasone in the prevention of respiratory distress syndrome. Am J Obstet Gynecol. 1980;136(3):313–20.
56. Economides DL, Nicolaides KH, Linton EA, Perry LA, Chard T. Plasma cortisol and adrenocorticotropin in appropriate and small for gestational age fetuses. Fetal Ther. 1988;3(3):158–64.
57. Edelmann MN, Sandman CA, Glynn LM, Wing DA, Davis EP. Antenatal glucocorticoid treatment is associated with diurnal cortisol regulation in term-born children. Psychoneuroendocrinology. 2016;72:106–12.
58. Elimian A, Verma U, Canterino J, Shah J, Visintainer P, Tejani N. Effectiveness of antenatal steroids in obstetric subgroups. Obstet Gynecol. 1999;93(2):174–9.
59. Fekih M, Chaieb A, Sboui H, Denguezli W, Hidar S, Khairi H. Value of prenatal corticother-

apy in the prevention of hyaline membrane disease in premature infants. Randomized prospective study. Tunis Med. 2002;80(5):260–5.
60. Field T, Diego M. Cortisol: the culprit prenatal stress variable. Int J Neurosci. 2008;118(8):1181.
61. Fillion A, Boutin A, Gareau-Leonard A, Labine L, Gasse C, Gaudreau C, Demers S, Bujold E. Use of antenatal corticosteroid therapy: a descriptive study of clinical practice trends. J Obstet Gynaecol Can. 2019;41(3):300–5.
62. Gamsu HR, Mullinger BM, Donnai P, Dash CH. Antenatal administration of betamethasone to prevent respiratory distress syndrome in preterm infants: report of a UK multicentre trial. Br J Obstet Gynaecol. 1989;96(4):401–10.
63. Garbrecht MR, Klein JM, Schmidt TJ, Snyder JM. Glucocorticoid metabolism in the human fetal lung: implications for lung development and the pulmonary surfactant system. Biol Neonate. 2006;89(2):109–19.
64. Garite TJ, Freeman RK, Linzey EM, Braly PS, Dorchester WL. Prospective randomized study of corticosteroids in the management of premature rupture of the membranes and the premature gestation. Am J Obstet Gynecol. 1981;141(5):508–15.
65. Garite TJ, Kurtzman J, Maurel K, Clark R, Obstetrix Collaborative Research Network. Impact of a 'rescue course' of antenatal corticosteroids: a multicenter randomized placebo-controlled trial. Am J Obstet Gynecol. 2009;200(3):248.e1–9.
66. Garite TJ, Rumney PJ, Briggs GG, Harding JA, Nageotte MP, Towers CV, Freeman RK. A randomized, placebo-controlled trial of betamethasone for the prevention of respiratory distress syndrome at 24 to 28 weeks' gestation. Am J Obstet Gynecol. 1992;166(2):646–51.
67. Goldenberg RL, Culhane JF, Iams JD, Romero R. Epidemiology and causes of preterm birth. Lancet. 2008;371(9606):75–84.
68. Goodfellow L, Care A, Sharp A, Ivandic J, Poljak B, Roberts D, Alfirevic Z. Effect of QUiPP prediction algorithm on treatment decisions in women with a previous preterm birth: a prospective cohort study. BJOG. 2019;126(13):1569–75.
69. Gunasekara L, Schurch S, Schoel WM, Nag K, Leonenko Z, Haufs M, Amrein M. Pulmonary surfactant function is abolished by an elevated proportion of cholesterol. Biochim Biophys Acta. 2005;1737(1):27–35.
70. Gyamfi-Bannerman C, Thom EA, Blackwell SC, Tita AT, Reddy UM, Saade GR, Rouse DJ, McKenna DS, Clark EA, Thorp JM Jr, Chien EK, Peaceman AM, Gibbs RS, Swamy GK, Norton ME, Casey BM, Caritis SN, Tolosa JE, Sorokin Y, VanDorsten JP, Jain L, NICHD Maternal–Fetal Medicine Units Network. Antenatal betamethasone for women at risk for late preterm delivery. N Engl J Med. 2016;374(14):1311–20.
71. Harding JE, Pang J, Knight DB, Liggins GC. Do antenatal corticosteroids help in the setting of preterm rupture of membranes? Am J Obstet Gynecol. 2001;184(2):131–9.
72. Hashimoto LN, Hornung RW, Lindsell CJ, Brewer DE, Donovan EF. Effects of antenatal glucocorticoids on outcomes of very low birth weight multifetal gestations. Am J Obstet Gynecol. 2002;187(3):804–10.
73. Higgins RD, Delivoria-Papadopoulos M, Raju TN. Executive summary of the workshop on the border of viability. Pediatrics. 2005;115(5):1392–6.
74. Hintz SR, Van Meurs KP, Perritt R, Poole WK, Das A, Stevenson DK, Ehrenkranz RA, Lemons JA, Vohr BR, Heyne R, Childers DO, Peralta-Carcelen M, Dusick A, Johnson YR, Morris B, Dillard R, Vaucher Y, Steichen J, Adams-Chapman I, Konduri G, Myers GJ, de Ungria M, Tyson JE, Higgins RD, NICHD Neonatal Research Network. Neurodevelopmental outcomes of premature infants with severe respiratory failure enrolled in a randomized controlled trial of inhaled nitric oxide. J Pediatr. 2007;151(1):16–22. 22 e11-13
75. Hubinont C, Nicolini U, Fisk NM, Tannirandorn Y, Rodeck CH. Endocrine pancreatic function in growth-retarded fetuses. Obstet Gynecol. 1991;77(4):541–4.
76. Iams JD, Talbert ML, Barrows H, Sachs L. Management of preterm prematurely ruptured membranes: a prospective randomized comparison of observation versus use of steroids and timed delivery. Am J Obstet Gynecol. 1985;151(1):32–8.
77. Imseis HM, Iams JD. Glucocorticoid use in patients with preterm premature rupture of the fetal membranes. Semin Perinatol. 1996;20(5):439–50.
78. Ishikawa H, Miyazaki K, Ikeda T, Murabayashi N, Hayashi K, Kai A, Ishikawa K, Miyamoto Y, Nishimura K, Kono Y, Kusuda S, Fujimura M, Neonatal Research Network of Japan. The effects of antenatal corticosteroids on short- and long-term outcomes in small-for-gestational-age infants. Int J Med Sci. 2015;12(4):295–300.
79. Jobe AH. Glucocorticoids, inflammation and the perinatal lung. Semin Neonatol. 2001;6(4):331–42.
80. Jobe AH, Goldenberg RL. Antenatal corticosteroids: an assessment of anticipated benefits and potential risks. Am J Obstet Gynecol. 2018;219(1):62–74.
81. Jobe AH, Ikegami M. Lung development and function in preterm infants in the surfactant treatment era. Annu Rev Physiol. 2000;62:825–46.
82. Jobe AH, Kemp M, Schmidt A, Takahashi T, Newnham J, Milad M. Antenatal corticosteroids: a reappraisal of the drug formulation and dose. Pediatr Res. 2021;89(2):318–25.
83. Kari MA, Hallman M, Eronen M, Teramo K, Virtanen M, Koivisto M, Ikonen RS. Prenatal

dexamethasone treatment in conjunction with rescue therapy of human surfactant: a randomized placebo-controlled multicenter study. Pediatrics. 1994;93(5):730–6.
84. Kuk JY, An JJ, Cha HH, Choi SJ, Vargas JE, Oh SY, Roh CR, Kim JH. Optimal time interval between a single course of antenatal corticosteroids and delivery for reduction of respiratory distress syndrome in preterm twins. Am J Obstet Gynecol. 2013;209(3):256 e251-257.
85. Levin HI, Friedman AM. Antenatal corticosteroids are currently used excessively and more stringent controls on their use should be established: AGAINST: current use of antenatal corticosteroids effectively reduces neonatal morbidity and mortality. BJOG. 2016;123(11):1788.
86. Lewis DF, Brody K, Edwards MS, Brouillette RM, Burlison S, London SN. Preterm premature ruptured membranes: a randomized trial of steroids after treatment with antibiotics. Obstet Gynecol. 1996;88(5):801–5.
87. Ley D, Wide-Swensson D, Lindroth M, Svenningsen N, Marsal K. Respiratory distress syndrome in infants with impaired intrauterine growth. Acta Paediatr. 1997;86(10):1090–6.
88. Liauw J, Foggin H, Socha P, Crane J, Joseph KS, Burrows J, Lacaze-Masmonteil T, Jain V, Boutin A, Hutcheon J. Technical update no. 439: antenatal corticosteroids at late preterm gestation. J Obstet Gynaecol Can. 2023;45(6):445–457 e442.
89. Liggins GC, Howie RN. A controlled trial of antepartum glucocorticoid treatment for prevention of the respiratory distress syndrome in premature infants. Pediatrics. 1972;50(4):515–25.
90. Loussert L, Dupuis N, Guerby P. Optimal antenatal corticosteroids timing in women with non-severe preeclampsia. Am J Obstet Gynecol. 2024;230(6):e123.
91. Magann EF, Haram K, Ounpraseuth S, Mortensen JH, Spencer HJ, Morrison JC. Use of antenatal corticosteroids in special circumstances: a comprehensive review. Acta Obstet Gynecol Scand. 2017;96(4):395–409.
92. Martins JG, Kawakita T, Barake C, Gould L, Baraki D, Connell P, Sinkovskaya E, Abuhamad A. Rate of deterioration of umbilical artery Doppler indices in fetuses with severe early-onset fetal growth restriction. Am J Obstet Gynecol MFM. 2024;6(3):101283.
93. McDougall ARA, Aboud L, Lavin T, Cao J, Dore G, Ramson J, Oladapo OT, Vogel JP. Effect of antenatal corticosteroid administration-to-birth interval on maternal and newborn outcomes: a systematic review. EClinicalMedicine. 2023;58:101916.
94. McGoldrick E, Stewart F, Parker R, Dalziel SR. Antenatal corticosteroids for accelerating fetal lung maturation for women at risk of preterm birth. Cochrane Database Syst Rev. 2020;12(12):CD004454.
95. McKinlay CJD, Alsweiler JM, Anstice NS, Burakevych N, Chakraborty A, Chase JG, Gamble GD, Harris DL, Jacobs RJ, Jiang Y, Paudel N, San Diego RJ, Thompson B, Wouldes TA, Harding JE, Children With Hypoglycemia and Their Later Development (CHYLD) Study Team. Association of Neonatal Glycemia with Neurodevelopmental Outcomes at 4.5 years. JAMA Pediatr. 2017;171(10):972–83.
96. McLaughlin KJ, Crowther CA, Walker N, Harding JE. Effects of a single course of corticosteroids given more than 7 days before birth: a systematic review. Aust N Z J Obstet Gynaecol. 2003;43(2):101–6.
97. McMillen IC, Adams MB, Ross JT, Coulter CL, Simonetta G, Owens JA, Robinson JS, Edwards LJ. Fetal growth restriction: adaptations and consequences. Reproduction. 2001;122(2):195–204.
98. McTernan CL, Draper N, Nicholson H, Chalder SM, Driver P, Hewison M, Kilby MD, Stewart PM. Reduced placental 11beta-hydroxysteroid dehydrogenase type 2 mRNA levels in human pregnancies complicated by intrauterine growth restriction: an analysis of possible mechanisms. J Clin Endocrinol Metab. 2001;86(10):4979–83.
99. Mei-Dan E, Jain V, Melamed N, Lim KI, Aviram A, Ryan G, Barrett J. Guideline no. 428: management of dichorionic twin pregnancies. J Obstet Gynaecol Can. 2022;44(7):819–834 e811.
100. Melamed N, Asztalos E. Antenatal betamethasone regimen for women at risk of preterm birth. Lancet. 2022;400(10352):541–3.
101. Melamed N, Asztalos E, Murphy K, Zaltz A, Redelmeier D, Shah BR, Barrett J. Neurodevelopmental disorders among term infants exposed to antenatal corticosteroids during pregnancy: a population-based study. BMJ Open. 2019;9(9):e031197.
102. Melamed N, Baschat A, Yinon Y, Athanasiadis A, Mecacci F, Figueras F, Berghella V, Nazareth A, Tahlak M, McIntyre HD, Da Silva Costa F, Kihara AB, Hadar E, McAuliffe F, Hanson M, Ma RC, Gooden R, Sheiner E, Kapur A, Divakar H, Ayres-de-Campos D, Hiersch L, Poon LC, Kingdom J, Romero R, Hod M. FIGO (international Federation of Gynecology and obstetrics) initiative on fetal growth: best practice advice for screening, diagnosis, and management of fetal growth restriction. Int J Gynaecol Obstet. 2021;152(Suppl 1):3–57.
103. Melamed N, Murphy K, Barrett J, Asztalos E, McDonald SD, Yoon EW, Shah PS, Canadian Neonatal Network (CNN), Canadian Preterm Birth Network (CPTBN) Investigators, Makary H, Chandra S, Mundle W, Whittle W. Benefit of antenatal corticosteroids by year of birth among preterm infants in Canada during 2003–2017: a

population-based cohort study. BJOG. 2020;128(3):521–31.

104. Melamed N, Pittini A, Barrett J, Shah J, Yoon EW, Lemyre B, Lee SK, Murphy KE, Shah PS. Antenatal corticosteroids and outcomes of small-for-gestational-age neonates. Obstet Gynecol. (Accepted for publication). 2016a;128:1001.
105. Melamed N, Shah J, Soraisham A, Yoon EW, Lee SK, Shah PS, Murphy KE. Association between antenatal corticosteroid administration-to-birth interval and outcomes of preterm neonates. Obstet Gynecol. 2015;125(6):1377–84.
106. Melamed N, Shah J, Yoon EW, Pelausa E, Lee SK, Shah PS, Murphy KE, Canadian Neonatal Network Investigators. The role of antenatal corticosteroids in twin pregnancies complicated by preterm birth. Am J Obstet Gynecol. 2016b;215(4):482.e1-9.
107. Mitsiakos G, Kovacs L, Papageorgiou A. Are antenatal steroids beneficial to severely growth restricted fetuses? J Matern Fetal Neonatal Med. 2013;26(15):1496–9.
108. Moisiadis VG, Matthews SG. Glucocorticoids and fetal programming part 1: outcomes. Nat Rev Endocrinol. 2014a;10(7):391–402.
109. Moisiadis VG, Matthews SG. Glucocorticoids and fetal programming part 2: mechanisms. Nat Rev Endocrinol. 2014b;10(7):403–11.
110. Morales WJ, Angel JL, O'Brien WF, Knuppel RA. Use of ampicillin and corticosteroids in premature rupture of membranes: a randomized study. Obstet Gynecol. 1989;73(5 Pt 1):721–6.
111. Mori R, Kusuda S, Fujimura M, Neonatal Research Network Japan. Antenatal corticosteroids promote survival of extremely preterm infants born at 22 to 23 weeks of gestation. J Pediatr. 2011;159(1):110–114 e111.
112. Morrison JL. Sheep models of intrauterine growth restriction: fetal adaptations and consequences. Clin Exp Pharmacol Physiol. 2008;35(7):730–43.
113. Mulder EJ, de Heus R, Visser GH. Antenatal corticosteroid therapy: short-term effects on fetal behaviour and haemodynamics. Semin Fetal Neonatal Med. 2009;14(3):151–6.
114. Mulder EJ, Derks JB, Visser GH. Effects of antenatal betamethasone administration on fetal heart rate and behavior in twin pregnancy. Pediatr Res. 2004;56(1):35–9.
115. Murphy DJ, Caukwell S, Joels LA, Wardle P. Cohort study of the neonatal outcome of twin pregnancies that were treated with prophylactic or rescue antenatal corticosteroids. Am J Obstet Gynecol. 2002;187(2):483–8.
116. Murphy KE, Hannah ME, Willan AR, Hewson SA, Ohlsson A, Kelly EN, Matthews SG, Saigal S, Asztalos E, Ross S, Delisle MF, Amankwah K, Guselle P, Gafni A, Lee SK, Armson BA, MACS Collaborative Group. Multiple courses of antenatal corticosteroids for preterm birth (MACS): a randomised controlled trial. Lancet. 2008;372(9656):2143–51.
117. Murphy KE, Willan AR, Hannah ME, Ohlsson A, Kelly EN, Matthews SG, Saigal S, Asztalos E, Ross S, Delisle MF, Amankwah K, Guselle P, Gafni A, Lee SK, Armson BA, Multiple Courses of Antenatal Corticosteroids for Preterm Birth Study Collaborative Group. Effect of antenatal corticosteroids on fetal growth and gestational age at birth. Obstet Gynecol. 2012;119(5):917–23.
118. Nelson LH, Meis PJ, Hatjis CG, Ernest JM, Dillard R, Schey HM. Premature rupture of membranes: a prospective, randomized evaluation of steroids, latent phase, and expectant management. Obstet Gynecol. 1985;66(1):55–8.
119. Ninan K, Gojic A, Wang Y, Asztalos EV, Beltempo M, Murphy KE, McDonald SD. The proportions of term or late preterm births after exposure to early antenatal corticosteroids, and outcomes: systematic review and meta-analysis of 1.6 million infants. BMJ. 2023;382:e076035.
120. Ninan K, Liyanage SK, Murphy KE, Asztalos EV, McDonald SD. Evaluation of long-term outcomes associated with preterm exposure to antenatal corticosteroids: a systematic review and meta-analysis. JAMA Pediatr. 2022;176(6):e220483.
121. Norberg H, Kowalski J, Marsal K, Norman M. Timing of antenatal corticosteroid administration and survival in extremely preterm infants: a national population-based cohort study. BJOG. 2017;124(10):1567–74.
122. Norman J, Shennan A, Jacobsson B, Stock SJ, FIGO Working Group for Preterm Birth. FIGO good practice recommendations on the use of prenatal corticosteroids to improve outcomes and minimize harm in babies born preterm. Int J Gynaecol Obstet. 2021;155(1):26–30.
123. Norman M, Piedvache A, Borch K, Huusom LD, Bonamy AE, Howell EA, Jarreau PH, Maier RF, Pryds O, Toome L, Varendi H, Weber T, Wilson E, Van Heijst A, Cuttini M, Mazela J, Barros H, Van Reempts P, Draper ES, Zeitlin J, Effective Perinatal Intensive Care in Europe (EPICE) Research Group. Association of short antenatal corticosteroid administration-to-birth intervals with survival and morbidity among very preterm infants: results from the EPICE cohort. JAMA Pediatr. 2017;171(7):678–86.
124. Nowik CM, Davies GA, Smith GN. We should proceed with caution when it comes to antenatal corticosteroids after 34 weeks. J Obstet Gynaecol Can. 2017;39(1):49–51.
125. Ohuma EO, Moller AB, Bradley E, Chakwera S, Hussain-Alkhateeb L, Lewin A, Okwaraji YB, Mahanani WR, Johansson EW, Lavin T, Fernandez DE, Dominguez GG, de Costa A, Cresswell JA, Krasevec J, Lawn JE, Blencowe H, Requejo J, Moran AC. National, regional, and global estimates of preterm birth in 2020, with

trends from 2010: a systematic analysis. Lancet. 2023;402(10409):1261–71.
126. Pattinson RC, Makin JD, Funk M, Delport SD, Macdonald AP, Norman K, Kirsten G, Stewart C, Woods D, Moller G, Coetzee E, Smith P, Anthony J, Schoon M, Grobler S. The use of dexamethasone in women with preterm premature rupture of membranes–a multicentre, double-blind, placebo-controlled, randomised trial. Dexiprom Study Group. S Afr Med J. 1999;89(8):865–70.
127. Perin J, Mulick A, Yeung D, Villavicencio F, Lopez G, Strong KL, Prieto-Merino D, Cousens S, Black RE, Liu L. Global, regional, and national causes of under-5 mortality in 2000-19: an updated systematic analysis with implications for the Sustainable Development Goals. Lancet Child Adolesc Health. 2022;6(2):106–15.
128. Piazze J, Dillon KC, Cerekja A. Betamethasone effects on umbilical arteries and ductus venosus Doppler velocity waveforms in growth-restricted fetuses. J Matern Fetal Neonatal Med. 2012;25(7):1179–82.
129. Qublan HS, Malkawi HY, Hiasat MS, Hindawi IM, Al-Taani MI, Abu-Khait SA, Al-Maaitah JF. The effect of antenatal corticosteroid therapy on pregnancies complicated by premature rupture of membranes. Clin Exp Obstet Gynecol. 2001;28(3):183–6.
130. Quinlivan JA, Beazley LD, Evans SF, Newnham JP, Dunlop SA. Retinal maturation is delayed by repeated, but not single, maternal injections of betamethasone in sheep. Eye (Lond). 2000;14(Pt 1):93–8.
131. Quist-Therson EC, Myhr TL, Ohlsson A. Antenatal steroids to prevent respiratory distress syndrome: multiple gestation as an effect modifier. Acta Obstet Gynecol Scand. 1999;78(5):388–92.
132. Raikkonen K, Gissler M, Kajantie E. Associations between maternal antenatal corticosteroid treatment and mental and behavioral disorders in children. JAMA. 2020;323(19):1924–33.
133. Raikkonen K, Gissler M, Tapiainen T, Kajantie E. Associations between maternal antenatal corticosteroid treatment and psychological developmental and neurosensory disorders in children. JAMA Netw Open. 2022;5(8):e2228518.
134. Razaz N, Skoll A, Fahey J, Allen VM, Joseph KS. Trends in optimal, suboptimal, and questionably appropriate receipt of antenatal corticosteroid prophylaxis. Obstet Gynecol. 2015;125(2):288–96.
135. Reynolds RM. Glucocorticoid excess and the developmental origins of disease: two decades of testing the hypothesis–2012 Curt Richter Award Winner. Psychoneuroendocrinology. 2013;38(1):1–11.
136. Ring AM, Garland JS, Stafeil BR, Carr MH, Peckman GS, Pircon RA. The effect of a prolonged time interval between antenatal corticosteroid administration and delivery on outcomes in preterm neonates: a cohort study. Am J Obstet Gynecol. 2007;196(5):457 e451-456.
137. Riskin-Mashiah S, Riskin A, Bader D, Kugelman A, Boyko V, Lerner-Geva L, Reichman B, Israel Neonatal Network. Antenatal corticosteroid treatment in singleton, small-for-gestational-age infants born at 24–31 weeks' gestation: a population-based study. BJOG. 2015;123(11):1779–86.
138. Rizzo G, Capponi A, Cavicchioni O, Vendola M, Arduini D. Low cardiac output to the placenta: an early hemodynamic adaptive mechanism in intrauterine growth restriction. Ultrasound Obstet Gynecol. 2008;32(2):155–9.
139. Roberts D, Brown J, Medley N, Dalziel SR. Antenatal corticosteroids for accelerating fetal lung maturation for women at risk of preterm birth. Cochrane Database Syst Rev. 2017;3:CD004454.
140. Roberts D, Dalziel S. Antenatal corticosteroids for accelerating fetal lung maturation for women at risk of preterm birth. Cochrane Database Syst Rev. 2006;3(3):CD004454.
141. Robertson MC, Murila F, Tong S, Baker LS, Yu VY, Wallace EM. Predicting perinatal outcome through changes in umbilical artery Doppler studies after antenatal corticosteroids in the growth-restricted fetus. Obstet Gynecol. 2009;113(3):636–40.
142. Rodriguez A, Wang Y, Ali Khan A, Cartwright R, Gissler M, Jarvelin MR. Antenatal corticosteroid therapy (ACT) and size at birth: a population-based analysis using the Finnish Medical Birth Register. PLoS Med. 2019;16(2):e1002746.
143. Saito K, Nishimura E, Ota E, Namba F, Swa T, Ramson J, Lavin T, Cao J, Vogel JP. Antenatal corticosteroids in specific groups at risk of preterm birth: a systematic review. BMJ Open. 2023;13(9):e065070.
144. Schaap AH, Wolf H, Bruinse HW, Smolders-De Haas H, Van Ertbruggen I, Treffers PE. Effects of antenatal corticosteroid administration on mortality and long-term morbidity in early preterm, growth-restricted infants. Obstet Gynecol. 2001;97(6):954–60.
145. Schmidt AF, Kemp MW, Rittenschober-Bohm J, Kannan PS, Usuda H, Saito M, Furfaro L, Watanabe S, Stock S, Kramer BW, Newnham JP, Kallapur SG, Jobe AH. Low-dose betamethasone-acetate for fetal lung maturation in preterm sheep. Am J Obstet Gynecol. 2018;218(1):132 e131–9.
146. Schmitz T, Doret-Dion M, Sentilhes L, Parant O, Claris O, Renesme L, Abbal J, Girault A, Torchin H, Houllier M, Le Sache N, Vivanti AJ, De Luca D, Winer N, Flamant C, Thuillier C, Boileau P, Blanc J, Brevaut V, Bouet PE, Gascoin G, Beucher G, Datin-Dorriere V, Bounan S, Bolot P, Poncelet C, Alberti C, Ursino M, Aupiais C, Baud O,

BETADOSE trial study group; Groupe de Recherche en Obstétrique et Gynécologie. Neonatal outcomes for women at risk of preterm delivery given half dose versus full dose of antenatal betamethasone: a randomised, multicentre, double-blind, placebo-controlled, non-inferiority trial. Lancet. 2022;400(10352):592–604.
147. Schutte MF, Treffers PE, Koppe JG, Breur W. The influence of betamethasone and orciprenaline on the incidence of respiratory distress syndrome in the newborn after preterm labour. Br J Obstet Gynaecol. 1980;87(2):127–31.
148. Seckl JR. Glucocorticoids, feto-placental 11 beta-hydroxysteroid dehydrogenase type 2, and the early life origins of adult disease. Steroids. 1997;62(1):89–94.
149. Sehdev HM, Abbasi S, Robertson P, Fisher L, Marchiano DA, Gerdes JS, Ludmir J. The effects of the time interval from antenatal corticosteroid exposure to delivery on neonatal outcome of very low birth weight infants. Am J Obstet Gynecol. 2004;191(4):1409–13.
150. Senat MV, Ville Y. Effect of steroids on arterial Doppler in intrauterine growth retardation fetuses. Fetal Diagn Ther. 2000;15(1):36–40.
151. Shams M, Kilby MD, Somerset DA, Howie AJ, Gupta A, Wood PJ, Afnan M, Stewart PM. 11Beta-hydroxysteroid dehydrogenase type 2 in human pregnancy and reduced expression in intrauterine growth restriction. Hum Reprod. 1998;13(4):799–804.
152. Sheibani L, Fong A, Henry DE, Norton ME, Truong YN, Anyikam A, Laurent LC, Rao R, Wing DA, University of California Fetal Consortium (UCfC). Maternal and neonatal outcomes after antenatal corticosteroid administration for PPROM at 32 to 33 6/7 weeks gestational age. J Matern Fetal Neonatal Med. 2017;30(14):1676–80.
153. Silver RK, Vyskocil C, Solomon SL, Ragin A, Neerhof MG, Farrell EE. Randomized trial of antenatal dexamethasone in surfactant-treated infants delivered before 30 weeks' gestation. Obstet Gynecol. 1996;87(5 Pt 1):683–91.
154. Simchen MJ, Alkazaleh F, Adamson SL, Windrim R, Telford J, Beyene J, Kingdom J. The fetal cardiovascular response to antenatal steroids in severe early-onset intrauterine growth restriction. Am J Obstet Gynecol. 2004;190(2):296–304.
155. Simon E, Permuy C, Sacristan L, Zamoro-Lorenci MJ, Villalain C, Galindo A, Herraiz I. sFlt-1/PlGF ratio for the prediction of delivery within 48 hours and adverse outcomes in expectantly managed early-onset preeclampsia. Pregnancy Hypertens. 2020;22:17–23.
156. Skoll A, Boutin A, Bujold E, Burrows J, Crane J, Geary M, Jain V, Lacaze-Masmonteil T, Liauw J, Mundle W, Murphy K, Wong S, Joseph KS. No. 364-antenatal corticosteroid therapy for improving Neonatal outcomes. J Obstet Gynaecol Can. 2018;40(9):1219–39.
157. Skoll A, Ferreira E, Pedneault L, Duchesne M, Letourneau G. Do we use too much antenatal betamethasone? J Obstet Gynaecol Can. 2002;24(4):330–4.
158. Smith J, Murphy KE, McDonald SD, Asztalos E, Aviram A, Ronzoni S, Mei-Dan E, Zaltz A, Barrett J, Melamed N. Timing of antenatal corticosteroids in relation to clinical indication. Arch Gynecol Obstet. 2022;306:997.
159. Socha P, McGee A, Bhattacharya S, Young C, Wang R. Antenatal corticosteroids and Neonatal outcomes in twins: a systematic review and meta-analysis. Obstet Gynecol. 2022;140(1):20–30.
160. Society for Maternal-Fetal Medicine (SMFM), Reddy UM, Deshmukh U, Dude A, Harper L, Osmundson SS. Society for Maternal-Fetal Medicine Consult Series #58: use of antenatal corticosteroids for individuals at risk for late preterm delivery: replaces SMFM statement #4, implementation of the use of antenatal corticosteroids in the late preterm birth period in women at risk for preterm delivery, August 2016. Am J Obstet Gynecol. 2021;225(5):B36–42.
161. Society for Maternal-Fetal Medicine (SMFM), Hamm RF, Combs CA, Aghajanian P, Friedman AM, Patient S, Quality C. Society for Maternal-Fetal Medicine Special Statement: quality metrics for optimal timing of antenatal corticosteroid administration. Am J Obstet Gynecol. 2022;226(6):B2–B10.
162. Sotiriadis A, McGoldrick E, Makrydimas G, Papatheodorou S, Ioannidis JP, Stewart F, Parker R. Antenatal corticosteroids prior to planned caesarean at term for improving neonatal outcomes. Cochrane Database Syst Rev. 2021;12(12):CD006614.
163. Sotiriadis A, Tsiami A, Papatheodorou S, Baschat AA, Sarafidis K, Makrydimas G. Neurodevelopmental outcome after a single course of antenatal steroids in children born preterm: a systematic review and meta-analysis. Obstet Gynecol. 2015;125(6):1385–96.
164. Spinillo A, Capuzzo E, Ometto A, Stronati M, Baltaro F, Iasci A. Value of antenatal corticosteroid therapy in preterm birth. Early Hum Dev. 1995;42(1):37–47.
165. Stock SJ, Thomson AJ, Papworth S, Royal College of Obstetricians and Gynaecologists. Antenatal corticosteroids to reduce neonatal morbidity and mortality: green-top guideline no. 74. BJOG. 2022;129(8):e35–60.
166. Stutchfield P, Whitaker R, Russell I, Antenatal Steroids for Term Elective Caesarean Section (ASTECS) Research Team. Antenatal betamethasone and incidence of neonatal respiratory dis-

tress after elective caesarean section: pragmatic randomised trial. BMJ. 2005;331(7518):662.
167. Stutchfield PR, Whitaker R, Gliddon AE, Hobson L, Kotecha S, Doull IJ. Behavioural, educational and respiratory outcomes of antenatal betamethasone for term caesarean section (ASTECS trial). Arch Dis Child Fetal Neonatal Ed. 2013;98(3):F195–200.
168. Taeusch HW Jr, Frigoletto F, Kitzmiller J, Avery ME, Hehre A, Fromm B, Lawson E, Neff RK. Risk of respiratory distress syndrome after prenatal dexamethasone treatment. Pediatrics. 1979;63(1):64–72.
169. Teramo K, Hallman M, Raivio KO. Maternal glucocorticoid in unplanned premature labor. Controlled study on the effects of betamethasone phosphate on the phospholipids of the gastric aspirate and on the adrenal cortical function of the newborn infant. Pediatr Res. 1980;14(4 Pt 1):326–9.
170. Torrance HL, Derks JB, Scherjon SA, Wijnberger LD, Visser GH. Is antenatal steroid treatment effective in preterm IUGR fetuses? Acta Obstet Gynecol Scand. 2009;88(10):1068–73.
171. Travers CP, Clark RH, Spitzer AR, Das A, Garite TJ, Carlo WA. Exposure to any antenatal corticosteroids and outcomes in preterm infants by gestational age: prospective cohort study. BMJ. 2017;356:j1039.
172. Turan S, Miller J, Baschat AA. Integrated testing and management in fetal growth restriction. Semin Perinatol. 2008;32(3):194–200.
173. Turrentine MA, Wilson PD, Wilkins IA. A retrospective analysis of the effect of antenatal steroid administration on the incidence of respiratory distress syndrome in preterm twin pregnancies. Am J Perinatol. 1996;13(6):351–4.
174. Tyson JE, Parikh NA, Langer J, Green C, Higgins RD, National Institute of Child Health and Human Development Neonatal Research Network. Intensive care for extreme prematurity–moving beyond gestational age. N Engl J Med. 2008;358(16):1672–81.
175. Usuda H, Fee EL, Carter S, Furfaro L, Takahashi T, Takahashi Y, Newnham JP, Milad MA, Saito M, Jobe AH, Kemp MW. Low-dose antenatal betamethasone treatment achieves preterm lung maturation equivalent to that of the World Health Organization dexamethasone regimen but with reduced endocrine disruption in a sheep model of pregnancy. Am J Obstet Gynecol. 2022;227(6):903 e901–16.
176. van Stralen G, van der Bos J, Lopriore E, Te Pas AB, Bloemenkamp KW, Walther FJ, Scherjon S. No short-term benefits of antenatal corticosteroid treatment in severely preterm growth restricted fetuses: a case-control study. Early Hum Dev. 2009;85(4):253–7.
177. Vermillion ST, Soper DE, Newman RB. Is betamethasone effective longer than 7 days after treatment? Obstet Gynecol. 2001;97(4):491–3.
178. Vidaeff AC, Ramin SM, Gilstrap LC 3rd, Alcorn JL. In vitro quantification of dexamethasone-induced surfactant protein B expression in human lung cells. J Matern Fetal Neonatal Med. 2004;15(3):155–9.
179. Villalain C, Herraiz I, Dominguez-Del Olmo P, Angulo P, Ayala JL, Galindo A. Prediction of delivery within 7 days after diagnosis of early onset preeclampsia using machine-learning models. Front Cardiovasc Med. 2022;9:910701.
180. Ville Y, Proudler A, Kuhn P, Nicolaides KH. Aldosterone concentration in normal, growth-retarded, anemic, and hydropic fetuses. Obstet Gynecol. 1994;84(4):511–4.
181. Vis JY, Wilms FF, Kuin RA, Reuvers JM, Stam MC, Pattinaja DA, Mol BW. Time to delivery after the first course of antenatal corticosteroids: a cohort study. Am J Perinatol. 2011;28(9):683–8.
182. Vogel JP, Ramson J, Darmstadt GL, Qureshi ZP, Chou D, Bahl R, Oladapo OT. Updated WHO recommendations on antenatal corticosteroids and tocolytic therapy for improving preterm birth outcomes. Lancet Glob Health. 2022;10(12):e1707–8.
183. Wallace EM, Baker LS. Effect of antenatal betamethasone administration on placental vascular resistance. Lancet. 1999;353(9162):1404–7.
184. Wapner RJ, Sorokin Y, Thom EA, Johnson F, Dudley DJ, Spong CY, Peaceman AM, Leveno KJ, Harper M, Caritis SN, Miodovnik M, Mercer B, Thorp JM, Moawad A, O'Sullivan MJ, Ramin S, Carpenter MW, Rouse DJ, Sibai B, Gabbe SG, National Institute of Child Health and Human Development Maternal Fetal Medicine Units Network. Single versus weekly courses of antenatal corticosteroids: evaluation of safety and efficacy. Am J Obstet Gynecol. 2006;195(3):633–42.
185. Waters TP, Mercer B. Impact of timing of antenatal corticosteroid exposure on neonatal outcomes. J Matern Fetal Neonatal Med. 2009;22(4):311–4.
186. Watson HA, Carter J, Seed PT, Shennan AH. Re: effect of QUiPP prediction algorithm on treatment decisions in women with a previous preterm birth: a prospective cohort study. BJOG. 2019;126(13):1642.
187. Watson HA, Carter J, Seed PT, Tribe RM, Shennan AH. The QUiPP App: a safe alternative to a treat-all strategy for threatened preterm labor. Ultrasound Obstet Gynecol. 2017;50(3):342–6.
188. Weitzner O, Barrett J, Murphy KE, Kingdom J, Aviram A, Mei-Dan E, Hiersch L, Ryan G, Van Mieghem T, Abbasi N, Fox NS, Rebarber A, Berghella V, Melamed N. National and interna-

tional guidelines on the management of twin pregnancies: a comparative review. Am J Obstet Gynecol. 2023;229(6):577–98.
189. Whitsett JA, Matsuzaki Y. Transcriptional regulation of perinatal lung maturation. Pediatr Clin N Am. 2006;53(5):873–87. viii
190. Wijnberger LD, Bilardo CM, Hecher K, Stigter RH, Visser GH. Effect of antenatal glucocorticoid therapy on arterial and venous blood flow velocity waveforms in severely growth-restricted fetuses. Ultrasound Obstet Gynecol. 2004;23(6):584–9.
191. Williams MJ, Ramson JA, Brownfoot FC. Different corticosteroids and regimens for accelerating fetal lung maturation for babies at risk of preterm birth. Cochrane Database Syst Rev. 2022;8(8):CD006764.
192. Wynne K, Rowe C, Delbridge M, Watkins B, Brown K, Addley J, Woods A, Murray H. Antenatal corticosteroid administration for foetal lung maturation. F1000Res. 2020;9:**219**.
193. Yu HY, Wang W, Benson CB, Doubilet P, Rouse DJ, Little SE. External validation of a prediction model assessing risk of delivery in fetuses with growth restriction after Diagnosis of Abnormal Umbilical Artery Doppler. Am J Perinatol. 2024;41(S 01):e1824–9.

Preeclampsia Screening and Prediction

Piya Chaemsaithong and Liona C. Poon

Contents

Y. Yogev, A. Khalil (eds.), *Prevention of Complications in Obstetrics*,
https://doi.org/10.1007/978-3-032-23479-7_13

Learning Objectives

- Explain principles of preeclampsia prediction and the limitations of maternal risk-factor–only screening
- Describe biophysical and biochemical markers used in first-, second-, and third-trimester prediction
- Compare major prediction approaches, including logistic regression, Bayes theorem, and competing risk models
- Evaluate validation evidence for different prediction algorithms, especially FMF models
- Understand the role of quality assurance in maintaining measurement accuracy and screening performance

13.1 Introduction

Preeclampsia is a heterogeneous, multi-organ disorder of pregnancy characterized by a new onset of hypertension with significant proteinuria or other maternal end-organ dysfunction, including neurological complications, pulmonary edema, hematologic complications, acute kidney injury, or uteroplacental dysfunction occurring after 20 weeks' gestation. This condition affects 2–8% of pregnancies globally and causes significant maternal and neonatal morbidity and mortality [1–10]. Approximately 76,000 women and 500,000 babies die annually from this disorder [11].

Screening women and identifying those at risk of developing preeclampsia allow early intervention and prophylactic administration of low-dose aspirin and therefore improve maternal and fetal outcomes [12–19]. Without a single test that can determine risk, many algorithms have been developed and modified in recent years. This review aims to describe methods to screen for preeclampsia to optimize patient care of women throughout all gestations of pregnancy.

13.2 Principle of Prediction of Preeclampsia

One of the major tasks in obstetrics is to estimate the risk for an individual patient: this can be done using a risk indicator or predictor or, more frequently, a combination of factors (e.g., Apgar scores and Bishop scores). In the particular case of preeclampsia, the American College of Obstetrics and Gynecologists (ACOG) has proposed a risk assessment method that classifies patients into high-risk or low-risk groups based on maternal characteristics (e.g., age, parity, body mass index, history of chronic hypertension, etc.) to consider aspirin administration to prevent preeclampsia [20]. New approaches for prediction consider not only historical information but also that derived from parameters observed during the ongoing pregnancy [e.g., mean arterial pressure, maternal circulating concentration of placental growth factor (PlGF), etc.]. When multiple predictors are available, the key question is how to combine them to arrive at an estimate of personalized risk for a given patient—mathematical models are used for this purpose and are now in daily use in obstetrics.

The key factors that define predictive model strategies are (1) the specific predictors considered (e.g., maternal characteristics, obstetrical history, and biophysical and biochemical biomarkers); (2) the method used to combine the information provided by the predictors into a risk estimate (e.g., via multivariate logistic regression or Bayes' theorem); and (3) the outcome (binary: preeclampsia vs. non-preeclampsia, or continuous: gestational age at delivery with preeclampsia). Other key aspects that can influence the generalizability of the findings include population characteristics and the method used to determine predictive performance. Such estimates have been reported using: (1) re-substitution, in which the same data set is used to develop and test the model; (2) internal cross-validation using a split-sample approach or bootstrap based on data collected from the same population; and (3) external validation, in which the model is applied to an independent data set, ideally by an independent investigator. Models should also be calibrated to estimate agreement between outcomes and predictors [21, 22].

A common approach in clinical medicine for combining multiple predictors into a disease risk score is the use of multivariate logistic regression, which allows calculation of the risk of preeclampsia (treated as a binary outcome—yes/no) or its clinical subtypes (early, late, preterm, or term). The log-odds of disease generated from such logistic regression models can be transformed into a probability of disease [p = odds/(1 + odds)], and women with a probability above a cutoff (e.g., 0.9) will be considered as being at risk. When this approach is used, the lack of independence of predictors is accounted for by assigning weights (i.e., coefficients) to the different parameters to maximize model fit [21, 22].

One advantage of multivariate logistic regression is that it can be implemented using standard statistical packages. However, this approach has limitations: it does not predict when preeclampsia will occur in gestation, and hence, separate models would need to be generated for early, preterm, and term preeclampsia. Another limitation is the requirement that all predictors be observed in the same patients; one solution would be to create separate prediction models based on data that is more available (e.g., maternal characteristics and obstetrical history) and another model using biophysical and biochemical markers (referred to as biomarkers), with each model generating a risk estimate for a given patient. The former is generally referred to as a *prior risk* model since it is based on information available before pregnancy (e.g., maternal age, parity, etc.) or early gestation (e.g., history of chronic hypertension). The Bayes Theorem is then used to combine the prior risk of preeclampsia derived from biomarkers; yet, the fundamental assumption of the Bayes Theorem is that the two risk estimates are independent. However, this requirement is not met because biomarker values (such as concentrations of an analyte or mean arterial blood pressure) also vary with some of the same maternal characteristics incorporated in the *prior risk* model. Therefore, to decouple the sources of evidence and render them independent, the biomarker data are first transformed into multiples of the mean (MoM) values for maternal characteristics and gestational age at measurement [23].

Different groups of investigators have used the concept of combining the risk estimate derived from a prior risk model (e.g., fit using logistic regression) and evidence from a biomarker-based model [24–30]. Differences among approaches include whether the a priori risk and biomarker-based risk are assigned equal weight (Fetal Medicine Foundation [31, 32]) or different weights [33] and the method to calculate biomarker-based risk.

The Fetal Medicine Foundation (FMF) proposed to frame the prediction of preeclampsia as a time-to-event model (or "survival time model") for gestational age at delivery with preeclampsia rather than whether or not the patient developed preeclampsia. Therefore, this approach, called the "competing risk model," captures disease severity via gestational age at delivery with preeclampsia, while approaches using a binary outcome are blind to that information. The 'competing risk model' also alleviates the need for separate models for early, preterm, and term phenotypes because it estimates the risk of delivering with preeclampsia at any gestational age [34–36]. Tarca et al. have proposed that instead of equal weighting of prior risk and biomarker risk calculations, more weight could be given to biomarker-derived risk, especially later in pregnancy, when it is more predictive of disease [33].

Serra et al. have proposed an alternative model to predict early-onset preeclampsia as a binary outcome by fitting the biomarker log MoM data to a multivariate normal distribution [32]. This approach is similar to logistic regression modeling in that it allows the calculation of risk for a specific binary outcome (e.g., early, preterm preeclampsia). The biomarker-derived risk and the prior risk are combined using Bayes Theorem just as the Fetal Medicine Foundation (FMF) approach does. However, Serra et al. [32] described that an advantage of their method is that the prior risk is based on knowledge accumulated from different sources via aggregate meta-analysis instead of being derived from individual patient data. Which modeling approach is best requires further investigation.

An important advantage of the FMF approach is that it has been internally and externally validated, although risk cut-offs may need to be customized depending on the target population. Indeed, when the FMF model was applied to an Asian population, the risk cut-offs were modified based on information derived from the population [37, 38].

13.3 Maternal Risk Factors

In 2008, the National Institute for Health and Care Excellence (NICE) reported maternal risk factors for the determination of a patient's risk for preeclampsia [39]. However, a subsequent study demonstrated that the use of maternal risk factors alone was inaccurate since this method had detection rates of 89.2%, 93.0%, and 85.0% for early preeclampsia, late preeclampsia, and gestational hypertension, respectively, at a false positive rate of 64.1% [28].

In 2010, maternal risk factors were subsequently classified into moderate- and high-risk for preeclampsia [40]. For example, the presence of one of the following risk factors is considered high-risk: hypertensive disease in a previous pregnancy, chronic hypertension, chronic renal disease, or diabetes mellitus (or autoimmune disease). The presence of more than one moderate risk factor (nulliparity, age ≥40 years, body mass index [BMI] ≥35 kg/m^2, family history of preeclampsia, or inter-pregnancy interval of >10 years) is also considered high-risk. Patients classified as high-risk are recommended to administer 75 mg of aspirin daily from 12 weeks of gestation until delivery. Subsequently, in 2019, such recommendations were modified and changed the dose of aspirin for high-risk patients to 75–150 mg daily; in addition, multiple pregnancies are included as a moderate risk factor [41].

Similarly, the American College of Obstetricians and Gynecologists (ACOG) in the U.S. Preventive Services Task Force (USPTF) has described maternal risk factors for preeclampsia in 2013 [42], and the administration of low-dose aspirin for the prevention of preeclampsia is recommended for patients with ≥1 high-risk factor or ≥2 moderate risk factors. The ACOG preeclampsia screening recommendation has updated USPSTF guidelines in 2018, and it includes the use of low-dose aspirin at 81 mg/day initiated between 12 and 28 weeks of gestation, although it is preferable to administer it at <16 weeks of gestation until delivery to high-risk patients [42]. A previous study demonstrated that the ACOG recommendation (2013) had detection rates of 5% (95% CI: 2–14) and 2% (95% CI: 0.3–5) for preterm and term preeclampsia, respectively, with a 0.2% false positive rate [28]. The expanded list of clinical risk factors included in the USPSTF 2018 recommendation has increased the detection rates to 90% (95% CI: 79–96) and 89% (95% CI: 84–94) for preterm and term preeclampsia, respectively; however, the false positive rate has increased to as high as 64% [43]. In fact, the recommendations by NICE and ACOG treat each maternal risk factor as a separate screening test with an additive detection rate and screen-positive rate. In addition, such maternal risk factors do not differentiate the severity of preeclampsia (i.e., preterm vs. term) [37]. Altogether, these factors underpin the suboptimal performance of preeclampsia screening based on maternal risk factors alone.

Other professional organizations, including the World Health Organization (2011) [44], the Society of Obstetric Medicine of Australia and New Zealand (2014) [45], the International Society for the Study of Hypertension in Pregnancy (2021) [46], and the International Federation of Gynecology and Obstetrics (FIGO) (2019) [47], have also proposed the use of maternal risk factors for the screening of preeclampsia. Table 13.1 demonstrates a summary of maternal risk factors for preeclampsia screening according to some professional organizations.

Table 13.1 Maternal Risk factors for preeclampsia according to common professional organizations [47]

NICE 2019	**ACOG 2020**	**FIGO 2019**	**ISSHP 2021**
One or more of the following: *High-risk factors* Hypertensive disease in a previous pregnancy Chronic kidney disease Autoimmune diseases such as SLE or antiphospholipid syndrome Type 1 or type 2 diabetes Chronic hypertension OR *Any two of the following:* *Moderate risk factors* First pregnancy Age $\geq$40 years Pregnancy interval >10 years BMI $\geq$35 kg/m^2 at first prenatal visit Family history of preeclampsia Multiple pregnancy	*One or more of the following:* *High-risk factors* History of preeclampsia Multiple pregnancy Chronic hypertension Type 1 or type 2 diabetes Kidney disease Autoimmune diseases, such as SLE or antiphospholipid syndrome OR *Any two of the following:* *Moderate risk factors* First pregnancy Obesity (BMI >30 kg/m^2) Family history of preeclampsia (mother or sister) African-American Age $\geq$35 years Personal history factors (i.e., LBW, SGA, previous adverse pregnancy outcome, >10-year pregnancy interval) IVF Pregnancy interval >10 years	Maternal characteristics Age Weight Height Ethnicity (white, Afro-Caribbean, South Asian, East Asian, Mixed) Past obstetric history (nulliparous, parous with and without prior preeclampsia) Inter-pregnancy interval Gestational age at delivery (weeks) and birthweight of previous pregnancy beyond 24 weeks Family history of pre-eclampsia (mother) Method of conception (spontaneous, ovulation induction, IVF) Smoking Chronic hypertension Diabetes type 1, type 2, insulin intake SLE or antiphospholipid syndrome	*One or more of the following:* *High-risk factors* Prior preeclampsia Chronic hypertension Pregestational diabetes mellitus Prepregnancy BMI >30 kg/m^2 Chronic kidney disease SLE or Antiphospholipid syndrome Assisted reproductive therapy (varies with the methods used) OR *≥ 2 of moderate risk factors* Maternal age >40 years Prior placental abruption Prior stillbirth Prior fetal growth restriction Nulliparity Multifetal pregnancy

(continued)

Table 13.1 (continued)

NICE 2019	ACOG 2020	FIGO 2019	ISSHP 2021
Aspirin 75–150 mg daily from 12 weeks until the birth of the baby in High risk ≥2 moderate risk factors	Aspirin 81 mg daily should be initiated between 12 and 28 weeks' gestation (optimally before 16 weeks) until the birth of the baby in High risk ≥2 moderate risk factors	Aspirin ~150 mg/night should be commenced at 11–14^{+6} weeks' gestation until 36 weeks' gestation in high-risk women according to the Fetal Medicine Foundation first-trimester combined preeclampsia screening test	Aspirin 100–162 mg/night should be given preferably before 16 until 36 weeks' gestation in High risk ≥2 moderate risk factors In addition, aspirin ~150 mg/night should be commenced at 11–14^{+6} weeks' gestation until 36 weeks' gestation in high-risk women according to the Fetal Medicine Foundation first-trimester combined preeclampsia screening test

IVF in vitro fertilization, *LBW* low birth weight, *SGA* small for gestational age, *SLE* systemic lupus erythematosus, *NICE* National Institute for Health and Care Excellence, *FIGO* The International Federation of Gynecology and Obstetrics, *ISSHP* The International Society for the Study of Hypertension in Pregnancy, *ACOG* American College of Obstetricians and Gynecologists, *BMI* body mass index, *BP* blood pressure, *hCG* human chorionic gonadotropin, *ISSHP* International Society for the Study of Hypertension in Pregnancy, *NICE* National Institute for Health and Care Excellence, *PAPP-A* pregnancy-associated plasma protein-A, *PE* preeclampsia, *SGA* small for gestational age, *SOGC* Society of Obstetricians and Gynaecologists of Canada, *SOMANZ* Society of Obstetric Medicine of Australia and New Zealand, *WHO* World Health Organization

The other alternative approach is to use a logistic regression for the combination of maternal risk factors. Specifically, in a study of 9149 singleton pregnancies with seven cases with early preeclampsia, 128 cases of late preeclampsia, and 140 with gestational hypertension, the presence of chronic hypertension (OR 8.70), ovulation induction (OR 4.75), a history of preeclampsia (OR 4.02), and women of Afro-Caribbean origin (OR 3.64) are associated with early preeclampsia [48]. In contrast, maternal risk factors of late preeclampsia include the presence of a family history of preeclampsia (OR 2.91), a history of preeclampsia (OR 2.18), maternal age (OR 1.04), BMI (OR 1.10), and Afro-Caribbean and South Asian women (OR 2.66–3.31). The detection rate of maternal risk factors alone achieved a detection rate of 37% and 29% for early- and late preeclampsia, respectively, at a 5% false positive rate. This approach differs from previous studies in that the maternal risk factors based on logistic regression were separated between early- and late- preeclampsia [48].

A recent large systematic review and meta-analysis, including 92 studies with over 25 million pregnancies, has been conducted to determine maternal risk factors at ≤16 weeks of gestation for a risk of preeclampsia [49]. The presence of antiphospholipid antibody syndrome had the highest risk of preeclampsia (RR 17.3, 95% CI: 6.8–31.4). The risk of other maternal factors was the following: a history of preeclampsia (RR 8.4) and chronic hypertension (RR 5.1), pregestational diabetes mellitus (RR 3.7), prepregnancy BMI of >30 kg/m^2 (RR 2.8), nulliparity (RR 2.1), chronic kidney disease (RR 1.8), conception by assisted reproductive technology (RR 1.8), and maternal age >35 years (RR 1.2) [49].

13.4 Biophysical Markers

13.4.1 Mean Arterial Pressure

Women who subsequently develop preeclampsia have higher blood pressure since the first and second trimesters of pregnancy [24].

Standardized blood pressure measurement is the key to early screening and diagnosis of preeclampsia. Variations in measurement techniques or incorrect protocol adherence lead to inaccuracy of screening performance.

Based on the protocol by the National Heart Foundation of Australia (NHFA) [50], women are asked to rest for 5 min in the sitting position with their backs leaning against the seat, their arms supported at the level of the heart, and their legs uncrossed. Appropriate cuff size is selected based on the mid-arm circumference (small <22 cm, normal 22–32 cm, or large 33–42 cm) (◘ Fig. 13.1). According to this protocol, blood pressure is measured in both arms, and at least two recordings are made at 1-min intervals until variations between consecutive readings fall to within 10 mmHg in systolic BP and 6 mmHg in diastolic blood pressure in both arms [50]. When this point of stability is achieved, the average of the last two stable measurements of the left and right arms is calculated, and it is recommended that the higher of these two measurements from the two arms be used [51]. However, to achieve the necessary point of blood pressure stability according to the NHFA protocol, it has been shown that it is necessary to perform two measurements in both arms in about 50% of cases, three measurements in 25% of cases, and four measurements in 25% [52]. In addition, whether blood pressure should be taken on the left or right arm remains a subject of discussion. The evidence supporting simultaneous measurement of both arms is derived from the study published by Poon et al. [53]. The prevalence of blood pressure inter-arm difference (IAD; defined as an IAD of >10 mmHg of systolic and diastolic blood pressure) was found in 8.3% of normal pregnant women (n = 5435) [53]. These observations suggest the importance of blood pressure measurement in both arms.

A simplified protocol for blood pressure measurement has been developed through a study of 25,505 singleton pregnancies where blood pressure measurements were made at 11–13 weeks of gestation by using a validated automatic device (3BTO-A2, Microlife, Taipei, Taiwan) [52]. The performance of preeclampsia screening by different combinations of mean arterial pressure has been compared to that derived from the NHFA protocol. The results have demonstrated that the performance of screening for preeclampsia by taking the average of a minimum of two measurements from both arms is comparable to the NHFA protocol. Our group has demonstrated that at 10–40 weeks of gesta-

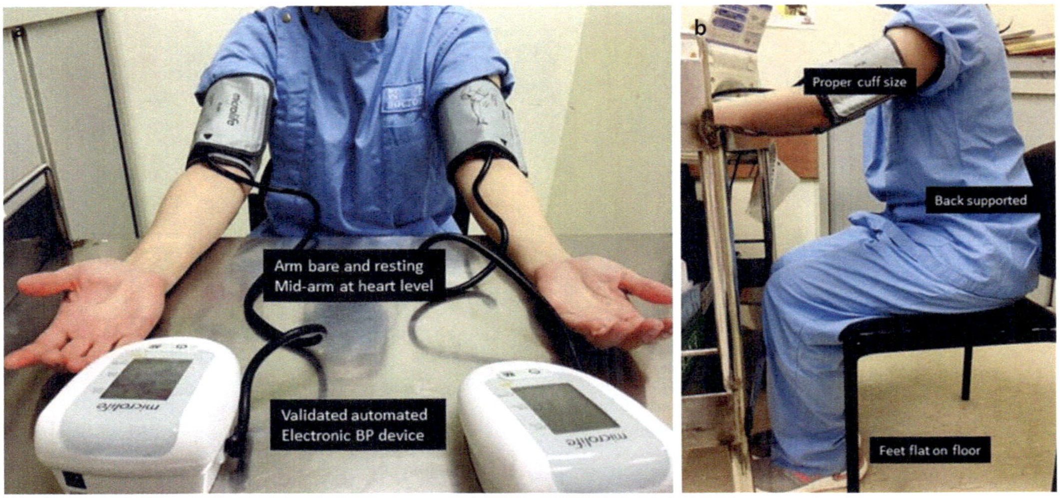

◘ **Fig. 13.1** Correct position for blood pressure measurement in pregnant women: **a** front view and **b** side view; from Chaemsaithong. First-trimester preeclampsia screening and prediction. (Am J Obstet Gynecol 2022). Measurement of uterine artery resistance indices in the first trimester tion, blood pressure recordings can be obtained by the same simplified protocol using the average of two measurements in both arms [54]. In conclusion, the blood pressure should be measured in both arms simultaneously with the correct positioning of patients, and the final mean arterial pressure is calculated from the average of the four measurements (◘ Fig. 13.1).

Mean arterial pressure is affected by several factors, including gestational age, maternal age, racial origin, BMI, smoking, family history of preeclampsia, history of preeclampsia, chronic hypertension, and diabetes mellitus [55]. Therefore, the mean arterial pressure should be converted to a multiple of the median (MoM), which measures how far an individual test result deviates from the median of the reference population (or normal population), adjusted for these variables in a multivariable prediction model.

Poon et al. reported the value of mean arterial pressure at 11–13^{+6} weeks of gestation in the prediction of preeclampsia [24]. Maternal blood pressure was determined in 5590 singleton pregnant women by automated devices (3BTO-A2 Microlife) and appropriately trained doctors. The measurement of blood pressure followed the NHFA protocol [52]. Mean arterial pressure alone and combined testing (history and mean arterial pressure) had the detection rates for preeclampsia of 37.5% and 62.5%, respectively, at a 10% false positive rate. A follow-up study of more than 9000 pregnancies at 11–13 weeks of gestation compared the screening performance of systolic blood pressure, diastolic blood pressure, and mean arterial pressure [25]. The mean arterial pressure is the best marker with a detection rate for early preeclampsia, increasing from 47% (based on maternal factors alone) to 76% (based on a combination of maternal risk factors and mean arterial pressure) at a false positive rate of 10% [25].

13

13.4.2 Uterine Artery Pulsatility Index (UtA-PI)

Impaired uteroplacental circulation can be observed as abnormal uterine artery Doppler velocimetry as early as the first trimester. A standardized measurement of uterine pulsatility index (UtA-PI) is required for reproducible, consistent, and accurate preeclampsia screening. The Fetal Medicine Foundation (FMF) recommends obtaining UtA-PI measurements at the cervical internal os level via a transabdominal ultrasound measurement (◘ Fig. 13.2). The measurement of UtA-PI at

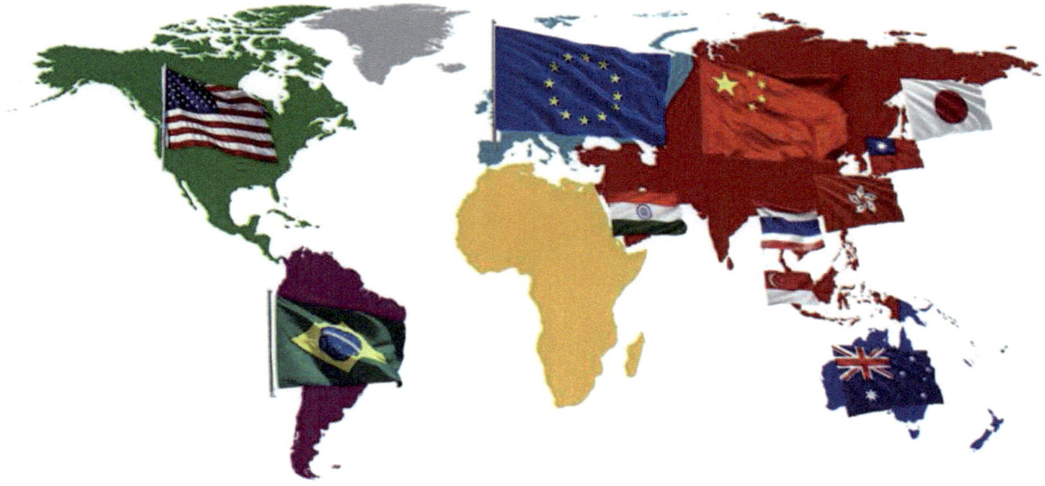

◘ **Fig. 13.2** Countries and regions with successful external validation of the first-trimester Fetal Medicine Foundation preeclampsia prediction models from Chaemsaithong. First-trimester preeclampsia screening and prediction. (Am J Obstet Gynecol 2022)

the level of internal os during the first trimester is more reproducible than those obtained at the level of external iliac vessels crossover [56]. In addition, a better correlation between the first- and second-trimester UtA-PI when the first-trimester measurement is taken at the level of the internal os rather than at the external iliac vessels crossover was observed [56].

UtA-PI is associated with several factors, including gestational age, maternal age at birth of the last pregnancy, and birthweight Z-score [57]. Hence, the UtA-PI value must be adjusted for the above variables and converted into MoM before comparing affected and unaffected groups. The detection rate by UtA-PI alone is 77% for early-onset preeclampsia and 27% for late-onset preeclampsia at a 10% false positive rate [58, 59]. The combination of maternal factors and UtA-PI achieved 77.3% (95% CI: 54.6–92.1%) and 42.3% (95% CI: 30.6–54.6%) for early and late-onset preeclampsia, respectively, at a 10% false positive rate. These findings were confirmed by the same group of authors in a follow-up study of 8366 women, including 165 cases of preeclampsia [60].

A large meta-analysis of first-trimester uterine artery Doppler measurement for the prediction of preeclampsia included eight studies in the prediction of early preeclampsia (n = 41,692 women) and 11 studies in the prediction of preeclampsia of any gestation (n = 39,179 women) [61]. The first-trimester abnormal uterine artery Doppler, defined as the UtA-resistance index or UtA-PI >90th centile, had a sensitivity of 47.8% at 92.1% specificity for the identification of early preeclampsia. The sensitivity for predicting late preeclampsia was reduced to 26.4% at 93.4% specificity. In a low-risk population with a prevalence of early-onset preeclampsia of 0.4–1.0%, the number needed to screen to prevent one case of early preeclampsia with aspirin ranges between 1000 and 2500. For the abnormal uterine artery Doppler, the number was decreased to 173–421, which is similar to screening performance for those with the presence of high-risk factors according to the NICE guideline [62]. The measurement of UtA-PI is under scrutiny because of its methodological challenges and moderate reproducibility [63, 64]. An alternative approach in the transverse plane obtains the UtA-PI comparable to that of the conventional sagittal approach in terms of reliability, reproducibility, and time required, but is easier to perform [65]. However, as the data used to develop prediction models was based on the sagittal approach, the transverse approach can only be considered complementary.

13.5 Maternal Circulating Biochemical Markers

The most informative biochemical biomarkers for the prediction of preeclampsia are the plasma/serum concentrations of angiogenic and anti-angiogenic factors, including PlGF, sFlt-1, and sEng [66–70]. The key observations that supported the use of these biomarkers for prediction were derived from longitudinal studies in normal pregnancies, preterm preeclampsia, term preeclampsia, and small for gestational age (SGA) [71–75]. The first longitudinal study to determine angiogenic and anti-angiogenic factors in women with preeclampsia was reported by Levine et al. [71]. Maternal serum Flt-1 concentration was higher in women who subsequently developed preeclampsia, and this change occurred approximately 5 weeks before the onset of preeclampsia. In contrast, maternal PlGF concentrations were significantly lower in women with preeclampsia compared to controls beginning from 13 to 16 weeks of gestation onward, and the greatest difference was observed weeks before the diagnosis of preeclampsia. Subsequently, Romero et al. reported angiogenic and anti-angiogenic factor profiles in women with preeclampsia (classified as term and preterm) and SGA [74]. The key observations were that (1) women who developed preterm or term preeclampsia and those who delivered SGA neonates had lower maternal plasma PlGF concentrations compared to normal pregnancy from 10 to 11 weeks of gestation onward; (2) maternal plasma sFlt-1 was higher in women destined to develop preterm and term preeclampsia than that of controls from 26 to 29 weeks of gestation onward.

However, there was no difference in maternal plasma sFlt-1 concentration between women destined to deliver an SGA neonate compared to controls [74]; (3) women who subsequently delivered an SGA neonate or developed preterm and term preeclampsia had significantly higher maternal plasma sEng than controls from 10, 23, and 30 weeks, respectively. These observations supported the concept that PlGF may have predictive value for the identification of preeclampsia starting in the first trimester, while sFlt-1 and sEng might be of value for the prediction of preeclampsia only in the second or third trimester onwards [74]. These findings provided the impetus to use angiogenic and anti-angiogenic factors for risk assessment and prediction of preeclampsia in early gestation and prior to the time of diagnosis.

For the first-trimester preeclampsia prediction, incorporating PlGF to maternal factors and UtA-PI increased the detection rate from 76% to 90% at a 10% false positive rate [76]. Hence, PlGF has shown promise for early prediction of preeclampsia, as it can be detected in the maternal circulation as early as 6 weeks of gestation [77]. Similar to mean arterial pressure and UtA-PI, the measurements of PlGF are affected by maternal and pregnancy characteristics [31]. In addition, there are several PlGF analyzers, and there were statistically significant inter-manufacturer immunoassay differences regarding assay sensitivities/recovery and cross-reactivity. The values should be validated against clinical outcomes and are not interchangeable and require separate clinical validation [78].

13.6 First Trimester Preeclampsia Prediction Algorithm

The search for the optimal algorithm to enable accurate and effective prediction of preeclampsia has been ongoing for more than one decade, as there is no single variable or biomarker that can be used for the prediction of preeclampsia, and maternal risk factors alone are insufficient for the effective prediction of preeclampsia. A systematic review has reported that among the 70 preeclampsia prediction models, a combined model (including measurements of mean arterial pressure, UtA-PI, and/or biochemical markers) had higher predictive performance in both early- and late-onset preeclampsia than the 22 simple models using only maternal risk factors [79]. In addition, another systematic review, including 68 preeclampsia prediction models from 70 studies with 425,125 participants, has demonstrated that the most frequently used predictors are maternal risk factors, blood pressure, and UtA-PI [80]. Notably, most models are neither internally nor externally validated. For example, there are only two combined first-trimester prediction models [26, 81] that have undergone external validation in an independent population with different demographics and geographic settings than those of the original models [28, 82–84].

The first-trimester effective preeclampsia prediction model using a combination of factors, including maternal factors and several biomarkers (mean arterial pressure, UtA-PI, pregnancy-associated plasma protein-A, and PlGF) based on a logistic regression approach, was developed in 2009 [85]. These models had a detection rate of 93% and 36% at 5% false positive rates for early-onset and late-onset preeclampsia, respectively [85]. Although the logistic regression approach allows the addition of biomarkers, this approach assumes a binary or dichotomous outcome and that separate models are needed for each subtype of preeclampsia. Importantly, the models derived from the logistic regression approach are prone to overfitting, which can overestimate screening performance [23].

The alternative approach for the development of a prediction model is to use Bayes' theorem. This approach describes the probability of the occurrence of an event related to any condition and allows us to express a conditional probability. The advantage of this approach is that it allows the assessment of individualized patient-specific risks of preeclampsia that require delivery before a specified gestation. In addition, the risk assessment can be updated when new biomarkers are available, thus providing a dynamic risk assessment [37].

Based on Bayes' theorem, the competing risk model has been developed. This approach is based on a survival-time model in which the assumption is that if the pregnancy were to continue indefinitely, all women would develop preeclampsia. The "competition" is whether delivery occurs before preeclampsia or vice versa. The advantage of this approach is that it allows for the personalization of risk assessment, incorporating both the risk factors and the protective factors, such as the presence of no history of preeclampsia [35].

Using a competing risk model approach, a study including 120,492 singleton pregnancies with 2704 cases of preeclampsia (2.2%) demonstrated that maternal factors had a 54% and 48% detection rate for early- and late-onset preeclampsia at a 10% false positive rate. These numbers are greater than the detection rates from the NICE approach [86].

The largest study for a first-trimester preeclampsia prediction model using the competing risk model was performed in 61,174 women with 1770 (2.9%) cases of preeclampsia [31]. The combination model, including maternal factors, UtA-PI, mean arterial pressure, and PlGF, achieved a 90% detection rate of early preeclampsia, 75% of preterm preeclampsia, and 41% of term preeclampsia at a false positive rate of 10%. The incorporation of pregnancy-associated plasma protein-A did not improve predictive performance [37].

Other first-trimester preeclampsia prediction models have been developed by several groups of investigators, mainly in Spain and the United States. Two Spanish cohort studies reported similar performances as the FMF model [87, 88], while the studies on American populations had lower detection rates [89–91].

The prediction model for early-onset preeclampsia using a multivariable Gaussian distribution approach was developed [92]. This approach allows flexibility and adaptation to various populations because of multiple approaches to biomarker acquisition. Specifically, a model consisting of maternal factors, mean arterial pressure, and UtA-PI at 11 to 13^{+6} weeks of gestation and PlGF at 8 to 13^{+6} weeks of gestation achieved a detection rate of 94.1% at a 10% false positive rate for the identification of early-onset preeclampsia [92]. The UtA-PI measurement can be performed either transabdominally or transvaginally, and the PlGF measurement can be done from as early as 8 weeks of gestation, which can be done at the same time as Down syndrome screening. Yet, the drawbacks of this approach are related to the lack of internal and external validation.

A prospective cohort study performed in a Spanish population included 10,110 women with 32 (0.3%), 72 (0.7%), and 230 (2.3%) cases of early preterm and any preeclampsia [93]. The authors compared the preeclampsia screening performance of (1) an FMF triple test, (2) a model developed by Crovetto et al., (3) a model developed by Serra et al., (4) NICE, and (5) the ACOG guideline. A combined model with maternal factors achieves the best performance of screening for preterm preeclampsia, mean arterial pressure, UtA-PI, and PlGF, as compared to risk-scoring systems such as those of NICE and ACOG. The three algorithms show similar results in terms of overall prediction; the FMF model showed the best performance at an individual level, in which the best correlation between predicted and observed cases was achieved by the FMF model, with an area under the curve (AUC) of 0.91, a slope of 0.98, and an intercept of 0.15 [93]. Thus far, preeclampsia prediction models derived from the Fetal Medicine Foundation are the only models successfully validated internally and externally.

13.7 The Fetal Medicine Foundation Preeclampsia Prediction Models

Originally, the first-trimester FMF preeclampsia prediction models were developed from the European population. The first version of the model was described by Poon et al. in 2009 [85]. A combined model consisting of maternal factors, mean arterial pressure, UtA-PI, pregnancy-associated plasma protein-A, and PlGF by the use of multivariate logistic regression analysis achieved detection rates of 93% and 36% for early- and late-onset preeclampsia, respectively, at a 5% false positive rate [85].

Subsequently, the combined model (maternal characteristics, biophysical, and biochemical markers) with the use of a competing risk algorithm (a survival-time model) yielded a detection rate of 96% and 54% of cases of early and late preeclampsia at a false positive rate of 10% [81]. Data from prospective screening, including 35,948 singleton pregnancies with 1058 pregnancies (2.9%) with preeclampsia, were used to update the original algorithm. Combined screening with a "triple test" had 75% and 47% detection rates for preterm and term preeclampsia, respectively, at a false positive rate of 10%. The incorporation of pregnancy-associated plasma protein-A did not improve the screening performance. These numbers are similar to the detection rates of an aspirin implementation study conducted in six countries [13].

In 2018, a large study on the development of the FMF first-trimester combination test using the competing risk model was reported by Tan et al. in 2018 [31, 94]. The best predictive performance was achieved by a combination of maternal factors with mean arterial pressure, UtA-PI, and serum PlGF (the FMF triple test), with detection rates of 90% for very early preeclampsia with delivery at <32 weeks, 75% for preterm, and 41% for term preeclampsia at a 10% false positive rate. The latest FMF triple test has undergone successful internal and external validation and calibration [94]. The addition of sFlt-1 does not improve the screening performance [95].

To further improve the detection rate of the FMF triple test, a recent study found that the addition of maternal serum glycosylated fibronectin (GlyFn), a biomarker associated with vascular remodeling, to the FMF triple test for preterm preeclampsia increased significantly the AUC from 0.86 to 0.89 ($p = 0.012$) with an increased detection rate at a 10% false positive rate from 64.9% (95% CI: 48.7–81.1%) to 82.9% (95% CI: 66.4–93.4%). The detection rates at a 10% false positive rate for any-onset preeclampsia were 52.5% (95% CI: 42.3–62.5%) and 65.4% (95% CI: 55.2–74.5%), respectively [96].

13.7.1 Validation of the First Trimester Fetal Medicine Foundation Preeclampsia Prediction Models

Effective first-trimester prediction models are developed to institute appropriate preventive strategies. However, past research has focused on specific populations and settings in formulating these prediction models. The differences in population characteristics, such as race, height, weight, prevalence of preeclampsia, and small study population sizes used for prediction models, can affect predictive performance.

External validation is necessary to determine a prediction model's reproducibility and generalizability to new and different patients [97, 98]. The best approach for evaluating a prediction model is to perform external validation, in which the population tested should be independent of the population used for the development of the model [99]. This approach reflects the generalizability of the prediction model [21].

The FMF algorithm model has been evaluated in several populations, including Italian, Australian, US, Brazilian, mixed European [26, 27, 82, 100–105], and Asian populations [19, 43]. Almost all validation studies have reported comparable predictive performance corresponding to the original studies [26, 82, 101, 104], except in the Italian and USA populations [100, 106]. Specifically, the validation study performed by Farina et al. [100] in 554 Italian pregnant women with 39 cases of late-onset preeclampsia (7%) showed that among the eight evaluated models, two models had lower detection rates, four models had similar detection rates, and two models had lower, similar, and higher detection rates, respectively, compared to the original studies. The model reported by Poon et al. (2010), which consisted of maternal factors, mean arterial pressure, UtA-PI, and maternal serum pregnancy-associated placental protein-A concentration at 11–13 weeks of gestation, achieved the highest detection rate (detection rate 84.6% at a 10% false positive rate) for the identification of late-onset preeclampsia. However, these detection rates deviate from the original study (57% at a 10% false positive rate), which might be attributed to the small sample size.

The validation study of the FMF model performed in the USA population demonstrated the discrepancies of prediction algorithms between validated and original studies [106]. Oliveira et al. evaluated the predictive performance of six first-trimester algorithms [59, 89, 107, 108] in 2969 women, with frequencies of early and late onset of preeclampsia of 1.0–1.2% and 4.1–5.0%, respectively. For the prediction of early-onset preeclampsia, observed detection rates at a fixed 10% false positive rate of all models except one [89] were lower than those derived from the original models. The detection rates obtained from validated cohorts ranged between 29% and 80% at a 10% false positive rate. Similar to the model for early-onset preeclampsia, the detection rates for late-onset preeclampsia in the validation studies were lower than the reported values. The differences in detection rates might be attributed to the origin of the population, as only the model derived from the USA population had better predictive values in the external validation study.

Several validation studies of first-trimester FMF preeclampsia prediction models have been performed in large populations. First, O'Gorman et al. conducted a European-wide multicenter, prospective, nonintervention study to validate the FMF first-trimester combined test in 8775 pregnant women, including 239 (2.7%) with preeclampsia. The screening performance was similar to that obtained from the original study and reported detection rates of 100%, 75%, and 43% at a 10% false positive rate for very early, preterm, and term preeclampsia, respectively [28]. Subsequently, in 2018, in a prospective study of 61,174 mixed European singleton pregnancies, including 1770 (2.9%) with preeclampsia, combined screening by maternal factors, UtA-PI, mean arterial pressure, and PlGF had detection rates of 90% of early preeclampsia, 75% of preterm preeclampsia, and 41% of term preeclampsia at a screen-positive rate of 10%. The incorporation of PAPP-A did not improve the screening performance. Such detection rates nearly doubled that of the 41.6% by NICE [31].

Recently, the FMF triple test was validated in a multicenter study in Asia, including 10,935 women with 73 cases (0.67%) of preterm preeclampsia [43]. The FMF triple test achieved detection rates of 64.0% at a 10% false positive rate for the prediction of preterm preeclampsia. The screening performance was comparable with that of East Asian women in previously published data from the FMF study [31] and was superior to the approach recommended by ACOG and NICE [43]. This study is considered a landmark study for the external validation of preeclampsia prediction models because the study population is different from the original population utilized for model development.

In a recent multicenter stepped wedge cluster randomized trial including 42,897 women from ten Asian regions, this trial started with a nonintervention phase in which all recruiting centers provided routine antenatal care without study-related intervention [19]. At regular 6-week intervals, one cluster was randomized to transition from the nonintervention phase to the intervention phase [19]. In the intervention phase, women underwent first-trimester FMF triple test screening for preterm preeclampsia. High-risk women (risk ≥1 in 100) received low-dose aspirin from <16 weeks until 36 weeks of gestation. In this study, the first-trimester FMF triple test achieved an AUC of 0.89 (95% CI: 0.85–0.93) and had a detection rate of 70.9% at a 10% false positive rate, respectively, for the prediction of preterm preeclampsia. On the calibration of the model, the intercept was 0.0002, and the calibration slope was 0.85 (95% CI: 0.84–0.85), which was close to 1.0, suggesting a good agreement between the predicted risks and observed incidence of preterm preeclampsia. The administration of aspirin prophylaxis was significantly associated with a 41% reduction in the incidence of preterm preeclampsia (aOR 0.59; 95% CI: 0.37–0.92) among high-risk women in the intervention phase. In addition, the administration of aspirin prophylaxis correlated with a 54%, 55%, and 64% reduction in the frequency of preeclampsia with delivery at <34 weeks (aOR 0.46; 95% CI: 0.23–0.93), spontaneous preterm birth <34 weeks (aOR 0.45; 95% CI: 0.22–0.92), and perinatal death (aOR 0.34; 95% CI:

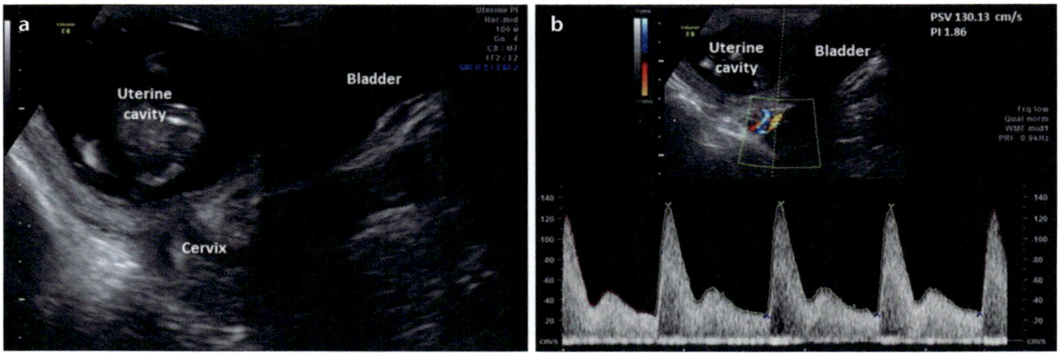

Fig. 13.3 Measurement of uterine artery resistance indices in the first trimester: **a** sagittal section of the cervix is identified. The ultrasound probe is tilted to see the uterine artery. **b** The uterine artery is identified at the level of the cervical os. From Chaemsaithong. First-trimester preeclampsia screening and prediction. (Am J Obstet Gynecol 2022)

0.12–0.91), respectively. These observations demonstrated a successful external validation of the FMF triple test and underscore the importance of the widespread implementation of the screen-and-prevent strategy for preterm preeclampsia [19].

In summary, the FMF first-trimester combined models are the only models that have successfully undergone internal and external validations (Fig. 13.3). Several professional organizations have endorsed first-trimester FMF preeclampsia prediction, including the International Society of Ultrasound in Obstetrics and Gynecology (ISUOG) and the International Federation of Gynecology and Obstetrics (FIGO) in 2019 [47, 109]. Other models developed by other investigators have not undergone successful or lacked validation studies, and this process is essential prior to clinical implementation [37].

13

13.7.2 Risk Assessment of Preeclampsia in the Second Trimester in Asymptomatic Pregnant Women

For risk assessment in the second trimester, Kusanovic et al. demonstrated that an imbalance in angiogenic and anti-angiogenic factors in early pregnancy (6–15 weeks) and mid-trimester (20–25 weeks of gestation) could be used for the identification of women who are destined to develop preeclampsia. The PlGF/sEng ratio at mid-trimester, its delta (change in maternal PlGF/sEng ratio between early pregnancy and mid-trimester), and its slope (difference between PlGF/sEng ratio between early pregnancy and mid-trimester divided by the number of weeks between the measurements) had a sensitivity of 100%; a specificity of 98–99%; and positive likelihood ratios of 57.6, 55.6, and 89.6 for the prediction of preeclampsia diagnosed at <34 weeks of gestation, respectively [110]. PlGF/sFlt-1 or PlGF/sEng-1 were used instead of sFlt-1/PlGF or sEng-1/PlGF because PlGF concentrations were occasionally undetectable with the available assays. In addition, the profile of PlGF/sFlt-1 throughout gestation resembles that of PlGF.

Subsequently, several studies have evaluated the use of sFlt-1 and/or PlGF for preeclampsia risk stratification in the second trimester either as a single predictor or combined with other biomarkers [38, 111]. The largest study to date was performed on 7748 unselected pregnant women at 19–24 weeks of gestation [112]. A competing risk model based on maternal factors, mean arterial pressure, UtA-PI, and maternal serum PlGF achieved detection rates of 99%, 85%, and 46% for the identification of preeclampsia with delivery at <32, <37, and ≥37 weeks of gestation, at a 10% false positive rate [112]. This prediction algorithm has been successfully validated in 16,254 unselected pregnant women [29]. Key findings from these observations are that (1) preeclampsia risk assessment at 19–24 weeks of gestation yields greater predictive performance for the identification of early and preterm preeclampsia compared to preeclampsia risk assessment determined in the first trimester, and (2) importantly, risk assessment for preeclampsia at the second trimester has limited value for the identification of women with late or term preeclampsia [29, 30, 110].

13.7.3 Risk Assessment of Preeclampsia in the Third Trimester in Asymptomatic Pregnant Women

Several prediction algorithms have been developed based on blood samples obtained between 31 and 34 and 35 and 37 weeks of gestation [105, 113–115]. Chaiworapongsa et al. were the first to demonstrate the use of maternal plasma angiogenic/anti-angiogenic factors in the third trimester of pregnancy (30–34 weeks of gestation) for the identification of late-onset preeclampsia [113]. In 1269 pregnancies, including 40 women with preeclampsia, the maternal plasma concentration of PlGF/sEng <0.3 MoM at 30–34 weeks of gestation was associated with the development of late-onset preeclampsia (aOR 7) and severe late-onset preeclampsia (aOR 16), respectively. In addition, PlGF/sEng and PlGF/sFlt-1 ratios had sensitivities of 78% and 74% for the identification of late-onset and severe late-onset preeclampsia, respectively, at a false positive rate of 16% [113].

Other studies have evaluated the value of angiogenic markers alone or in combination with maternal factors or biophysical markers for predicting term or impending preeclampsia [111]. Tan et al. reported that a competing risk model based on a combination of maternal factors, maternal serum PlGF, and sFlt-1 measured at 31–34 weeks of gestation had an area under the curve (AUC) of 0.99 for the prediction of preeclampsia delivery within 4 weeks from assessment [115]. This predictive performance is equivalent to the performance obtained from sFlt-1/PlGF measurement [115]. In contrast, the predictive performance of the combined model was greater for delivery at ≥4 weeks after the assessment when compared to that of sFlt-1/PlGF alone [AUC 0.88 (95% CI: 0.85–0.91) vs. AUC 0.82 (95% CI: 0.78–0.86); $p < 0.0001$] [115].

The same group of investigators has also developed a competing risk model to predict impending preeclampsia within 2–4 weeks of the assessment based on the combination of maternal factors, mean arterial pressure, maternal serum PlGF, and sFlt-1 at 35–37 weeks of gestation [114]. This combined model achieved detection rates of 90% and 70% for the prediction of preeclampsia within 2–4 weeks of assessment, respectively, at a false positive rate of 8%. Such performance is greater than performance derived from PlGF alone or the sFlt-1/PlGF ratio [114].

Collectively, the findings suggested that: (1) risk assessment of late-onset preeclampsia is possible with the evaluation of angiogenic and anti-angiogenic factors; (2) testing performed closer to the event of disease diagnosis yields better results than tests performed in earlier gestation; (3) risk assessment of preeclampsia in the third trimester for late-onset or term preeclampsia outperforms risk assessment obtained from the first or second trimester; and (4) the strategy of testing at the beginning of the third trimester to assess the risk of disease could be considered for patients who did not receive earlier prenatal care. An important question is whether detection in the second or third trimester could improve maternal or neonatal outcomes. It is possible that labor induction as soon as term is reached (i.e., 39 weeks) may reduce the rate of term preeclampsia. Validation of the predictive models in the second and third trimesters and randomized studies of interventions (e.g., aspirin, statins, metformin, and/or induction of labor) will be required to determine if these strategies can reduce the rate of term preeclampsia or adverse outcomes.

13.7.4 Quality Assurance Assessment

In general, there is a certain amount of natural variability (background noise) around an established value (target). This variability is due to “chance or common causes,” which cannot be avoided. However, sometimes a process might be affected by causes that are not from a chance pattern, also known as “special causes.” A process that is under common causes is considered to be “in control.” In contrast, a process affected by special causes is labeled as “out of control,” and such a process demonstrates a deviation from the target. Generally, one should never expect that a process will be in control forever, and at a particular time, a deviation to an out-of-control state will happen due to the sudden special causes [116]. In other words, there will be small but sustained shifts throughout a period of time [116].

In prenatal care, early advances in quality control originated from the fetal nuchal translucency measurements for the screening program of Down syndrome [117, 118]. This is the consequence of a large variation in screening efficiency between centers, illustrating that the conditions under which the measurement is performed should be clearly defined. This approach has led to both quantitative and qualitative forms of control. The quantitative approach compares the distributions of measurements taken with reference values [117, 118]. A qualitative control mechanism assesses an individual’s performance through an audit process. Such an audit involves both assessments of the distributions of measurements for a given sonographer and the examination of the quality of random images from each sonographer. If the criteria are met, the sonographer will be given a certification of competence and a license to practice until the next audit [117, 119–121]. The use of quality assurance tools, cumulative sums (CUSUM), and target plots has been used as quality control for fetal nuchal translucency measurement [122] and serum biochemical markers [123] in Down syndrome screening. Figures 13.4 and 13.5 demonstrate the CUSUM and target plot.

This particular aspect is also relevant in the context of screening for preeclampsia, as each of the biophysical and biochemical markers is susceptible to inaccurate measurements, thus impacting the risk given to the patient and the performance of screening [124]. The biophysical markers mean arterial pressure and UtA-PI are equally susceptible to extensive variability in their measurements, mainly as a result of poor adherence to well-defined protocols. The quality control of the UtA-PI measurement by using CUSUM and target plots has demonstrated that the mea-

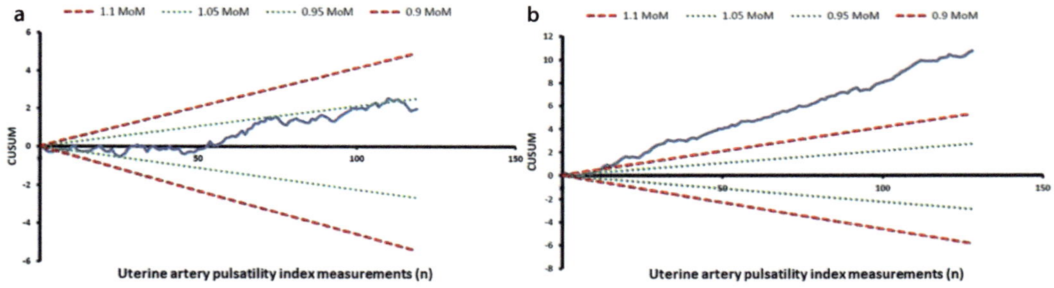

Fig. 13.4 Cumulative sums (CUSUM): The reference value (mean or common reference point) is selected, and this value is subtracted from each data point in succession. The successive deviations of the data from the reference value are then added to the previous sum. Changes in the CUSUM indicate changes in the mean or trend of data from the baseline (mean or reference point), which allow the detection of small but sustained changes that are obscured by conventional methods. **a** The measurements are within 0.95–1.05 MoM. **b** The overmeasurement requires biomarker acquisition reassessment or a biomarker adjustment factor. CUSUM, cumulative sum; MoM, multiples of the median. From Chaemsaithong. First-trimester preeclampsia screening and prediction. (Am J Obstet Gynecol 2022)

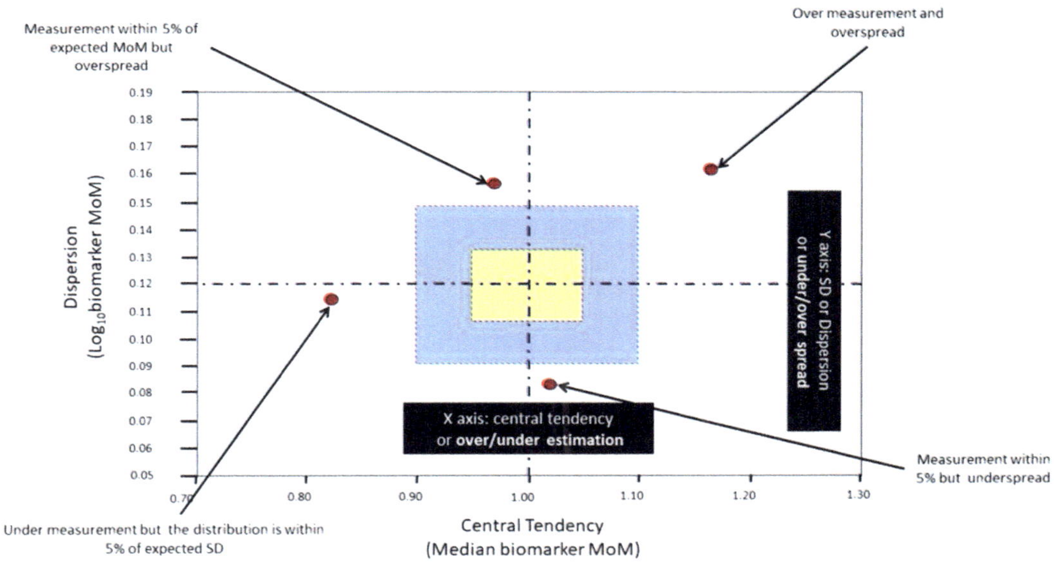

Fig. 13.5 Target plot: The target plot is a common tool to evaluate central tendency (deviation from expected median MoM) and dispersion (deviation from expected median SD). Central tendency is plotted against the *X*-axis, and dispersion is plotted against the *Y*-axis. Acceptable performance is considered if the central tendency and dispersion are within 10% of the expected median MoM and SD (represented as the outer square box, blue). The inner square box (yellow) corresponds to the central tendency and dispersion that are within 5% of the expected median MoM and SD. From Chaemsaithong. First-trimester preeclampsia screening and prediction. (Am J Obstet Gynecol 2022)

surement of UtA-PI is more accurate in the group of sonographers who receive feedback on their performance than those without any feedback [124]. In addition, the authors have demonstrated that the screen-positive rate is also significantly higher (4.3% vs. 6.8%; $p = 0.012$) in the no-feedback group. Other studies have demonstrated that measurements distal to the correct sampling site [125] result in lower pulsatility index values [126]. Operators with a low central tendency (median MoM <0.95) may be sampling the uterine artery too distally in a significant proportion of patients. In contrast, for operators who tend to overestimate the MoM (>1.05), the measurement acquisition is unknown, and although never formally tested, it is suspected that the UtA-PI value is from a sampling site proximal to the recommended site. Similarly, inaccurate biochemical marker results may occur as a result of a change in batch of reagent used, a change in temperature [122], deviation from the manufacturer's protocol, and failure to implement a continuous quality control process. Proposed model for screening, prediction, and management of preeclampsia starting from the first trimester throughout pregnancy (Fig. 13.6).

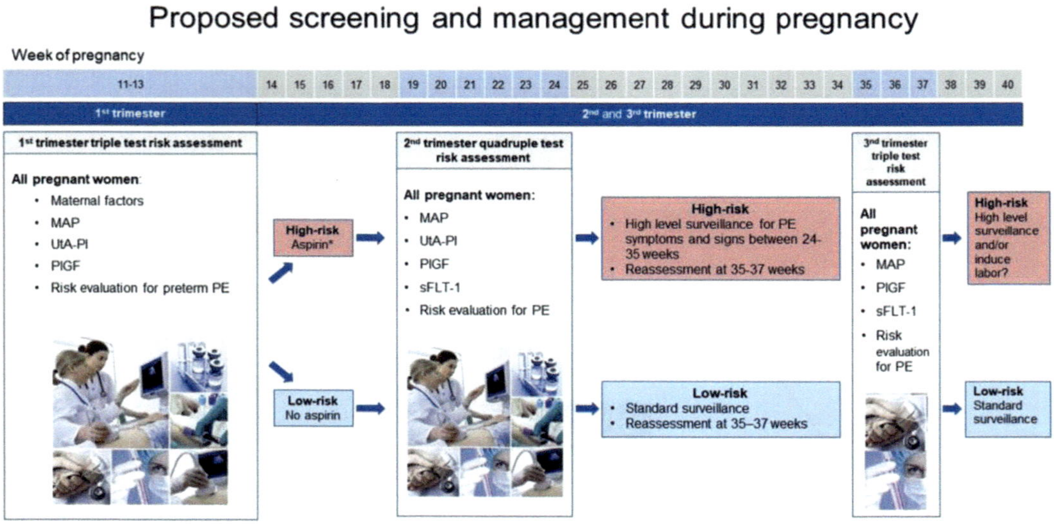

Fig. 13.6 Proposed model for screening, prediction, and management of preeclampsia starting from the first trimester throughout pregnancy; Preeclampsia risk assessment is based on the FMF algorithms. FMF, Fetal Medicine Foundation; MAP, mean arterial pressure; PE, preeclampsia; PlGF, placental growth factor; sFLT-1, soluble fms-like tyrosine kinase-1; UtA-PI, uterine artery pulsatility index. Chaemsaithong. First-trimester preeclampsia screening and prediction. (Am J Obstet Gynecol 2022). *Aspirin 100 or 160 mg nightly from <16 weeks until 36 weeks' gestation. From Chaemsaithong. First-trimester preeclampsia screening and prediction. (Am J Obstet Gynecol 2022)

13.8 Conclusions

Preeclampsia is a syndrome caused by multiple pathological processes leading to a common manifestation. As in other obstetrical syndromes, it is unlikely that a single method for risk assessment and a single intervention during pregnancy (e.g., aspirin) will be able to prevent both early and late preeclampsia. Recent data suggesting that aspirin and other agents may have a role in the prevention of preeclampsia is important because they open the door for the prevention of obstetrical disease. This door has been closed for decades. A key to their effective use is correctly identifying women at risk for effective interventions. The era of administering only aspirin to all nulliparous or parous patients at risk for preeclampsia solely based on obstetrical history (i.e., prior preeclampsia, diabetes, history of chronic hypertension, etc.) has ended. Evidence suggests the risk assessment of preeclampsia with a combination of maternal factors, mean arterial pressure, UtA-PI, and PlGF (the FMF triple test) in the first trimester achieved 90% and 41% for early and preterm preeclampsia, respectively, at a 10% false positive rate. Women classified as high risk will be administered low-dose aspirin prophylaxis from 11–13^{+6} weeks until 36 weeks of gestation. A similar risk assessment can also be performed during the second and third trimesters in all pregnant women, irrespective of first-trimester screening results. The use of PlGF, UtA-PI, and sFlt-1 combined with other biomarkers is part of risk assessment. Quality assurance assessment is an essential process to maintain an effective screening strategy.

Chapter Key Points

- Preeclampsia is a major cause of maternal and perinatal morbidity and mortality; early identification enables prevention with aspirin
- FMF triple test (maternal risk factors, MAP, UtA-PI, PlGF) is the most validated and effective first-trimester screening model

13

- Prediction models must be validated; FMF models uniquely have extensive internal and external validation
- Quality assurance in measuring MAP, UtA-PI and biomarkers is essential to maintain screening accuracy
- Angiogenic biomarkers (PlGF, sFlt-1, sEng) play increasing roles in second- and third-trimester risk assessment
- Competing risk models provide personalized risk and outperform traditional binary models

Chapter-End Summary

This chapter reviews prediction and screening strategies for preeclampsia across pregnancy. Maternal risk-factor–based screening alone has limited accuracy, whereas combined models incorporating mean arterial pressure, uterine artery Doppler indices, and biochemical markers—especially PlGF—substantially improve prediction. The Fetal Medicine Foundation competing risk model demonstrates the best validated performance, with high detection rates for early and preterm preeclampsia. Second- and third-trimester angiogenic marker profiles further refine risk assessment, particularly for imminent disease. Accurate measurement techniques and structured quality assurance programs are critical to maintaining robust screening performance.

References

1. Redman CW. Current topic: pre-eclampsia and the placenta. Placenta. 1991;12(4):301–8.
2. Duley L. The global impact of pre-eclampsia and eclampsia. Semin Perinatol. 2009;33(3):130–7.
3. Chaiworapongsa T, Chaemsaithong P, Yeo L, Romero R. Pre-eclampsia part 1: current understanding of its pathophysiology. Nat Rev Nephrol. 2014;10(8):466–80.
4. Roberts JM. The perplexing pregnancy disorder preeclampsia: what next? Physiol Genomics. 2018;50(6):459–67.
5. Phipps EA, Thadhani R, Benzing T, Karumanchi SA. Pre-eclampsia: pathogenesis, novel diagnostics and therapies. Nat Rev Nephrol. 2019;15(5):275–89.
6. Chappell LC, Cluver CA, Kingdom J, Tong S. Pre-eclampsia. Lancet. 2021;398(10297):341–54.
7. Erez O, Romero R, Jung E, Chaemsaithong P, Bosco M, Suksai M, et al. Preeclampsia and eclampsia: the conceptual evolution of a syndrome. Am J Obstet Gynecol. 2022;226(2s):S786–803.
8. Jung E, Romero R, Yeo L, Gomez-Lopez N, Chaemsaithong P, Jaovisidha A, et al. The etiology of preeclampsia. Am J Obstet Gynecol. 2022;226(2s):S844–66.
9. Bisson C, Dautel S, Patel E, Suresh S, Dauer P, Rana S. Preeclampsia pathophysiology and adverse outcomes during pregnancy and postpartum. Front Med (Lausanne). 2023;10:1144170.
10. Dimitriadis E, Rolnik DL, Zhou W, Estrada-Gutierrez G, Koga K, Francisco RPV, et al. Pre-eclampsia. Nat Rev Dis Primers. 2023;9(1):8.
11. Kuklina EV, Ayala C, Callaghan WM. Hypertensive disorders and severe obstetric morbidity in the United States. Obstet Gynecol. 2009;113(6):1299–306.
12. Masotti G, Galanti G, Poggesi L, Abbate R, Neri Serneri GG. Differential inhibition of prostacyclin production and platelet aggregation by aspirin. Lancet. 1979;2(8154):1213–7.
13. Rolnik DL, Wright D, Poon LC, O'Gorman N, Syngelaki A, de Paco Matallana C, et al. Aspirin versus placebo in pregnancies at high risk for preterm preeclampsia. N Engl J Med. 2017;377(7):613–22.
14. Wright D, Rolnik DL, Syngelaki A, de Paco Matallana C, Machuca M, de Alvarado M, et al. Aspirin for Evidence-Based Preeclampsia Prevention trial: effect of aspirin on length of stay in the neonatal intensive care unit. Am J Obstet Gynecol. 2018;218(6):612.e1–6.
15. Seidler AL, Askie L, Ray JG. Optimal aspirin dosing for preeclampsia prevention. Am J Obstet Gynecol. 2018;219(1):117–8.
16. Roberge S, Bujold E, Nicolaides KH. Aspirin for the prevention of preterm and term preeclampsia: systematic review and metaanalysis. Am J Obstet Gynecol. 2018;218(3):287–93.e1.
17. Rolnik DL, Nicolaides KH, Poon LC. Prevention of preeclampsia with aspirin. Am J Obstet Gynecol. 2022;226(2s):S1108–19.
18. Foisy MA, Marchant I, Lessard L, Caron L, Bujold E. Aspirin for the prevention of preeclampsia. J Perinat Med. 2022;50(9):1271–2.
19. Nguyen-Hoang L, Dinh LT, Tai AST, Nguyen DA, Pooh RK, Shiozaki A, et al. Implementation of first-trimester screening and prevention of preeclampsia: a stepped wedge cluster-randomized trial in Asia. Circulation. 2024;150(16):1223–35.
20. Cheong-See F, Allotey J, Marlin N, Mol BW, Schuit E, Ter Riet G, et al. Prediction models in obstetrics: understanding the treatment paradox

and potential solutions to the threat it poses. BJOG. 2016;123(7):1060–4.
21. Altman DG, Royston P. What do we mean by validating a prognostic model? Stat Med. 2000;19(4):453–73.
22. Kleinrouweler CE, Cheong-See FM, Collins GS, Kwee A, Thangaratinam S, Khan KS, et al. Prognostic models in obstetrics: available, but far from applicable. Am J Obstet Gynecol. 2016;214(1):79–90.e36.
23. Efthimiou O, Seo M, Chalkou K, Debray T, Egger M, Salanti G. Developing clinical prediction models: a step-by-step guide. BMJ. 2024;386:e078276.
24. Poon LC, Kametas NA, Pandeva I, Valencia C, Nicolaides KH. Mean arterial pressure at 11(+0) to 13(+6) weeks in the prediction of preeclampsia. Hypertension. 2008;51(4):1027–33.
25. Poon LC, Kametas NA, Valencia C, Chelemen T, Nicolaides KH. Hypertensive disorders in pregnancy: screening by systolic diastolic and mean arterial pressure at 11–13 weeks. Hypertens Pregnancy. 2011;30(1):93–107.
26. O'Gorman N, Wright D, Syngelaki A, Akolekar R, Wright A, Poon LC, et al. Competing risks model in screening for preeclampsia by maternal factors and biomarkers at 11–13 weeks gestation. Am J Obstet Gynecol. 2016;214(1):103.e1–12.
27. O'Gorman N, Wright D, Poon LC, Rolnik DL, Syngelaki A, Wright A, et al. Accuracy of competing-risks model in screening for pre-eclampsia by maternal factors and biomarkers at 11–13 weeks' gestation. Ultrasound Obstet Gynecol. 2017;49(6):751–5.
28. O'Gorman N, Wright D, Poon LC, Rolnik DL, Syngelaki A, de Alvarado M, et al. Multicenter screening for pre-eclampsia by maternal factors and biomarkers at 11–13 weeks' gestation: comparison with NICE guidelines and ACOG recommendations. Ultrasound Obstet Gynecol. 2017;49(6):756–60.
29. Litwinska M, Syngelaki A, Wright A, Wright D, Nicolaides KH. Management of pregnancies after combined screening for pre-eclampsia at 19–24 weeks' gestation. Ultrasound Obstet Gynecol. 2018;52(3):365–72.
30. Poon LC, Galindo A, Surbek D, Chantraine F, Stepan H, Hyett J, et al. From first-trimester screening to risk stratification of evolving preeclampsia in second and third trimesters of pregnancy: comprehensive approach. Ultrasound Obstet Gynecol. 2020;55(1):5–12.
31. Tan MY, Syngelaki A, Poon LC, Rolnik DL, O'Gorman N, Delgado JL, et al. Screening for pre-eclampsia by maternal factors and biomarkers at 11–13 weeks' gestation. Ultrasound Obstet Gynecol. 2018;52(2):186–95.
32. Serra B, Mendoza M, Scazzocchio E, Meler E, Nolla M, Sabrià E, et al. A new model for screening for early-onset preeclampsia. Am J Obstet Gynecol. 2020;222(6):608.e1–18.
33. Tarca AL, Taran A, Romero R, Jung E, Paredes C, Bhatti G, et al. Prediction of preeclampsia throughout gestation with maternal characteristics and biophysical and biochemical markers: a longitudinal study. Am J Obstet Gynecol. 2022;226(1):126.e1–22.
34. Wright D, Tan MY, O'Gorman N, Poon LC, Syngelaki A, Wright A, et al. Predictive performance of the competing risk model in screening for preeclampsia. Am J Obstet Gynecol. 2019;220(2):199.e1–13.
35. Wright D, Wright A, Nicolaides KH. The competing risk approach for prediction of preeclampsia. Am J Obstet Gynecol. 2020;223(1):12–23.e7.
36. Syngelaki A, Magee LA, von Dadelszen P, Akolekar R, Wright A, Wright D, et al. Competing-risks model for pre-eclampsia and adverse pregnancy outcomes. Ultrasound Obstet Gynecol. 2022;60(3):367–72.
37. Chaemsaithong P, Sahota DS, Poon LC. First trimester preeclampsia screening and prediction. Am J Obstet Gynecol. 2022;226(2S):S1071–97.e2.
38. Lee NMW, Chaemsaithong P, Poon LC. Prediction of preeclampsia in asymptomatic women. Best Pract Res Clin Obstet Gynaecol. 2024;92:102436.
39. National Collaborating Centre for Women's and Children's Health (UK). Antenatal care: routine care for the healthy pregnant woman. National Institute for Health and Clinical Excellence: Guidance. London: RCOG Press; 2021.
40. National Collaborating Centre for Women's and Children's Health (UK). Hypertension in pregnancy: the management of hypertensive disorders during pregnancy. London: RCOG Press; 2010.
41. Hypertension in pregnancy: diagnosis and management. https://www.nice.org.uk/guidance/NG133.
42. ACOG Committee Opinion No. 743: low-dose aspirin use during pregnancy. Obstet Gynecol. 2018;132(1):e44–52.
43. Chaemsaithong P, Pooh RK, Zheng M, Ma R, Chaiyasit N, Tokunaka M, et al. Prospective evaluation of screening performance of first-trimester prediction models for preterm preeclampsia in an Asian population. Am J Obstet Gynecol. 2019;221(6):650.e1–16.
44. WHO recommendations for prevention and treatment of pre-eclampsia and eclampsia. Geneva: WHO Guidelines Approved by the Guidelines Review Committee; 2011.
45. Magee LA, Pels A, Helewa M, Rey E, von Dadelszen P, Canadian Hypertensive Disorders of Pregnancy Working G. Diagnosis, evaluation, and management of the hypertensive disorders of pregnancy. Pregnancy Hypertens. 2014;4(2):105–45.
46. Brown MA, Magee LA, Kenny LC, Karumanchi SA, McCarthy FP, Saito S, et al. Hypertensive disorders of pregnancy: ISSHP classification, diagnosis, and management recommendations for

international practice. Hypertension. 2018;72(1):24–43.
47. Poon LC, Shennan A, Hyett JA, Kapur A, Hadar E, Divakar H, et al. The International Federation of Gynecology and Obstetrics (FIGO) initiative on pre-eclampsia: a pragmatic guide for first-trimester screening and prevention. Int J Gynaecol Obstet. 2019;145 Suppl 1(Suppl 1):1–33.
48. Poon LC, Kametas NA, Chelemen T, Leal A, Nicolaides KH. Maternal risk factors for hypertensive disorders in pregnancy: a multivariate approach. J Hum Hypertens. 2010;24(2):104–10.
49. Bartsch E, Medcalf KE, Park AL, Ray JG. Clinical risk factors for pre-eclampsia determined in early pregnancy: systematic review and meta-analysis of large cohort studies. BMJ. 2016;353:i1753.
50. National Heart Foundation of Australia. Hypertension management guide for doctors. 2004. http://www.heartfoundation.org.au.
51. Gabb GM, Mangoni AA, Anderson CS, Cowley D, Dowden JS, Golledge J, et al. Guideline for the diagnosis and management of hypertension in adults – 2016. Med J Aust. 2016;205(2):85–9.
52. Poon LC, Zymeri NA, Zamprakou A, Syngelaki A, Nicolaides KH. Protocol for measurement of mean arterial pressure at 11–13 weeks' gestation. Fetal Diagn Ther. 2012;31(1):42–8.
53. Poon LC, Kametas N, Strobl I, Pachoumi C, Nicolaides KH. Inter-arm blood pressure differences in pregnant women. BJOG. 2008;115(9):1122–30.
54. Roberts L, Chaemsaithong P, Sahota DS, Nicolaides KH, Poon LCY. Protocol for measurement of mean arterial pressure at 10–40 weeks' gestation. Pregnancy Hypertens. 2017;10:155–60.
55. Wright A, Wright D, Ispas CA, Poon LC, Nicolaides KH. Mean arterial pressure in the three trimesters of pregnancy: effects of maternal characteristics and medical history. Ultrasound Obstet Gynecol. 2015;45(6):698–706.
56. Lefebvre J, Demers S, Bujold E, Nicolaides KH, Girard M, Brassard N, et al. Comparison of two different sites of measurement for transabdominal uterine artery Doppler velocimetry at 11–13 weeks. Ultrasound Obstet Gynecol. 2012;40(3):288–92.
57. Tayyar A, Guerra L, Wright A, Wright D, Nicolaides KH. Uterine artery pulsatility index in the three trimesters of pregnancy: effects of maternal characteristics and medical history. Ultrasound Obstet Gynecol. 2015;45(6):689–97.
58. Plasencia W, Maiz N, Poon L, Yu C, Nicolaides KH. Uterine artery Doppler at 11 + 0 to 13 + 6 weeks and 21 + 0 to 24 + 6 weeks in the prediction of pre-eclampsia. Ultrasound Obstet Gynecol. 2008;32(2):138–46.
59. Poon LC, Maiz N, Valencia C, Plasencia W, Nicolaides KH. First-trimester maternal serum pregnancy-associated plasma protein-A and pre-eclampsia. Ultrasound Obstet Gynecol. 2009;33(1):23–33.
60. Poon LC, Staboulidou I, Maiz N, Plasencia W, Nicolaides KH. Hypertensive disorders in pregnancy: screening by uterine artery Doppler at 11–13 weeks. Ultrasound Obstet Gynecol. 2009;34(2):142–8.
61. Velauthar L, Plana MN, Kalidindi M, Zamora J, Thilaganathan B, Illanes SE, et al. First-trimester uterine artery Doppler and adverse pregnancy outcome: a meta-analysis involving 55,974 women. Ultrasound Obstet Gynecol. 2014;43(5):500–7.
62. Milne F, Redman C, Walker J, Baker P, Black R, Blincowe J, et al. Assessing the onset of pre-eclampsia in the hospital day unit: summary of the pre-eclampsia guideline (PRECOG II). BMJ. 2009;339:b3129.
63. Ridding G, Hyett JA, Sahota D, McLennan AC. Assessing quality standards in measurement of uterine artery pulsatility index at 11 to 13 + 6 weeks' gestation. Ultrasound Obstet Gynecol. 2015;46(3):299–305.
64. Chaemsaithong P, Ting YH, Cheng KYY, Poon CYL, Leung TY, Sahota DS. Uterine artery pulsatility index in the first trimester: assessment of intersonographer and intersampling site measurement differences. J Matern Fetal Neonatal Med. 2018;31(17):2276–83.
65. Drouin O, Johnson JA, Chaemsaithong P, Metcalfe A, Huber J, Schwarzenberger J, et al. Transverse technique: complementary approach to measurement of first-trimester uterine artery Doppler. Ultrasound Obstet Gynecol. 2018;52(5):639–47.
66. Rana S, Lemoine E, Granger JP, Karumanchi SA. Preeclampsia: pathophysiology, challenges, and perspectives. Circ Res. 2019;124(7):1094–112.
67. Stepan H, Hund M, Andraczek T. Combining biomarkers to predict pregnancy complications and redefine preeclampsia: the angiogenic-placental syndrome. Hypertension. 2020;75(4):918–26.
68. Rana S, Burke SD, Karumanchi SA. Imbalances in circulating angiogenic factors in the pathophysiology of preeclampsia and related disorders. Am J Obstet Gynecol. 2022;226(2S):S1019–S34.
69. Burwick RM, Rodriguez MH. Angiogenic biomarkers in preeclampsia. Obstet Gynecol. 2024;143(4):515–23.
70. Roberts JM. Preeclampsia epidemiology(ies) and pathophysiology(ies). Best Pract Res Clin Obstet Gynaecol. 2024;94:102480.
71. Levine RJ, Maynard SE, Qian C, Lim KH, England LJ, Yu KF, et al. Circulating angiogenic factors and the risk of preeclampsia. N Engl J Med. 2004;350(7):672–83.
72. Levine RJ, Lam C, Qian C, Yu KF, Maynard SE, Sachs BP, et al. Soluble endoglin and other circulating antiangiogenic factors in preeclampsia. N Engl J Med. 2006;355(10):992–1005.

73. Erez O, Romero R, Espinoza J, Fu W, Todem D, Kusanovic JP, et al. The change in concentrations of angiogenic and anti-angiogenic factors in maternal plasma between the first and second trimesters in risk assessment for the subsequent development of preeclampsia and small-for-gestational age. J Matern Fetal Neonatal Med. 2008;21(5):279–87.
74. Romero R, Nien JK, Espinoza J, Todem D, Fu W, Chung H, et al. A longitudinal study of angiogenic (placental growth factor) and anti-angiogenic (soluble endoglin and soluble vascular endothelial growth factor receptor-1) factors in normal pregnancy and patients destined to develop preeclampsia and deliver a small for gestational age neonate. J Matern Fetal Neonatal Med. 2008;21(1):9–23.
75. Romero R, Jung E, Chaiworapongsa T, Erez O, Gudicha DW, Kim YM, et al. Toward a new taxonomy of obstetrical disease: improved performance of maternal blood biomarkers for the great obstetrical syndromes when classified according to placental pathology. Am J Obstet Gynecol. 2022;227(4):615.e1–25.
76. Akolekar R, Zaragoza E, Poon LC, Pepes S, Nicolaides KH. Maternal serum placental growth factor at 11 + 0 to 13 + 6 weeks of gestation in the prediction of pre-eclampsia. Ultrasound Obstet Gynecol. 2008;32(6):732–9.
77. Wortelboer EJ, Koster MP, Kuc S, Eijkemans MJ, Bilardo CM, Schielen PC, et al. Longitudinal trends in fetoplacental biochemical markers, uterine artery pulsatility index and maternal blood pressure during the first trimester of pregnancy. Ultrasound Obstet Gynecol. 2011;38(4):383–8.
78. Cheng YKY, Poon LCY, Shennan A, Leung TY, Sahota DS. Inter-manufacturer comparison of automated immunoassays for the measurement of soluble FMS-like tyrosine kinase-1 and placental growth factor. Pregnancy Hypertens. 2019;17:165–71.
79. Al-Rubaie Z, Askie LM, Ray JG, Hudson HM, Lord SJ. The performance of risk prediction models for pre-eclampsia using routinely collected maternal characteristics and comparison with models that include specialised tests and with clinical guideline decision rules: a systematic review. BJOG. 2016;123(9):1441–52.
80. De Kat AC, Hirst J, Woodward M, Kennedy S, Peters SA. Prediction models for preeclampsia: a systematic review. Pregnancy Hypertens. 2019;16:48–66.
81. Akolekar R, Syngelaki A, Poon L, Wright D, Nicolaides KH. Competing risks model in early screening for preeclampsia by biophysical and biochemical markers. Fetal Diagn Ther. 2013;33(1):8–15.
82. Skråstad RB, Hov GG, Blaas HG, Romundstad PR, Salvesen K. Risk assessment for preeclampsia in nulliparous women at 11–13 weeks gestational age: prospective evaluation of two algorithms. BJOG. 2015;122(13):1781–8.
83. Mosimann B, Pfiffner C, Amylidi-Mohr S, Risch L, Surbek D, Raio L. First trimester combined screening for preeclampsia and small for gestational age – a single centre experience and validation of the FMF screening algorithm. Swiss Med Wkly. 2017;147:w14498.
84. Lobo GAR, Nowak PM, Panigassi AP, Lima AIF, Araujo Júnior E, Nardozza LMM, et al. Validation of Fetal Medicine Foundation algorithm for prediction of pre-eclampsia in the first trimester in an unselected Brazilian population. J Matern Fetal Neonatal Med. 2019;32(2):286–92.
85. Poon LC, Kametas NA, Maiz N, Akolekar R, Nicolaides KH. First-trimester prediction of hypertensive disorders in pregnancy. Hypertension. 2009;53(5):812–8.
86. Wright D, Syngelaki A, Akolekar R, Poon LC, Nicolaides KH. Competing risks model in screening for preeclampsia by maternal characteristics and medical history. Am J Obstet Gynecol. 2015;213(1):62.e1–10.
87. Scazzocchio E, Figueras F, Crispi F, Meler E, Masoller N, Mula R, et al. Performance of a first-trimester screening of preeclampsia in a routine care low-risk setting. Am J Obstet Gynecol. 2013;208(3):203.e1–10.
88. Crovetto F, Figueras F, Triunfo S, Crispi F, Rodriguez-Sureda V, Dominguez C, et al. First trimester screening for early and late preeclampsia based on maternal characteristics, biophysical parameters, and angiogenic factors. Prenat Diagn. 2015;35(2):183–91.
89. Odibo AO, Zhong Y, Goetzinger KR, Odibo L, Bick JL, Bower CR, et al. First-trimester placental protein 13, PAPP-A, uterine artery Doppler and maternal characteristics in the prediction of pre-eclampsia. Placenta. 2011;32(8):598–602.
90. Baschat AA, Magder LS, Doyle LE, Atlas RO, Jenkins CB, Blitzer MG. Prediction of preeclampsia utilizing the first trimester screening examination. Am J Obstet Gynecol. 2014;211(5):514.e1–7.
91. Sonek J, Krantz D, Carmichael J, Downing C, Jessup K, Haidar Z, et al. First-trimester screening for early and late preeclampsia using maternal characteristics, biomarkers, and estimated placental volume. Am J Obstet Gynecol. 2018;218(1):126.e1–13.
92. Serra B, Mendoza M, Scazzocchio E, Meler E, Nolla M, Sabria E, et al. A new model for screening for early-onset preeclampsia. Am J Obstet Gynecol. 2020;222(6):608.e1–18.
93. Cuenca-Gómez D, De Paco Matallana C, Rolle V, Mendoza M, Valiño N, Revello R, et al. Comparison of different methods of first-trimester screening for preterm pre-eclampsia: cohort study. Ultrasound Obstet Gynecol. 2024;64(1):57–64.

94. Tan MY, Wright D, Syngelaki A, Akolekar R, Cicero S, Janga D, et al. Comparison of diagnostic accuracy of early screening for pre-eclampsia by NICE guidelines and a method combining maternal factors and biomarkers: results of SPREE. Ultrasound Obstet Gynecol. 2018;51(6):743–50.
95. Chaiyasit N, Sahota DS, Ma R, Choolani M, Wataganara T, Sim WS, et al. Prospective evaluation of international prediction of pregnancy complications collaborative network models for prediction of preeclampsia: role of serum sFlt-1 at 11–13 weeks' gestation. Hypertension. 2022;79(2):314–22.
96. Moungmaithong S, Wang X, Lau CSL, Tse AWT, Lee NMW, Leung HHY, et al. Glycosylated fibronectin improves first-trimester prediction of pre-eclampsia. Ultrasound Obstet Gynecol. 2023;62(4):512–21.
97. Moons KG, Altman DG, Reitsma JB, Ioannidis JP, Macaskill P, Steyerberg EW, et al. Transparent Reporting of a multivariable prediction model for Individual Prognosis or Diagnosis (TRIPOD): explanation and elaboration. Ann Intern Med. 2015;162(1):W1–73.
98. Ramspek CL, Jager KJ, Dekker FW, Zoccali C, van Diepen M. External validation of prognostic models: what, why, how, when and where? Clin Kidney J. 2021;14(1):49–58.
99. Justice AC, Covinsky KE, Berlin JA. Assessing the generalizability of prognostic information. Ann Intern Med. 1999;130(6):515–24.
100. Farina A, Rapacchia G, Freni Sterrantino A, Pula G, Morano D, Rizzo N. Prospective evaluation of ultrasound and biochemical-based multivariable models for the prediction of late pre-eclampsia. Prenat Diagn. 2011;31(12):1147–52.
101. Park FJ, Leung CH, Poon LC, Williams PF, Rothwell SJ, Hyett JA. Clinical evaluation of a first trimester algorithm predicting the risk of hypertensive disease of pregnancy. Aust N Z J Obstet Gynaecol. 2013;53(6):532–9.
102. Park F, Russo K, Williams P, Pelosi M, Puddephatt R, Walter M, et al. Prediction and prevention of early-onset pre-eclampsia: impact of aspirin after first-trimester screening. Ultrasound Obstet Gynecol. 2015;46(4):419–23.
103. Allen RE, Zamora J, Arroyo-Manzano D, Velauthar L, Allotey J, Thangaratinam S, et al. External validation of preexisting first trimester preeclampsia prediction models. Eur J Obstet Gynecol Reprod Biol. 2017;217:119–25.
104. Guizani M, Valsamis J, Dutemeyer V, Kang X, Ceccotti V, Khalife J, et al. First-trimester combined multimarker prospective study for the detection of pregnancies at a high risk of developing preeclampsia using the Fetal Medicine Foundation-algorithm. Fetal Diagn Ther. 2018;43(4):266–73.
105. Panaitescu A, Ciobanu A, Syngelaki A, Wright A, Wright D, Nicolaides KH. Screening for pre-eclampsia at 35–37 weeks' gestation. Ultrasound Obstet Gynecol. 2018;52(4):501–6.
106. Oliveira N, Magder LS, Blitzer MG, Baschat AA. First-trimester prediction of pre-eclampsia: external validity of algorithms in a prospectively enrolled cohort. Ultrasound Obstet Gynecol. 2014;44(3):279–85.
107. Poon LC, Stratieva V, Piras S, Piri S, Nicolaides KH. Hypertensive disorders in pregnancy: combined screening by uterine artery Doppler, blood pressure and serum PAPP-A at 11–13 weeks. Prenat Diagn. 2010;30(3):216–23.
108. Parra-Cordero M, Rodrigo R, Barja P, Bosco C, Rencoret G, Sepúlveda-Martinez A, et al. Prediction of early and late pre-eclampsia from maternal characteristics, uterine artery Doppler and markers of vasculogenesis during first trimester of pregnancy. Ultrasound Obstet Gynecol. 2013;41(5):538–44.
109. Sotiriadis A, Hernandez-Andrade E, da Silva Costa F, Ghi T, Glanc P, Khalil A, et al. ISUOG Practice Guidelines: role of ultrasound in screening for and follow-up of pre-eclampsia. Ultrasound Obstet Gynecol. 2019;53(1):7–22.
110. Kusanovic JP, Romero R, Chaiworapongsa T, Erez O, Mittal P, Vaisbuch E, et al. A prospective cohort study of the value of maternal plasma concentrations of angiogenic and anti-angiogenic factors in early pregnancy and midtrimester in the identification of patients destined to develop preeclampsia. J Matern Fetal Neonatal Med. 2009;22(11):1021–38.
111. Chaemsaithong P, Gil MM, Chaiyasit N, Cuenca-Gomez D, Plasencia W, Rolle V, et al. Accuracy of placental growth factor alone or in combination with soluble fms-like tyrosine kinase-1 or maternal factors in detecting preeclampsia in asymptomatic women in the second and third trimesters: a systematic review and meta-analysis. Am J Obstet Gynecol. 2023;229(3):222–47.
112. Gallo DM, Wright D, Casanova C, Campanero M, Nicolaides KH. Competing risks model in screening for preeclampsia by maternal factors and biomarkers at 19–24 weeks' gestation. Am J Obstet Gynecol. 2016;214(5):619.e1–17.
113. Chaiworapongsa T, Romero R, Korzeniewski SJ, Kusanovic JP, Soto E, Lam J, et al. Maternal plasma concentrations of angiogenic/antiangiogenic factors in the third trimester of pregnancy to identify the patient at risk for stillbirth at or near term and severe late preeclampsia. Am J Obstet Gynecol. 2013;208(4):287.e1–15.
114. Ciobanu A, Wright A, Panaitescu A, Syngelaki A, Wright D, Nicolaides KH. Prediction of imminent preeclampsia at 35–37 weeks gestation. Am J Obstet Gynecol. 2019;220(6):584.e1–11.
115. Tan MY, Koutoulas L, Wright D, Nicolaides KH, Poon LCY. Protocol for the prospective validation study: 'screening programme for pre-

eclampsia' (SPREE). Ultrasound Obstet Gynecol. 2017;50(2):175–9.

116. Biau DJ, Porcher R, Salomon LJ. CUSUM: a tool for ongoing assessment of performance. Ultrasound Obstet Gynecol. 2008;31(3):252–5.
117. Wøjdemann KR, Larsen SO, Shalmi A, Sundberg K, Christiansen M, Tabor A. First trimester screening for Down syndrome and assisted reproduction: no basis for concern. Prenat Diagn. 2001;21(7):563–5.
118. Snijders R, Smith E. The role of fetal nuchal translucency in prenatal screening. Curr Opin Obstet Gynecol. 2002;14(6):577–85.
119. Herman A, Maymon R, Dreazen E, Caspi E, Bukovsky I, Weinraub Z. Nuchal translucency audit: a novel image-scoring method. Ultrasound Obstet Gynecol. 1998;12(6):398–403.
120. McLennan A, Schluter PJ, Pincham V, Hyett J. First-trimester fetal nasal bone audit: evaluation of a novel method of image assessment. Ultrasound Obstet Gynecol. 2009;34(6):623–8.
121. Chalouhi GE, Salomon LJ, Fontanges M, Althuser M, Haddad G, Scemama O, et al. Formative assessment based on an audit and feedback improves nuchal translucency ultrasound image quality. J Ultrasound Med. 2013;32(9):1601–5.
122. Sahota DS, Pooh RK, Choy KW, Leung TY, Lau TK. First trimester serum markers stability during sample transportation from the obstetrical site to the screening laboratory. J Matern Fetal Neonatal Med. 2012;25(7):966–9.
123. Knight GJ. Quality assessment of a prenatal screening program. Early Hum Dev. 1996;47(Suppl):S49–53.
124. Rolnik DL, da Silva Costa F, Sahota D, Hyett J, McLennan A. Quality assessment of uterine artery Doppler measurement in first-trimester combined screening for pre-eclampsia. Ultrasound Obstet Gynecol. 2019;53(2):245–50.
125. Khalil A, Nicolaides KH. How to record uterine artery Doppler in the first trimester. Ultrasound Obstet Gynecol. 2013;42(4):478–9.
126. Ridding G, Schluter PJ, Hyett JA, McLennan AC. Influence of sampling site on uterine artery Doppler indices at $11–13^{+6}$ weeks gestation. Fetal Diagn Ther. 2015;37(4):310–5.

The Role of Magnesium Sulfate in Prevention of Eclampsia

Zakaria Doughan and Baha M. Sibai

Contents

Y. Yogev, A. Khalil (eds.), *Prevention of Complications in Obstetrics*,
https://doi.org/10.1007/978-3-032-23479-7_14

Learning Objectives
- To describe risk factors and pathophysiology of eclampsia
- To summarize evidence-based trials regarding the use of magnesium sulfate for the prevention of eclamptic seizures
- To discuss the benefits and risks of magnesium sulfate regimens
- To emphasize the need for further research regarding the optimal dose, duration, and timing of magnesium sulfate prophylaxis

14.1 Introduction

Eclampsia is a major cause of maternal mortality and morbidity worldwide. Magnesium sulfate is considered the cornerstone for the prevention and treatment of eclamptic seizures. However, the exact dose and the indications for administration remain controversial. Our objective is to describe risk factors, symptoms, and time of onset of eclampsia, as well as to summarize randomized trials dealing with indications for magnesium sulfate and duration of its administration, particularly as it plays to its indications in the postpartum period.

14.2 Definition

The term "eclampsia" was first formally introduced in 1619 by Varandaeus in a treatise on gynecology. However, descriptions of pregnancy-related convulsions can be traced back to earlier civilizations. Hippocrates observed that symptoms such as headaches, convulsions, and drowsiness were significant warning signs during pregnancy [1]. Eclampsia is considered to be the most severe acute complication of pregnancy, as it is associated with increased risk of maternal mortality in developed countries (0–1.8%) and up to 15% in developing countries [2]. It is also associated with increased rates of maternal morbidities such as pulmonary edema, abruptio placentae, acute renal injury, and aspiration. Eclampsia is defined as the development of generalized tonic-clonic convulsions in patients with a hypertensive disorder in pregnancy, where the seizures are not attributable to any other underlying medical disorder.

14.3 Pathophysiology

Several hypotheses have been proposed to explain the pathogenesis of eclamptic seizures, although none have been definitively proven. One such hypothesis is an alteration in the autoregulation in the cerebral circulation, similar to that occurring in hypertensive encephalopathy. This hypothesis suggests that a disruption in the blood-brain barrier allows the passage of fluids, ions, and plasma proteins into the brain parenchyma [2]. Cerebral autoregulation is a mechanism that ensures stable cerebral blood flow despite fluctuations in blood pressure, with vasoconstriction occurring during elevated pressure and vasodilation occurring during lowered pressure. This process is mediated by myogenic, neurogenic, metabolic, or endothelial mechanisms [2]. Failure of autoregulation can result in increased hydrostatic pressure, decreased cerebral vascular resistance, and ultimately cerebral edema, neuroinflammation, and neuronal damage [3–6]. The classic neuroimaging finding following an eclamptic seizure is posterior reversible encephalopathy syndrome (PRES), a reversible neurologic disorder that manifests with a range of symptoms including headaches, visual dysfunction such as impaired visual acuity or visual field defects, altered consciousness, confusion, seizures, and focal neurologic deficits. PRES typically presents on neuroimaging as vasogenic edema, which can either be focal or confluent, often involving the posterior parietal or occipital lobes [2] (Fig. 14.1).

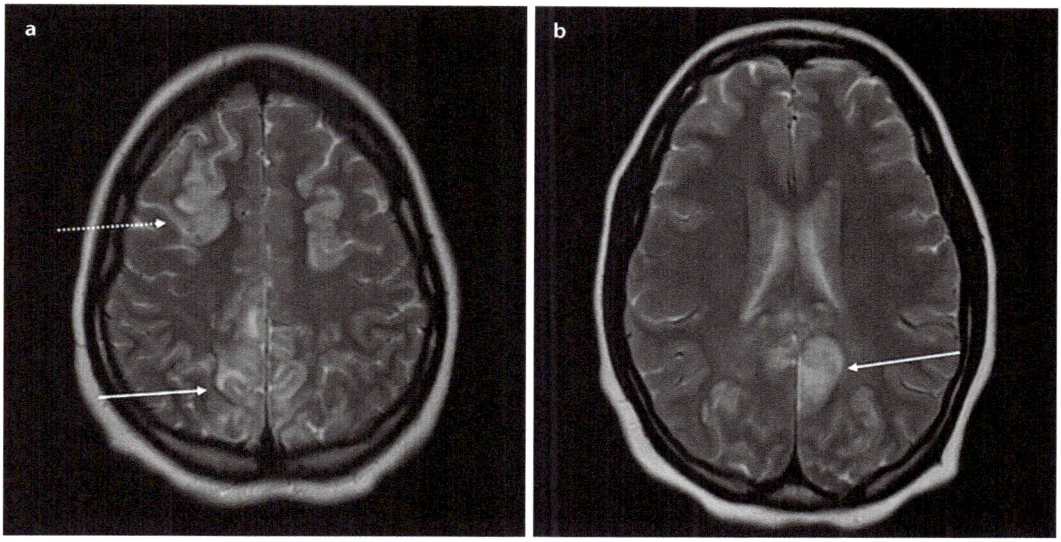

Fig. 14.1 MRI of the brain showing posterior reversible encephalopathy syndrome in a woman with eclampsia. **a**, the dotted line points at an area of vasogenic edema occurring at the level of the frontal-temporal region, and the solid line points at an area of vasogenic edema occurring at the level of the occipital region. **b**, the solid line points at an area of subcortical white matter edema. *MRI, magnetic resonance imaging*

Table 14.1 Time of onset of eclampsia in relation to delivery

	Yorkshire [16] (n = 82)[a]	UKOSS [15] (n = 214)	Mattar and Sibai [14] (n = 399)	Katz et al. [17] (n = 53)
Antepartum	45 (55%)	96 (45%)	212	28 (53%)
At home	18 (22%)	44 (21%)	NR	NR
In-hospital	27 (33%)	52 (24%)	NR	10[b]
During labor	11 (13%)	41 (19%)	77	19 (36%)
Postpartum	26 (32%)	77 (36%)	110 (28%)	6 (11%)

[a]73 (89%) were considered not candidates for magnesium sulfate, 1005 with severe preeclampsia (no magnesium sulfate)
[b]8 were intrapartum, and 2 were ≤48 h postpartum while receiving magnesium sulfate

14.4 Time of Onset

Eclampsia can present at any time during pregnancy and the postpartum period, including antepartum, during labor and delivery, immediately postpartum (within 48 h after delivery), late-onset postpartum (3–7 days after delivery), and even extremely late-onset postpartum (beyond 7 days postpartum). The rates of onset of eclampsia in relation to delivery reported in various series are summarized in Table 14.1.

14.5 Risk Factors and Clinical Symptoms

In general, the risk factors for eclampsia are similar to those of preeclampsia (Table 14.2). Patients with eclampsia may present with a broad spectrum of clinical premonitory manifestations, including visual disturbances such as blurred vision, persistent headaches primarily localized to the occipital and frontal regions, epigastric pain,

Table 14.2 Risk factors for eclampsia

Nulliparity
Prior history of eclampsia
Prior history of severe preeclampsia
Current pregnancy with severe preeclampsia
Preexisting chronic hypertension or diabetes mellitus
Hypertensive disorder of pregnancy in association with headaches, blurred vision, or epigastric pain
Multifetal gestation
Nonimmune hydrops fetalis
Partial molar pregnancy

and altered mental status that usually precede the development of convulsions. These symptoms often occur in association with hypertension, proteinuria, and tonic-clonic convulsions.

14.6 Prevention of Eclampsia

There are three main approaches discussed in literature for preventing eclampsia: (1) primary prevention, which focuses on stopping the development and/or progression of preeclampsia with timely diagnosis and delivery; (2) secondary prevention, involving the use of pharmacologic agents such as prophylaxis in patients with established preeclampsia; and (3) tertiary prevention, aimed at preventing recurrent convulsions in patients who have already developed eclampsia [1]. Among these strategies, the use of magnesium sulfate prophylaxis has been extensively debated, given its potential advantages and disadvantages. These considerations, particularly in the context of its universal administration in all patients with preeclampsia, are outlined in Table 14.3, which compares its potential benefits and limitations for clinical practice.

Table 14.3 Advantages and disadvantages of universal magnesium sulfate prophylaxis

Advantages	Disadvantages
Potential to reduce eclampsia only	*Requires intensive monitoring*
During labor and delivery Within 48 h postpartum Less than 40% of all eclampsia if 100% effective	Nurses Physicians Space
Does not prevent morbidity and mortality due to severe preeclampsia	*Maternal side effects*
Pulmonary edema/ARDS Stroke Acute renal failure Liver hemorrhage Disseminated intravascular coagulopathy Sepsis	Minor (15–50%) Serious (<1%): Respiratory depression/arrest Cardiac arrest
Does not prevent morbidity and mortality due to eclampsia that occurs	*Neonatal depression*
Antepartum Outside the hospital Beyond 48 hours postpartum	Low Apgar scores Floppy infant Need for respiratory support/intubation

14.7 Magnesium Sulfate Toxicity and Its Management

The use of magnesium sulfate necessitates vigilant monitoring due to the potential for toxicity at varying serum levels, particularly when these levels exceed the therapeutic threshold. This toxicity can result in a range of adverse effects, which are directly related to the serum concentration of magnesium. Following administration of parenteral magnesium sulfate (IV or IM), serum levels of

Table 14.4 Signs and management of magnesium sulfate toxicity

Signs **Manifestations**	**Level (mg/dl)**
Loss of patellar reflexes	8–12
Double vision	8–12
Feeling of warmth, flushing, nausea	9–12
Somnolence	10–12
Slurred speech	10–12
Muscular paralysis	15–17
Respiratory arrest	15–17
Cardiac arrest	20–25
Management	
Discontinuation of magnesium sulfate	
Obtain magnesium level	
Restart or reduce the dose according to the magnesium level	
For respiratory compromise:	
Give 1 g of IV calcium gluconate	
Intubate if needed	
Assisted ventilation	

magnesium will depend on the volume of distribution as well as renal excretion. Therefore, the dose should be adjusted based on body mass index (BMI), which correlates with volume of distribution as well as serum creatinine levels that reflect renal function. If serum creatinine levels are more than or equal to 1.2 mg/dl, we recommend administration of the loading dose and then checking serum magnesium levels 2–4 h after initiation of the maintenance dose. The goal of monitoring magnesium levels is to ensure that serum magnesium levels are maintained between 4 and 8 mg/dl. If serum creatinine levels are more than 2.5 mg/dl and/or in the presence of end-stage renal disease, we recommend administration of the loading dose only. Subsequent management should depend on serum magnesium levels. The need for maintenance therapy or adjusting the dose will depend on magnesium levels. In addition, monitoring urine output, leg reflexes, and respiratory rate should occur in all patients receiving magnesium sulfate. Early detection and intervention are crucial to preventing severe complications (Table 14.4).

14.8 Effect of Magnesium Sulfate on Eclampsia Prevention

For almost a century, parenteral magnesium sulfate has been utilized in the US for the prevention of recurrent seizures in eclamptic patients and as a prophylaxis for the prevention of eclamptic seizures in hypertensive disorders of pregnancy [6, 7]. During this time period, multiple protocols and regimens have been recommended for use in preeclampsia and eclampsia. At the present time, most protocols recommend IV administration in moderate- and high-resource countries, whereas intramuscular regimens are recommended in low-resource countries. The most popular regimens are summarized in Table 14.5. Although magnesium sulfate has been used for nearly a hundred years in the prevention

Table 14.5 Magnesium sulfate prophylaxis for eclampsia: Current popular protocols for magnesium sulfate administration

IV Magnesium sulfate protocols
4 g bolus over 20 min as loading dose followed by 1 g/h maintenance 6 g bolus over 20 min as loading dose followed by 2 g/h maintenance
IM Magnesium sulfate protocols
4 g IV bolus over 5 min plus 10 g intramuscular as a loading dose, followed by 5 g IM every 4 h as maintenance

Table 14.6 Rate of eclampsia and number needed to treat (NNT) by subgroup in the Magpie trial

	Magnesium sulfate	Placebo	RR (95% C.I)	NNT
Imminent eclampsia	8/810 (1.0)	31/829 (3.1)	0.26 (0.12–0.57)	36
No imminent eclampsia	32/4245 (0.7)	65/4226 (1.5)	0.49 (0.32–0.75)	127
Low PMR country	4/778 (0.5)	6/782 (0.8)	0.67 (0.19–2037)	385

of preeclampsia and eclampsia, its precise mechanism of action remains undetermined to this date [7]. In making decisions about giving magnesium sulfate prophylaxis, it is important to take into consideration the severity of preeclampsia, the presence or absence of symptoms, and the time of onset of preeclampsia. Multiple randomized trials have evaluated the effectiveness of magnesium sulfate compared with other anticonvulsants in women with eclampsia. The findings consistently demonstrated that magnesium sulfate significantly reduces the incidence of recurrent seizures and is associated with lower maternal mortality rates compared to other anticonvulsants [7, 8]. The primary goal of magnesium sulfate prophylaxis in preeclampsia is to prevent or minimize the progression to eclampsia and mitigate complications associated with the condition [9]. Moreover, secondary benefits include reducing maternal and perinatal morbidity and mortality, even in cases where seizures do not develop [10, 11].

The Magpie trial, a large-scale, multicenter study conducted across 33 countries, involved 10,110 women with preeclampsia who were randomized into treatment groups receiving either magnesium sulfate (IV or IM regimens) or placebo. Some patients received magnesium sulfate antepartum during expectant management for 24 h without subsequent dosing during labor or postpartum. Others were treated during labor and delivery, while a subset was randomized in the postpartum period. The trial revealed a significant reduction in rates of eclampsia in those randomized to magnesium sulfate as compared to placebo (40/5055 (0.8%) versus 96/5055 (1.9%), RR 0.29–0.60; 95% confidence interval). The trial also demonstrated that magnesium sulfate significantly reduced the incidence of eclampsia, particularly in low-income and middle-income countries. However, no significant reduction was observed in high-income countries, which had a smaller sample size compared to the former [7, 10]. Table 14.6 summarizes the results of the trial according to the presence or absence of imminent eclampsia prior to randomization, as well as to those enrolled in moderate- to high-resource countries. It also provides the number of patients needed to treat to prevent one case of eclampsia according to various subgroups. Despite its strengths, the trial revealed variability in clinical management. Some patients received magnesium sulfate antepartum during expectant management for 24 hours without subsequent dosing during labor or postpartum. Others were treated during labor and delivery, while a subset was randomized in the postpartum period. A trial by Belfort et al. compared the efficacy of magnesium sulfate to nimodipine in preventing eclamptic seizures. In this study, 1650 women were randomized into two groups, with one group receiving nimodipine and the other receiving magnesium sulfate from enrollment until 24 hours postpartum. The study found that magnesium sulfate was superior to nimodipine in preventing eclamptic convulsions, particularly in women with severe preeclampsia. It also showed a significant reduction in rates of postpartum convulsions [11].

14.9 Effect on Maternal Mortality and Morbidity

Mattar et al. investigated the risk factors linked to the adverse maternal outcomes in pregnancies complicated by eclampsia. The cohort included 399 eclamptic patients treated with an intravenous magnesium sulfate loading dose of 4 g over 15–30 min, which was later adjusted to 6 g, followed by a maintenance dose of 2 g/h, unless renal compromise was evident. Antihypertensive therapy was used to manage severe ranges of blood pressure. Two maternal deaths occurred, with both presenting after 30 weeks' gestation, one presenting at 39 weeks and the other presenting with no prenatal care. In addition to maternal mortality, many percent had abruption, pulmonary edema, renal failure, stroke, etc. The Magpie trial documented 11 maternal deaths in the magnesium sulfate group compared to 20 in the placebo group (RR 0.55, 95% CI 0.26–1.14). Analysis revealed that 40% of the maternal deaths in the placebo group were due to renal failure ($n = 3$), pulmonary embolism ($n = 3$), and infection ($n = 2$). These causes were unrelated to the primary effects of magnesium sulfate, which focuses on preventing status epilepticus and aspiration. In addition, there were no differences in rates of stroke or other maternal complications. These findings emphasize that the excess mortality in the placebo group cannot be attributed to magnesium sulfate but highlight other factors influencing maternal outcome. Hall et al. investigated the necessity of prophylactic magnesium sulfate and its complications in women with preeclampsia prior to labor. The study involved careful blood pressure monitoring and withholding magnesium sulfate unless eclampsia occurred. During labor, magnesium sulfate was selectively administered, based on clinician judgment or in response to eclampsia. The findings demonstrated that among women with antepartum preeclampsia who did not receive magnesium sulfate but had well-controlled blood pressure, the incidence of eclampsia was lower, and eclampsia did not worsen maternal or fetal prognosis [9].

14.10 Magnesium Sulfate in the Postpartum Period

The optimal duration for postpartum magnesium sulfate administration remains a subject for ongoing research, particularly regarding its benefits when continued for 24 hours after delivery in women who received intrapartum magnesium sulfate [2]. Several protocols were initiated throughout the years to determine the ideal protocol for magnesium sulfate prophylaxis for eclampsia in the postpartum period [14–17].

In the Magpie trial, a total of 1337 women were enrolled in the postpartum period: 639 were assigned to magnesium and 696 were assigned to placebo. In the group of women who were randomized in the postpartum period, there was no significant difference in the rate of eclampsia between magnesium vs. placebo (RR 0.54, 95% CI 0.16–1.8) [10].

Vigil-DeGarcia et al. conducted a randomized trial involving 1113 women with preeclampsia. Participants were randomized into two groups: one group received magnesium sulfate for 24 h postpartum ($n = 555$), while the other group discontinued it immediately after delivery (n = 558). All the women enrolled in the study were given a uniform magnesium sulfate regimen: a 4 g loading dose of IV magnesium sulfate and a maintenance dose of 1 g per hour intravenously. The study evaluated the incidence of postpartum eclampsia, maternal morbidity and mortality, time to initiate breastfeeding, and ambulation onset [2, 12]. This trial showed that there was no difference in the rate of eclampsia between the two groups; the incidence of eclampsia in the group that continued magnesium sulfate was 0.18% compared to 0.35% in the other group (1 in 555 vs. 2 in 558) [2, 12]. However, the sample size was based on an expected eclampsia rate that exceeded the observed rate in the control group [2]. Livingston et al. assessed the efficacy of magnesium sulfate in preventing the progression of mild preeclampsia. Participants were randomized into two groups, with the experimental group receiving magnesium sulfate as a 6 g bolus in 100 ml normal saline over 20 min, followed by a maintenance dose of 2 g/h initiated within an hour of randomization and continued for 12 h postpartum. For those who developed mild preeclampsia postpartum, magnesium sulfate was administered for a total of 12 h. The study demonstrated that no women in either group developed eclampsia [13].

14.11 Conclusion

Magnesium sulfate remains a cornerstone in the management of preeclampsia with severe features as prophylaxis for prevention of eclamptic convulsions. Extensive research has consistently demonstrated its efficacy in reducing the incidence of recurrent seizures, particularly in women with severe preeclampsia. Despite its widespread use, several questions remain unanswered, particularly regarding the ideal candidates for magnesium sulfate prophylaxis, the optimal timing for administration—whether antepartum, intrapartum, or postpartum—the appropriate dosing regimen (loading, maintenance), and the ideal duration of prophylaxis. Further research is necessary to address these gaps in knowledge, particularly to identify which patient populations benefit the most from magnesium sulfate, the best timing for intervention, and how to balance potential risks of toxicity with therapeutic effectiveness. Until these questions are resolved, magnesium sulfate continues to be a key therapeutic agent, but its use should be guided by individualized clinical assessment and careful monitoring to optimize maternal and fetal outcomes.

Major Pearls and Pitfalls

- Based on our review of the literature and our experience with the use of magnesium sulfate as prophylaxis for eclamptic seizures, there are still pitfalls about the ideal candidate with preeclampsia who will benefit from its use. In addition, there are gaps regarding the timing of administration in relation to delivery and duration of administration.
- The risk-to-benefit ratio does not justify the administration of magnesium sulfate in patients with non-severe preeclampsia.
- There is no data that demonstrates a beneficial role of magnesium sulfate in patients with severe gestational hypertension only.
- There is minimal to no data demonstrating its benefit when administered in the postpartum period.

Chapter Key Points

- Magnesium sulfate is the gold standard for preventing and treating eclamptic seizures.
- Evidence does not support prophylactic magnesium sulfate for non-severe preeclampsia or isolated severe gestational hypertension.
- Optimal timing, dosing, and duration—especially postpartum—remain uncertain.
- Monitoring for toxicity is essential; serum levels, reflexes, respiration, and urine output must guide dosing.

- Randomized trials such as Magpie show significant seizure-risk reduction, largely in low- and middle-income settings.
- Postpartum benefit is minimal when magnesium sulfate is continued routinely after delivery.

Chapter-End Summary

This chapter reviews the role of magnesium sulfate as the primary intervention for preventing eclamptic seizures in women with hypertensive disorders of pregnancy. Evidence strongly supports its use in severe preeclampsia and in women with eclampsia, with large trials demonstrating meaningful reductions in seizure risk and maternal morbidity. However, data do not support routine use in non-severe preeclampsia or isolated severe gestational hypertension. Key controversies persist regarding ideal candidates, optimal dosing strategies, and the value of postpartum continuation. Close clinical monitoring is critical to avoid toxicity. Continued research is needed to refine indications and maximize maternal safety while minimizing unnecessary intervention.

References

1. Sibai BM. 38 – Preeclampsia and hypertensive disorders. In: Gabbe's obstetrics: normal and problem pregnancies. 8th ed. Elsevier Inc; 2021. p. 708–750. e7. https://doi.org/10.1016/B978-0-323-60870-1.00038-1.
2. Fishel Bartal M, Sibai BM. Eclampsia in the 21st century. Am J Obstet Gynecol [Internet]. 2020;226(2). Available from: https://www.sciencedirect.com/science/article/pii/S0002937820311285.
3. Jones-Muhammad W. Cerebral blood flow regulation in pregnancy, hypertension, and hypertensive disorders of pregnancy. Brain Sci. 2019;9(9):224.
4. Cipolla MJ, Bishop N, Chan SL. Effect of pregnancy on autoregulation of cerebral blood flow in anterior versus posterior cerebrum. Hypertension. 2012;60(3):705–11.
5. Veen van, Panerai RB, Haeri S, Griffioen AC, Zeeman GG, Belfort MA. Cerebral autoregulation in normal pregnancy and preeclampsia. Obstet Gynecol. 2013;122(5):1064–9.
6. Friedman A, Kaufer D, Heinemann U. Blood–brain barrier breakdown-inducing astrocytic transformation: novel targets for the prevention of epilepsy. Epilepsy Res. 2009;85(2–3):142–9.
7. Sibai BM. Magnesium sulfate prophylaxis in preeclampsia: lessons learned from recent trials. Am J Obstet Gynecol. 2004;190(6):1520–6.
8. Witlin AG, Sibai BM. Magnesium sulfate therapy in preeclampsia and eclampsia. Obstet Gynecol. 1998;92(5):883–9.
9. Hall D, Odendaal HJ, Smith M. Is the prophylactic administration of magnesium sulphate in women with pre-eclampsia indicated prior to labour? BJOG. 2000;107(7):903–8.
10. Altman D, Carroli G, Duley L, Farrell B, Moodley J, Neilson J, et al. Do women with pre-eclampsia, and their babies, benefit from magnesium sulphate? The magpie trial: a randomised placebo-controlled trial. Lancet (London, England) [Internet]. 2002;359(9321):1877–90. Available from: https://www.ncbi.nlm.nih.gov/pubmed/12057549.
11. Belfort MA, Anthony J, Saade GR, Allen JC. A comparison of magnesium sulfate and nimodipine for the prevention of eclampsia. N Engl J Med. 2003;348(4):304–11.
12. Vigil-DeGracia P, Ludmir J, Ng J, Reyes-Tejada O, Nova C, Beltré A, et al. Is there benefit to continue magnesium sulphate postpartum in women receiving magnesium sulphate before delivery? A randomised controlled study. BJOG. 2018;125(10):1304–11.
13. Livingston JC, Livingston LW, Ramsey R, Mabie BC, Sibai BM. Magnesium sulfate in women with mild preeclampsia: a randomized controlled trial. Obstet Gynecol [Internet]. 2003;101(2):217–20. Available from: https://www.sciencedirect.com/science/article/abs/pii/S0029784402030533?via%3Dihub.
14. Mattar F, Sibai BM. Eclampsia. VIII. Risk factors for maternal morbidity. Am J Obstet Gynecol. 2000;182(2):307–12. https://doi.org/10.1016/S0002-9378(00)70216-X.
15. Knight M, UKOSS. Eclampsia in the United Kingdom 2005. BJOG [Internet]. 2007;114(9):1072–8. Available from: https://pubmed.ncbi.nlm.nih.gov/17617191/.
16. Tuffnell DJ, Jankowicz D, Lindow SW, Lyons G, Mason GC, Russell IF, et al. Outcomes of severe pre-eclampsia/eclampsia in Yorkshire 1999/2003. BJOG. 2005;112(7):875–80.
17. Katz VL, Farmer R, Kuller JA. Preeclampsia into eclampsia: toward a new paradigm. Am J Obstet Gynecol. 2000;182(6):1389–96.

Prevention of Fetal Growth Restriction

Emmanuel Attali, Nir Melamed, and Liran Hiersch

Contents

Y. Yogev, A. Khalil (eds.), *Prevention of Complications in Obstetrics*,
https://doi.org/10.1007/978-3-032-23479-7_15

Learning Objectives

- Describe major etiologies and mechanisms underlying FGR.
- Identify lifestyle, nutritional, and environmental factors influencing fetal growth.
- Explain maternal comorbidities associated with increased FGR risk and preventive strategies.
- Summarize evidence supporting aspirin and other pharmacologic interventions.
- Discuss limitations of current predictive and preventive tools for placenta-mediated FGR.

15.1 Introduction

Fetal growth restriction (FGR), or intrauterine growth restriction (IUGR), implies the failure of a fetus to meet its growth potential [1, 2]. The most commonly used approach with regard to screening for FGR is sonographic fetal weight estimation (EFW) to detect fetuses small for gestational age (SGA), most commonly defined as EFW <10th percentile for gestational age [3, 4].

However, the detection of FGR does not imply a specific etiology, but rather an obstetric condition that warrants further investigation. Several causes have been related to FGR, including fetal conditions [5, 6] (e.g., chromosomal anomalies, genetic syndromes, structural anomalies), maternal comorbidities [7–12] (e.g., environmental toxins exposure, uterine anomalies, infections, malnutrition), and most commonly placental dysfunction (Table 15.1) [13].

FGR is associated with various short- and long-term morbidities such as perinatal mortality, neonatal metabolic and electrolyte imbalance [14], neurodevelopmental delay [15], and metabolic syndrome in adulthood [16–18].

At present, there is no effective treatment for FGR, and the main approach involves identifying the most probable etiology, fetal surveillance, and finally, determining the optimal timing for delivery to prevent intrauterine demise [1]. Nevertheless, preterm birth may also increase the risk for complications, and this widely used strategy failed to reduce morbidities, especially childhood neurodevelopmental adverse outcomes [19]. Hence, there is a necessity to identify those most susceptible to developing FGR and offer them primary or secondary preventive strategies.

In the current chapter, we review available evidence regarding various strategies for the prevention of FGR.

Table 15.1 Common etiologies of fetal growth restriction

Maternal factors:
Hypoxemia (chronic lung disease, high altitude)
Anemia
Smoking and substance abuse (cocaine, methamphetamines)
Malabsorption and poor weight gain
Environmental toxins: air pollution, heavy metals
Placental factors:
Maternal vascular malperfusion pathology (infarction, chronic abruption)
Chronic placental inflammation
Confined placental mosaicism
Umbilical cord factors:
True cord knot
Single umbilical artery
Velamentous cord insertion
Fetal disorders:
Genetic disorders
Structural anomalies (congenital heart disease, gastroschisis)
Congenital infections (cytomegalovirus, toxoplasmosis, herpes, rubella, syphilis, Zika, malaria)
Teratogen exposure (drugs, toxins)

15.2 Lifestyle Modifications

15.2.1 Smoking, Alcohol, and Recreational Drugs

Maternal use of various recreational agents and addictive substances is associated with FGR [20–22], although specific causality is often difficult to establish due to associated cofounders and the often-simultaneous use of multiple substances. The impact of active and passive cigarette smoking on pregnancy outcomes is well-studied. A French perinatal survey published in 2022 revealed a decline in the prevalence of smoking among pregnant women, although it remained notably elevated at 12.2% [23]. Delcroix-Gomez et al. published a well-conducted prospective study on the impact of smoking and cessation at different trimesters on the development of FGR [20], defined as reported smoking status and exhaled carbon monoxide (CO) at delivery. The risk of FGR in women who smoked through pregnancy or stopped smoking in the third trimester was about twice the risk in nonsmokers. On the other hand, the authors observed a decrease in the rate of FGR among women who quit smoking early in pregnancy, reducing it to the level observed in the nonsmoker population. Those findings highlight the importance of smoking cessation guidance to mitigate the risk of FGR, preferably as early in gestation as possible. Psychological interventions to support women to stop smoking during pregnancy increase the proportion of women who stop smoking and decrease the proportion of low-birth-weight infants [24].

Most recreational drugs can easily cross the placenta, not only leading to an SGA fetus but also causing malformations and impaired neurocognitive development [22, 25–27]. Thus, it is important to emphasize that maternal cannabis, cocaine, and amphetamine use during pregnancy should be avoided. Alcohol consumption during pregnancy can result in fetal alcohol syndrome or fetal alcohol spectrum disorders. Although a meta-analysis found that women who consumed low-moderate amounts of alcohol (1 drink/day) during pregnancy were at no increased risk for SGA [21] compared to abstainers, alcohol intake is also related to dysmorphic features and cognitive impairments [28].

15.2.2 Maternal Weight, Diet, and Nutrition

Numerous studies confirmed the association of maternal diet and caloric intake with intrauterine fetal growth [10, 12, 29–35].The effect of maternal malnutrition and undernutrition on fetal development is well established, with several major studies conducted on mothers exposed to famine and nutrition intervention trials in developing countries. During the harsh Dutch famine of 1944–1955, daily average caloric intake below 1500 during the third trimester was associated with significant reductions in birth weight [36, 37].

Maternal weight and body mass index (BMI) are also important factors of fetal growth and are associated with the risk of FGR. In a meta-analysis including more than 1,000,000 patients with singleton pregnancies, underweight women had a higher risk of low birth weight (LBW) than those born to women of normal weight [38]. Thus, maternal nutrition and prepregnancy BMI should be taken into consideration in risk stratification for FGR, and dietary counseling should be recommended not only to overweight but also to underweight women. For the latter group, it is important to advise a higher gestational weight gain to reduce the risk of LBW and FGR, as suggested by the World Health Organization (WHO) guidelines [39, 40].

Maternal diet and the consumption of specific micro- and macronutrients may also play a role in intrauterine fetal growth [31, 32]. Several long-term cohort studies emphasize the relation of the pre- and peri-conceptual diet with SGA infants. The "Generation R Study" [41] investigated the association of dietary habits early in pregnancy (before 18 weeks) with fetal growth and birthweight in a prospective observational study of 3207 Caucasian women in the Netherlands. In this study, low adherence to the Mediterranean diet (high intake of vegetables, fish, pasta, and rice, and low intake of meat, potatoes, and fatty sauces) was associated with a lower birth weight. Those findings are in accordance with a Danish study that assessed the association between maternal diet during pregnancy and fetal growth [42]. A maternal diet that was based on red and processed meat was found to be associated with a higher risk of SGA (OR 0.74: 95% CI 0.64–0.86) as compared to those with a diet characterized by the intake of vegetables, fruits, poultry, and fish.

It is important to note that the association of maternal diet and specific use of micro- and macronutrients on intrauterine growth is not uniform across all populations. In low-income countries, supplementations with multiple maternal micronutrients are associated with a lower incidence of LBW and SGA [43]. While maternal anemia is another known risk factor for LBW [44], and routine iron supplementation with or without folic acid reduces the risk of maternal anemia, the effect on fetal growth is less clear [45].

15.3 Maternal Comorbidities and Preexisting Diseases

15.3.1 Maternal Autoimmune Disorders

Maternal autoimmune and collagen disorders, especially those with vascular involvement, are associated with adverse perinatal outcomes and specifically with aberrant fetal growth [46–49].

15

About 10–30% of pregnancies in women with Systemic Lupus Erythematosus (SLE) are complicated by FGR or SGA [49]. The risk is higher in the presence of active disease [50] and lupus nephritis [51]. Thus, optimizing the control of the disease is crucial in women with SLE before and during pregnancy. Hydroxychloroquine treatment in pregnancy has been shown to decrease disease flares and several adverse pregnancy outcomes [52, 53], but its impact on preeclampsia and FGR remains unclear [54, 55].

SLE in pregnancy is associated with an almost 3-fold rise in adverse neonatal outcomes, especially in the presence of antiphospholipid antibodies (APLA) [56]. APLA syndrome is clearly and strongly related to low birth weight. A meta-analysis of twenty-two studies showed that APLA increased the risk of FGR, which was more prominent in women with anticardiolipin (OR 2.25 95% CI 1.55–2.94) and anti-beta2Glycoprotein1 (OR 1.31 95% CI 1.12–1.49) antibodies [57].

Pregnancy outcomes in women with well-controlled rheumatoid arthritis (RA) are similar to those in the general population, but those with active disease are at higher risk for SGA and FGR [58]. A recent study tried to explore the association of maternal RA with pregnancy outcomes in relation to disease activity and antirheumatic treatment before and during pregnancy [59]. It seems that disease activity rather than maternal treatment is the most important risk factor for SGA.

15.3.2 Hypertensive Disorders

In women with mild-moderate chronic hypertension, a 2018 Cochrane review showed that antihypertensive medications halve the risk of severe hypertension but have no clear effect on SGA [60]. Recently, two major randomized controlled trials have been published on this topic. In the CHIP (Control of Hypertension in Pregnancy) trial, tight control of hypertension (diastolic blood pressure targets of 85 mmHg compared to 100 mmHg) did not reduce the risk of delivering an SGA infant [61]. Moreover, the CHAP (Chronic Hypertension and Pregnancy) trial consortium [62], assessed the impact of targeting a blood pressure of less than 140/90 mmHg on adverse pregnancy outcomes and reported a lower primary outcome (composite of preeclampsia with severe features, medically indicated preterm birth, placental abruption, and perinatal deaths) in the study group, without any changes in SGA rates. Thus, while strict blood pressure control may be beneficial for some pregnancy-related complications, its effect on the prevention of FGR is limited [63].

15.3.3 Pregestational Diabetes Mellitus

Pregnancies complicated by maternal pregestational diabetes are often associated with accelerated growth and macrosomia [63]. However, in those who also suffer from nephropathy or vasculopathy, often developing after more than a decade from the diagnosis of diabetes, the risk of FGR is increased [64]. Thus, women with pregestational diabetes in their reproductive periods should be advised regarding the need to maintain good glycemic control to minimize the development of long-term end-organ damage and the subsequent adverse effects on pregnancy outcomes [66–68].

15.3.4 Epilepsy

Infants born to women with epilepsy face a greater risk of SGA, likely stemming from prenatal exposure to antiepileptic drugs. The risk seems particularly notable when using topiramate, although it is also evident with other antiepileptic medications [65, 66]. Additionally, the use of multiple antiepileptic drugs concurrently is linked to a greater risk of FGR [67]. Genetic factors may also play a role in FGR among this population [67].

A population-based study from Taiwan found an increased risk for SGA in women with uncontrolled epilepsy and repeated seizures during pregnancy. However, the study could not determine whether the increased risk was due to multiple seizures or antiepileptic medications [65]. Therefore, women with epilepsy should undergo prepregnancy consults, including the consideration of reducing the anti-seizure medications to the minimum needed for seizure prophylaxis. In addition, agents with a high safety profile during pregnancy should be preferred when possible.

15.4 Perinatal Infections

About 5–10% of FGR cases can be attributed to in-utero viral or protozoan infections [68].

The most common viral agents implicated in FGR are rubella, cytomegalovirus (CMV), varicella-zoster (VZV), Zika, and human immunodeficiency virus (HIV) [13]. The pathophysiology is not entirely clear but has been suggested to involve placentitis, vascular endothelial lesions, and direct inhibition of cell multiplication. Protozoan infections that can cause FGR include toxoplasmosis [69] and malaria. The adverse effects of malaria on fetal health are profound and are mainly due to maternal anemia [70].

Although the most important intervention remains prevention, some antiviral and anti-protozoan prenatal treatments are available. The maternal treatment of toxoplasmosis by anti-protozoan medications, such as pyrimethamine, sulfadiazine, and spiramycin, is well established and has demonstrated a reduction in maternal-to-fetal transmission but also congenital clinical sequelae [71–73]. Similarly, level 1 evidence suggests that maternal administration of high-dose valacyclovir for primary CMV infection substantially reduces the risk of congenital CMV infection, especially if begun before 14 weeks of gestation and within 4–8 weeks of the maternal infections [74].

15.5 Placental Factors

Uteroplacental insufficiency stands as a primary contributor to FGR. In the initial stage of pregnancy, the trophoblast invasion of the maternal spiral arteries and subsequent remodeling of the smooth muscle layer result in decreased arterial resistance and, consequently, high-flow uteroplacental circulation. Those hemodynamic changes are pivotal and facilitate efficient gaseous and nutrient exchange necessary for optimal fetal growth [75]. In contrast, inadequate or abnormal trophoblast invasion is associated with reduced placental perfusion and increased oxidative stress and can lead to placenta-mediated complications such as FGR and preeclampsia [76].

Numerous interventions have been explored for the prevention and management of FGR attributed to uteroplacental insufficiency, and the main ones are discussed below.

15.5.1 Aspirin

Aspirin exerts various vascular effects that could potentially prevent FGR (◘ Fig. 15.1). First, it suppresses the production of prostaglandins and thromboxane by inactivating the cyclooxygenase enzyme. Thromboxane, known for its potent vasoconstrictive properties, is inhibited by low doses of aspirin. Second, recent data suggest that aspirin also acts as an antioxidant and may induce the release of nitric oxide from the vascular endothelium [77]. Finally, aspirin increases the activity of heme oxygenase-1, which leads to a reduction in oxidative stress, injury, and inflammation [78].

Most studies on the administration of aspirin for the prevention of placenta-mediated complications focused on preeclampsia as a primary outcome, with FGR being considered as a secondary one. However, the volume and quality of evidence available permit a meaningful interpretation also for the effect of aspirin on the prevention of SGA or FGR. A systematic review based on a study-level meta-analysis including 20,909 women [79], and individual patient data-based meta-analyses including 32,217 women [80] conclude that aspirin provides a modest risk reduction for SGA and FGR (RR 0.56; 95% CI 0.44–0.70 and 0.76; 95% CI 0.61–0.94). Furthermore, the systemic and study-level meta-analyses support earlier initiation (<16 weeks) and favor a dose of 100–150 mg per day [79].

Regarding the time during the day when aspirin is most effective, a small ($n = 350$) randomized control trial has found that at bedtime, but not upon waking, administration of aspirin reduces the incidence of FGR (3.4% vs. 17.2%, p-value 0.011) and hypertensive disorders of pregnancy [81].

However, it should be noticed that in the ASPRE TRIAL, the largest trial on the use of aspirin for the prevention of preeclampsia, aspirin administration was not associated with a reduction in the risk of FGR [82].

Patient selection and accurate identification of those who can benefit from this treatment are not clear. One important limitation of most studies on early prediction of FGR is the lack of a gold standard for the antenatal and postnatal diagnosis of FGR. Studies that considered SGA at birth as the primary outcome failed to differentiate between infants who are constitutionally small and healthy and those who are small due to FGR.

15

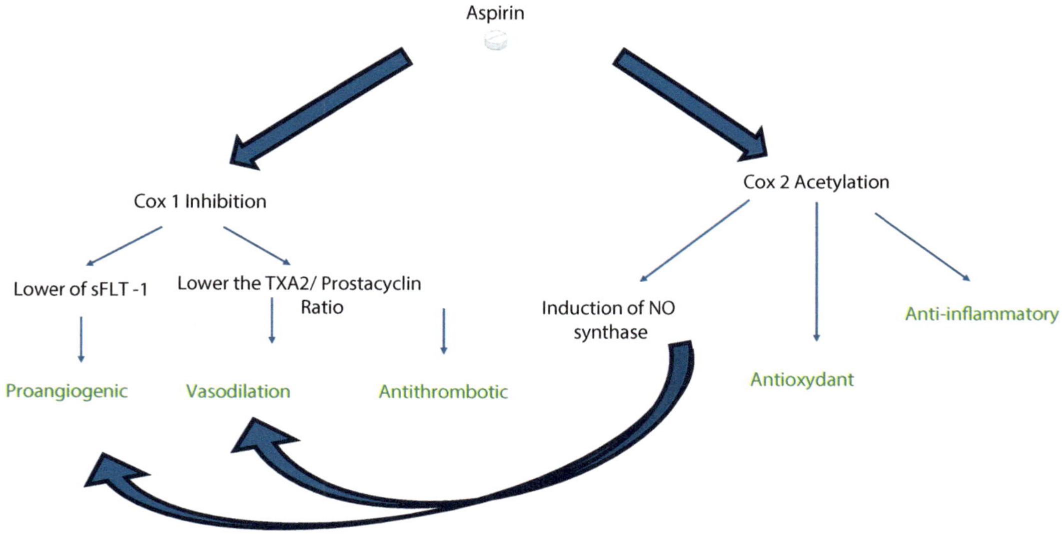

◘ **Fig. 15.1** Mechanism of action of Aspirin with regard to preventing placenta-mediated complications

Prediction models for placental insufficiency mainly focus on preeclampsia and have not been sufficiently validated for FGR. In a prospective cohort of 4970 women, the combination of first-trimester serum Pregnancy-Associated Plasma Protein A (PAPP-A), beta-Human Chorionic Gonadotropin (HCG), maternal blood pressure, and uterine artery Doppler had a detection rate of 73% for early SGA (<34 weeks) but only 32% for late SGA (>34 weeks) [83]. Another model, which was evaluated in a larger cohort (9150 women) and included Placental Growth Factor (PLGF) and soluble Fms-like tyrosine kinase 1 (sFlt-1), achieved a better detection rate of 86% for early SGA and 66% for late SGA [84].

Yet, given the safety of aspirin and the overlap in the risk factors and pathogenesis of preeclampsia and FGR, most national and international guidelines recommend a 100–150 mg aspirin dose to prevent FGR and SGA in women at high risk (Table 15.2) [1, 3].

Table 15.2 National and international guidelines of aspirin use for fetal growth prevention [104]

Society (country)	Date of publication	Recommendation
FIGO	2021	Low-dose Aspirin, starting between 12 and 16 weeks may be considered in selected cases such as women who are at high risk of preeclampsia or those with a history of placenta-mediated FGR—dose 100–150 mg
ACOG (United States)	2021	Insufficient evidence
RCOG (United Kingdom)	2024	Low-dose Aspirin, starting between 12 and 16 weeks for FGR prevention in women at risk for PET or with a history of placenta-mediated FGR—dose 150 mg
CNGOF (France)	2015	Low-dose Aspirin before 16 weeks for FGR prevention in women with a history of "severe" FGR (<5th percentile) or previous PET before 34 weeks—dose 100–160 mg
SOGC (Canada)	2013	Low-dose Aspirin before 16 weeks for FGR prevention in women with prior preeclampsia, growth restriction or two or more risk factors for SGA

FIGO International Federation of Gynecology and Obstetrics, *ACOG* American College of Obstetricians and Gynecologists, *RCOG* Royal College of Obstetricians and Gynecologists, *CNGOF* College National des Gynecologues et Obstetriciens, *SOGC* Society of Obstetricians and Gynecologists of Canada, *FGR* Fetal Growth Restriction, *PET* Preeclampisa

15.5.2 Heparin and Low-Molecular-Weight Heparin

Unfractionated heparin and low-molecular-weight heparin (LMWH) are commonly used in pregnancy for thromboprophylaxis and treatment of venous thromboembolism. The anticoagulant properties and the presumed ability to prevent placental thrombosis and infarction were first thought to be able to further prevent placental-mediated pathology, including pregnancy loss and preeclampsia. However, in vitro and in vivo data suggest heparin has additional biological properties, including anti-inflammatory and pro-angiogenic effects [85–87]. For example, heparin use during pregnancy for anticoagulation leads to an increase in serum PLGF concentration and a decrease in the sFlt-1/PLGF ratio [88].

However, the impact of heparin on the risk of preeclampsia and FGR remains controversial. The EPPI trial (enoxaparin for preeclampsia and intrauterine growth restriction) included women at high risk for placental-mediated complications and showed no difference in the rate of the composite outcome (defined as preeclampsia or SGA <5th percentile) in treated women compared to those who were not [89]. On the other hand, a study-level meta-analysis of six trials (848 women) showed that LMWH was associated with a reduction of placental-mediated morbidities, including preeclampsia, SGA, placental abruption, and late abortion [90]. In contrast, a subsequent individual patient data meta-analysis found no beneficial effect of the treatment [91]. The latest meta-analysis on this topic was published in 2022 [92] and included a total of 15 studies (2795 participants). In high-risk women (defined as either a history of preeclampsia, FGR, fetal demise, or miscarriage, or being at high risk after the first-trimester screening of preeclampsia), treatment with LMWH was associated with a reduction in the development of preeclampsia and SGA. Subgroup analysis by type of heparin showed that Dalteparin was associated with a significant reduction in the development of SGA, whereas in patients treated by Enoxaparin, such reduction did not reach statistical significance (**Dalteparin**: 6 RCTs, 1103 participants; OR, 0.48: 95% CI, 0.28–0.82, $P = 0.007$; **Exoxaparin**: 7 RCTs, 1532 participants; OR, 0.75; 95% CI, 0.50–1.11; $P = 0.150$).

Therefore, due to the controversial data (◘ Table 15.3), the FIGO guidelines for the management of FGR [1] stated that LMWH cannot be recommended for the prevention of FGR in high-risk women. Of note, those guidelines were published in 2021 and before the publication of the previously described meta-analysis from 2022.

15.5.3 Statins, Proton Pump Inhibitors, and Others

Recently, statins have been proposed to prevent preeclampsia and improve pregnancy outcomes [93] by increasing the activity of HO-l/carbon monoxide and inhibiting the release of sFlt-1 [94, 95]. The therapeutic use of statins in preeclampsia has been examined in a few human trials with an overall low number of participants [96, 97] and failed to draw a clear conclusion.

Since preeclampsia and FGR may share a common pathophysiological pathway, some suggest that statins should be studied as a potential preventive agent for FGR. To date, no human trials have been conducted to investigate the effect of statins on FGR prevention. A systematic review and meta-analysis of animal data demonstrate that statins only induce lower maternal pressure in rodent pregnancies complicated by preeclampsia but have no effect on birth weight [98].

In vitro studies show that proton pump inhibitors (PPIs) decrease sFlt-1 and soluble endoglin, while esomeprazole reduces blood pressure in a preeclampsia transgenic mouse model that overexpresses sFlt-1 [99]. In vivo, trials on PPI and FGR, or PPI and preeclampsia, that studied birthweight as a secondary outcome have not been published yet. A large Australian RCT that aims to investigate the effect of esomeprazole on outcomes in women at high risk of preeclampsia (ANZCTR12618001755224) is still recruiting.

Sildenafil citrate, a phosphodiesterase-5 competitive inhibitor that activates the effects of nitric oxide, has been approved by the Food and Drug Administration for the treatment of erectile dysfunction. The activation of nitric oxide and secondary relaxation of vascular smooth muscle cells and vasodilation can reduce vascular resistance in the uterine and umbilical arteries and prevent or treat FGR [100, 101]. Sildenafil was first studied as an intervention in cases of early FGR. A large RCT conducted in the Netherlands investigated whether sildenafil reduces perinatal mortality and major morbidity (defined as the primary outcome) in women with severe FGR between 20 and 30 weeks of gestation [102]. The trial was discontinued prematurely due to safety concerns, whereas the benefit on the primary outcome was unlikely. Furthermore, pulmonary hypertension occurred in 18.8% of the neonates in the sildenafil-treated group, in comparison to 5.1% in the control group, suggesting that sildenafil may increase the risk of neonatal pulmonary hypertension.

Table 15.3 Major studies on low molecular weight heparin and fetal growth restriction prevention

Reference	Study population	GA at inclusion	Interventions		Use of Aspirin	Outcome	Main findings
Rey et al. [105]	History of PET, SGA, PA, or IUFD without thrombophilia	<16 weeks	Dalteparin, daily ($n = 57$)	No intervention ($n = 57$)	Yes	Preeclampsia, Fetal Growth Restriction	Reduction of recurrence of placental-mediated complications in women without thrombophilia
Gris et al. [106]	History of PA without APS	At positive pregnancy test	Enoxaparin ($n = 80$)	Standard high-risk care	Yes	Composite of placental-mediated complications (SGA <5th percentile)	Reduction of the composite outcome
Gris et al. [107]	History of PET without APS	At positive pregnancy test	Enoxaparin + Aspirin ($n = 112$)	Aspirin ($n = 112$)	Yes	PET, SGA, Stillbirth, and PA reported as secondary outcomes	No significant differences
Mertinelli et al. [108]	History of PET, SGA, PA, or IUFD without thrombophilia	<12 weeks	Nadroparin ($n = 63$)	Standard high-risk care	Yes	Composite of placental-mediated complications	No significant differences
Haddad et al. [108]	History of PET diagnosed <34 weeks gestation	<14 weeks	Enoxaparin + Aspirin ($n = 124$)	Aspirin ($n = 125$)	Yes	Composite of placental-mediated complications	No significant differences
Groom et al. [89]	Women at high risk of PE or/and SGA based on history	6–16 weeks	Enoxaparin ($n = 73$)	Standard high-risk care	Yes	Composite of PET and/or SGA < 5th percentile	No significant differences

In 2023, a meta-analysis was performed including nine trials that studied the effect of sildenafil treatment on birthweight and prolongation of gestation in pregnancies complicated by FGR [103]. The authors found that sildenafil treatment increased birthweight and prolonged gestation but did not affect the rate of stillbirth, neonatal deaths, and NICU admission. The rate of neonatal pulmonary hypertension was not reported. Currently, data are scarce regarding the effect of sildenafil on SGA and FGR in high-risk populations.

15.6 Summary and Clinical Implications

Currently, clinicians have limited ability to prevent FGR. The main interventions remain lifestyle modifications, avoiding smoking, alcohol, and recreational drug use, along with prepregnancy optimization of chronic conditions and adequate nutrition and gestational weight gain (◘ Table 15.4).

The capability to enhance placentation and prevent placental dysfunction and subsequent FGR also remains limited, partly due to the lack of proven therapeutic options but also the challenge in identifying women at risk.

◘ **Table 15.4** Summary of intervention for prevention of Fetal Growth Restriction

Intervention	Recommendation
Smoking cessation	Smoking cessation in recommended at any stage of pregnancy, especially in the first trimester
Dietary supplementation	As standard pregnancy care
Anemia: screening and treatment	As standard pregnancy care
Low-dose Aspirin	Before week 16 in women with risk factors for preeclampsia. Some also recommend it in women with previous history of severe fetal growth restriction
Low molecular weight Heparin	Not sufficient data to make a recommendation

15

A 100–150 mg bedtime aspirin, commenced before 16 weeks of gestation, may provide a modest risk reduction in women at high risk for placenta-mediated complications based on conventional obstetric history-based risk factors. The addition of LMWH (dalteparin, to be specific) could lead to a further reduction in the risk of SGA in this population, but before formal recommendations can be given, more studies are needed to support it.

Chapter Key Points

- FGR is multifactorial with maternal, fetal, and placental contributors; prevention focuses on modifiable risks.
- Lifestyle modifications—smoking cessation, avoidance of alcohol and drugs, optimal nutrition—reduce risk.
- Optimization of maternal comorbidities (autoimmune disease, hypertension, diabetes) is essential.
- Aspirin 100–150 mg before 16 weeks provides a modest reduction in placenta-mediated FGR in high-risk women.
- LMWH evidence remains inconsistent; routine use is not recommended.
- No proven placentation-enhancing therapy exists; preventive strategies remain limited.

Chapter-End Summary

This chapter reviews evidence-based strategies to prevent fetal growth restriction. While most cases are related to placental dysfunction, prevention remains limited to modifying maternal risk factors, optimizing nutrition, encouraging smoking and substance cessation, and controlling chronic conditions. Aspirin initiated before 16 weeks offers a modest benefit in high-risk populations, whereas data for LMWH, statins, PPIs, and other agents remain inconclusive. Current predictive tools insufficiently identify women at risk, underscoring the need for improved screening and effective placental therapies.

References

1. Melamed N, Baschat A, Yinon Y, et al. FIGO (international Federation of Gynecology and obstetrics) initiative on fetal growth: best practice advice for screening, diagnosis, and management of fetal growth restriction. Int J Gynaecol Obstet. 2021;152(Suppl 1):3–57. https://doi.org/10.1002/IJGO.13522.
2. Hiersch L, Melamed N. Fetal growth velocity and body proportion in the assessment of growth. Am J Obstet Gynecol. 2018;218(2):S700-S711.e1. https://doi.org/10.1016/j.ajog.2017.12.014.
3. McCowan LM, Figueras F, Anderson NH. Evidence-based national guidelines for the management of suspected fetal growth restriction: comparison, consensus, and controversy. Am J Obstet Gynecol. 2018;218(2) https://doi.org/10.1016/j.ajog.2017.12.004.
4. Martins JG, Biggio JR, Abuhamad A. Society for Maternal-Fetal Medicine Consult Series #52: diagnosis and management of fetal growth restriction: (replaces clinical guideline number 3, April 2012). Am J Obstet Gynecol. 2020;223(4) https://doi.org/10.1016/j.ajog.2020.05.010.
5. Dall'Asta A, Stampalija T, Mecacci F, et al. Incidence, clinical features and perinatal outcome in anomalous fetuses with late-onset growth restriction: cohort study. Ultrasound Obstet Gynecol. 2022;60(5) https://doi.org/10.1002/uog.24961.
6. Meler E, Sisterna S, Borrell A. Genetic syndromes associated with isolated fetal growth restriction. Prenat Diagn. 2020;40(4) https://doi.org/10.1002/pd.5635.
7. Proctor LK, Kfouri J, Hiersch L, et al. Association between hypertensive disorders and fetal growth restriction in twin compared with singleton gestations. Am J Obstet Gynecol. 2019;221(3):251.e1–8. https://doi.org/10.1016/j.ajog.2019.04.022.
8. Hiersch L, Yeoshoua E, Miremberg H, et al. The association between Mullerian anomalies and short-term pregnancy outcome. J Matern Fetal Neonatal Med. 2016;29(16) https://doi.org/10.3109/14767058.2015.1098613.
9. Melamed N, Hiersch L, Peled Y, Hod M, Wiznitzer A, Yogev Y. The association between low 50g glucose challenge test result and fetal growth restriction. J Matern Fetal Neonatal Med. 2013;26(11) https://doi.org/10.3109/14767058.2013.770460.
10. Anteby M, Yogev Y, Hiersch L. Pregnancy: impact of maternal nutrition on intrauterine fetal growth. World Rev Nutr Diet. 2022:125. https://doi.org/10.1159/000521799.
11. Kesary Y, Avital K, Hiersch L. Maternal plant-based diet during gestation and pregnancy outcomes. Arch Gynecol Obstet. 2020;302(4) https://doi.org/10.1007/s00404-020-05689-x.
12. Hiersch L, Yogev Y. Pregnancy: impact of maternal nutrition on intrauterine fetal growth. World Rev Nutr Diet. 2016:114. https://doi.org/10.1159/000441824.
13. Nardozza LMM, Caetano ACR, Zamarian ACP, et al. Fetal growth restriction: current knowledge. Arch Gynecol Obstet. 2017;295(5) https://doi.org/10.1007/s00404-017-4341-9.
14. Wang LY, Wang LY, Wang YL, Ho CH. Early neonatal hypoglycemia in term and late preterm small for gestational age newborns. Pediatr Neonatol. 2023;64(5):538–46. https://doi.org/10.1016/J.PEDNEO.2022.09.021.
15. Sacchi C, Marino C, Nosarti C, Vieno A, Visentin S, Simonelli A. Association of intrauterine growth restriction and small for gestational age status with childhood cognitive outcomes: a systematic review and meta-analysis. JAMA Pediatr. 2020;174(8):772–81. https://doi.org/10.1001/JAMAPEDIATRICS.2020.1097.
16. Barker DJP. Fetal origins of coronary heart disease. BMJ. 1995;311(6998):171. https://doi.org/10.1136/BMJ.311.6998.171.
17. Malin GL, Morris RK, Riley R, Teune MJ, Khan KS. When is birthweight at term abnormally low? A systematic review and meta-analysis of the association and predictive ability of current birthweight standards for neonatal outcomes. BJOG. 2014;121(5):515–26. https://doi.org/10.1111/1471-0528.12517.
18. Zeitlin J, El Ayoubi M, Jarreau PH, et al. Impact of fetal growth restriction on mortality and morbidity in a very preterm birth cohort. J Pediatr. 2010;157(5) https://doi.org/10.1016/J.JPEDS.2010.05.002.
19. Andreasen LA, Tabor A, Nørgaard LN, Rode L, Gerds TA, Tolsgaard MG. Detection of growth-restricted fetuses during pregnancy is associated with fewer intrauterine deaths but increased adverse childhood outcomes: an observational study. BJOG. 2021;128(1):77–85. https://doi.org/10.1111/1471-0528.16380.
20. Delcroix-Gomez C, Delcroix MH, Jamee A, Gauthier T, Marquet P, Aubard Y. Fetal growth restriction, low birth weight, and preterm birth: effects of active or passive smoking evaluated by maternal expired CO at delivery, impacts of cessation at different trimesters. Tob Induc Dis. 2022;20(August) https://doi.org/10.18332/TID/152111.

21. Patra J, Bakker R, Irving H, Jaddoe VWV, Malini S, Rehm J. Dose-response relationship between alcohol consumption before and during pregnancy and the risks of low birthweight, preterm birth and small for gestational age (SGA)-a systematic review and meta-analyses. BJOG. 2011;118(12) https://doi.org/10.1111/j.1471-0528.2011.03050.x.
22. Gouin K, Murphy K, Shah PS. Effects of cocaine use during pregnancy on low birthweight and preterm birth: systematic review and metaanalyses. Am J Obstet Gynecol. 2011;204(4) https://doi.org/10.1016/j.ajog.2010.11.013.
23. Le Ray, Camille, et al. Results of the 2021 French National Perinatal Survey and trends in perinatal health in metropolitan France since 1995. J Gynecol Obstet Hum Reprod. 2022;51(10):102509.
24. Chamberlain C, O'Mara-Eves A, Porter J, et al. Psychosocial interventions for supporting women to stop smoking in pregnancy. Cochrane Database Syst Rev. 2017;2(2) https://doi.org/10.1002/14651858.CD001055.PUB5.
25. Lo JO, Hedges JC, Girardi G. Impact of cannabinoids on pregnancy, reproductive health, and offspring outcomes. Am J Obstet Gynecol. 2022;227(4):571–81. https://doi.org/10.1016/J.AJOG.2022.05.056.
26. Ladhani NNN, Shah PS, Murphy KE. Prenatal amphetamine exposure and birth outcomes: a systematic review and metaanalysis. Am J Obstet Gynecol. 2011;205(3) https://doi.org/10.1016/j.ajog.2011.04.016.
27. Fergusson DM, Horwood LJ, Northstone K. Maternal use of cannabis and pregnancy outcome. BJOG. 2002;109(1) https://doi.org/10.1111/j.1471-0528.2002.01020.x.
28. Sokol RJ, Delaney-Black V, Nordstrom B. Fetal alcohol spectrum disorder. JAMA. 2003;290(22):2996–9. https://doi.org/10.1001/JAMA.290.22.2996.
29. Wu G, Bazer FW, Cudd TA, Meininger CJ, Spencer TE. Maternal nutrition and fetal development. J Nutr. 2004;134(9) https://doi.org/10.1093/jn/134.9.2169.
30. Yogev Y, Hiersch L. Pregnancy: impact of maternal nutrition on intrauterine fetal growth. World Rev Nutr Diet. 2014:109. https://doi.org/10.1159/000356110.
31. Anteby M, Yogev Y, Hiersch L. Pregnancy: impact of maternal nutrition on intrauterine fetal growth. World Rev Nutr Diet. 2021:123. https://doi.org/10.1159/000516447.
32. Anteby M, Yogev Y, Hiersch L. Pregnancy: the impact of maternal nutrition on intrauterine fetal growth. World Rev Nutr Diet. 2023;126 https://doi.org/10.1159/000527922.
33. Hiersch L, Yogev Y. Pregnancy: impact of maternal nutrition on intrauterine fetal growth. World Rev Nutr Diet. 2017:116. https://doi.org/10.1159/000452191.
34. Hiersch L, Yogev Y. Pregnancy: impact of maternal nutrition on intrauterine fetal growth. World Rev Nutr Diet. 2019:119. https://doi.org/10.1159/000494314.
35. Hiersch L, Yogev Y. Pregnancy: impact of maternal nutrition on intrauterine fetal growth. World Rev Nutr Diet. 2018:117. https://doi.org/10.1159/000484504.
36. Stein AD, Zybert PA, van de Bor M, Lumey LH. Intrauterine famine exposure and body proportions at birth: the Dutch Hunger Winter. Int J Epidemiol. 2004;33(4):831–6. https://doi.org/10.1093/ije/dyh083.
37. Stein Z, Susser M. The Dutch famine, 1944–1945, and the reproductive process. I. Effects on six indices at birth. Pediatr Res. 1975;9(2):70–6. https://doi.org/10.1203/00006450-197502000-00003.
38. Han Z, Mulla S, Beyene J, Liao G, McDonald SD. Maternal underweight and the risk of preterm birth and low birth weight: a systematic review and meta-analyses. Int J Epidemiol. 2011;40(1) https://doi.org/10.1093/ije/dyq195.
39. Rasmussen KM, Yaktine AL. Weight gain during pregnancy: reexamining the guidelines. National Academies Press. 2009;184(3) https://doi.org/10.1067/mob.2001.109591.
40. Nohr EA, Vaeth M, Baker JL, Sørensen TIA, Olsen J, Rasmussen KM. Combined associations of prepregnancy body mass index and gestational weight gain with the outcome of pregnancy. Am J Clin Nutr. 2008;87(6) https://doi.org/10.1093/ajcn/87.6.1750.
41. Timmermans S, Steegers-Theunissen RP, Vujkovic M, et al. The Mediterranean diet and fetal size parameters: the Generation R Study. Br J Nutr. 2012;108(8) https://doi.org/10.1017/S000711451100691X.
42. Knudsen VK, Orozova-Bekkevold IM, Mikkelsen TB, Wolff S, Olsen SF. Major dietary patterns in pregnancy and fetal growth. Eur J Clin Nutr. 2008;62(4) https://doi.org/10.1038/sj.ejcn.1602745.
43. Keats EC, Haider BA, Tam E, Bhutta ZA. Multiple-micronutrient supplementation for women during pregnancy. Cochrane Database Syst Rev. 2019;3(3) https://doi.org/10.1002/14651858.CD004905.PUB6.
44. Figueiredo ACMG, Gomes-Filho IS, Silva RB, et al. Maternal anemia and low birth weight: a systematic review and meta-analysis. Nutrients. 2018;10(5) https://doi.org/10.3390/nu10050601.
45. Peña-Rosas JP, De-Regil LM, Garcia-Casal MN, Dowswell T. Daily oral iron supplementation during pregnancy. Cochrane Database Syst Rev. 2015;2015(7) https://doi.org/10.1002/14651858.CD004736.pub5.
46. Abou-Nassar K, Carrier M, Ramsay T, Rodger MA. The association between antiphospholipid antibodies and placenta mediated complications: a systematic review and meta-analysis. Thromb

Res. 2011;128(1) https://doi.org/10.1016/j.thromres.2011.02.006.
47. Andreoli L, Bertsias GK, Agmon-Levin N, et al. EULAR recommendations for women's health and the management of family planning, assisted reproduction, pregnancy and menopause in patients with systemic lupus erythematosus and/or antiphospholipid syndrome. Ann Rheum Dis. 2017;76(3) https://doi.org/10.1136/annrheumdis-2016-209770.
48. Cohen-Sela E, Brener A, Raviv O, et al. Outcomes in maternal Graves' disease: a population-based mother–infant dyad cohort study. Thyroid. 2024;34(1) https://doi.org/10.1089/thy.2023.0291.
49. Smyth A, Oliveira GHM, Lahr BD, Bailey KR, Norby SM, Garovic VD. A systematic review and meta-analysis of pregnancy outcomes in patients with systemic lupus erythematosus and lupus nephritis. Clin J Am Soc Nephrol. 2010;5(11) https://doi.org/10.2215/CJN.00240110.
50. Clowse MEB. Lupus activity in pregnancy. Rheum Dis Clin North Am. 2007;33(2) https://doi.org/10.1016/j.rdc.2007.01.002.
51. Saavedra MA, Cruz-Reyes C, Vera-Lastra O, et al. Impact of previous lupus nephritis on maternal and fetal outcomes during pregnancy. Clin Rheumatol. 2012;31(5) https://doi.org/10.1007/s10067-012-1941-4.
52. Clowse MEB, Magder L, Witter F, Petri M. Hydroxychloroquine in lupus pregnancy. Arthritis Rheum. 2006;54:11. https://doi.org/10.1002/art.22159.
53. Levy RA, Vilela VS, Cataldo MJ, et al. Hydroxychloroquine (HCQ) in lupus pregnancy: double-blind and placebo-controlled study. Lupus. 2001;10(6) https://doi.org/10.1191/096120301678646137.
54. Silver R, Craigo S, Porter F, Osmundson SS, Kuller JA, Norton ME. Society for Maternal-Fetal Medicine Consult Series #64: systemic lupus erythematosus in pregnancy. Am J Obstet Gynecol. 2023;228(3) https://doi.org/10.1016/j.ajog.2022.09.001.
55. Seo MR, Chae J, Kim YM, et al. Hydroxychloroquine treatment during pregnancy in lupus patients is associated with lower risk of preeclampsia. Lupus. 2019;28(6) https://doi.org/10.1177/0961203319843343.
56. McNeil HP. Immunology and clinical importance of antiphospholipid antibodies. Adv Immunol. 1991:49. https://doi.org/10.1016/s0065-2776(08)60777-4.
57. Xu J, Chen D, Tian Y, Wang X, Peng B. Antiphospholipid antibodies increase the risk of fetal growth restriction: a systematic meta-analysis. Int J Clin Pract. 2022;2022 https://doi.org/10.1155/2022/4308470.
58. Chakravarty EF, Nelson L, Krishnan E. Obstetric hospitalizations in the United States for women with systemic lupus erythematosus and rheumatoid arthritis. Arthritis Rheum. 2006;54(3) https://doi.org/10.1002/art.21663.
59. Hellgren K, Secher AE, Glintborg B, et al. Pregnancy outcomes in relation to disease activity and anti-rheumatic treatment strategies in women with rheumatoid arthritis: a matched cohort study from Sweden and Denmark. Rheumatology (United Kingdom). 2022;61(9) https://doi.org/10.1093/rheumatology/keab894.
60. Abalos E, Duley L, Steyn DW, Gialdini C. Antihypertensive drug therapy for mild to moderate hypertension during pregnancy. Cochrane Database Syst Rev. 2018;2018(10) https://doi.org/10.1002/14651858.CD002252.pub4.
61. Magee LA, von Dadelszen P, Rey E, et al. Less-tight versus tight control of hypertension in pregnancy. N Engl J Med. 2015;372(5) https://doi.org/10.1056/nejmoa1404595.
62. Tita AT, Szychowski JM, Boggess K, et al. Treatment for mild chronic hypertension during pregnancy. N Engl J Med. 2022;386(19) https://doi.org/10.1056/nejmoa2201295.
63. Lampl M, Jeanty P. Exposure to maternal diabetes is associated with altered fetal growth patterns: a hypothesis regarding metabolic allocation to growth under hyperglycemic-hypoxemic conditions. Am J Hum Biol. 2004;16(3) https://doi.org/10.1002/ajhb.20015.
64. Klemetti MM, Laivuori H, Tikkanen M, Nuutila M, Hiilesmaa V, Teramo K. White's classification and pregnancy outcome in women with type 1 diabetes: a population-based cohort study. Diabetologia. 2016;59(1) https://doi.org/10.1007/s00125-015-3787-1.
65. Chen YH, Chiou HY, Lin HC, Lin HL. Affect of seizures during gestation on pregnancy outcomes in women with epilepsy. Arch Neurol. 2009;66(8) https://doi.org/10.1001/archneurol.2009.142.
66. Kilic D, Pedersen H, Kjaersgaard MIS, et al. Birth outcomes after prenatal exposure to antiepileptic drugs – a population-based study. Epilepsia. 2014;55(11) https://doi.org/10.1111/epi.12758.
67. Tomson T, Battino D, Bromley R, et al. Management of epilepsy in pregnancy: a report from the International League Against Epilepsy Task Force on Women and Pregnancy. Epilept Disord. 2019;21(6) https://doi.org/10.1684/epd.2019.1105.
68. Maulik D. Fetal growth restriction: the etiology. Clin Obstet Gynecol. 2006;49(2) https://doi.org/10.1097/00003081-200606000-00006.
69. Hampton MM. Congenital toxoplasmosis: a review. Neonatal Netw. 2015;34:5. https://doi.org/10.1891/0730-0832.34.5.274.
70. Shulman CE, Marshall T, Dorman EK, et al. Malaria in pregnancy: adverse effects on haemoglobin levels and birthweight in primigravidae and multigravidae. Trop Med Int Health.

2001;6(10) https://doi.org/10.1046/j.1365-3156.2001.00786.x.
71. Cortina-Borja M, Tan HK, Wallon M, et al. Prenatal treatment for serious neurological sequelae of congenital toxoplasmosis: an observational prospective cohort study. PLoS Med. 2010;7(10) https://doi.org/10.1371/journal.pmed.1000351.
72. Mandelbrot L, Kieffer F, Sitta R, et al. Prenatal therapy with pyrimethamine + sulfadiazine vs spiramycin to reduce placental transmission of toxoplasmosis: a multicenter, randomized trial. Am J Obstet Gynecol. 2018;219(4) https://doi.org/10.1016/j.ajog.2018.05.031.
73. Effectiveness of prenatal treatment for congenital toxoplasmosis: a meta-analysis of individual patients' data. Lancet. 2007;369(9556) https://doi.org/10.1016/S0140-6736(07)60072-5.
74. D'Antonio F, Marinceu D, Prasad S, Khalil A. Effectiveness and safety of prenatal valacyclovir for congenital cytomegalovirus infection: systematic review and meta-analysis. Ultrasound Obstet Gynecol. 2023;61(4) https://doi.org/10.1002/uog.26136.
75. Pijnenborg R, Bland JM, Robertson WB, Brosens I. Uteroplacental arterial changes related to interstitial trophoblast migration in early human pregnancy. Placenta. 1983;4(4) https://doi.org/10.1016/S0143-4004(83)80043-5.
76. Khong TY, De Wolf F, Robertson WB, Brosens I. Inadequate maternal vascular response to placentation in pregnancies complicated by preeclampsia and by small-for-gestational age infants. BJOG. 1986;93(10) https://doi.org/10.1111/j.1471-0528.1986.tb07830.x.
77. Taubert D, Berkels R, Grosser N, Schröder H, Gründemann D, Schömig E. Aspirin induces nitric oxide release from vascular endothelium: a novel mechanism of action. Br J Pharmacol. 2004;143(1) https://doi.org/10.1038/sj.bjp.0705907.
78. Grosser N, Abate A, Oberle S, et al. Heme oxygenase-1 induction may explain the antioxidant profile of aspirin. Biochem Biophys Res Commun. 2003;308(4) https://doi.org/10.1016/S0006-291X(03)01504-3.
79. Roberge S, Nicolaides K, Demers S, Hyett J, Chaillet N, Bujold E. The role of aspirin dose on the prevention of preeclampsia and fetal growth restriction: systematic review and meta-analysis. Am J Obstet Gynecol. 2017;216 https://doi.org/10.1016/j.ajog.2016.09.076.
80. Meher S, Duley L, Hunter K, Askie L. Antiplatelet therapy before or after 16 weeks' gestation for preventing preeclampsia: an individual participant data meta-analysis. Am J Obstet Gynecol. 2017;216(2) https://doi.org/10.1016/j.ajog.2016.10.016.
81. Ayala DE, Ucieda R, Hermida RC. Chronotherapy with low-dose aspirin for prevention of complications in pregnancy. Chronobiol Int. 2013;(1–2):30. https://doi.org/10.3109/07420528.2012.717455.
82. Rolnik DL, Wright D, Poon LC, et al. Aspirin versus placebo in pregnancies at high risk for preterm preeclampsia. N Engl J Med. 2017;377(7):613–22. https://doi.org/10.1056/NEJMOA1704559.
83. Crovetto F, Crispi F, Scazzocchio E, et al. First-trimester screening for early and late small-for-gestational-age neonates using maternal serum biochemistry, blood pressure and uterine artery Doppler. Ultrasound Obstet Gynecol. 2014;43(1) https://doi.org/10.1002/uog.12537.
84. McCowan LME, Thompson JMD, Taylor RS, et al. Prediction of small for gestational age infants in healthy nulliparous women using clinical and ultrasound risk factors combined with early pregnancy biomarkers. PLoS One. 2017;12(1) https://doi.org/10.1371/journal.pone.0169311.
85. Sobel ML, Kingdom J, Drewlo S. Angiogenic response of placental villi to heparin. Obstet Gynecol. 2011;117(6) https://doi.org/10.1097/AOG.0b013e31821b5384.
86. McLaughlin K, Baczyk D, Potts A, Hladunewich M, Parker JD, Kingdom JCP. Low molecular weight heparin improves endothelial function in pregnant women at high risk of preeclampsia. Hypertension. 2017;69(1) https://doi.org/10.1161/HYPERTENSIONAHA.116.08298.
87. Bose P, Black S, Kadyrov M, et al. Adverse effects of lupus anticoagulant positive blood sera on placental viability can be prevented by heparin in vitro. Am J Obstet Gynecol. 2004;191(6) https://doi.org/10.1016/j.ajog.2004.05.014.
88. Yinon Y, Ben Meir E, Margolis L, et al. Low molecular weight heparin therapy during pregnancy is associated with elevated circulatory levels of placental growth factor. Placenta. 2015;36(2) https://doi.org/10.1016/j.placenta.2014.12.008.
89. Groom KM, McCowan L, Mackay L, et al. Enoxaparin for the prevention of preeclampsia and intrauterine growth restriction in women with a history: a randomized trial. Am J Obstet Gynecol. 2017;216 https://doi.org/10.1016/j.ajog.2017.01.014.
90. Rodger MA, Carrier M, Le Gal G, et al. Meta-analysis of low-molecular-weight heparin to prevent recurrent placenta-mediated pregnancy complications. Blood. 2014;123(6) https://doi.org/10.1182/blood-2013-01-478958.
91. Rodger MA, Gris JC, de Vries JIP, et al. Low-molecular-weight heparin and recurrent placenta-mediated pregnancy complications: a meta-analysis of individual patient data from randomised controlled trials. Lancet. 2016;388(10060) https://doi.org/10.1016/S0140--6736(16)31139-4.

92. Cruz-Lemini M, Vázquez JC, Ullmo J, Llurba E. Low-molecular-weight heparin for prevention of preeclampsia and other placenta-mediated complications: a systematic review and meta-analysis. Am J Obstet Gynecol. 2022;226(2) https://doi.org/10.1016/j.ajog.2020.11.006.
93. Bauer AJ, Banek CT, Needham K, et al. Pravastatin attenuates hypertension, oxidative stress, and angiogenic imbalance in rat model of placental ischemia-induced hypertension. Hypertension. 2013;61(5) https://doi.org/10.1161/HYPERTENSIONAHA.111.00226.
94. Wang K, Ahmad S, Cai M, et al. Dysregulation of hydrogen sulfide producing enzyme cystathionine γ-lyase contributes to maternal hypertension and placental abnormalities in preeclampsia. Circulation. 2013;127(25) https://doi.org/10.1161/CIRCULATIONAHA.113.001631.
95. Kumasawa K, Ikawa M, Kidoya H, et al. Pravastatin induces placental growth factor (PGF) and ameliorates preeclampsia in a mouse model. Proc Natl Acad Sci USA. 2011;108(4) https://doi.org/10.1073/pnas.1011293108.
96. Ahmed A, Williams DJ, Cheed V, et al. Pravastatin for early-onset preeclampsia: a randomised, blinded, placebo-controlled trial. BJOG. 2020;127(4) https://doi.org/10.1111/1471-0528.16013.
97. Costantine MM, Cleary K, Hebert MF, et al. Safety and pharmacokinetics of pravastatin used for the prevention of preeclampsia in high-risk pregnant women: a pilot randomized controlled trial. Am J Obstet Gynecol. 2016;214(6) https://doi.org/10.1016/j.ajog.2015.12.038.
98. Meijerink L, Wever KE, Terstappen F, Ganzevoort W, Lely AT, Depmann M. Statins in preeclampsia or fetal growth restriction: a systematic review and meta-analysis on maternal blood pressure and fetal growth across species. BJOG. 2023;130(6) https://doi.org/10.1111/1471-0528.17393.
99. Onda K, Tong S, Beard S, et al. Proton pump inhibitors decrease soluble fms-like tyrosine kinase-1 and soluble endoglin secretion, decrease hypertension, and rescue endothelial dysfunction. Hypertension. 2017;69(3) https://doi.org/10.1161/HYPERTENSIONAHA.116.08408.
100. Thaler I, Amit A, Kamil D, Itskovitz-Eldor J. The effect of isosorbide dinitrate on placental blood flow and maternal blood pressure in women with pregnancy induced hypertension. Am J Hypertens. 1999;12(4 I) https://doi.org/10.1016/S0895-7061(98)00249-0.
101. El-Sayed MA, Saleh SAA, Maher MA, Khidre AM. Utero-placental perfusion Doppler indices in growth restricted fetuses: effect of sildenafil citrate. J Matern Fetal Neonatal Med. 2018;31(8) https://doi.org/10.1080/14767058.2017.1306509.
102. Pels A, Derks J, Elvan-Taspinar A, et al. Maternal sildenafil vs placebo in pregnant women with severe early-onset fetal growth restriction: a randomized clinical trial. JAMA Netw Open. 2020;3(6) https://doi.org/10.1001/jamanetworkopen.2020.5323.
103. Rakhanova Y, Almawi WY, Aimagambetova G, Riethmacher D. The effects of sildenafil citrate on intrauterine growth restriction: a systematic review and meta-analysis. BMC Pregnancy Childbirth. 2023;23(1) https://doi.org/10.1186/s12884-023-05747-7.
104. Giouleka S, Tsakiridis I, Mamopoulos A, Kalogiannidis I, Athanasiadis A, Dagklis T. Fetal growth restriction: a comprehensive review of major guidelines. Obstet Gynecol Surv. 2023;78(11) https://doi.org/10.1097/OGX.0000000000001203.
105. Rey E, Garneau P, David M, et al. Dalteparin for the prevention of recurrence of placental-mediated complications of pregnancy in women without thrombophilia: a pilot randomized controlled trial. J Thromb Haemost. 2009;7(1) https://doi.org/10.1111/j.1538-7836.2008.03230.x.
106. Gris JC, Chauleur C, Faillie JL, et al. Enoxaparin for the secondary prevention of placental vascular complications in women with abruptio placentae: the pilot randomised controlled NOH-AP trial. Thromb Haemost. 2010;104(4) https://doi.org/10.1160/TH10-03-0167.
107. Martinelli I, Ruggenenti P, Cetin I, et al. Heparin in pregnant women with previous placenta-mediated pregnancy complications: a prospective, randomized, multicenter, controlled clinical trial. Blood. 2012;119(14) https://doi.org/10.1182/blood-2011-11-391383.
108. Demers S, Bujold E, Roberge S. Enoxaparin and aspirin compared with aspirin alone to prevent placenta-mediated pregnancy complications: a randomized controlled trial. Obstet Gynecol. 2017;129(2) https://doi.org/10.1097/AOG.0000000000001882.

Prevention of Obesity and Excessive Gestational Weight Gain in Pregnancy

Itamar Gilboa and Yariv Yogev

Contents

Y. Yogev, A. Khalil (eds.), *Prevention of Complications in Obstetrics*,
https://doi.org/10.1007/978-3-032-23479-7_16

Learning Objectives
- Understand maternal and fetal risks associated with obesity and excessive GWG.
- Describe evidence-based lifestyle, pharmacologic, and surgical strategies before and during pregnancy.
- Explain IOM GWG guidance and emerging data challenging recommendations for higher obesity classes.
- Recognize safety considerations for anti-obesity medications and metformin use.
- Identify intergenerational metabolic impacts and long-term outcomes linked to maternal obesity.

16.1 Introduction

Obesity is a significant global health issue characterized by excessive fat accumulation that poses serious risks to health. It is associated with numerous comorbidities, including cardiovascular diseases, diabetes, and certain types of cancer, which can lead to increased morbidity and mortality [1]. The prevalence of obesity is rising worldwide, affecting individuals across all age groups, including women of reproductive age [1, 2]. This demographic is particularly concerning due to the implications of obesity on fertility, pregnancy, and long-term health outcomes for both mother and child [2, 3].

In the context of pregnancy, obesity presents unique challenges and risks. Maternal obesity is linked to an increased risk of fertility complications, gestational diabetes mellitus (GDM), hypertensive disorders such as preeclampsia, and a higher likelihood of cesarean delivery (CD), labor, and postpartum complications. For the fetus, maternal obesity is associated with a higher risk of congenital anomalies, macrosomia, and stillbirth. In the long term, children born to obese mothers are at a higher risk of developing obesity and metabolic disorders themselves. This intergenerational transmission of obesity can be influenced by genetic, environmental, and lifestyle factors [2–4].

Pregnancy is recognized as a teachable moment, encouraging women to adopt healthier lifestyle behaviors that lead to positive outcomes. It serves as an ideal time to promote healthy habits not only among expectant mothers but also for their children, partners, and extended family [5]. To achieve the best possible results for both mother and newborn, a collaborative approach involving obstetricians, nutritionists, and other healthcare professionals is essential. This chapter will outline the complications related to obesity during pregnancy and explore management strategies during both the preconception period and pregnancy, highlighting the significance and potential risks associated with this condition.

16.2 Epidemiology

The World Health Organization (WHO) estimated in the year 2022 that as many as 890 million people worldwide were clinically overweight, with as many as 16% of adults classified as obese [6]. To classify individuals as underweight, normal weight, overweight, or obese, the body mass index (BMI) is utilized. This index is determined by dividing an individual's weight in kilograms by their height in meters squared. In the case of nonpregnant adults, a BMI of 25 kg/m^2 or more indicates overweight, and a BMI of 30 kg/m^2 or more indicates obesity. Obesity is further characterized by BMI into class I (30–34.9), class II (35–39.9), and class III (greater than 40) [7].

Nevertheless, this classification does not consider personal differences in body frame and lean mass, nor does it examine the distribution of fat, which is significant since visceral fat poses more metabolic risks compared to subcutaneous fat [8].

Over the past few decades, the prevalence of obesity has risen significantly among women of reproductive age in the United States [2]. However, according to the National Center for Health Statistics (NCHS), the most recent report indicated that from 2013–2014 to August 2023, the age-adjusted prevalence of obesity among adults did not show significant changes, with the obesity rate among women aged 20–39 years reported at 36.8% [9].

16.3 Antepartum Complications

16.3.1 Fertility and Reproduction

Obese women generally experience more menstrual irregularities and are less likely to conceive within a year after stopping contraception compared to women of normal weight [10]. Overweight and obesity are commonly linked to ovulatory dysfunction, posing a three-fold higher risk of anovulatory infertility compared to those with a normal BMI [11]. Various mechanisms have been proposed to explain how obesity contributes to ovulatory dysfunction [12–17].

Obesity also impacts the success rates of assisted reproductive technology (ART) and in vitro fertilization (IVF) through multiple pathways. Obese women often show lower responsiveness to ovulation induction and ovarian stimulation medications [18, 19] and have poorer outcomes in terms of oocyte and embryo quality and cycle success [20]. Obesity is associated with altered follicular molecular content and changes in granulosa cells, indicating multiple mechanisms may impede oocyte development [21–23]. Additionally, obesity is believed to adversely affect endometrial receptivity [24]. Although studies using donor oocytes found no significant differences in outcomes [25], research on third-party surrogates showed that women with higher BMI had lower live birth rates [26].

16.3.2 Miscarriages

The role of obesity in miscarriage and pregnancy loss remains a subject of debate. While some studies have not identified obesity as a significant risk factor for pregnancy loss [27, 28], others have shown a marked association between obesity and increased rates of miscarriage [24, 29, 30]. Notably, a meta-analysis of 33 IVF studies indicated that overweight or obese women experienced a higher miscarriage rate compared to women of normal weight, with a relative risk (RR) of 1.31 ($p < 0.001$) [31].

16.3.3 Gestational Diabetes Mellitus

According to the Centers for Disease Control and Prevention (CDC), rates of gestational diabetes mellitus (GDM) rose by 30% between 2016 and 2020, reaching 7.8 cases per 100 women [32]. Various factors contribute to the risk of GDM, including ethnicity and obstetrical and family history [33, 34]. However, the link between obesity and the risk of developing gestational diabetes is well documented, with numerous studies indicating that obesity raises the risk of GDM by 2–5 times [35–38].

In 2009, the Institute of Medicine (IOM) issued guidelines for managing and preventing GDM, particularly with regard to gestational weight gain (GWG). The IOM advises that women adhere to specific weight gain targets during pregnancy based on their prepregnancy body mass index (BMI) to lower the risk of GDM and other complications [39].

Further studies examining the influence of early gestational weight gain on the likelihood of developing GDM have found that excessive GWG is a significant risk factor for GDM [40–42].

Several mechanisms contribute to the relationship between obesity, excessive GWG, and GDM. These conditions are linked to chronic low-grade inflammation and elevated levels of circulating free fatty acids, which promote insulin resistance. This insulin resistance is further exacerbated during pregnancy due to the hormonal changes that occur, such as increased levels of placental hormones like human placental lactogen, which counteract insulin action [35, 43].

16.3.4 Hypertensive Disorders

Several studies have found increased risk in obese women with hypertensive disorders of pregnancy (HDP), including preeclampsia [38, 44–46]. In a recent large population-based cohort study of 14.0 million women, Bicocca et al. found that the risk of early-onset and late-onset hypertensive disorders of pregnancy is significantly and progressively increased with higher classes of obesity. According to O'brien et al., the risk of preeclampsia doubles for every increase of 5–7 in the BMI [47]. A recent meta-analysis and Mendelian randomization study revealed that maternal obesity significantly increases the risk of gestational hypertension and preeclampsia, with odds ratios (OR) of 1.98 (95% CI: 1.83–2.15) and 3.77 (95% CI: 3.45–4.13), respectively [45].

It is thought that the pathogenesis of HDP and preeclampsia in obesity involve several key mechanisms, which include a chronic inflammatory state with elevated levels of pro-inflammatory cytokines and adipokines, which further exacerbate placental dysfunction and promote the expression of anti-angiogenic factors [48, 49]. In addition, metabolic abnormalities associated with obesity, including hyperinsulinemia, insulin resistance, and dyslipidemia, contribute to oxidative stress and endothelial dysfunction, further increasing the risk of preeclampsia [49].

16.4 Fetal Complications

16.4.1 Birth Defects

Maternal obesity is associated with increased risk for congenital anomalies with a dose-response relationship, primarily heart and neural tube defects [50–52]. For neural tube defects, the associations meet three criteria for causality, which indicates a moderate level of uncertainty about the link, while for congenital heart defects, the associations potentially meet only two criteria, pointing to a lower level of certainty regarding the associations [53].

16.4.2 Preterm Delivery

The relationship between preterm birth and obesity remains a subject of debate [35, 54–56]. A meta-analysis and systematic review by Torloni et al. found that overweight and class I obese women had a lower risk of preterm birth, with odds ratios (OR) of 0.85 (95% CI: 0.80–0.92) and 0.83 (95% CI: 0.75–0.92), respectively. Conversely, women classified as class II and III obese exhibited a higher risk of preterm birth, with ORs of 1.30 (95% CI: 1.12–1.57) and 2.27 (95% CI: 1.76–2.94), respectively [57]. However, another systematic review and meta-analysis indicated that both overweight and obesity were significant risk factors for preterm birth [55].

In a large population cohort study, Liu et al. reported that maternal prepregnancy obesity was associated with an increased risk of preterm birth across various maternal age groups and racial/ethnic backgrounds [56]. Additionally, Liu et al. found that maternal prepregnancy obesity was significantly linked to all phenotypes of preterm birth, with the highest association observed for extremely preterm birth (OR 3.4, 95% CI: 1.07–10.97) [58].

The effects of excessive gestational weight gain also remain contentious. While Goldstein et al. demonstrated that excessive weight gain is associated with a lower risk of preterm delivery (OR 0.77, 95% CI: 0.69–0.86) [59], Liu et al. reported a contrary relationship, indicating that excessive gestational weight gain is linked to an increased risk of preterm birth (OR 2.51, 95% CI: 1.83–3.45) [60].

16.4.3 Post-term Pregnancy

Several studies have explored the relationship between obesity and post-term pregnancy. A systematic review and meta-analysis by Heslehurst et al. found a nonlinear association between maternal BMI and post-term birth (≥42 weeks), with increasing odds ratios for obesity classes I-III (OR 1.42, 95% CI 1.27–1.58), (OR 1.55, 95% CI 1.37–1.75), and (OR 1.65, 95% CI 1.44–1.87), respectively [61]. Additionally, Akselsson et al. confirmed in a study of 64,632 women that overweight and obese women had a higher risk of prolonged pregnancy (≥42 weeks) compared to normal weight women [62].

The relationship between excessive GWG and post-term pregnancy is debated. Some studies found that excessive GWG increased the odds of prolonged pregnancy [63], while others, like Zhu et al., reported that higher GWG z scores were associated with a decreased risk of post-term birth, with OR 0.84 (95% CI 0.83–0.85) and OR 0.59 (95% CI 0.58–0.60) for the third and fourth quartiles of GWG, respectively [64].

Overall, these findings underline the increased risk of post-term pregnancy linked to higher maternal BMI, raising important questions about the optimal timing for labor induction in this population.

16.4.4 Stillbirth and Intrauterine Fetal Demise

Obesity poses a major risk factor for stillbirth [37, 38, 65]. Auene et al. showed in their meta-analysis that even after excluding participants with conditions like pregestational diabetes and hypertension, the relative risk (RR) remained significant at 1.57 per 5 BMI units [65]. Other factors may also impact these outcomes, such as the difficulty in perceiving fetal movements, particularly in cases of severe obesity [66], as well as post-term pregnancy [62, 67] and the presence of congenital anomalies [68].

Excessive GWG is also associated with an increased risk of stillbirth, particularly among obese women and morbidly obese women [69, 70]. Yao et al. found that excessive weight gain was associated with a higher risk of stillbirth among obese and morbidly obese women (hazard ratio [HR] 2.00 (95% CI 1.55–2.58) for obese and HR 3.16 (95% CI 2.17–4.62) for morbidly obese) [69].

16.4.5 Fetal Overgrowth

Obesity and excessive GWG were previously linked in several studies as risk factors for macrosomia and large for gestational age [59, 71–73]. Gaudet et al. performed a systematic review and meta-analysis that demonstrated maternal obesity is associated with fetal overgrowth. The ORs for birth weight ≥4000 g, ≥4500 g, and ≥90th percentile for gestational age were 2.17 (95% CI 1.92–2.45), 2.77 (95% CI 2.22–3.45), and 2.42 (95% CI 2.16–2.72), respectively [72].

Goldstein et al. conducted a systematic review and meta-analysis that included over 1.3 million women. The study found that GWG above the Institute of Medicine (IOM) guidelines was associated with a higher risk of LGA (OR 1.85, 95% CI 1.76–1.95) and macrosomia (OR 1.95, 95% CI 1.79–2.11) [59]. In addition, excessive GWG greater than the IOM guidelines was previously related to increased neonatal adiposity in normal weight women [74].

16.5 Labor, Delivery, and Postpartum Conditions

16.5.1 Anesthesia in Obese Women

Obesity significantly increases the risk of anesthesia complications in obstetrics. It is linked to several comorbidities, including sleep apnea, hypertension, coronary artery disease, pulmonary hypertension, diabetes mellitus, and various other conditions that can complicate anesthesia management [75]. The risk for an epidural failure is significantly greater in obese women [76]. Furthermore, airway management is particularly challenging in obese patients due to anatomical changes and increased risk of difficult or failed intubation [77]. Therefore, the American College of Obstetricians and Gynecologists (ACOG) advises an anesthesia consultation for obese women before labor and for early labor epidural catheter placement [2].

16.5.2 Cesarean Delivery

Compared to women of normal weight, women with obesity bear an elevated risk for cesarean delivery (CD) [78, 79] with a relatively higher prevalence of maternal morbidity following CD in women with obesity [80, 81]. Consequently, Gabbai et al. have developed a predictive model for intrapartum CD among obese women in order to identify those at high risk, showing that the risk increases with higher body mass index (BMI) [82].

A meta-analysis by Su et al. found that women with GWG above the 2009 IOM guidelines had higher odds of CD across all classes of obesity, with ORs of 1.27 (95% CI 1.20–1.33) for obesity class I, OR 1.22 (95% CI 1.20–1.23) for class II, and OR 1.17 (95% CI 1.15–1.19) for class III [83].

16.5.3 Shoulder Dystocia

Obesity has been linked as a risk factor for shoulder dystocia. A meta-analysis by Zhang et al. indicated that maternal prepregnancy obesity significantly raises the risk of shoulder dystocia, revealing a pooled RR of 1.63 (95% CI 1.33–1.99) when comparing obese to non-obese women. This elevated risk is consistent across various obesity classes, with the highest risks seen in the more severe obesity categories [84]. Cheedalla et al. further noted that higher maternal BMI correlates with an increased number of maneuvers required to address shoulder dystocia, which may lead to greater neonatal morbidity [85]. The elevated risk was also linked to excessive GWG. Kominiarek et al. found that GWG exceeding the IOM guidelines was associated with a higher risk of shoulder dystocia [86].

One proposed mechanism for these complications is the increase in soft tissue within the pelvis, which narrows the birth canal and complicates delivery, particularly for larger infants, which in turn increases the risk for shoulder dystocia [78].

16.5.4 Postpartum Hemorrhage

Postpartum hemorrhage (PPH) is another obstetric complication linked to obesity. Blomberg found that the risk of atonic uterine hemorrhage rises with increasing BMI [87]. Women with a BMI of 40 or higher faced a significantly elevated risk of PPH after normal delivery (OR 1.23, 95% CI 1.04–1.45) and an even greater risk following instrumental delivery (OR 1.69, 95% CI 1.22–2.34). A recent systematic review and meta-analysis also indicated that the risk of PPH is heightened for overweight and obese women, with an OR of 1.67 (95% CI 1.42–1.96) for overweight women and 1.88 (95% CI 1.55–2.29) for obese women [88].

It is possible that the increased volume of distribution for uterotonics in obese women, along with the challenges in identifying the fundus and performing bimanual massage, likely contribute to the heightened risk of postpartum hemorrhage [89]

16.5.5 Infection

Maternal obesity is associated with a higher risk of postpartum infections. Axelsson et al. identified a dose-dependent relationship between rising maternal BMI and an increased likelihood of postpartum infections. Specifically, women in obesity classes II and III faced an elevated risk for endometritis following normal vaginal delivery, OR 1.45 (95% CI 1.29–1.63), and for wound infections after cesarean delivery, OR 3.83 (95% CI 3.39–4.32) [90]. Additionally, another study found that obese women had a twofold increased risk of postpartum sepsis compared to women of normal weight [91].

However, excessive weight gain beyond the IOM guidelines does not seem to be a risk factor for postpartum infection. Kawakita and Covello conducted a retrospective study involving 2376 obese women who underwent cesarean delivery, categorizing them based on whether their gestational weight gain was below, within, or above the IOM guidelines. The study found no significant differences in the rates of surgical site infections among these groups [92].

16.5.6 Thromboembolic Complications

A recent systematic review and meta-analysis revealed a positive association between BMI and the risk of venous thromboembolism (VTE), indicating that obese patients have a hazard ratio (HR) of 1.62 (95% CI: 1.29–2.04) compared to those with a normal BMI [93]. Additionally, Butwick et al. found that the prevalence of antepartum and postpartum VTE increases with higher BMI. Specifically, the risk of antepartum VTE in women classified as obesity class III (BMI $\geq$ 40) was found to be 2.9 (95% CI: 2.2–3.8) compared to women with normal BMI, while the odds ratio (OR) for postpartum VTE was 3.6 (95% CI: 2.9–4.6) [94].

Furthermore, a retrospective study of 196 women with VTE assessed the relationship between maternal weight gain during pregnancy and the risk of VTE. The findings indicated that greater total weight gain elevates the risks of pulmonary embolism (PE) and VTE, particularly among underweight and normal weight women [95].

16.6 Long-Term Complications

Obesity and excessive GWG during pregnancy are linked to various long-term health outcomes for mothers. Specifically, maternal obesity increases the risk of cardiovascular events and premature mortality [96, 97]. Both obesity and excessive GWG contribute to greater postpartum weight retention, leading to long-term obesity and related health issues [97, 98]. Catalano and Shankar also noted that weight retention after childbirth raises future cardio-metabolic risks and the likelihood of prepregnancy obesity in subsequent pregnancies [97]. Furthermore, women with excessive GWG are at an increased risk of developing type 2 diabetes later in life [98], as some have linked excessive GWG to higher levels of abdominal fat and waist circumference, both of which are significant risk factors for cardio-metabolic diseases. [99].

Addressing the psychosocial aspects of obesity is also crucial, particularly the roles of depression and anxiety, which are associated with obesity before and after pregnancy [100, 101]. Additionally, an individual's perception of their ability to engage in healthy eating and goal-oriented behaviors, despite challenges, is inversely related to body weight in both early pregnancy and two years postpartum [102].

16.6.1 Offspring Susceptibility to Obesity and Metabolic Syndrome

Obesity is associated with metabolic and endocrine disruptions influenced by genetic, epigenetic, and lifestyle factors that impact weight gain, adiposity, and metabolism. Several studies have identified mechanisms associating maternal obesity with increased adiposity and metabolic issues in offspring, suggesting that dietary changes or exposure to obesity-related metabolites during critical developmental phases can lead to greater fat accumulation [103–105].

Maternal obesity and excessive GWG are associated with increased risks of obesity and metabolic dysfunction in offspring. It appears that maternal obesity leads to hypothalamic inflammation and structural damage to the blood-brain barrier (BBB) in the offspring, affecting neurons that regulate food intake and energy expenditure [106].

Boney et al. investigated the association between maternal obesity, GDM, and the development of metabolic syndrome in childhood. The study focused on LGA and appropriate-for-gestational-age (AGA) children, revealing that both LGA status and maternal obesity were correlated with insulin resistance, and LGA children exposed to maternal GDM exhibited a 3.6-fold greater risk of developing metabolic syndrome by age

11. These findings highlight that children of obese or diabetic mothers are at increased risk for obesity and metabolic dysfunction, underscoring the implications for intergenerational health [107].

Excessive GWG plays a role in negatively affecting a child's long-term health and increasing their risk of obesity. Studies indicate that higher GWG correlates with increased offspring risk for obesity, hypertension, hyperglycemia, insulin resistance, and coronary artery disease [108–110].

16.7 Prevention

16.7.1 Prepregnancy

According to the American Association of Clinical Endocrinologists and the American College of Endocrinology, women with obesity or overweight who are planning to conceive should aim for a 10% reduction in body weight before the preconception period [111].

Nevertheless, it is important to note that preconception weight loss has been associated with potential adverse outcomes. Lecorguillé et al. noted that women who lost weight before pregnancy tended to gain more weight during pregnancy, which could offset the benefits of prepregnancy weight loss [112]. In addition, some have suggested that prepregnancy weight loss and a low-protein diet may negatively impact the nutritional status of the mother and therefore impair fetal growth and development [113, 114].

16.7.2 Prepregnancy Lifestyle Weight Loss

Several studies have explored the effects of nonsurgical preconception weight loss on fertility and pregnancy outcomes in women with overweight or obesity. In a randomized trial by Wadden et al., 224 obese adults participated and found that a combination of medication and lifestyle modification resulted in greater weight loss compared to either intervention alone [115].

The Look AHEAD (Action for Health in Diabetes) trial demonstrated that an intensive lifestyle intervention in individuals with type 2 diabetes mellitus led to significant long-term weight loss and improvements in cardiovascular risk factors over four years. Participants in the intensive lifestyle intervention group achieved a mean weight loss of 4.7% compared to 1.1% in the standard care group. This weight loss was associated with lower HbA1c levels, reduced need for diabetes medications, lower blood pressure, improved lipid profiles, and enhanced quality of life [116]. Other small randomized controlled trials indicated that low-energy or low-glycemic-index diets led to more significant BMI reductions than the control group [117, 118], especially when combined with behavioral therapy and psychotherapy [118, 119]. A larger randomized trial involving 577 women assessed the impact of a 6-month lifestyle intervention before 18 months of infertility treatment. The intervention group, consisting of 290 women, did not achieve higher rates of vaginal birth of a healthy singleton at term compared to 287 women assigned to prompt infertility treatment for 24 months, nor did they experience improved pregnancy outcomes [120]. On the other hand, a recent systematic review and meta-analysis of 20 studies examined the link between preconception maternal weight loss and hypertensive disorders in pregnancy. The review found that weight loss from lifestyle interventions and bariatric surgery significantly reduced the incidence of conditions such as hypertensive disorders of pregnancy (OR 0.45, 95% CI 0.32–0.63) and preeclampsia (OR 0.67, 95% CI 0.51–0.88) [121]. Additionally, a randomized controlled trial involving 164 obese women evaluated the impact of a nonsurgical preconception weight loss intervention on pregnancy outcomes among those with a BMI of 30–55 kg/m^2. Women in the very low-energy diet group lost significantly more weight than those in the control group and experienced fewer adverse pregnancy outcomes. However, no differences were observed in fasting glucose levels between 26 and 28 weeks or in singleton live birth rates [122].

16.7.3 Prepregnancy Pharmacological Treatment

Metformin during the preconception period in obese women has been associated with modest weight loss and improved pregnancy outcomes. This drug primarily acts by decreasing hepatic glucose production and improving insulin sensitivity. Several studies have demonstrated that metformin can lead to modest weight reduction in obese women [123–125].

In a multicenter, double-blind, placebo-controlled randomized trial involving 320 women with polycystic ovarian syndrome (PCOS), Morin-Papunen et al. found that metformin significantly improved pregnancy rates and live birth rates compared to placebo, particularly benefiting obese women [124]. In addition, a systematic review and meta-analysis found that metformin use was associated with lower gestational weight gain compared to other treatments [125]. Additionally, metformin has been shown to reduce the risk of preeclampsia in pregnant women with severe obesity [126].

In women with polycystic ovary syndrome (PCOS), metformin has been shown to improve ovulation rates and pregnancy outcomes. The American Society for Reproductive Medicine recommends metformin for ovulation induction in obese women with PCOS, as it can improve pregnancy rates and live birth rates when combined with other treatments [4]. However, it is important to note that metformin should be discontinued prior to conception due to limited safety data during pregnancy. The American Diabetes Association highlights that metformin crosses the placenta, and while it is associated with less maternal weight gain and a lower risk of preeclampsia, it may also lead to smaller neonates and increased postnatal growth [127].

Glucagon-like peptide 1 (GLP-1) receptor agonists (RAs) are Federal Drug Administration (FDA) approved antidiabetic and anti-obesity medications [128]. These medications are classified as pregnancy category C due to their ability to cross the placenta, which has been associated with fetal growth restrictions and congenital abnormalities in animal studies. Therefore, their use during pregnancy is not recommended, and effective contraception is advised while taking these medications [129]. A meta-analysis involving eight randomized controlled trials found that in patients with polycystic ovarian syndrome (PCOS), GLP-1 RAs are more effective than metformin in reducing insulin resistance, BMI, and abdominal circumference [130]. There is limited data available regarding the appropriate timing for discontinuing GLP-1 RAs prior to conception. Further research on pregnancy and neonatal outcomes is needed to determine a safe washout period. Current literature suggests considering a washout period of four weeks before attempting to conceive [131].

16.7.4 Prepregnancy Surgical Treatment

Bariatric surgery is regarded as the most effective treatment for morbid obesity, leading to significantly better weight loss outcomes and improvement in obesity-related comorbidities than nonsurgical methods, regardless of the surgical procedure type employed [132]. Beyond the primary mechanisms of restriction and malabsorption, bariatric surgeries assist with weight loss through several additional pathways: by altering gut hormonal modulation, insulin secretion, bile acid, and microbiome, resulting in significant weight loss [133].

Numerous studies have demonstrated that substantial weight loss achieved through bariatric surgery significantly reduces the rates of adverse maternal and neonatal outcomes [134–137]. A systematic review and meta-analysis found that bariatric surgery reduced risk for GDM (OR 0.20, 95% CI 0.11–0.37), LGA (OR 0.31, 95% CI 0.17–0.59), and gestational hypertension (OR 0.38, 95% CI 0.19–0.76) [135]. Another large retrospective study of more than 20,000 women by Getahun et al. found reduced risk for GDM (OR 0.60, 95% CI 0.53–0.69) and preeclampsia (OR 0.53, 95% CI 0.46–0.61) [134]. Nevertheless, some studies found an association between bariatric surgery and adverse perinatal outcomes such as increased risk for preterm birth and small-for-gestational-age (SGA) infants [135, 138] and, in some, for stillbirth and neonatal death [137, 138]. In addition, bariatric surgery can be accompanied by micronutrient deficiencies and metabolic and endocrine disorders, which all should be addressed and monitored accordingly [139]. These findings underscore the need for careful monitoring and management of pregnancies following bariatric surgery to mitigate potential risks.

16.7.5 Timing of Bariatric Surgery

The timing of bariatric surgery in relation to pregnancy has a significant impact on maternal and neonatal outcomes. Pregnancies occurring within 12 months following bariatric surgery are associated with elevated risks of adverse outcomes due to continued weight loss and potential nutritional deficiencies. Research indicates that early pregnancies (≤12 months post-surgery) are correlated with inadequate gestational weight gain, lower neonatal birth weight, and increased rates of preterm birth [140, 141]. In contrast, pregnancies occurring 12–24 months after bariatric surgery generally exhibit improved outcomes compared to those in the first year. This interval apparently allows for the stabilization of weight and nutritional status, which helps decrease the risks of small-for-gestational-age (SGA) infants and preterm deliveries. Nevertheless, some studies still report heightened risks of SGA infants and neonatal intensive care unit (NICU) admissions within this timeframe [142, 143]. Pregnancies that occur more than 24 months after bariatric surgery tend to show the most favorable outcomes. Longer intervals between surgery and conception are associated with decreased risks of prematurity, NICU admissions, and SGA status. For example, Parent et al. found that intervals of more than four years from surgery to birth were linked to lower risks of prematurity and NICU admissions compared to intervals of less than two years [142].

16.7.6 Antepartum

As previously mentioned, obesity and excessive weight gain are linked to a higher risk of adverse maternal and neonatal outcomes, making interventions during pregnancy crucial for enhancing immediate outcomes for women and their children, as well as having long-term effects.

In 2009, the Institute of Medicine (IOM) revised its guidelines on gestational weight gain, advising that obese women should gain between 5 and 9 kg during pregnancy to support necessary physiological change. Nevertheless, it is important to mention that the IOM guidelines are not stratified for the level of obesity [39]. Catalano et al. reinforced this recommendation, finding that obese women who gained 5 kg or less during pregnancy had neonates with significantly lower birthweight, lean body mass, fat mass, body fat percentage, and length compared to those of overweight and obese women who gained more than 5 kg [144]. However, in addition to previous studies that suggested that minimal weight gain or even weight loss during pregnancy might improve pregnancy outcomes [145, 146], a recent large study by Johansson et al. found that in pregnancies involving class 1 or 2 obesity, achieving gestational weight gain below the lower limit of the IOM recommendations or experiencing weight loss did not increase the risk of adverse composite outcomes. Additionally, in pregnancies classified as class 3 obesity, weight gain below the IOM limit or weight loss was associated with a reduced risk of adverse composite outcomes (RR 0.81, 95% CI: 0.71–0.89). Based on these findings, the authors concluded that the lower limit of current IOM recommendations for pregnant women with obesity should be reconsidered or removed [147].

16.7.7 Antepartum Lifestyle Weight Loss

Lifestyle interventions during pregnancy can be divided into physical activity, dietary, and mixed weight loss. The US Preventive

Services Task Force found that counseling and active behavioral interventions to limit GWG were associated with decreased risks of GDM, emergent CD, macrosomia, and LGA infants [148].

Recent studies emphasize the critical role of lifestyle interventions in managing GWG and improving pregnancy outcomes. A systematic review and meta-analysis demonstrated that antenatal lifestyle interventions, which include dietary changes and physical activity, are linked to a reduction in GWG (−1.15 kg), a lower risk of GDM (OR 0.79, 95% CI 0.70–0.89), and fewer adverse maternal outcomes (OR 0.89, 95% CI 0.84–0.94) compared to routine care [149]. Moreover, a systematic review by Farpour-Lambert et al. showed that lifestyle interventions significantly reduced GWG and improved several pregnancy outcomes, including decreased risks of GDM, pregnancy-induced hypertension, and cesarean delivery [150]. These findings suggest that structured lifestyle interventions can be beneficial in managing GWG and improving maternal and neonatal health. In contrast, large-scale randomized controlled trials (RCTs), such as LIMIT and UPBEAT, reported modest or negligible improvements in pregnancy outcomes despite enhanced maternal diet and physical activity. The LIMIT trial found no significant reduction in the risk of large-for-gestational-age infants or other adverse maternal outcomes, although it did report a decrease in the incidence of infants with a birth weight exceeding 4000 g [151]. Similarly, the UPBEAT trial noted improvements in maternal dietary habits and physical activity but did not achieve a significant impact on the primary outcome of gestational diabetes risk [152]. Catalano et al. highlighted that metabolic alterations occurring in early pregnancy, often before the majority of interventions are implemented, may limit the effectiveness of lifestyle changes initiated later in pregnancy [153]. This finding suggests that initiating lifestyle modifications earlier, potentially even before conception, could yield more favorable pregnancy outcomes. Furthermore, a recent systematic review and Bayesian network meta-analysis comparing various intervention modalities for managing GWG among overweight or obese women included 60 randomized controlled trials, encompassing over 16,000 participants. The interventions were categorized as remote (R), in-person (I), or a combination of both (R+I). The study identified five intervention categories: education (E), physical activity (PA), dietary changes (D), behavior modification (B), and combinations thereof. Notably, the in-person dietary (I-D) intervention was found to be the most effective method for managing GWG in obese pregnancies, while the in-person combined approach (I-PADB) closely followed in effectiveness. However, the authors advise caution in drawing definitive conclusions from these results due to the low quality of the supporting evidence and the lack of direct comparative studies [154].

In conclusion, while structured lifestyle interventions demonstrate promise in managing GWG and improving maternal and neonatal health outcomes, further research is needed to refine these strategies and enhance their efficacy, particularly regarding the optimal timing for interventions.

16.7.8 Antepartum Pharmacological Weight Loss

Pharmacological treatments for managing obesity during pregnancy, such as Orlistat, Topiramate, and Phentermine, are generally not recommended because of potential risks to both maternal and neonatal health. These medications should be avoided during pregnancy, in women who are planning to become pregnant, or while breastfeeding [2, 4, 111].

Metformin has been used to treat gestational diabetes mellitus [155] and has not been associated with an increased incidence of birth defects linked to its use [156]. Research involving women with gestational diabetes has demonstrated that metformin can help reduce gestational weight gain [155, 157]. In light of this, Syngelaki et al. conducted a double-blind, placebo-controlled trial in 2016, enrolling 400 women with a

BMI exceeding 35 kg/m^2. Participants received either 3.0 g of metformin per day or a placebo from 12 to 18 weeks of gestation until delivery. The primary outcome of the study was to assess a reduction in the median neonatal birth weight z-score by 0.3 standard deviations (SD). The authors found that the median GWG was lower in the metformin group than in the placebo group (4.6 kg vs. 6.3, $p < 0.001$) and reduced risk for pre-eclampsia (OR = 0.24, 95% CI 0.10–0.61). Nevertheless, they did not find differences in rates of the primary outcomes with neonatal birth weight z scores of 0.05 in the metformin group and 0.17 in the placebo group [158]. In another large multicenter, randomized, double-blind, placebo-controlled trial, pregnant women between 10 and 20 weeks of gestation with a BMI of 25 kg/m^2 or higher were assigned to receive either metformin or a placebo. The study found no significant difference in the proportion of infants born with a birth weight over 4000 g. However, women who received metformin had a lower average weekly gestational weight gain and were more likely to have GWG below the recommended levels (RR 1.46, 95% CI 1.10–1.94). There were no significant differences between the groups in terms of total gestational weight gain, pregnancy and birth outcomes, maternal diet and physical activity, or maternal quality of life and emotional well-being [159].

16.7.9 Inter-pregnancy Weight Loss

Inter-pregnancy weight loss has several effects on subsequent pregnancy outcomes. A systematic review and meta-analysis by Teulings et al. found that inter-pregnancy weight loss was associated with a lower risk of delivering an LGA neonate [160]. Similarly, Oteng-Ntim et al. reported that inter-pregnancy BMI decrease was associated with a decreased risk of LGA births (OR 0.70, 95% CI 0.55–0.90) [161]. Some have also reported a decreased incidence of LGA in overweight and obese women who had an inter-pregnancy weight loss of only 1–2 BMI units [162, 163]. However, inter-pregnancy weight loss also has potential adverse effects. Oteng-Ntim et al. found that it was associated with an increased risk of SGA infants (OR 1.31, 95% CI 1.06–1.63) [161]. Wallace et al. also reported that weight loss between pregnancies increased the risk of spontaneous preterm delivery and SGA birth [164]. A recent meta-analysis of 11 studies evaluated the effectiveness of lifestyle modification control trials that utilized exercise interventions, with or without dietary intervention, on weight loss among postpartum women. This study found a significant mean weight loss of −2.57 kg (−3.6 to −1.5) in the intervention group. Subgroup analysis indicated that the most effective interventions were those that included objective goals, such as the use of heart rate monitors, pedometers, and exercise combined with intensive dietary intervention, leading to a weight loss of −4.1 kg [165].

Supervised lifestyle interventions during the inter-pregnancy period are effective in reducing the risks of LGA infants and GDM, with mixed effects on SGA infants and preterm birth. These findings underscore the importance of balanced and structured weight management strategies to optimize subsequent pregnancy outcomes [166].

16.8 Conclusion

Obesity and excessive gestational weight gain during pregnancy significantly heighten the risk of adverse maternal and fetal outcomes in both the short and long term. In order to improve outcomes for both mothers and children, effective interventions promoting healthy weight management before, during, and after pregnancy are crucial. By focusing on the psychosocial aspects of obesity and adopting structured lifestyle changes, healthcare providers can better assist women in achieving healthier pregnancies and reducing long-term risks. Ultimately, a comprehensive strategy that includes medical guidance and community support is vital to address the growing prevalence of obesity and its associated health consequences.

Chapter Key Points

- Obesity and excessive GWG increase risks across fertility, pregnancy, delivery, and long-term maternal–offspring health.
- Early lifestyle intervention—including diet, activity, and behavioral support—reduces GWG and improves outcomes.
- IOM GWG targets may be too high for class II–III obesity; minimal gain or loss may be safe.
- Pharmacologic weight loss agents are unsafe in pregnancy; metformin shows selective benefit but no impact on neonatal size.
- Preconception and inter-pregnancy weight reduction improve outcomes but require careful monitoring.
- Bariatric surgery reduces GDM and hypertensive disorders but raises SGA/preterm risks if conception occurs <12 months post-op.

Chapter-End Summary

Obesity and excessive gestational weight gain substantially elevate risks of maternal complications (GDM, hypertensive disorders, cesarean delivery, and PPH), fetal complications (congenital anomalies, stillbirth, and macrosomia), and long-term metabolic disease in mother and child. Effective prevention spans preconception, pregnancy, and inter-pregnancy periods. Lifestyle interventions remain the cornerstone, with modest effects on GWG and metabolic outcomes; early initiation improves efficacy. Pharmacologic agents are generally contraindicated, though metformin can reduce GWG and preeclampsia risk in selected populations. Bariatric surgery offers meaningful risk reduction but requires attention to timing and nutritional surveillance. A comprehensive, multidisciplinary, and individualized approach is essential.

References

1. Obesity and overweight [Internet]. [cited 2024 Dec 8]. Available from: https://www.who.int/en/news-room/fact-sheets/detail/obesity-and-overweight
2. Obesity in pregnancy. ACOG practice bulletin, number 230. Obstet Gynecol. 2021;137(6):e128–44.
3. Yogev Y, Catalano PM. Pregnancy and obesity. Obstet Gynecol Clin North Am. 2009;36(2):285–300. viii
4. Practice Committee of the American Society for Reproductive Medicine. Obesity and reproduction: a committee opinion. Fertil Steril. 2015;104(5):1116–26.
5. Phelan S. Pregnancy: a "teachable moment" for weight control and obesity prevention. Am J Obstet Gynecol. 2010;202(2):135.e1–8.
6. Obesity and overweight [Internet]. [cited 2024 Dec 8]. Available from: https://www.who.int/news-room/fact-sheets/detail/obesity-and-overweight
7. WHO. Obesity: preventing and managing the global epidemic. Report of a WHO consultation. World Health Organ Tech Rep Ser. 2000;894:i–xii. 1
8. Liu J, Fox CS, Hickson DA, May WD, Hairston KG, Carr JJ, et al. Impact of abdominal visceral and subcutaneous adipose tissue on cardiometabolic risk factors: the Jackson Heart Study. J Clin Endocrinol Metab. 2010;95(12):5419–26.
9. Emmerich S, Fryar C, Stierman B, Ogden C. Obesity and severe obesity prevalence in adults: united states, august 2021–august 2023. Atlanta: Centers for Disease Control and Prevention; 2024.
10. Douchi T, Kuwahata R, Yamamoto S, Oki T, Yamasaki H, Nagata Y. Relationship of upper body obesity to menstrual disorders. Acta Obstet Gynecol Scand. 2002;81(2):147–50.
11. Rich-Edwards JW, Goldman MB, Willett WC, Hunter DJ, Stampfer MJ, Colditz GA, et al. Adolescent body mass index and infertility caused by ovulatory disorder. Am J Obstet Gynecol. 1994;171(1):171–7.
12. Pasquali R, Casimirri F, Platè L, Capelli M. Characterization of obese women with reduced sex hormone-binding globulin concentrations. Horm Metab Res. 1990;22(5):303–6.
13. McCartney CR, Blank SK, Prendergast KA, Chhabra S, Eagleson CA, Helm KD, et al. Obesity and sex steroid changes across puberty: evidence for marked hyperandrogenemia in pre- and early pubertal obese girls. J Clin Endocrinol Metab. 2007;92(2):430–6.
14. Agarwal SK, Vogel K, Weitsman SR, Magoffin DA. Leptin antagonizes the insulin-like growth factor-I augmentation of steroidogenesis in gran-

ulosa and theca cells of the human ovary. J Clin Endocrinol Metab. 1999;84(3):1072–6.
15. Greisen S, Ledet T, Møller N, Jørgensen JO, Christiansen JS, Petersen K, et al. Effects of leptin on basal and FSH stimulated steroidogenesis in human granulosa luteal cells. Acta Obstet Gynecol Scand. 2000;79(11):931–5.
16. Jain A, Polotsky AJ, Rochester D, Berga SL, Loucks T, Zeitlian G, et al. Pulsatile luteinizing hormone amplitude and progesterone metabolite excretion are reduced in obese women. J Clin Endocrinol Metab. 2007;92(7):2468–73.
17. Santoro N, Lasley B, McConnell D, Allsworth J, Crawford S, Gold EB, et al. Body size and ethnicity are associated with menstrual cycle alterations in women in the early menopausal transition: the Study of Women's Health across the Nation (SWAN) Daily Hormone Study. J Clin Endocrinol Metab. 2004;89(6):2622–31.
18. Imani B, Eijkemans MJC, te Velde ER, Habbema JDF, Fauser BCJM. A nomogram to predict the probability of live birth after clomiphene citrate induction of ovulation in normogonadotropic oligoamenorrheic infertility. Fertil Steril. 2002;77(1):91–7.
19. Mulders AGMGJ, Laven JSE, Eijkemans MJC, Hughes EG, Fauser BCJM. Patient predictors for outcome of gonadotrophin ovulation induction in women with normogonadotrophic anovulatory infertility: a meta-analysis. Hum Reprod Update. 2003;9(5):429–49.
20. Shah DK, Missmer SA, Berry KF, Racowsky C, Ginsburg ES. Effect of obesity on oocyte and embryo quality in women undergoing in vitro fertilization. Obstet Gynecol. 2011;118(1):63–70.
21. La Vignera S, Condorelli R, Bellanca S, La Rosa B, Mousaví A, Busà B, et al. Obesity is associated with a higher level of pro-inflammatory cytokines in follicular fluid of women undergoing medically assisted procreation (PMA) programs. Eur Rev Med Pharmacol Sci. 2011;15(3):267–73.
22. Bausenwein J, Serke H, Eberle K, Hirrlinger J, Jogschies P, Hmeidan FA, et al. Elevated levels of oxidized low-density lipoprotein and of catalase activity in follicular fluid of obese women. Mol Hum Reprod. 2010;16(2):117–24.
23. Valckx SDM, Arias-Alvarez M, De Pauw I, Fievez V, Vlaeminck B, Fransen E, et al. Fatty acid composition of the follicular fluid of normal weight, overweight and obese women undergoing assisted reproductive treatment: a descriptive cross-sectional study. Reprod Biol Endocrinol. 2014;12:13.
24. Bellver J, Pellicer A, García-Velasco JA, Ballesteros A, Remohí J, Meseguer M. Obesity reduces uterine receptivity: clinical experience from 9,587 first cycles of ovum donation with normal weight donors. Fertil Steril. 2013;100(4):1050–8.
25. Luke B, Brown MB, Stern JE, Missmer SA, Fujimoto VY, Leach R, et al. Female obesity adversely affects assisted reproductive technology (ART) pregnancy and live birth rates. Hum Reprod. 2011;26(1):245–52.
26. DeUgarte DA, DeUgarte CM, Sahakian V. Surrogate obesity negatively impacts pregnancy rates in third-party reproduction. Fertil Steril. 2010;93(3):1008–10.
27. Turner MJ, Fattah C, O'Connor N, Farah N, Kennelly M, Stuart B. Body Mass Index and spontaneous miscarriage. Eur J Obstet Gynecol Reprod Biol. 2010;151(2):168–70.
28. Veleva Z, Tiitinen A, Vilska S, Hydén-Granskog C, Tomás C, Martikainen H, et al. High and low BMI increase the risk of miscarriage after IVF/ICSI and FET. Hum Reprod. 2008;23(4):878–84.
29. Lashen H, Fear K, Sturdee DW. Obesity is associated with increased risk of first trimester and recurrent miscarriage: matched case-control study. Hum Reprod. 2004;19(7):1644–6.
30. Metwally M, Ong KJ, Ledger WL, Li TC. Does high body mass index increase the risk of miscarriage after spontaneous and assisted conception? A meta-analysis of the evidence. Fertil Steril. 2008;90(3):714–26.
31. Rittenberg V, Seshadri S, Sunkara SK, Sobaleva S, Oteng-Ntim E, El-Toukhy T. Effect of body mass index on IVF treatment outcome: an updated systematic review and meta-analysis. Reprod Biomed Online. 2011;23(4):421–39.
32. Gregory CWE, Danielle ME. Trends and characteristics in gestational diabetes: United States, 2016–2020. Atlanta: Centers for Disease Control and Prevention; 2022.
33. American College of Obstetricians and Gynecologists. ACOG practice bulletin no. 190: gestational diabetes mellitus. Obstet Gynecol. 2018;131(2):e49–64.
34. Lee KW, Ching SM, Ramachandran V, Yee A, Hoo FK, Chia YC, et al. Prevalence and risk factors of gestational diabetes mellitus in Asia: a systematic review and meta-analysis. BMC Pregnancy Childbirth. 2018;18(1):494.
35. Torloni MR, Betrán AP, Horta BL, Nakamura MU, Atallah AN, Moron AF, et al. Prepregnancy BMI and the risk of gestational diabetes: a systematic review of the literature with meta-analysis. Obes Rev. 2009;10(2):194–203.
36. Alwash SM, McIntyre HD, Mamun A. The association of general obesity, central obesity and visceral body fat with the risk of gestational diabetes mellitus: evidence from a systematic review and meta-analysis. Obes Res Clin Pract. 2021;15(5):425–30.
37. Vats H, Saxena R, Sachdeva MP, Walia GK, Gupta V. Impact of maternal pre-pregnancy body mass index on maternal, fetal and neonatal adverse outcomes in the worldwide populations: a systematic review and meta-analysis. Obes Res Clin Pract. 2021;15(6):536–45.
38. D'Souza R, Horyn I, Pavalagantharajah S, Zaffar N, Jacob C-E. Maternal body mass index and

pregnancy outcomes: a systematic review and metaanalysis. Am J Obstetr Gynecol MFM. 2019;1(4):100041.
39. Rasmussen KM, Yaktine AL, editors. Institute of Medicine (US) and National Research Council (US) Committee to Reexamine IOM Pregnancy Weight Guidelines. Weight gain during pregnancy: reexamining the guidelines. Washington, DC: National Academies Press (US); 2009.
40. Morisset A-S, Tchernof A, Dubé M-C, Veillette J, Weisnagel SJ, Robitaille J. Weight gain measures in women with gestational diabetes mellitus. J Womens Health (Larchmt). 2011;20(3):375–80.
41. Brunner S, Stecher L, Ziebarth S, Nehring I, Rifas-Shiman SL, Sommer C, et al. Excessive gestational weight gain prior to glucose screening and the risk of gestational diabetes: a meta-analysis. Diabetologia. 2015;58(10):2229–37.
42. Hedderson MM, Gunderson EP, Ferrara A. Gestational weight gain and risk of gestational diabetes mellitus. Obstet Gynecol. 2010;115(3):597–604.
43. Bozkurt L, Göbl CS, Pfligl L, Leitner K, Bancher-Todesca D, Luger A, et al. Pathophysiological characteristics and effects of obesity in women with early and late manifestation of gestational diabetes diagnosed by the International Association of Diabetes and Pregnancy Study Groups criteria. J Clin Endocrinol Metab. 2015;100(3):1113–20.
44. Bicocca MJ, Mendez-Figueroa H, Chauhan SP, Sibai BM. Maternal obesity and the risk of early-onset and late-onset hypertensive disorders of pregnancy. Obstet Gynecol. 2020;136(1):118–27.
45. Sun M, Gao M, Luo M, Wang T, Ruan X, Tang J, et al. Impact of multiple obesity metrics on hypertensive disorders of pregnancy: a meta-analysis and Mendelian randomisation study. Heart. 2024;110(20):1216–22.
46. Xiang C, Sui L, Ding X, Cao M, Li G, Du Z. Maternal adiposity measures and hypertensive disorders of pregnancy: a meta-analysis. BMC Pregnancy Childbirth. 2024;24(1):675.
47. O'Brien TE, Ray JG, Chan W-S. Maternal body mass index and the risk of preeclampsia: a systematic overview. Epidemiology. 2003;14(3):368–74.
48. Lopez-Jaramillo P, Barajas J, Rueda-Quijano SM, Lopez-Lopez C, Felix C. Obesity and preeclampsia: common pathophysiological mechanisms. Front Physiol. 2018;9:1838.
49. Spradley FT. Metabolic abnormalities and obesity's impact on the risk for developing preeclampsia. Am J Physiol Regul Integr Comp Physiol. 2017;312(1):R5–12.
50. Vena F, D'Ambrosio V, Paladini V, Saluzzi E, Di Mascio D, Boccherini C, et al. Risk of neural tube defects according to maternal body mass index: a systematic review and meta-analysis. J Matern Fetal Neonatal Med. 2022;35(25):7296–305.
51. Zheng Z, Yang T, Chen L, Wang L, Zhang S, Wang T, et al. Increased maternal Body Mass Index is associated with congenital heart defects: an updated meta-analysis of observational studies. Int J Cardiol. 2018;273:112–20.
52. Brite J, Laughon SK, Troendle J, Mills J. Maternal overweight and obesity and risk of congenital heart defects in offspring. Int J Obes (Lond). 2014;38(6):878–82.
53. Correa A, Marcinkevage J. Prepregnancy obesity and the risk of birth defects: an update. Nutr Rev. 2013;71(Suppl 1):S68–77.
54. Aly H, Hammad T, Nada A, Mohamed M, Bathgate S, El-Mohandes A. Maternal obesity, associated complications and risk of prematurity. J Perinatol. 2010;30(7):447–51.
55. McDonald SD, Han Z, Mulla S, Beyene J, Knowledge Synthesis Group. Overweight and obesity in mothers and risk of preterm birth and low birth weight infants: systematic review and meta-analyses. BMJ. 2010;341:c3428.
56. Liu B, Xu G, Sun Y, Du Y, Gao R, Snetselaar LG, et al. Association between maternal pre-pregnancy obesity and preterm birth according to maternal age and race or ethnicity: a population-based study. Lancet Diabetes Endocrinol. 2019;7(9):707–14.
57. Torloni MR, Betrán AP, Daher S, Widmer M, Dolan SM, Menon R, et al. Maternal BMI and preterm birth: a systematic review of the literature with meta-analysis. J Matern Fetal Neonatal Med. 2009;22(11):957–70.
58. Liu K, Chen Y, Tong J, Yin A, Wu L, Niu J. Association of maternal obesity with preterm birth phenotype and mediation effects of gestational diabetes mellitus and preeclampsia: a prospective cohort study. BMC Pregnancy Childbirth. 2022;22(1):459.
59. Goldstein RF, Abell SK, Ranasinha S, Misso M, Boyle JA, Black MH, et al. Association of gestational weight gain with maternal and infant outcomes: a systematic review and meta-analysis. JAMA. 2017;317(21):2207–25.
60. Liu L, Hong Z, Zhang L. Associations of prepregnancy body mass index and gestational weight gain with pregnancy outcomes in nulliparous women delivering single live babies. Sci Rep. 2015;5:12863.
61. Heslehurst N, Vieira R, Hayes L, Crowe L, Jones D, Robalino S, et al. Maternal body mass index and post-term birth: a systematic review and meta-analysis. Obes Rev. 2017;18(3):293–308.
62. Akselsson A, Rossen J, Storck-Lindholm E, Rådestad I. Prolonged pregnancy and stillbirth among women with overweight or obesity – a population-based study in Sweden including 64,632 women. BMC Pregnancy Childbirth. 2023;23(1):21.
63. Ornaghi S, Fumagalli S, Galimberti S, Ornago AM, Brivio V, Lambicchi L, et al. Adverse childbirth and perinatal outcomes among healthy, low-

16

risk pregnant women with abnormal total gestational weight gain. J Womens Health (Larchmt). 2023;32(5):521–8.
64. Zhu Y, Zhang J, Li Q, Lin M. Association between gestational weight gain and preterm birth and post-term birth: a longitudinal study from the National Vital Statistics System database. BMC Pediatr. 2023;23(1):127.
65. Aune D, Saugstad OD, Henriksen T, Tonstad S. Maternal body mass index and the risk of fetal death, stillbirth, and infant death: a systematic review and meta-analysis. JAMA. 2014;311(15):1536–46.
66. Marchi J, Berg M, Dencker A, Olander EK, Begley C. Risks associated with obesity in pregnancy, for the mother and baby: a systematic review of reviews. Obes Rev. 2015;16(8):621–38.
67. Aedla NR, Mahmood T, Ahmed B, Konje JC. Challenges in timing and mode of delivery in morbidly obese women. Best Pract Res Clin Obstet Gynaecol. 2024;92:102425.
68. Lawn JE, Blencowe H, Pattinson R, Cousens S, Kumar R, Ibiebele I, et al. Stillbirths: Where? When? Why? How to make the data count? Lancet. 2011;377(9775):1448–63.
69. Yao R, Park BY, Foster SE, Caughey AB. The association between gestational weight gain and risk of stillbirth: a population-based cohort study. Ann Epidemiol. 2017;27(10):638–644.e1.
70. Nohr EA, Vaeth M, Baker JL, Sørensen TI, Olsen J, Rasmussen KM. Combined associations of prepregnancy body mass index and gestational weight gain with the outcome of pregnancy. Am J Clin Nutr. 2008;87(6):1750–9.
71. Liu P, Xu L, Wang Y, Zhang Y, Du Y, Sun Y, et al. Association between perinatal outcomes and maternal pre-pregnancy body mass index. Obes Rev. 2016;17(11):1091–102.
72. Gaudet L, Ferraro ZM, Wen SW, Walker M. Maternal obesity and occurrence of fetal macrosomia: a systematic review and meta-analysis. Biomed Res Int. 2014;2014:640291.
73. Dai R-X, He X-J, Hu C-L. Maternal pre-pregnancy obesity and the risk of macrosomia: a meta-analysis. Arch Gynecol Obstet. 2018;297(1):139–45.
74. Waters TP, Huston-Presley L, Catalano PM. Neonatal body composition according to the revised institute of medicine recommendations for maternal weight gain. J Clin Endocrinol Metab. 2012;97(10):3648–54.
75. Tan HS, Habib AS. Peri-operative anaesthetic management of women with obesity. Best Pract Res Clin Obstet Gynaecol. 2023;89:102335.
76. Dresner M, Brocklesby J, Bamber J. Audit of the influence of body mass index on the performance of epidural analgesia in labour and the subsequent mode of delivery. BJOG. 2006;113(10):1178–81.
77. Mhyre JM. Anesthetic management for the morbidly obese pregnant woman. Int Anesthesiol Clin. 2007;45(1):51–70.
78. Chu SY, Kim SY, Schmid CH, Dietz PM, Callaghan WM, Lau J, et al. Maternal obesity and risk of cesarean delivery: a meta-analysis. Obes Rev. 2007;8(5):385–94.
79. Weiss JL, Malone FD, Emig D, Ball RH, Nyberg DA, Comstock CH, et al. Obesity, obstetric complications and cesarean delivery rate – a population-based screening study. Am J Obstet Gynecol. 2004;190(4):1091–7.
80. Machado LS. Cesarean section in morbidly obese parturients: practical implications and complications. N Am J Med Sci. 2012;4(1):13–8.
81. Nivatpumin P, Lertbunnaphong T, Maneewan S, Vittayaprechapon N. Comparison of perioperative outcomes and anesthetic-related complications of morbidly obese and super-obese parturients delivering by cesarean section. Ann Med. 2023;55(1):1037–46.
82. Gabbai D, Gilboa I, Attali E, Yogev Y, Lavie A. Prediction of intrapartum cesarean delivery among women with obesity: a retrospective cohort study. Int J Gynaecol Obstet. 2024;
83. Su L, Zhang Y, Chen C, Lu L, Sutton D, D'Alton M, et al. Gestational weight gain and mode of delivery by the class of obesity: a meta-analysis. Obes Rev. 2022;23(12):e13509.
84. Zhang C, Wu Y, Li S, Zhang D. Maternal prepregnancy obesity and the risk of shoulder dystocia: a meta-analysis. BJOG. 2018;125(4):407–13.
85. Cheedalla A, Thompson A, Fortman E, Grasch JL, Venkatesh KK, Landon MB, et al. Maternal body mass index, maneuvers, and neonatal morbidity associated with shoulder dystocia. Am J Obstet Gynecol. 2024;
86. Kominiarek MA, Saade G, Mele L, Bailit J, Reddy UM, Wapner RJ, et al. Association between gestational weight gain and perinatal outcomes. Obstet Gynecol. 2018;132(4):875–81.
87. Blomberg M. Maternal obesity and risk of postpartum hemorrhage. Obstet Gynecol. 2011;118(3):561–8.
88. Zhang Y, Lu M, Yi Y, Xia L, Zhang R, Li C, et al. Influence of maternal body mass index on pregnancy complications and outcomes: a systematic review and meta-analysis. Front Endocrinol (Lausanne). 2024;15:1280692.
89. Mission JF, Marshall NE, Caughey AB. Pregnancy risks associated with obesity. Obstet Gynecol Clin North Am. 2015;42(2):335–53.
90. Axelsson D, Brynhildsen J, Blomberg M. Maternal obesity and the risk of postpartum infections according to mode of delivery. J Matern Fetal Neonatal Med. 2023;36(2):2245102.
91. Axelsson D, Blomberg M. Maternal obesity, obstetric interventions and post-partum anaemia

increase the risk of post-partum sepsis: a population-based cohort study based on Swedish medical health registers. Infect Dis (Lond). 2017;49(10):765–71.
92. Kawakita T, Coviello E. The association between surgical site infections and gestational weight gain in obese women. Arch Gynecol Obstet. 2020;301(6):1411–6.
93. Rahmani J, Haghighian Roudsari A, Bawadi H, Thompson J, Khalooei Fard R, Clark C, et al. Relationship between body mass index, risk of venous thromboembolism and pulmonary embolism: a systematic review and dose-response meta-analysis of cohort studies among four million participants. Thromb Res. 2020;192:64–72.
94. Butwick AJ, Bentley J, Leonard SA, Carmichael SL, El-Sayed YY, Stephansson O, et al. Prepregnancy maternal body mass index and venous thromboembolism: a population-based cohort study. BJOG. 2019;126(5):581–8.
95. Wu Y, Pei J, Dong L, Zhou Z, Zhou T, Zhao X, et al. Association between maternal weight gain in different periods of pregnancy and the risk of venous thromboembolism: a retrospective case-control study. Front Endocrinol (Lausanne). 2022;13:858868.
96. Lee KK, Raja EA, Lee AJ, Bhattacharya S, Bhattacharya S, Norman JE, et al. Maternal obesity during pregnancy associates with premature mortality and major cardiovascular events in later life. Hypertension. 2015;66(5):938–44.
97. Catalano PM, Shankar K. Obesity and pregnancy: mechanisms of short term and long term adverse consequences for mother and child. BMJ. 2017;356:j1.
98. Mamun AA, Kinarivala M, O'Callaghan MJ, Williams GM, Najman JM, Callaway LK. Associations of excess weight gain during pregnancy with long-term maternal overweight and obesity: evidence from 21 y postpartum follow-up. Am J Clin Nutr. 2010;91(5):1336–41.
99. McClure CK, Catov JM, Ness R, Bodnar LM. Associations between gestational weight gain and BMI, abdominal adiposity, and traditional measures of cardiometabolic risk in mothers 8 y postpartum. Am J Clin Nutr. 2013;98(5):1218–25.
100. Dachew BA, Ayano G, Betts K, Alati R. The impact of pre-pregnancy BMI on maternal depressive and anxiety symptoms during pregnancy and the postpartum period: a systematic review and meta-analysis. J Affect Disord. 2021;281:321–30.
101. Molyneaux E, Poston L, Ashurst-Williams S, Howard LM. Obesity and mental disorders during pregnancy and postpartum: a systematic review and meta-analysis. Obstet Gynecol. 2014;123(4):857–67.
102. Lipsky LM, Strawderman MS, Olson CM. Weight-related self-efficacy in relation to maternal body weight from early pregnancy to 2 years post-partum. Matern Child Nutr. 2016;12(3):569–78.
103. Godfrey KM, Reynolds RM, Prescott SL, Nyirenda M, Jaddoe VWV, Eriksson JG, et al. Influence of maternal obesity on the long-term health of offspring. Lancet Diabetes Endocrinol. 2017;5(1):53–64.
104. Crume TL, Brinton JT, Shapiro A, Kaar J, Glueck DH, Siega-Riz AM, et al. Maternal dietary intake during pregnancy and offspring body composition: the Healthy Start Study. Am J Obstet Gynecol. 2016;215(5):609.e1–8.
105. Crume TL, Shapiro AL, Brinton JT, Glueck DH, Martinez M, Kohn M, et al. Maternal fuels and metabolic measures during pregnancy and neonatal body composition: the healthy start study. J Clin Endocrinol Metab. 2015;100(4):1672–80.
106. Haddad-Tóvolli R, Morari J, Barbizan R, Bóbbo VC, Carraro RS, Solon C, et al. Maternal obesity damages the median eminence blood-brain barrier structure and function in the progeny: the beneficial impact of cross-fostering by lean mothers. Am J Physiol Endocrinol Metab. 2023;324(2):E154–66.
107. Boney CM, Verma A, Tucker R, Vohr BR. Metabolic syndrome in childhood: association with birth weight, maternal obesity, and gestational diabetes mellitus. Pediatrics. 2005;115(3):e290–6.
108. Mamun AA, O'Callaghan M, Callaway L, Williams G, Najman J, Lawlor DA. Associations of gestational weight gain with offspring body mass index and blood pressure at 21 years of age: evidence from a birth cohort study. Circulation. 2009;119(13):1720–7.
109. Kislal S, Shook LL, Edlow AG. Perinatal exposure to maternal obesity: lasting cardiometabolic impact on offspring. Prenat Diagn. 2020;40(9):1109–25.
110. Ludwig DS, Rouse HL, Currie J. Pregnancy weight gain and childhood body weight: a within-family comparison. PLoS Med. 2013;10(10):e1001521.
111. Garvey WT, Mechanick JI, Brett EM, Garber AJ, Hurley DL, Jastreboff AM, et al. American association of clinical endocrinologists and american college of endocrinology comprehensive clinical practice guidelines for medical care of patients with obesity. Endocr Pract. 2016;22(Suppl 3):1–203.
112. Lecorguillé M, Jacota M, de Lauzon-Guillain B, Forhan A, Cheminat M, Charles M-A, et al. An association between maternal weight change in the year before pregnancy and infant birth weight: ELFE, a French national birth cohort study. PLoS Med. 2019;16(8):e1002871.
113. Matusiak K, Barrett HL, Callaway LK, Nitert MD. Periconception weight loss: common sense for mothers, but what about for babies? J Obes. 2014;2014:204295.

114. Lou M-F, Shen W, Fu R-S, Zhang X-Y, Wang D-H. Maternal dietary protein supplement confers long-term sex-specific beneficial consequences of obesity resistance and glucose tolerance to the offspring in Brandt's voles. Comp Biochem Physiol Part A Mol Integr Physiol. 2015;182:38–44.
115. Wadden TA, Berkowitz RI, Womble LG, Sarwer DB, Phelan S, Cato RK, et al. Randomized trial of lifestyle modification and pharmacotherapy for obesity. N Engl J Med. 2005;353(20):2111–20.
116. Look AHEAD Research Group, Wing RR. Long-term effects of a lifestyle intervention on weight and cardiovascular risk factors in individuals with type 2 diabetes mellitus: four-year results of the Look AHEAD trial. Arch Intern Med. 2010;170(17):1566–75.
117. Becker GF, Passos EP, Moulin CC. Short-term effects of a hypocaloric diet with low glycemic index and low glycemic load on body adiposity, metabolic variables, ghrelin, leptin, and pregnancy rate in overweight and obese infertile women: a randomized controlled trial. Am J Clin Nutr. 2015;102(6):1365–72.
118. Sim KA, Dezarnaulds GM, Denyer GS, Skilton MR, Caterson ID. Weight loss improves reproductive outcomes in obese women undergoing fertility treatment: a randomized controlled trial. Clin Obes. 2014;4(2):61–8.
119. Galletly C, Clark A, Tomlinson L, Blaney F. Improved pregnancy rates for obese, infertile women following a group treatment program. An open pilot study. Gen Hosp Psychiatry. 1996;18(3):192–5.
120. Mutsaerts MAQ, van Oers AM, Groen H, Burggraaff JM, Kuchenbecker WKH, Perquin DAM, et al. Randomized trial of a lifestyle program in obese infertile women. N Engl J Med. 2016;374(20):1942–53.
121. Schenkelaars N, Rousian M, Hoek J, Schoenmakers S, Willemsen S, Steegers-Theunissen R. Preconceptional maternal weight loss and hypertensive disorders in pregnancy: a systematic review and meta-analysis. Eur J Clin Nutr. 2021;75(12):1684–97.
122. Price SAL, Sumithran P, Nankervis AJ, Permezel M, Prendergast LA, Proietto J. Impact of preconception weight loss on fasting glucose and pregnancy outcomes in women with obesity: a randomized trial. Obesity (Silver Spring). 2021;29(9):1445–57.
123. Pasquali R, Gambineri A, Biscotti D, Vicennati V, Gagliardi L, Colitta D, et al. Effect of long-term treatment with metformin added to hypocaloric diet on body composition, fat distribution, and androgen and insulin levels in abdominally obese women with and without the polycystic ovary syndrome. J Clin Endocrinol Metab. 2000;85(8):2767–74.
124. Morin-Papunen L, Rantala AS, Unkila-Kallio L, Tiitinen A, Hippeläinen M, Perheentupa A, et al. Metformin improves pregnancy and live-birth rates in women with polycystic ovary syndrome (PCOS): a multicenter, double-blind, placebo-controlled randomized trial. J Clin Endocrinol Metab. 2012;97(5):1492–500.
125. Tarry-Adkins JL, Ozanne SE, Aiken CE. Impact of metformin treatment during pregnancy on maternal outcomes: a systematic review/meta-analysis. Sci Rep. 2021;11(1):9240.
126. Alqudah A, McKinley MC, McNally R, Graham U, Watson CJ, Lyons TJ, et al. Risk of pre-eclampsia in women taking metformin: a systematic review and meta-analysis. Diabet Med. 2018;35(2):160–72.
127. American Diabetes Association Professional Practice Committee. 15. Management of Diabetes in Pregnancy: standards of care in diabetes-2024. Diabetes Care. 2024;47(Suppl 1):S282–94.
128. Drucker DJ. Mechanisms of Action and Therapeutic Application of Glucagon-like Peptide-1. Cell Metab. 2018;27(4):740–56.
129. Papaetis GS, Kyriacou A. GLP-1 receptor agonists, polycystic ovary syndrome and reproductive dysfunction: Current research and future horizons. Adv Clin Exp Med. 2022;31(11):1265–74.
130. Han Y, Li Y, He B. GLP-1 receptor agonists versus metformin in PCOS: a systematic review and meta-analysis. Reprod Biomed Online. 2019;39(2):332–42.
131. Minis E, Stanford FC, Mahalingaiah S. Glucagon-like peptide-1 receptor agonists and safety in the preconception period. Curr Opin Endocrinol Diabetes Obes. 2023;30(6):273–9.
132. Colquitt JL, Pickett K, Loveman E, Frampton GK. Surgery for weight loss in adults. Cochrane Database Syst Rev. 2014;2014(8):CD003641.
133. Xu G, Song M. Recent advances in the mechanisms underlying the beneficial effects of bariatric and metabolic surgery. Surg Obes Relat Dis. 2021;17(1):231–8.
134. Getahun D, Fassett MJ, Jacobsen SJ, Sacks DA, Murali SB, Peltier MR, et al. Perinatal outcomes after bariatric surgery. Am J Obstet Gynecol. 2022;226(1):121.e1–121.e16.
135. Kwong W, Tomlinson G, Feig DS. Maternal and neonatal outcomes after bariatric surgery; a systematic review and meta-analysis: do the benefits outweigh the risks? Am J Obstet Gynecol. 2018;218(6):573–80.
136. Balestrin B, Urbanetz AA, Barbieri MM, Paes A, Fujie J. Pregnancy after bariatric surgery: a comparative study of post-bariatric pregnant women versus non-bariatric obese pregnant women. Obes Surg. 2019;29(10):3142–8.
137. Johansson K, Cnattingius S, Näslund I, Roos N, Trolle Lagerros Y, Granath F, et al. Outcomes of pregnancy after bariatric surgery. N Engl J Med. 2015;372(9):814–24.
138. Akhter Z, Rankin J, Ceulemans D, Ngongalah L, Ackroyd R, Devlieger R, et al. Pregnancy after

bariatric surgery and adverse perinatal outcomes: a systematic review and meta-analysis. PLoS Med. 2019;16(8):e1002866.
139. Shawe J, Ceulemans D, Akhter Z, Neff K, Hart K, Heslehurst N, et al. Pregnancy after bariatric surgery: consensus recommendations for periconception, antenatal and postnatal care. Obes Rev. 2019;20(11):1507–22.
140. Solaiman S, Al-Baghdadi OO, Thin Hla T, Abdulmajid Kapadia S, Elbiss HM. Maternal and perinatal outcomes in women conceiving after bariatric surgery: a cohort study. Medicine (Baltimore). 2023;102(24):e33913.
141. Heusschen L, Krabbendam I, van der Velde JM, Deden LN, Aarts EO, Merién AER, et al. A matter of timing-pregnancy after bariatric surgery. Obes Surg. 2021;31(5):2072–9.
142. Parent B, Martopullo I, Weiss NS, Khandelwal S, Fay EE, Rowhani-Rahbar A. Bariatric surgery in women of childbearing age, timing between an operation and birth, and associated perinatal complications. JAMA Surg. 2017;152(2):128–35.
143. Carreira A, Araújo B, Lavrador M, Vieira I, Rodrigues D, Paiva S, et al. From bariatric surgery to conception: the ideal timing to optimize fetal weight. Obes Surg. 2023;33(9):2859–65.
144. Catalano PM, Mele L, Landon MB, Ramin SM, Reddy UM, Casey B, et al. Inadequate weight gain in overweight and obese pregnant women: what is the effect on fetal growth? Am J Obstet Gynecol. 2014;211(2):137.e1–7.
145. Oken E, Kleinman KP, Belfort MB, Hammitt JK, Gillman MW. Associations of gestational weight gain with short- and longer-term maternal and child health outcomes. Am J Epidemiol. 2009;170(2):173–80.
146. Bodnar LM, Siega-Riz AM, Simhan HN, Himes KP, Abrams B. Severe obesity, gestational weight gain, and adverse birth outcomes. Am J Clin Nutr. 2010;91(6):1642–8.
147. Johansson K, Bodnar LM, Stephansson O, Abrams B, Hutcheon JA. Safety of low weight gain or weight loss in pregnancies with class 1, 2, and 3 obesity: a population-based cohort study. Lancet. 2024;403(10435):1472–81.
148. Cantor AG, Jungbauer RM, McDonagh M, Blazina I, Marshall NE, Weeks C, et al. Counseling and behavioral interventions for healthy weight and weight gain in pregnancy: evidence report and systematic review for the US preventive services task force. JAMA. 2021;325(20):2094–109.
149. Teede HJ, Bailey C, Moran LJ, Bahri Khomami M, Enticott J, Ranasinha S, et al. Association of antenatal diet and physical activity-based interventions with gestational weight gain and pregnancy outcomes: a systematic review and meta-analysis. JAMA Intern Med. 2022;182(2):106–14.
150. Farpour-Lambert NJ, Ells LJ, Martinez de Tejada B, Scott C. Obesity and weight gain in pregnancy and postpartum: an evidence review of lifestyle interventions to inform maternal and child health policies. Front Endocrinol (Lausanne). 2018;9:546.
151. Dodd JM, Turnbull D, McPhee AJ, Deussen AR, Grivell RM, Yelland LN, et al. Antenatal lifestyle advice for women who are overweight or obese: LIMIT randomised trial. BMJ. 2014;348:g1285.
152. Mills HL, Patel N, White SL, Pasupathy D, Briley AL, Santos Ferreira DL, et al. The effect of a lifestyle intervention in obese pregnant women on gestational metabolic profiles: findings from the UK Pregnancies Better Eating and Activity Trial (UPBEAT) randomised controlled trial. BMC Med. 2019;17(1):15.
153. Catalano P, deMouzon SH. Maternal obesity and metabolic risk to the offspring: why lifestyle interventions may have not achieved the desired outcomes. Int J Obes (Lond). 2015;39(4):642–9.
154. Yu H, Li M, Qian G, Yue S, Ossowski Z, Szumilewicz A. A systematic review and Bayesian network meta-analysis comparing in-person, remote, and blended interventions in physical activity, diet, education, and behavioral modification on gestational weight gain among overweight or obese pregnant individuals. Adv Nutr. 2024;15(7):100253.
155. Rowan JA, Hague WM, Gao W, Battin MR, Moore MP, Investigators MGT. Metformin versus insulin for the treatment of gestational diabetes. N Engl J Med. 2008;358(19):2003–15.
156. Cassina M, Donà M, Di Gianantonio E, Litta P, Clementi M. First-trimester exposure to metformin and risk of birth defects: a systematic review and meta-analysis. Hum Reprod Update. 2014;20(5):656–69.
157. Balani J, Hyer SL, Rodin DA, Shehata H. Pregnancy outcomes in women with gestational diabetes treated with metformin or insulin: a case-control study. Diabet Med. 2009;26(8):798–802.
158. Syngelaki A, Nicolaides KH, Balani J, Hyer S, Akolekar R, Kotecha R, et al. Metformin versus placebo in obese pregnant women without diabetes mellitus. N Engl J Med. 2016;374(5):434–43.
159. Dodd JM, Louise J, Deussen AR, Grivell RM, Dekker G, McPhee AJ, et al. Effect of metformin in addition to dietary and lifestyle advice for pregnant women who are overweight or obese: the GRoW randomised, double-blind, placebo-controlled trial. Lancet Diabetes Endocrinol. 2019;7(1):15–24.
160. Teulings NEWD, Masconi KL, Ozanne SE, Aiken CE, Wood AM. Effect of interpregnancy weight change on perinatal outcomes: systematic review and meta-analysis. BMC Pregnancy Childbirth. 2019;19(1):386.
161. Oteng-Ntim E, Mononen S, Sawicki O, Seed PT, Bick D, Poston L. Interpregnancy weight change and adverse pregnancy outcomes: a systematic

review and meta-analysis. BMJ Open. 2018;8(6):e018778.
162. Bogaerts A, Van den Bergh BRH, Ameye L, Witters I, Martens E, Timmerman D, et al. Interpregnancy weight change and risk for adverse perinatal outcome. Obstet Gynecol. 2013;122(5):999–1009.
163. Jain AP, Gavard JA, Rice JJ, Catanzaro RB, Artal R, Hopkins SA. The impact of interpregnancy weight change on birthweight in obese women. Am J Obstet Gynecol. 2013;208(3):205.e1–7.
164. Wallace JM, Bhattacharya S, Campbell DM, Horgan GW. Inter-pregnancy weight change impacts placental weight and is associated with the risk of adverse pregnancy outcomes in the second pregnancy. BMC Pregnancy Childbirth. 2014;14:40.
165. Nascimento SL, Pudwell J, Surita FG, Adamo KB, Smith GN. The effect of physical exercise strategies on weight loss in postpartum women: a systematic review and meta-analysis. Int J Obes (Lond). 2014;38(5):626–35.
166. Rönö K, Stach-Lempinen B, Klemetti MM, Kaaja RJ, Pöyhönen-Alho M, Eriksson JG, et al. Prevention of gestational diabetes through lifestyle intervention: study design and methods of a Finnish randomized controlled multicenter trial (RADIEL). BMC Pregnancy Childbirth. 2014;14:70.

Prevention of Multifetal Pregnancy: The Role of Elective Single Embryo Transfer Policy

Yuval Fouks and Yariv Yogev

Contents

Y. Yogev, A. Khalil (eds.), *Prevention of Complications in Obstetrics*,
https://doi.org/10.1007/978-3-032-23479-7_17

Learning Objectives

- Explain the benefits and limitations of eSET versus DET.
- Describe patient-centered factors influencing embryo transfer decisions.
- Summarize evidence on maternal–fetal risks of multiple gestation.
- Identify clinical predictors for eSET suitability.
- Discuss the role of PGT-A in embryo selection for eSET.

17.1 Essentials

1. National eSET Programs: Accumulating evidence supports well-constructed national elective single embryo transfer (eSET) programs.
2. Emotional, Physical, and Financial Burdens: While cumulative cycles with cryopreservation maintain success rates, they also bring emotional, physical, and substantial financial burdens.
3. Patient-Centered Decisions: It is crucial for doctors to consider the specific needs and preferences of each patient, providing full disclosure of the short- and long-term consequences of multiple pregnancies.
4. Patient Preference for Twins: Despite the potential to maintain overall live birth rates (LBR) with an eSET strategy, many patients still express a preference for twin pregnancies.
5. Cost-Effectiveness in Older Women: The cost-effectiveness of double embryo transfer (DET) may improve with age. An extended treatment duration in a complete eSET program can be particularly disadvantageous for older women due to declining fertility and increased oocyte aneuploidy.
6. Reducing Multiple Birth Rates: eSET, combined with frozen embryo transfer, is effective in decreasing multiple birth rates while still achieving acceptable live birth rates compared to DET.
7. Insufficient Evidence for Routine PGT-A: Currently, there is insufficient evidence to recommend the routine use of embryo biopsy with preimplantation genetic testing for aneuploidy (PGT-A) to enhance eSET and reduce the risk of twinning.
8. Need for Further Research: Further research is needed to explore outcomes following eSET in women of advanced age.
9. Challenges to eSET Use: Main challenges include clinician and patient education, out-of-pocket cycle costs, and effective embryo selection methods.
10. Risks of Twin Pregnancies: Fertility specialists should recognize the considerable risks associated with twin pregnancies, emphasizing that the optimal outcome of an in vitro fertilization (IVF) cycle is the birth of a healthy singleton newborn.
11. Avoiding DET with Donor Oocytes and Embryos: DET should be avoided in treatments involving donor oocytes, donated embryos, or gestational carriers due to the increased risk of pregnancy complications.

17.2 Introduction

Over the last three decades, there has been a significant enhancement in Assisted Reproductive Technology (ART) outcomes, as evidenced by the marked increase in the live birth rate per embryo transfer. Initially, live birth rates were below 15% in the mid-1980s [1–3], but by 2014, they had risen to over 35% [4, 5]. This upward trend is attributed to multiple advancements: an increase in the effectiveness and number of cryopreservation cycles [6, 7], advancements in embryo selection processes [8, 9], improvements in the quality of culture media [10], the introduction of Intracytoplasmic Sperm Injection (ICSI) [11], and the use of donor eggs and surrogacy. Additionally, the adoption of elective single embryo transfer (eSET) has become more common [12, 13], leading to fewer multi-embryo transfers and a significant reduction in multiple pregnancies [14–16].

The increased pregnancy rates in IVF have raised concerns about the morbidity and mortality associated with multiple pregnancies, prompting efforts to limit the number of embryos transferred. National guidelines have adopted eSET to varying degrees, with uptake ranging from 2.8% in the USA to 69.4% in some European countries [17, 18]. Some countries have taken proactive measures, issuing guidelines on the number of embryos to be transferred and, in some cases, enacting legislation to restrict this number. In countries like Sweden, the United Kingdom, Germany, and Switzerland [13, 18, 21–23], physicians who exceed the mandated number of transferred embryos risk losing their licenses.

These measures have contributed to a gradual reduction in the acceptable number of transferred embryos, particularly in younger women [24]. Notably, the percentage of triplet births from ART in the US has dramatically declined from 11.4% in 1995 to 0.9% in 2014 [5, 25, 26], while the rate of singleton pregnancies and deliveries has gradually increased [27–29]. However, nearly 25% of all ART-related live births in the United States are still multiple gestations [28, 30]. These high rates of multiple pregnancies often result in short- and long-term complications, including prematurity, low birth weight, gestational hypertension, gestational diabetes, birth defects, and increased perinatal mortality.

The 2024 ESHRE guidelines, encompassing 35 recommendations—25 evidence-based and 10 good practice points—strongly endorse eSET as the standard in IVF/ICSI procedures, particularly when multiple embryos are available. This preference for eSET, highlighted in cases involving donor oocytes, donated embryos, or gestational carriers, is driven by its equivalence in cumulative live birth rates to DET and a significantly lower risk of multiple births. The overall direction of recent guidelines promotes a personalized approach to embryo transfer, taking into account various prognostic factors and the history of previous unsuccessful treatments and transfers, to maximize successful outcomes and minimize complications.

17.3 Evaluating Safety and Efficacy of Embryo Transfer Strategies

Numerous studies have compared pregnancy outcomes between eSET and DET or multiple embryo transfers. These studies consistently show that obstetric and neonatal complications are significantly increased with multiple gestations [31, 32]. Proponents of eSET argue that success should be defined as the birth of a healthy single-term baby, focusing not only on outcomes from fresh cycles but also on cumulative live-term birth rates. There is no significant difference in cumulative live birth rates when comparing a single DET cycle with two consecutive SET cycles [33]. From a cross-sectional perspective, fertility outcomes after eSET are higher when considering the subsequent cryopreserved embryos from the first oocyte retrieval [34, 35]. In a study by Gerris et al. [31], patients with a good prognosis and at least two embryos available were randomized to either eSET or DET. Women in the DET group achieved a higher ongoing pregnancy rate than those in the eSET group (74.0% vs. 38.5%, $P = .013$); however, the multiple gestation rate was 30% in the DET group compared to only 4% in the eSET group. Montfoort et al. [34] reported comparable cumulative live birth rates between patients receiving either DET or eSET when embryo quality was good. They found pregnancy rates of 62.4% in the SET group and 62.6% in the DET group, with twin pregnancy rates of 10.1% and 13.4%, respectively.

These studies indicate that the cumulative live birth rate (LBR) following the subsequent replacement of a single frozen embryo in the eSET group is comparable to that of the DET group. A meta-analysis [36] comparing cleavage-stage eSET versus DET demonstrated similar cumulative LBRs from two pairs of eSET (fresh and frozen) cycles compared to DET, with a slight, insignificant advantage in LBR after a single DET cycle (38% vs. 42%). Another study examining birth rates before and after the implementation of an eSET policy found a significant reduction in multiple pregnancy rates among oocyte donors allocated to SET, with no impact on delivery rates [37]. This finding was supported by another subsequent study suggesting that when three embryos are available and eSET is performed, the cumulative LBR is not compromised [38]. A study comparing the outcomes of twin pregnancies to women having two singleton pregnancies after IVF [39] showed higher rates of various morbidities, including preeclampsia, preterm premature rupture of membranes, cesarean section, respiratory complications, jaundice, and sepsis in the twin group. Additionally, perinatal mortality was significantly reduced with eSET compared to DET [32].

Most studies reporting eSET results focus on patients with a good prognosis. However, patients with advanced maternal age and/or low ovarian reserve undergoing embryo transfers face a more challenging dilemma. An analysis of over 800 frozen embryo transfer cycles in women aged 36 to 39 years found no significant difference in pregnancy and live birth rates between the eSET and DET groups, with similar cumulative live birth rates in the eSET group [40]. However, studies focusing on older age groups have contradicted these findings, concluding that clinical pregnancy rates and live birth rates are significantly lower following eSET than DET [41].

As many studies are retrospective and lack randomization, there are inherent biases, especially when the decision to transfer embryos is based on prognostic factors. Some researchers argue that the eSET policy might be overadopted. They assert that the widespread implementation of eSET can be seen as an "add-on" treatment [42] to IVF, adversely affecting how IVF is practiced. A recent clinical perspective by Glacier et al. stated that the international acceptance of eSET occurred without proper prior validation of an unproven hypothesis and that the current practice is necessary only in a small number of selected cases [43]. Clearly, there are conflicting views on this issue, and the adoption of eSET in some patient subgroups requires better-quality evidence.

17.4 Patient Preferences and Autonomy in Embryo Transfer Decisions

Terms like "singleton live births" and "term singleton live birth" are well-received by obstetricians and perinatologists but may not always resonate with patients. Patients with a history of long-standing or repeatedly unsuccessful treatments often focus on the short-term goal of achieving a clinical pregnancy, finding it difficult to consider the broader implications. While higher-order pregnancies carry more significant risks and complications compared to singleton pregnancies [44], patients undergoing treatment may perceive these risks differently, often underestimating or disregarding them.

A significant factor contributing to the high rate of multiple gestations is patient pressure on physicians to transfer multiple embryos to increase the chances of a successful cycle. From the patient's perspective, a twin pregnancy can seem desirable [45], as the associated risks might be viewed as acceptable. Ezugwu and Van der Berg [46] reported that 58% of ART patients preferred having twins, with this preference rising to as high as 89% in some populations.

Patients often underestimate the risks involved, and misinformation frequently contributes to couples rejecting eSET recommendations [46]. Miscommunication between infertility care providers and patients, particularly regarding the risks of multiple pregnancies [47, 48], can also influence patient expectations and decisions. Even when fully informed about eSET, many patients opt for multiple embryos in a single transfer, believing it increases their chances of success. Some studies have shown that patients who are well-informed about the risks of DET are more likely to accept eSET [49].

A study assessing patient attitudes toward eSET policy [50] identified measures to improve its acceptance. It revealed that many patients perceive SET as unfair and view the risks of twins from DET as acceptable within their personal circumstances. These conflicting views on family planning may stem from concerns about treatment failure, the psychological impact of infertility, and worries about the time and costs associated with additional treatments. From the patient's perspective, the expected risks of multiple pregnancies are often less concerning and not considered in their short-term objectives [51].

Another challenge in promoting eSET is that IVF clinic success rates, especially in the United States [52], are typically reported as success per cycle start or per transfer, rather than capturing cumulative success rates from subsequent frozen embryo transfers derived from the same cycle. Consequently, promoting eSET is challenging because it appears to have lower "success" rates compared to transferring multiple embryos simultaneously, even though the total "success" rates are similar.

Finally, the belief that having twins is a more cost-effective way to achieve family planning may lead patients to accept obstetrical risks to achieve a pregnancy. This approach is more common among patients paying out-of-pocket for fertility treatments than among those covered by national policies and insurance. A US study examining SET versus multiple embryo transfer across over 260,000 fertility cycles found that the rate of single embryo transfer was significantly higher among patients with adequate insurance coverage. In Australia, where IVF is funded in part by healthcare insurance, there was a high rate of eSET (78.9% in 2013) and a notably low multiple pregnancy rate [53]. It is clear that providing patients with detailed information about associated risks is essential to help them make informed decisions about eSET.

17.5 Suitability Measures

Recent research has focused on identifying the patients most suitable for single embryo transfer (SET) [20]. Women of advanced age, who have lower chances of live birth, often receive multiple embryos during transfer. Applying an indiscriminate policy of multiple embryo transfers (ET) in this group may increase the risk of complications associated with multiple pregnancies [54]. Therefore, careful consideration should be given before transferring multiple embryos in these cases. A cohort study comparing outcomes following eSET and double embryo transfer (DET) in women over 40 years old [55] found that both eSET and DET resulted in comparable live birth rates (LBR) when transferring blastocysts in this age group. However, when more blastocysts were available for cryopreservation, DET was associated with both higher LBR and a greater number of twin pregnancies.

Clinical guidelines have evolved, gradually reducing the acceptable number of transferred embryos, particularly in women aged 37 and younger [29]. This policy change has led to a decline in the percentage of multiple pregnancies, especially triplet births from ART, from 11.4% to 0.9% over ten years. However, a later report by the CDC covering 2005–2014 indicated that although the rates of twin and triplet births have decreased significantly, nearly 1 in 4 live births resulting from ART in the United States is still a multiple gestation (Centers for Disease Control and Prevention, American Society for Reproductive Medicine (ASRM), Society for Assisted Reproductive Technology: 2014). Assisted Reproductive Technology National Summary Report. Atlanta (GA): US Department of Health and Human Services, 2016.

Fertility clinical societies such as the American Society for Reproductive Medicine (ASRM) [56] and the Association of Clinical Embryologists (ACE) [19] have issued guidelines to select appropriate candidates for eSET. These guidelines use various factors such as maternal age, obstetrical and gynecological history, previous treatment history, ovarian response, number of embryos created, embryo quality, blastocysts available for transfer, and cryopreservation to identify patients at the greatest risk of multiple pregnancies. The available data suggest that the likelihood of a twin pregnancy is similar for all patients regardless of the usual prognostic factors [57], with no specific attributable risk factors for multiple pregnancies. This indicates that the absolute risk of twins is greatest in patients with the best prognosis, making eSET most effective for this subgroup.

Despite these guidelines, there is still a lack of high-quality evidence on the best candidates for eSET and which groups would benefit the most. Clear predictors of twin likelihood, other than embryo development stage and quality at transfer, are still not well-defined. Therefore, the decision on the number of embryos to transfer often relies on local practices, lower-level evidence, or financial considerations.

17.6 PGT-A for eSET

Chromosomal abnormalities in human embryos often result in failed IVF cycles. Therefore, selecting the embryo with the highest implantation potential can significantly shorten the time to achieve pregnancy, especially in younger patients [58]. Both embryo quality and ploidy are crucial for embryo selection and are key components of a successful eSET strategy aimed at reducing multiple pregnancies [20].

Selecting embryos with higher morphological scores, whether by direct microscopy or time-lapse imaging, is essential for a successful eSET strategy, as these scores often indicate the embryos most likely to implant, thus shortening the time to pregnancy. Ploidy assessment has become an integral part of the criteria used to determine the number of embryos to transfer according to ASRM guidelines [56]. Studies assessing the impact of comprehensive chromosome screening after blastocyst biopsy have favored the use of preimplantation genetic screening (PGS) to reduce twinning. In the BEST trial, patients aged 42 years or younger with at least two blastocysts available were allocated to receive either DET of unscreened embryos or SET of one euploid embryo [9]. The results were notable. The ongoing pregnancy rate per first transfer was similar between the groups (euploid SET: 60.7% vs. untested DET: 65.1%; RR 0.9, 95% CI 0.7 to 1.2). However, there were no multiple gestations following euploid SET. Additionally, patients in the euploid SET group had a significantly higher chance of having an ongoing singleton pregnancy (60.7% vs. 33.7%; RR, 1.8; 95% CI 1.3 to 2.5). Neonatal risks such as preterm delivery (13% vs. 29%, $P = .03$), low birth weight (11% vs. 33%, $P = .002$), and NICU admission (11% vs. 26%, $P = .04$) were all significantly lower in the PGT SET group. This study demonstrated that applying PGT in patients with a good prognosis can improve the ongoing pregnancy rate and reduce the incidence of DET and multiple gestations.

A systematic review concluded that PGT-A is associated with higher implantation rates when comparable numbers of embryos are transferred and that screening improves embryo selection in patients undergoing eSET. While the review found that pregnancy rates in eSET after preimplantation genetic screening are maintained, the study groups mostly consisted of good-prognosis patients, making it difficult to determine if similar results would be observed in patients with poor prognosis [59]. Utilizing both morphology-based selection and PGT-A for embryo selection may enhance the accuracy of eSET, allowing clinicians to extend this approach to a broader range of patients.

17.7 Summary

In vitro fertilization (IVF) aims to increase birth rates while reducing pregnancy-related complications, which are significantly higher in multiple pregnancies. Multiple gestations not only elevate the risk of fetal issues such as prematurity and infant mortality but also increase maternal morbidity and impose a substantial burden on healthcare costs.

Elective single embryo transfer (eSET) is often beneficial for patients with good prognoses, as the cumulative live birth rate per fresh cycle remains equivalent when followed by consecutive frozen embryo transfers (FETs), given the current success rates of embryo cryopreservation [60]. While collective regulations on the number of embryos allowed for transfer can reduce multiple pregnancies, they may not account for individual patient circumstances, medical and fertility history, and family planning needs. Strict approaches that overlook the unique circumstances of individual women are more likely to reduce the chances of pregnancy [61].

The ASRM guidelines issued in 2017 categorize patients into those with a favorable prognosis and those without. Favorable prognosis characteristics include (1) expectation of one or more high-quality embryos available for cryopreservation, (2) euploid embryos, (3) previous live birth after an IVF cycle, and (4) availability of vitrified, high-quality blastocysts for transfer. The recommended number of embryos to be transferred at one time is based on the woman's age, the presence or absence of favorable characteristics, and the developmental stage of the embryos.

The recently published ESHRE guidelines strongly advocate for eSET, particularly in scenarios involving donor oocytes, donated embryos, or gestational carriers, to minimize the risks of pregnancy complications relative to DET. They further endorse the transfer of a single blastocyst to reduce the risks associated with monozygotic twins and multiple pregnancies. Although there are few randomized controlled trials, cohort study findings support a tailored approach that considers various prognostic factors for different patient cases. The ESHRE guidelines emphasize the significance of accounting for previous unsuccessful treatments, which affect the chances of successful implantation and live birth. In instances where multiple adverse prognostic indicators exist, DET might be an option, though it is crucial to thoroughly inform patients about the heightened risks, such as a substantially greater likelihood of ectopic pregnancy.

Chapter Key Points

- eSET reduces multiple gestations, lowering maternal and neonatal morbidity.
- Cumulative live birth rates with eSET+FET are comparable to DET.
- Twin pregnancies carry substantially higher risks than two singleton IVF pregnancies.
- Patient counseling and autonomy are central to improving eSET acceptance.
- PGT-A can enhance eSET effectiveness in good-prognosis patients.
- Older or poor-prognosis patients may still benefit from DET in select scenarios.

Chapter-End Summary

Elective single embryo transfer is a key strategy to prevent complications related to multiple gestations in ART. Evidence shows that cumulative live birth rates remain comparable to DET when FET cycles are included, while morbidity is significantly lower. eSET is most effective in good-prognosis patients, though clinical judgment is required in advanced age or poor prognosis. Patient education, counseling, and autonomy strongly influence acceptance. PGT-A and improved embryo selection support safer, individualized transfer decisions.

References

1. Wang J, Sauer MV. In vitro fertilization (IVF): a review of 3 decades of clinical innovation and technological advancement. Ther Clin Risk Manag. 2006;2(4):355–64.
2. Asch RH, Ellsworth LR, Balmaceda JP, Wong PC. Pregnancy after translaparoscopic gamete intrafallopian transfer. Lancet. 1984;2(8410):1034–5.
3. Henriksen T, Abyholm T, Tanbo T, Magnus O. Pregnancies after intrafallopian transfer of embryos. J In Vitro Fert Embryo Transf. 1988;5(5):296–8.
4. Forman EJ, Hong KH, Franasiak JM, Scott RT. Obstetrical and neonatal outcomes from the BEST Trial: single embryo transfer with aneuploidy screening improves outcomes after in vitro fertilization without compromising delivery rates. Am J Obstet Gynecol. 2014;210(2):157.e1–6.
5. Jain T, Missmer SA, Hornstein MD. Trends in embryo-transfer practice and in outcomes of the use of assisted reproductive technology in the United States. N Engl J Med. 2004;350(16):1639–45.

6. Cobo A, Kuwayama M, Pérez S, Ruiz A, Pellicer A, Remohí J. Comparison of concomitant outcome achieved with fresh and cryopreserved donor oocytes vitrified by the Cryotop method. Fertil Steril. 2008;89(6):1657–64.
7. Cobo A, Kuwayama M, Pérez S, Ruiz A, Pellicer A, Remohí J. Reprint of: Comparison of concomitant outcome achieved with fresh and cryopreserved donor oocytes vitrified by the Cryotop method. Fertil Steril. 2019;112(4 Suppl 1):e85–e92.
8. Wang L, Wang X, Zhang J, Song Z, Wang S, Gao Y, et al. Detection of chromosomal aneuploidy in human preimplantation embryos by next-generation sequencing. Biol Reprod. 2014;90(5):95.
9. Forman EJ, Hong KH, Ferry KM, Tao X, Taylor D, Levy B, et al. In vitro fertilization with single euploid blastocyst transfer: a randomized controlled trial. Fertil Steril. 2013;100(1):100–7.e1.
10. Gardner DK, Vella P, Lane M, Wagley L, Schlenker T, Schoolcraft WB. Culture and transfer of human blastocysts increases implantation rates and reduces the need for multiple embryo transfers. Fertil Steril. 1998;69(1):84–8.
11. Tesarik J, Junca AM, Hazout A, Aubriot FX, Nathan C, Cohen-Bacrie P, et al. Embryos with high implantation potential after intracytoplasmic sperm injection can be recognized by a simple, non-invasive examination of pronuclear morphology. Hum Reprod. 2000;15(6):1396–9.
12. Ryan GL, Sparks AE, Sipe CS, Syrop CH, Dokras A, Van Voorhis BJ. A mandatory single blastocyst transfer policy with educational campaign in a United States IVF program reduces multiple gestation rates without sacrificing pregnancy rates. Fertil Steril. 2007;88(2):354–60.
13. Harbottle S, Hughes C, Cutting R, Roberts S, Brison D, (BFS) AOCETABFS. Elective Single Embryo Transfer: an update to UK best practice guidelines. Hum Fertil (Camb). 2015;18(3):165–83.
14. Steinberg ML, Boulet S, Kissin D, Warner L, Jamieson DJ. Elective single embryo transfer trends and predictors of a good perinatal outcome – United States, 1999 to 2010. Fertil Steril. 2013;99(7):1937–43.
15. Luke B, Brown MB, Grainger DA, Cedars M, Klein N, Stern JE, et al. Practice patterns and outcomes with the use of single embryo transfer in the United States. Fertil Steril. 2010;93(2):490–8.
16. Pennings G. Avoiding multiple pregnancies in ART: multiple pregnancies: a test case for the moral quality of medically assisted reproduction. Hum Reprod. 2000;15(12):2466–9.
17. Chambers GM, Wand H, Macaldowie A, Chapman MG, Farquhar CM, Bowman M, et al. Population trends and live birth rates associated with common ART treatment strategies. Hum Reprod. 2016;31(11):2632–41.
18. Maheshwari A, Griffiths S, Bhattacharya S. Global variations in the uptake of single embryo transfer. Hum Reprod Update. 2011;17(1):107–20.
19. Cutting R, Morroll D, Roberts SA, Pickering S, Rutherford A, Ba ACE. Elective single embryo transfer: guidelines for practice British Fertility Society and Association of Clinical Embryologists. Hum Fertil (Camb). 2008;11(3):131–46.
20. Cutting R. Single embryo transfer for all. Best Pract Res Clin Obstet Gynaecol. 2018;53:30–7.
21. Källén B, Finnström O, Lindam A, Nilsson E, Nygren KG, Otterblad OP. Trends in delivery and neonatal outcome after in vitro fertilization in Sweden: data for 25 years. Hum Reprod. 2010;25(4):1026–34.
22. Mayor S. UK authority sets limit on number of embryos transferred. BMJ. 2004;328(7431):65.
23. Karlström PO, Bergh C. Reducing the number of embryos transferred in Sweden-impact on delivery and multiple birth rates. Hum Reprod. 2007;22(8):2202–7.
24. Sunderam S, Kissin DM, Zhang Y, Jewett A, Boulet SL, Warner L, et al. Assisted reproductive technology surveillance – United States, 2017. MMWR Surveill Summ. 2020;69(9):1–20.
25. Kissin DM, Kulkarni AD, Mneimneh A, Warner L, Boulet SL, Crawford S, et al. Embryo transfer practices and multiple births resulting from assisted reproductive technology: an opportunity for prevention. Fertil Steril. 2015;103(4):954–61.
26. Stern JE, Cedars MI, Jain T, Klein NA, Beaird CM, Grainger DA, et al. Assisted reproductive technology practice patterns and the impact of embryo transfer guidelines in the United States. Fertil Steril. 2007;88(2):275–82.
27. Styer AK, Luke B, Vitek W, Christianson MS, Baker VL, Christy AY, et al. Factors associated with the use of elective single-embryo transfer and pregnancy outcomes in the United States, 2004–2012. Fertil Steril. 2016;106(1):80–9.
28. Sunderam S, Kissin DM, Crawford SB, Folger SG, Jamieson DJ, Warner L, et al. Assisted reproductive technology surveillance – United States, 2013. MMWR Surveill Summ. 2015;64(11):1–25.
29. Sunderam S, Kissin DM, Crawford SB, Folger SG, Jamieson DJ, Warner L, et al. Assisted reproductive technology surveillance – United States, 2014. MMWR Surveill Summ. 2017;66(6):1–24.
30. Jones HW, Cooke I, Kempers R, Brinsden P, Saunders D. International federation of fertility societies surveillance 2010: preface. Fertil Steril. 2011;95(2):491.
31. Gerris J, De Neubourg D, Mangelschots K, Van Royen E, Van de Meerssche M, Valkenburg M. Prevention of twin pregnancy after in-vitro fertilization or intracytoplasmic sperm injection based on strict embryo criteria: a prospective randomized clinical trial. Hum Reprod. 1999;14(10):2581–7.

32. Sullivan EA, Wang YA, Hayward I, Chambers GM, Illingworth P, McBain J, et al. Single embryo transfer reduces the risk of perinatal mortality, a population study. Hum Reprod. 2012;27(12):3609–15.
33. Pandian Z, Marjoribanks J, Ozturk O, Serour G, Bhattacharya S. Number of embryos for transfer following in vitro fertilisation or intra-cytoplasmic sperm injection. Cochrane Database Syst Rev. 2013;(7):CD003416.
34. van Montfoort AP, Fiddelers AA, Land JA, Dirksen CD, Severens JL, Geraedts JP, et al. eSET irrespective of the availability of a good-quality embryo in the first cycle only is not effective in reducing overall twin pregnancy rates. Hum Reprod. 2007;22(6):1669–74.
35. Lukassen HG, Braat DD, Wetzels AM, Zielhuis GA, Adang EM, Scheenjes E, et al. Two cycles with single embryo transfer versus one cycle with double embryo transfer: a randomized controlled trial. Hum Reprod. 2005;20(3):702–8.
36. McLernon DJ, Harrild K, Bergh C, Davies MJ, de Neubourg D, Dumoulin JC, et al. Clinical effectiveness of elective single versus double embryo transfer: meta-analysis of individual patient data from randomised trials. BMJ. 2010;341:c6945.
37. Söderström-Anttila V, Vilska S, Mäkinen S, Foudila T, Suikkari AM. Elective single embryo transfer yields good delivery rates in oocyte donation. Hum Reprod. 2003;18(9):1858–63.
38. Clua E, Tur R, Coroleu B, Boada M, Rodríguez I, Barri PN, et al. Elective single-embryo transfer in oocyte donation programmes: Should it be the rule? Reprod Biomed Online. 2012;25(6):642–8.
39. Sazonova A, Källen K, Thurin-Kjellberg A, Wennerholm UB, Bergh C. Neonatal and maternal outcomes comparing women undergoing two in vitro fertilization (IVF) singleton pregnancies and women undergoing one IVF twin pregnancy. Fertil Steril. 2013;99(3):731–7.
40. Veleva Z, Vilska S, Hydén-Granskog C, Tiitinen A, Tapanainen JS, Martikainen H. Elective single embryo transfer in women aged 36–39 years. Hum Reprod. 2006;21(8):2098–102.
41. Fujimoto A, Morishima K, Harada M, Hirata T, Osuga Y, Fujii T. Elective single-embryo transfer improves cumulative pregnancy outcome in young patients but not in women of advanced reproductive age. J Assist Reprod Genet. 2015;32(12):1773–9.
42. Kamath MS, Mascarenhas M, Franik S, Liu E, Sunkara SK. Clinical adjuncts in in vitro fertilization: a growing list. Fertil Steril. 2019;112(6):978–86.
43. Gleicher N, Orvieto R. Transferring more than 1 embryo simultaneously is justifiable in most patients. Reprod Biomed Online. 2021;
44. Santana DS, Cecatti JG, Surita FG, Silveira C, Costa ML, Souza JP, et al. Twin pregnancy and severe maternal outcomes: the World Health Organization Multicountry Survey on Maternal and newborn health. Obstet Gynecol. 2016;127(4):631–41.
45. Goldfarb JM, Austin C, Lisbona H, Peskin B, Clapp M. Cost-effectiveness of in vitro fertilization. Obstet Gynecol. 1996;87(1):18–21.
46. Ezugwu E, der Burg SV. Debating elective single embryo transfer after in vitro fertilization: a plea for a context-sensitive approach. Ann Med Health Sci Res. 2015;5(1):1–7.
47. Klitzman L, R. Reducing the number of fetuses in a pregnancy: providers' and patients' views of challenges. Hum Reprod. 2016;31(11):2570–6.
48. Klitzman R. Impediments to communication and relationships between infertility care providers and patients. BMC Womens Health. 2018;18(1):84.
49. Rai V, Betsworth A, Beer C, Ndukwe G, Glazebrook C. Comparing patients' and clinicians' perceptions of elective single embryo transfer using the attitudes to a twin IVF pregnancy scale (ATIPS). J Assist Reprod Genet. 2011;28(1):65–72.
50. Leese B, Denton J. Attitudes towards single embryo transfer, twin and higher order pregnancies in patients undergoing infertility treatment: a review. Hum Fertil (Camb). 2010;13(1):28–34.
51. Pinborg A, Loft A, Schmidt L, Andersen AN. Attitudes of IVF/ICSI-twin mothers towards twins and single embryo transfer. Hum Reprod. 2003;18(3):621–7.
52. Technology PCoSfAR, Medicine PCoASfR. Elective single-embryo transfer. Fertil Steril. 2012;97(4):835–42.
53. Dyer S, Chambers GM, de Mouzon J, Nygren KG, Zegers-Hochschild F, Mansour R, et al. International Committee for Monitoring Assisted Reproductive Technologies world report: assisted reproductive technology 2008, 2009 and 2010. Hum Reprod. 2016;31(7):1588–609.
54. Sundhararaj UM, Madne MV, Biliangady R, Gurunath S, Swamy AG, Gopal IST. Single blastocyst transfer: the key to reduce multiple pregnancy rates without compromising the live birth rate. J Hum Reprod Sci. 2017;10(3):201–7.
55. Tannus S, Son WY, Dahan MH. Elective single blastocyst transfer in advanced maternal age. J Assist Reprod Genet. 2017;34(6):741–8.
56. ASRM@asrm.org PCotASfRMatPCftSfARTEa. Guidance on the limits to the number of embryos to transfer: a committee opinion. Fertil Steril. 2021;116(3):651–654.
57. Roberts SA, McGowan L, Mark Hirst W, Vail A, Rutherford A, Lieberman BA, et al. Reducing the incidence of twins from IVF treatments: predictive modelling from a retrospective cohort. Hum Reprod. 2011;26(3):569–75.
58. Goldman RH, Racowsky C, Farland LV, Munné S, Ribustello L, Fox JH. Predicting the likelihood of live birth for elective oocyte cryopreservation: a

counseling tool for physicians and patients. Hum Reprod. 2017;32(4):853–9.

59. Dahdouh EM, Balayla J, García-Velasco JA. Impact of blastocyst biopsy and comprehensive chromosome screening technology on preimplantation genetic screening: a systematic review of randomized controlled trials. Reprod Biomed Online. 2015;30(3):281–9.

60. Mancuso AC, Boulet SL, Duran E, Munch E, Kissin DM, Van Voorhis BJ. Elective single embryo transfer in women less than age 38 years reduces multiple birth rates, but not live birth rates, in United States fertility clinics. Fertil Steril. 2016;106(5):1107–14.

61. Schieve LA, Peterson HB, Meikle SF, Jeng G, Danel I, Burnett NM, et al. Live-birth rates and multiple-birth risk using in vitro fertilization. JAMA. 1999;282(19):1832–8.

Prevention of Alloimmunization

Misgav Rottenstreich and Eran Ashwal

Contents

Y. Yogev, A. Khalil (eds.), *Prevention of Complications in Obstetrics*,
https://doi.org/10.1007/978-3-032-23479-7_18

Learning Objectives

- Understand mechanisms and consequences of red cell alloimmunization.
- Identify preventive strategies, including RhIG, ccffDNA testing, and paternal/fetal antigen typing.
- Describe diagnostic tools for fetal anemia, particularly MCA Doppler velocimetry.
- Explain the indications, technique, and risks of intrauterine transfusion.
- Apply evidence-based management strategies for sensitized pregnancies, including those with prior severe HDFN.

18.1 Introduction

Exposure to foreign red cell antigens invariably results in the production of anti-red cell antibodies in the process known as red cell alloimmunization, which was formerly termed isoimmunization. The expression "sensitization" can be used interchangeably with alloimmunization. The active transport of these antibodies across the placenta during pregnancy results in fetal anemia, hyperbilirubinemia, and ultimately, hydrops fetalis. Before the advent of obstetric ultrasound, the perinatal effects of maternal red cell alloimmunization could be recognized only after the birth of an affected neonate. Thus, the neonatal consequences of maternal red cell alloimmunization came to be known as hemolytic disease of the newborn (HDN). Today, ultrasound and cordocentesis make the detection of the severely anemic fetus a reality. For this reason, the term "hemolytic disease of the fetus and newborn" (HDFN) would appear to be more appropriate for describing this disorder. This chapter describes the prevention and management of red cell alloimmunization.

Learning Objectives

1. Understand the concept of alloimmunization in the context of pregnancy.
2. Recognize the risk factors associated with alloimmunization.
3. Comprehend the impact of alloimmunization on maternal and fetal health.
4. Learn effective preventive measures to minimize the risk of alloimmunization.

18.2 Case Studies

1. Case Question

Why is it recommended that all pregnant patients undergo blood type determination and an antibody screen at the first prenatal visit?

- **Answer:**

It is recommended that all pregnant patients undergo blood type determination and an antibody screen at the first prenatal visit to assess Rh and ABO compatibility. This helps identify potential risks such as hemolytic disease of the fetus and newborn (HDFN). Early detection allows for timely interventions, such as administering antenatal and postpartum rhesus immune globulin (RhIG) in cases of Rh incompatibility, leading to improved maternal and fetal health outcomes [1, 2].

2. Case Question

What is the impact of routine administration of antenatal and postpartum rhesus immune globulin (RhIG) on the incidence of red cell alloimmunization secondary to the RhD antigen, and how have the rates of maternal Rh sensitization evolved with the adoption of this treatment in industrialized countries?

- **Answer:**

The routine administration of antenatal and postpartum rhesus immune globulin (RhIG) has significantly reduced the cases of red cell alloimmunization secondary to the RhD antigen in industrialized countries. Prior to the introduction of Rh immunoglobulin, approximately 9–10% of patients negative for Rh became sensitized with each full-term pregnancy [3]. With the adoption of routine treatment at delivery, this maternal Rh sensitization rate decreased to a range of 1.1–1.6%.

The introduction of additional prophylaxis in the third trimester further lowered the rate to approximately 0.2% in the USA, Canada, the UK, Europe, Australia, and New Zealand [4].

Despite the success of RhIG in reducing Rh HDFN (hemolytic disease of the fetus and newborn), the unavailability of RhIG in certain countries, like India and China, has led to ongoing perinatal morbidity and mortality. According to estimates, in these countries, Rh HDFN contributes to 41,000 stillbirths, 90,000 neonatal deaths, and 48,000 cases of kernicterus annually [5].

It is noteworthy that even in developed countries, cases of Rh HDFN still occur. These cases are attributed to maternal sensitization in the first two trimesters of pregnancy, inadvertent omission of RhIG, and inadequate dosing after delivery, especially in situations involving a large fetomaternal hemorrhage (FMH). Thus, while the routine administration of RhIG has been highly effective in reducing sensitization rates, challenges persist, necessitating continued attention to proper implementation and adherence to prophylactic measures.

3. Case Question

Given the implementation of antenatal and postpartum rhesus immune globulin (RhIG), leading to a decline in RhD alloimmunization, what challenges arise from the shift to other red cell antibodies in the context of hemolytic disease of the fetus and newborn (HDFN)? Additionally, how does this impact the risk for patients with known Rh-positive status?

- **Answer:**

The implementation of antenatal and postpartum rhesus immune globulin (RhIG) has effectively reduced the incidence of RhD alloimmunization. However, this success has resulted in a notable shift to other red cell antibodies, such as anti-E, anti-M, anti-K, and anti-C, contributing to complications associated with hemolytic disease of the fetus and newborn (HDFN). Notably, the RhD antibody, although accounting for only 19% of significant antibodies, continues to pose a risk [6].

Even patients with known Rh-positive status are not immune to complications, as the focus on RhD alloimmunization may overshadow the potential threat from other antibodies. Given the unlikelihood of developing immune globulins for all red cell antigens by pharmaceutical companies, red cell alloimmunization is expected to persist as a challenge in pregnancies.

4. Case Question

What are the implications for Rh immune globulin (RhIG) administration in the context of potential alloimmunization risk during pregnancy?

- **Answer:**

For RhD-negative pregnant women without evidence of anti-D alloimmunization, the recommendation is to administer 300 μg of RhIG at 28 weeks' gestation, reducing the background incidence of RhD alloimmunization from 2% to 0.1% [4]. The United Kingdom follows a protocol involving 100 μg (500 IU) of RhIG at 28 and 34 weeks in primigravidae [7].

Despite the slow absorption of exogenous anti-D from intramuscular injection, a repeat antibody screen at the time of the antenatal RhIG is recommended [8]. This cautious approach ensures monitoring for potential alloimmunization before subsequent RhIG administration, contributing to effective management of RhD-negative pregnant individuals at risk of RhD alloimmunization.

5. Case Question

What is the management of patients classified as weak Rh-positive, and what are the current recommendations regarding Rh immune globulin (RhIG) administration, considering the subgroups of weak D individuals and the potential for rhesus alloimmunization during pregnancy?

- **Answer:**

In the past, individuals classified as weak Rh-positive, particularly those with reduced expression of D antigens or variant D antigen expression, were initially considered Rh-positive, and RhIG administration was not recommended [8]. However, subsequent research identified two groups within weak D individuals: one with intact but reduced D antigens and another with missing D antigen epitopes, putting them at risk for rhesus alloimmunization [9].

Recent recommendations suggest that all weak D individuals should receive antenatal and appropriate postpartum RhIG, despite conflicting guidelines [8]. A work group proposed managing these cases as RhD-positive, emphasizing the importance of RhD genotyping in pregnant patients to identify the subgroup with weak D [10]. Although not universally adopted, this approach aims to prevent alloimmunization to missing D antigen epitopes.

6. Case Question

How does cell-free fetal DNA (ccffDNA) screening play a role in determining the need for antepartum Rh immune globulin (RhIG) administration?

▪ **Answer:**

An evolving paradigm in antenatal prophylaxis involves the use of cell-free fetal DNA (ccffDNA) screening to determine the fetal RhD status in Rh-negative pregnant women. Studies have shown that a portion of the maternal circulation's free DNA is of fetal origin, ranging from 3% in the first trimester to 6% in the third trimester [11], primarily originating from apoptosis of placental villi. The rapid clearance of fetal DNA occurs with a mean half-life of 16 minutes after cesarean delivery and 100 hours after vaginal delivery [12, 13].

18

Clinical assays have been developed to detect fetal RhD DNA sequences in maternal circulation, allowing for accurate determination of the fetal RhD status [14]. Approximately 40% of Rh-negative pregnant women are found to carry an Rh-negative fetus. In countries like Denmark, the Netherlands, Sweden, and France, routine screening of Rh-negative pregnant patients for fetal RhD status is practiced to guide the use of antenatal RhIG [15–17]. England's National Institute for Health and Care Excellence has recommended nationwide adoption of this practice [18], and Canada is planning to implement a similar program.

In contrast to some countries where RhIG availability is limited, the United States has unrestricted access to RhIG, which is manufactured from plasma collected from sensitized male volunteer donors. Ethical considerations, including the potential for infection with prions and other viruses, have led to debates about restricting antenatal RhIG to those patients who truly need it [19]. A cost-neutral strategy has been proposed, with studies indicating break-even costs for ccffDNA testing to range from $29 to $119 for the saved doses of RhIG [20, 21].

However, concerns have been raised about the potential increase in Rh alloimmunization if ccffDNA screening were to replace the universal use of RhIG. In the U.S., where over 500,000 RhD-negative women give birth to more than 350,000 RhD-positive infants annually, the adoption of ccffDNA for antenatal RhIG triage could result in 1 to 57 new cases of Rh alloimmunization each year. Despite ongoing debates, as of now, the use of ccffDNA to guide antenatal RhIG administration is not endorsed by any major U.S. organization [22].

7. Case Question

What are the indications for antepartum administration of Rh immune globulin (RhIG), and why is there a challenge in implementing a smaller dose (50 μg) for certain indications?

▪ **Answer:**

Several additional indications for the antepartum administration of Rh immune globulin (RhIG) were identified, supported by level A scientific evidence. These indications include spontaneous miscarriage, elective abortion, ectopic pregnancy, genetic amniocentesis, chorionic villus sampling, and cordocentesis [8]. Although some studies argued that the risk for Rh sensitization following first-trimester elective abortion is minor [23], later guidelines still support the offering of both RhD testing and RhIg administration for spontaneous and induced abortion at <12 weeks of gestation in unsensitized, RhD-negative individuals [24].

For pregnancies up to 13 weeks' gestation, a lower dose of 50 µg of RhIG is considered effective, given the small volume of red cells in the fetoplacental circulation during this early stage. However, a challenge arises in the implementation of this smaller dose, as most hospitals and offices typically do not stock it. This reluctance is attributed to the equivalent cost of the 50 µg dose compared to the standard 300 µg dose, making it less practical from a resource perspective. Despite the efficacy of the smaller dose for certain indications, the widespread availability and use of the 300 µg dose remain more common in clinical settings.

8. Case Question

What is the current stance on evaluating persistent maternal anti-D titers as an indication for withholding additional Rh immune globulin (RhIG) after an antenatal event, and what factors contribute to the recommendation of administering RhIG in cases of doubt?

- **Answer:**

The current practice discourages the evaluation of persistent maternal anti-D titers as an indication for withholding additional Rh immune globulin (RhIG) after an antenatal event [1]. Although the exact protective mechanism of RhIG is not fully understood, effective prophylaxis relies on an excess amount of exogenous antibody relative to the volume of RhD-positive red cells in the maternal circulation. Both animal and human studies have demonstrated that a low level of RhIG can potentially enhance the chance for alloimmunization [25]. The rule of thumb is to administer RhIG when in doubt rather than withholding it.

Given that the half-life of RhIG is approximately 16 days, 15–20% of patients receiving it at 28 weeks' gestation may have a very low anti-D titer at the time of admission for term labor [26]. In North America, the recommendation is to administer 300 µg of RhIG within 72 hours of delivery if umbilical cord blood typing reveals an RhD-positive infant, providing protection from sensitization due to an FMH of 30 mL of fetal whole blood [8].

The AABB recommends routine screening for excessive FMH in all women at delivery. The rosette test is performed first, with a positive or negative result. A negative result warrants the administration of a standard 300 µg dose of RhIG. If the rosette is positive, a quantitative assessment is undertaken, multiplying the percentage of fetal blood cells by a factor of 50 to estimate the volume of the FMH. The calculated dose may include an additional vial due to the estimation of maternal blood volume.

While guidelines exist for RhIG dosing, a survey by the American College of Pathologists noted that, even following these guidelines, inadequate doses were recommended in 9% of cases and excessive doses in 12% of cases [27]. No more than 5 mL RhIG should be administered intramuscularly in one 24-hour period. Larger doses can be given via intravenous preparations of RhIG, up to 600 µg every 8 hours until the total dose is achieved.

If RhIG is inadvertently omitted after delivery, some protection has been proven with administration within 13 days, with recommendations extending it up to 28 days post-delivery [28].

In cases when the administration of RhIG was done for antenatal indications close to delivery, such as amniocentesis for fetal lung maturity within 48 hours of delivery or external cephalic version in less than 3 weeks before delivery, the administration of a repeat dose of RhIG is unnecessary unless a large FMH is detected at the time of delivery [8].

Failed prophylaxis after the appropriate RhIG dose is rare. Persistent anti-D antibody screens beyond 6 months postpartum are likely the result of sensitization rather than inadequate RhIG administration.

9. Case Question

In cases where a maternal antibody screen reveals the presence of an anti-D antibody, what is the initial step in evaluating the RhD-sensitized patient during her first affected pregnancy, and how is the degree of alloimmunization determined?

- **Answer:**

Upon the detection of an anti-D antibody through a maternal antibody screen, the initial step in evaluating the RhD-sensitized patient during her first affected pregnancy involves titer determination. The human antiglobulin titer, assessed through the indirect Coombs test, is employed to measure the maternal IgG response and determine the degree of alloimmunization. Titer values, often reported as dilutions (e.g., 1:2, 1:4, 1:8, 1:16, 1:32, etc.), are common in obstetric literature.

A critical titer, defined as the anti-red cell titer associated with a significant risk for hydrops fetalis, serves as a pivotal indicator. The threshold for this critical titer varies across institutions and methodologies. However, in many centers, a critical titer for anti-D, ranging between 8 and 32, is frequently utilized. When a critical titer is identified, it signals the need for further fetal surveillance due to the heightened risk of hydrops fetalis associated with increased maternal alloimmunization. The precise value of the critical titer may differ, but it plays a crucial role in guiding subsequent management and monitoring protocols for RhD-sensitized pregnancies.

10. <u>Case Question</u>

What techniques are employed for determining the fetal blood type, particularly when the patient's partner is heterozygous for the involved red cell antigen, and what considerations and methods are associated with assessing the fetal RhD type?

- **Answer:**

In cases where the patient's partner is determined to be heterozygous for the involved red cell antigen, several techniques are utilized to determine the fetal blood type. If the fetus is found to be antigen-negative in half of the cases, further maternal and fetal testing becomes unnecessary.

1. Serology on blood obtained by ultrasound-directed cordocentesis—was no longer used for fetal testing due to a 1–2% risk of procedure-related loss.
2. Chorionic villus sampling—for detecting the RhD gene; however, its major disadvantage includes the potential for fetomaternal hemorrhage (FMH) and a rise in maternal titer, worsening fetal disease, making this procedure discouraged unless the patient plans to terminate all antigen-positive fetuses [29].
3. Amniocentesis—the most reliable method for assessing fetal blood type through DNA testing for the last three decades [30].
4. Fetal RhD determination using cell-free fetal DNA (ccffDNA)—a more advanced and less invasive approach. This method replaces amniocentesis where available. The initial steps involve assessing paternity and paternal zygosity, with molecular techniques accurately determining the paternal genotype at the RhD locus [31]. Some authorities suggest omitting the paternity step and testing every pregnancy with ccffDNA for fetal RhD determination to avoid issues with paternity. ccffDNA, typically obtained between 10 and 12 weeks' gestation, is a crucial tool for determining the fetal RhD type [15–17]. While availability is still limited, studies have shown high reliability [32], with minimal false negatives and inconclusive results. An RhD-positive ccffDNA result is considered reliable, confirming the absence of RhD DNA in maternal circulation. In the case of an RhD-negative ccffDNA result, the detection of the SRY gene from a male fetus confirms the presence of fetal DNA. An RhD-negative female result, however, may present challenges, and further validation using single-nucleotide polymorphisms (SNPs) is common in Europe. In the absence of SNPs in the US assay, an RhD-negative female result is reported with a qualifying statement. If a critical maternal anti-D titer of 32 or more is present and the ccffDNA result returns RhD-negative, female, or indeterminate, the fetal RhD status should be determined by amniocentesis, or, alternatively, surveil-

lance with serial MCA-peak systolic velocity (PSV) Dopplers can be undertaken.

11. Case Question:

How has ultrasound been instrumental in advancing the management of alloimmunized pregnancies, particularly concerning the prediction and surveillance of fetal anemia, and what key parameters are evaluated through Doppler ultrasound studies?

- **Answer:**

Ultrasound has become essential in improving the management of alloimmunized pregnancies, particularly in predicting and monitoring fetal anemia. After accurately determining the gestational age, ultrasound allows for the assessment of fetal parameters, such as the peak systolic velocity (PSV) in the middle cerebral artery (MCA) [33].

Hydrops fetalis, characterized by the accumulation of fluid in at least two fetal compartments, is a crucial indicator. Ascites often appear as the initial sign of impending hydrops, followed by scalp edema and pleural effusions as anemia worsens. When hydrops is detected, fetal hemoglobin levels are typically 7–10 g/dL below the average for the corresponding gestational age, indicating severe fetal anemia [34]. However, fetuses with severe anemia may show increased cardiac output and reduced blood viscosity, leading to higher blood velocities.

Doppler ultrasound, especially the measurement of PSV in the fetal MCA, has become vital for predicting fetal anemia [35]. A PSV reading exceeding 1.5 multiples of the median (MoM) for the corresponding gestational age predicts moderate to severe fetal anemia with an 88% sensitivity and an 89% negative predictive rate [33].

Serial MCA Doppler studies are now the main method for monitoring fetal anemia in pregnancies affected by red cell alloimmunization [8]. Proper technique is critical, requiring precise placement of the ultrasound transducer on the maternal abdomen to maintain an insonation angle close to zero. Measurements are taken at the proximal MCA, ensuring the fetus is in a quiescent state to avoid inaccuracies. Care should be taken to avoid any unnecessary pressure on the fetal head, as this may lead to increased PSV [36].

Reliable MCA measurements can be obtained as early as 18 weeks' gestation, with follow-up studies conducted every 1–2 weeks based on trends. The values are converted to MoM using calculators for thorough monitoring of fetal anemia in alloimmunized pregnancies.

12. Case Question

How is the clinical management approach structured for RhD-sensitized pregnancies, specifically focusing on the first affected pregnancy, and what diagnostic tools and monitoring strategies are employed to assess the severity of hemolytic disease of the fetus and newborn (HDFN)?

- **Answer:**

The clinical management of RhD-sensitized pregnancies is based on the patient's history of fetal or neonatal hemolytic disease of the fetus and newborn (HDFN). Generally, the first affected pregnancy tends to exhibit mild-to-moderate fetal or neonatal disease, with subsequent pregnancies experiencing progressively severe anemia.

In the initial affected pregnancy, upon detection of sensitization to the RhD antigen, maternal antibody titers are checked monthly until around 24 weeks, then every two weeks thereafter. If paternity is confirmed, the father's RhD status and zygosity are determined through DNA testing. Serial middle cerebral artery (MCA) Doppler studies begin at approximately 24 weeks' gestation and are repeated every 1–2 weeks, depending on the trend. Once a critical maternal titer, typically 32, is reached, MCA Doppler studies become essential for monitoring fetal anemia.

When the father's phenotype is heterozygous, or paternity is uncertain, cell-free fetal DNA (ccffDNA) testing is conducted at a DNA reference laboratory to determine the fetal RhD status. If the father or the fetus is RhD-negative, and paternity is assured, further maternal and fetal monitoring is unnecessary. Conversely, if an RhD-positive fetus is confirmed, ongoing fetal surveillance is required. If an MCA Doppler measurement exceeds 1.5 multiples of the median (MoM), cordocentesis should be performed at an experienced referral center, with preparations for intrauterine transfusion (IUT) if the fetal hematocrit is below 30%. This structured approach is designed to customize monitoring and interventions according to the severity of HDFN, ensuring timely and appropriate management for RhD-sensitized pregnancies.

Summary of the Decision Points Involved in the Process:

Detection of RhD Sensitization

- Initial monthly checks of maternal antibody titers until 24 weeks.
- Bi-weekly checks of maternal antibody titers after 24 weeks.

Determination of Father's RhD Status and Zygosity

- Confirm paternity.
- Conduct DNA testing for RhD status and zygosity.

Fetal RhD Status Determination

- If the father is heterozygous or paternity is uncertain, perform cell-free fetal DNA (ccffDNA) testing.

Monitoring and Interventions Based on Results

- **If the fetus is RhD-negative:** No further monitoring is needed.
- **If the fetus is RhD-positive:** Start serial MCA Doppler studies from 24 weeks, conducted every 1–2 weeks.

Critical Maternal Titer Reached (Typically 32)

- MCA Doppler studies become crucial for monitoring fetal anemia.

Monitoring Fetal Anemia

- **If MCA Doppler > 1.5 MoM:** Perform cordocentesis.
- Prepare for intrauterine transfusion (IUT) if fetal hematocrit is below 30%.

18

13. Case Question

How does the clinical management differ for patients with a history of a previous perinatal loss related to hemolytic disease of the fetus and newborn (HDFN), a need for intrauterine transfusion (IUT), or a need for neonatal exchange transfusion, and what diagnostic tools and monitoring strategies are recommended in such cases?

- **Answer:**

For patients with a history of perinatal loss due to HDFN, a previous need for intrauterine transfusion (IUT), or neonatal exchange transfusion, a specialized clinical management approach is required. These cases should be managed at a tertiary care center experienced in handling severely alloimmunized pregnancies.

In contrast to first affected pregnancies, maternal titers are not reliable indicators of the severity of fetal anemia in these situations. Nevertheless, obtaining a baseline titer is recommended to evaluate eligibility for immunomodulation. If the father's RhD phenotype is heterozygous or paternity is uncertain, cell-free fetal DNA (ccffDNA) analysis or amniocentesis when ccffDNA is not available should be performed to determine the fetal RhD status.

For cases involving other maternal antibodies, such as anti-Kell, amniocentesis is recommended after 15 weeks' gestation to determine the fetal red cell antigen status. Serial middle cerebral artery (MCA) Doppler measurements should begin at 18 weeks' gestation and continue every 1–2 weeks. This thorough approach ensures that patients with a history of severe alloimmunization receive specialized care and monitoring, focusing on diagnostic accuracy and timely interventions based on their specific previous HDFN experiences.

14. Case Question

How are intrauterine transfusions (IUTs) performed in the management of severe alloimmunization during pregnancy, and what factors influence the frequency and timing of these procedures?

▪ **Answer:**

In managing severe alloimmunization during pregnancy, intrauterine transfusions (IUTs) are conducted under continuous ultrasound guidance. This procedure involves directly infusing fresh, cytomegalovirus (CMV)-negative, type O, RhD-negative red blood cells into the umbilical cord vessels or the intrahepatic portion of the fetal umbilical vein [37]. A 20-gauge needle (or a 22-gauge needle for pregnancies less than 22 weeks) is inserted into the amniotic cavity and subsequently into the umbilical vein, all under constant ultrasound guidance. When dealing with an anterior placenta, the needle is passed through the placental tissue into the cord root. For posterior placentation, it is preferable to insert the needle at the cord's insertion point into the placenta, as puncturing a "floating" loop of the cord has been linked to a twofold increase in complication risk [38].

The red blood cell unit is cross-matched with the maternal blood sample, with extended cross-matching sometimes used to minimize the risk of new antibody formation. The blood unit is leukoreduced, irradiated, washed, and packed to achieve a final hematocrit of approximately 75–80%, preventing volume overload in the fetus.

Typically performed in the operating room, especially at viable gestational ages to allow for emergency delivery if necessary, the procedure involves administering a long-acting local anesthetic and possibly conscious sedation. A procedure needle is inserted into the amniotic cavity and then into the umbilical vein under continuous ultrasound guidance. Fetal blood is drawn to determine the initial hematocrit, and a short-term paralytic agent is given to temporarily halt fetal movement.

The amount of packed red blood cells to be infused is based on the estimated fetal weight (EFW) determined by ultrasound. The dose is calculated to increase the fetal hematocrit by 10% [39]. This procedure is repeated at scheduled intervals until fetal erythropoiesis suppression is observed, typically by the third IUT. Subsequent procedures depend on the individual fetus's hematocrit decline, usually at 3- to 4-week intervals. A recent study showed that MCA-PSV Doppler is not superior in the prediction of the need for the next IUT compared to the use of the predicted decline in fetal hematocrit to time subsequent procedures [40].

The final IUT generally occurs before 35 weeks' gestation, with delivery planned approximately 3 weeks later. Administering oral phenobarbital before delivery has been shown to reduce the need for neonatal exchange transfusions [41]. For severely anemic fetuses in the early second trimester, who cannot tolerate an acute correction of their hematocrit to normal levels [42], the initial hematocrit should not be increased by more than fourfold during the first procedure [43]. A repeat intravascular transfusion is performed within 48 hours to bring the fetal hematocrit to normal levels.

15. <u>Case Question</u>

What are the complications associated with intrauterine transfusions (IUTs) in the management of severe alloimmunization during pregnancy, and how do these complications impact perinatal outcomes?

▪ **Answer:**

Complications from intrauterine transfusions (IUTs) in managing severe alloimmunization during pregnancy are rare but can vary depending on the center's experience and the presence of hydrops fetalis. The overall survival rate after IUT is high, with one series from a center in the Netherlands reporting a 97% survival rate for over 900 procedures [38].

Complications can include the rare occurrences of preterm premature rupture of membranes (PPROM) and chorioamnionitis. Fetal bradycardia, often transient, may occur, especially if the umbilical artery is inadvertently punctured, and it typically resolves with the removal of the procedure needle. The procedure-related complication rate is approximately 1.2% [44, 45].

The presence of fetal hydrops, particularly if it persists after several IUTs, is associated with lower perinatal survival rates. The likelihood of fetal distress necessitating emergency delivery increases with advancing gestation, complicating up to 5% of procedures after 32 weeks' gestation. It is important to note that survival rates and complications can vary between centers based on their expertise and experience in managing severe alloimmunization cases.

16. Case Question

For patients with high anti-red cell titers and a history of recurrent perinatal loss in the second trimester due to severe alloimmunization, what are the current therapeutic options available, and what potential future therapeutic options are mentioned in the literature?

- **Answer:**

At present, patients with high anti-red cell titers and repeated perinatal losses in the second trimester have limited treatment options. These options include using red cell antigen-negative donor semen for artificial insemination, opting for surrogate pregnancy, or employing preimplantation genetic diagnosis if the father is heterozygous. These methods aim to prevent or mitigate the risk of severe complications related to alloimmunization.

Future prospects may include targeted immunotherapy with monoclonal antibodies to achieve placental blockade. This novel approach could potentially replace intrauterine transfusions by addressing the underlying alloimmunization, thereby improving outcomes for these high-risk pregnancies. However, it is important to recognize that these potential therapies are currently theoretical and will require extensive research and clinical trials before they can be validated and implemented.

Major Pearls/Pitfalls

- **Pearls:**

1. Early Detection Is Key: Timely identification of red cell alloimmunization is crucial for effective management.
2. Risk Assessment: Evaluate the risk factors, including anti-red cell titers and paternal phenotypes, to tailor the management plan.
3. Advances in Ultrasound: Utilize ultrasound for gestational age determination and fetal monitoring, providing valuable insights into the severity of hemolytic disease.
4. Individualized Approach: Recognize the need for an individualized approach in cases of weak Rh positivity and consider RhIG administration based on current recommendations.
5. Antenatal RhIG Use: Understand the indications and controversies surrounding antenatal RhIG use, taking into account the latest guidelines and research.

- **Pitfalls:**

1. Incomplete Paternal Assessment: Failure to accurately determine paternal RhD status may lead to uncertainties in the fetal RhD status.
2. Overreliance on Titers: While maternal titers provide essential information, they may not predict the degree of fetal anemia accurately.
3. Inadequate Monitoring: Insufficient monitoring of alloimmunized pregnancies, especially in cases of previous HDFN, may result in missed complications.
4. Limited Therapeutic Options: Acknowledge the limited current therapeutic options for high anti-red cell titers and recurrent perinatal loss, emphasizing the need for future developments.

How-to-Guides/Recipes

- **Managing Weak Rh Positivity:**
  - Confirm Rh status using current monoclonal reagents.
  - Assess the risk of alloimmunization, considering weak D types 1, 2, and 3.
  - Administer antenatal and appropriate postpartum RhIG based on the latest guidelines.

- **Implementing ccffDNA Screening:**
  - Understand the advantages and limitations of cell-free fetal DNA (ccffDNA) screening.
  - Evaluate the cost-neutral strategy for incorporating ccffDNA testing.
  - Navigate potential ethical concerns and considerations in implementing ccffDNA in antenatal RhIG triage.

Worked-Out Examples

- **Case: Management of Severe Alloimmunization:**
  - Patient with a history of severe HDFN and high anti-red cell titers.
    - Initiate serial MCA Doppler studies and assess fetal hematocrit.
    - Consider intrauterine transfusion if indicated, with a step-by-step guide to the procedure.
    - Administer oral phenobarbital for neonatal hyperbilirubinemia prevention.

Chapter-End Summaries

- **Key Takeaways:**
  1. Early detection is crucial for effective management.
  2. Individualize the approach based on risk factors and the severity of alloimmunization.
  3. Stay updated on guidelines for RhIG administration and other interventions.

- **Application in Practice:**
  1. Apply ultrasound for accurate gestational age determination and monitoring.
  2. Use MCA Doppler studies judiciously to predict and manage fetal anemia.

- **Looking Ahead:**
  1. Acknowledge the limited current therapeutic options for severe alloimmunization.
  2. Emphasize the potential of future immunotherapeutic approaches discussed in the literature.

Chapter Key Points

- Early detection and routine screening for alloimmunization are essential to prevent HDFN complications.
- RhD prophylaxis with antenatal and postpartum RhIG remains the cornerstone of prevention, reducing sensitization to ~0.1%.

- Non-RhD antibodies (e.g., anti-K, anti-C, anti-E) are increasingly relevant contributors to HDFN.
- MCA-PSV Doppler is the primary non-invasive tool for diagnosing fetal anemia, with >1.5 MoM indicating moderate–severe anemia.
- Intrauterine transfusion (IUT) is an effective intervention with high survival rates when performed in experienced centers.
- ccffDNA can determine fetal RhD status, reducing unnecessary RhIG use, but adoption varies globally.
- Weak D phenotypes require genotype-based management to prevent missed prophylaxis needs.

Chapter-End Summary

Red cell alloimmunization remains a significant preventable cause of fetal anemia and HDFN. Universal first-trimester screening, appropriate RhIG use, and targeted approaches—such as ccffDNA for fetal RhD status—are essential components of prevention. Management of sensitized pregnancies requires structured surveillance using MCA Doppler studies, timely cordocentesis, and intrauterine transfusions when indicated. With high survival rates in experienced centers, IUT remains the primary therapy for severe fetal anemia. As non-RhD antibodies become more clinically relevant, individualized care, improved diagnostic tools, and potential future immunotherapies will shape evolving prevention and treatment strategies.

18

References

1. Sperling JD, Dahlke JD, Sutton D, Gonzalez JM, Chauhan SP. Prevention of RhD alloimmunization: a comparison of four national guidelines. Am J Perinatol. 2018;35:110–9.
2. Moise KJ Jr, Argoti PS. Management and prevention of red cell alloimmunization in pregnancy: a systematic review. Obstet Gynecol. 2012;120:1132–9.
3. Klein HG, Anstee DJ. Mollison's blood transfusion in clinical medicine. Wiley; 2013.
4. Urbaniak SJ. The scientific basis of antenatal prophylaxis. BJOG An Int J Obstet Gynaecol. 1998;105:11–8.
5. Zipursky A, Paul VK. The global burden of Rh disease. Arch Dis Childhood-Fetal Neonatal Ed. 2011;96:F84–5.
6. Smith HM, Shirey RS, Thoman SK, Jackson JB. Prevalence of clinically significant red blood cell alloantibodies in pregnant women at a large tertiary-care facility. Immunohematology. 2013;29:127–30.
7. Urbaniak SJ. Consensus conference on anti-D prophylaxis, April 7 & 8, 1997: final consensus statement. Royal College of Physicians of Edinburgh/Royal College of Obstetricians and Gynaecologists. Transfusion. 1998;38:97–9.
8. ACOG Practice Bulletin No. 192: Management of Alloimmunization during Pregnancy. Obstet Gynecol. 2018;131:e82–90. https://doi.org/10.1097/AOG.0000000000002528.
9. Cannon M, Pierce R, Taber EB, Schucker J. Fatal hydrops fetalis caused by anti-D in a mother with partial D. Obstet Gynecol. 2003;102:1143–5.
10. Sandler SG, Roseff SD, Domen RE, Shaz B, Gottschall JL. Policies and procedures related to testing for weak D phenotypes and administration of Rh immune globulin: results and recommendations related to supplemental questions in the Comprehensive Transfusion Medicine survey of the College of American Pathologists. Arch Pathol Lab Med. 2014;138:620–5.
11. Lo YMD, Tein MSC, Lau TK, Haines CJ, Leung TN, Poon PMK, et al. Quantitative analysis of fetal DNA in maternal plasma and serum: implications for noninvasive prenatal diagnosis. Am J Hum Genet. 1998;62:768–75.
12. Lo YMD, Zhang J, Leung TN, Lau TK, Chang AMZ, Hjelm NM. Rapid clearance of fetal DNA from maternal plasma. Am J Hum Genet. 1999;64:218–24.
13. Nelson M, Eagle C, Langshaw M, Popp H, Kronenberg H. Genotyping fetal DNA by non-invasive means: extraction from maternal plasma. Vox Sang. 2001;80:112–6.
14. Lo Y-M, Bowell PJ, Selinger M, Mackenzie IZ, Chamberlain P, Gillmer MDG, et al. Prenatal determination of fetal RhD status by analysis of peripheral blood of rhesus negative mothers. Lancet. 1993;341:1147–8.
15. Clausen FB, Christiansen M, Steffensen R, Jørgensen S, Nielsen C, Jakobsen MA, et al. Report of the first nationally implemented clinical routine screening for fetal RHD in D− pregnant women to ascertain the requirement for antenatal RhD prophylaxis. Transfusion. 2012;52:752–8.

16. de Haas M, Thurik FF, van der Ploeg CPB, Veldhuisen B, Hirschberg H, Soussan AA, et al. Sensitivity of fetal RHD screening for safe guidance of targeted anti-D immunoglobulin prophylaxis: prospective cohort study of a nationwide programme in The Netherlands. BMJ. 2016;355:i5789.
17. Wikman AT, Tiblad E, Karlsson A, Olsson ML, Westgren M, Reilly M. Noninvasive single-exon fetal RHD determination in a routine screening program in early pregnancy. Obstet Gynecol. 2012;120:227–34.
18. Saramago Goncalves PR, Yang H, Llewellyn A, Palmer SJ, Simmonds MC, Griffin S. High-throughput, non-invasive prenatal testing for fetal RHD genotype to guide antenatal prophylaxis with anti-D immunoglobulin: a cost-effectiveness analysis. BJOG an Int J Obstet Gynaecol. 2018;125:1414–22.
19. Kent J, Farrell A-M, Soothill P. Routine administration of Anti-D: the ethical case for offering pregnant women fetal RHD genotyping and a review of policy and practice. BMC Pregnancy Childbirth. 2014;14:1–4.
20. Teitelbaum L, Metcalfe A, Clarke G, Parboosingh JS, Wilson RD, Johnson JM. Costs and benefits of non-invasive fetal RhD determination. Ultrasound Obstet Gynecol. 2015;45:84–8.
21. Hawk AF, Chang EY, Shields SM, Simpson KN. Costs and clinical outcomes of noninvasive fetal RhD typing for targeted prophylaxis. Obstet Gynecol. 2013;122:579–85.
22. Ma KK, Rodriguez MI, Cheng YW, Norton ME, Caughey AB. Should cell-free DNA testing be used to target antenatal rhesus immune globulin administration? J Matern Neonatal Med. 2016;29:1866–70.
23. Horvath S, Huang Z-Y, Koelper NC, Martinez C, Tsao PY, Zhao L, et al. Induced abortion and the risk of Rh sensitization. JAMA. 2023;330:1167–74.
24. Prabhu M, Louis JM, Kuller JA, Medicine S for M-F, Committee SP. Society for Maternal-Fetal Medicine Statement: RhD immune globulin after spontaneous or induced abortion at less than 12 weeks of gestation. Am J Obstet Gynecol. 2024;230:B2–5.
25. Pollack W, Gorman JG, Hager HJ, Freda VJ, Tripodi D. Antibody-mediated immune suppression to the Rh factor: animal models suggesting mechanism of action. Transfusion. 1968;8:134–45.
26. Goodrick J, Kumpel B, Pamphilon D, Fraser I, Chapman G, Dawes B, et al. Plasma half-lives and bioavailability of human monoclonal Rh D antibodies BRAD-3 and BRAD-5 following intramuscular injection into Rh D-negative volunteers. Clin Exp Immunol. 1994;98:17–20.
27. Ramsey G. Inaccurate doses of Rh immune globulin after Rh-incompatible fetomaternal hemorrhage: survey of laboratory practice. Arch Pathol Lab Med. 2009;133:465–9.
28. Bowman JM. Controversies in Rh prophylaxis: who needs Rh immune globulin and when should it be given? Am J Obstet Gynecol. 1985;151:289–94.
29. Moise KJ Jr, Carpenter RJ Jr. Chorionic villus sampling for Rh typing: clinical implications. Am J Obstet Gynecol. 1993;168:1002–3.
30. Bennett PR, Van Kim CL, Colin Y, Warwick RM, Cherif-Zahar B, Fisk NM, et al. Prenatal determination of fetal RhD type by DNA amplification. N Engl J Med. 1993;329:607–10.
31. Pirelli KJ, Pietz BC, Johnson ST, Pinder HL, Bellissimo DB. Molecular determination of RHD zygosity: predicting risk of hemolytic disease of the fetus and newborn related to anti-D. Prenat Diagn. 2010;30:1207–12.
32. Moise JKJ, Gandhi M, Boring NH, O'Shaughnessy R, Simpson LL, Wolfe HM, et al. Circulating cell-free DNA to determine the fetal RHD status in all three trimesters of pregnancy. Obstet Gynecol. 2016;128:1340–6.
33. Mari G, Deter RL, Carpenter RL, Rahman F, Zimmerman R, Moise KJ Jr, et al. Noninvasive diagnosis by Doppler ultrasonography of fetal anemia due to maternal red-cell alloimmunization. N Engl J Med. 2000;342:9–14.
34. Nicolaides KH, Clewell WH, Mibashan RS, Soothill PW, Rodeck CH, Campbell S. Fetal haemoglobin measurement in the assessment of red cell isoimmunisation. Lancet. 1988;331:1073–5.
35. Copel JA, Grannum PA, Green JJ, Belanger K, Hanna N, Jaffe CC, et al. Fetal cardiac output in the isoimmunized pregnancy: a pulsed Doppler-echocardiographic study of patients undergoing intravascular intrauterine transfusion. Am J Obstet Gynecol. 1989;161:361–5.
36. Bhide A, Acharya G, Baschat A, Bilardo CM, Brezinka C, Cafici D, et al. ISUOG practice guidelines (updated): use of Doppler velocimetry in obstetrics. Ultrasound Obstet Gynecol Off J Int Soc Ultrasound Obstet Gynecol. 2021;58:331–9. https://doi.org/10.1002/uog.23698.
37. Nicolini U, Santolaya J, Ojo OE, Fisk NM, Hubinont C, Tonge M, et al. The fetal intrahepatic umbilical vein as an alternative to cord needling for prenatal diagnosis and therapy. Prenat Diagn. 1988;8:665–71.
38. Zwiers C, Lindenburg ITM, Klumper FJ, De Haas M, Oepkes D, Van Kamp IL. Complications of intrauterine intravascular blood transfusion: lessons learned after 1678 procedures. Ultrasound Obstet Gynecol. 2017;50:180–6.
39. Giannina G, Moise KJ Jr, Dorman K. A simple method to estimate volume for fetal intravascular transfusions. Fetal Diagn Ther. 1998;13:94–7.
40. Dodd JM, Andersen C, Dickinson JE, Louise J, Deussen A, Grivell RM, et al. Fetal middle cerebral artery Doppler to time intrauterine transfusion in red-cell alloimmunization: a randomized

trial. Ultrasound Obstet Gynecol. 2018;51(3):306–12.
41. Trevett TN Jr, Dorman K, Lamvu G, Moise KJ Jr. Antenatal maternal administration of phenobarbital for the prevention of exchange transfusion in neonates with hemolytic disease of the fetus and newborn. Am J Obstet Gynecol. 2005;192:478–82.
42. Moise KJ Jr, Mari G, Fisher DJ, Huhta JC, Cano LE, Carpenter RJ Jr. Acute fetal hemodynamic alterations after intrauterine transfusion for treatment of severe red blood cell alloimmunization. Am J Obstet Gynecol. 1990;163:776–84.
43. Radunovic N, Lockwood CJ, Alvarez M, Plecas D, Chitkara U, Berkowitz RL. The severely anemic and hydropic isoimmune fetus: changes in fetal hematocrit associated with intrauterine death. Obstet Gynecol. 1992;79:390–3.
44. van Kamp IL, Klumper FJCM, Bakkum RSLA, Oepkes D, Meerman RH, Scherjon SA, et al. The severity of immune fetal hydrops is predictive of fetal outcome after intrauterine treatment. Am J Obstet Gynecol. 2001;185:668–73.
45. Klumper FJ, van Kamp IL, Vandenbussche FPHA, Meerman RH, Oepkes D, Scherjon SA, et al. Benefits and risks of fetal red-cell transfusion after 32 weeks gestation. Eur J Obstet Gynecol Reprod Biol. 2000;92:91–6.

Prevention of Intrapartum Neonatal Neurological Injuries

Tim Draycott, Chloe De Souza, and Andrew Demetri

Contents

Y. Yogev, A. Khalil (eds.), *Prevention of Complications in Obstetrics*,
https://doi.org/10.1007/978-3-032-23479-7_19

Learning Objectives

- Describe mechanisms and risk factors for intrapartum neurological injury.
- Apply combined foetal monitoring strategies beyond CTG interpretation.
- Explain prevention and management principles for shoulder dystocia and BPI.
- Recognise IFH, its complications, and evidence-based management manoeuvres.
- Evaluate the value of multidisciplinary simulation training in reducing harm.

19.1 Introduction

Intrapartum neurological injuries, particularly those resulting in hypoxic-ischaemic encephalopathy (HIE) and cerebral palsy, represent some of the most serious complications associated with childbirth, and their prevention is a global priority.

Women [1], their families and insurers [2] value safety in labour the highest. However, multiple national UK investigations have consistently reported that, although the overwhelming majority of births are safe, some births are less safe than they could and should be [3–5]. This observation accurately summarises almost the last century of obstetric care in the UK, and there is a severe danger of admiring the problem rather than acting to prevent avoidable intrapartum harm. Ethnicity and socio-economic background disparities in maternal and perinatal outcomes are particularly concerning and again consistently reported for at least 20 years [6].

The devastating human costs of avoidable intrapartum neurological injury notwithstanding, the NHS paid £2.8 bn on compensation and associated costs in 2023–24, but the 'estimated annual cost of harm' was £5.1 bn [6]. Maternity claims account for 13% of clinical claims but account for 41% of total clinical payments, which equates to £1.2 bn [6], the majority of which are related to avoidable intrapartum neurological injury.

Not all maternity harm is preventable, but the best way to control costs is to improve care so that both patient harm and subsequent litigation are reduced to a minimum. However, maternity safety is a crowded landscape and has not been lacking in initiatives; there have been 15 large national maternity improvement initiatives since 2010 in England alone, but there has been little in the way of improvement and generally poor reporting and evaluation [7]. Furthermore, the current multiplicity of incident investigations does not appear to be improving systemic learning [8–10] nor addressing all the wider needs of families [11] and may even be compounding harm [12]. There is emerging evidence that the use of restorative approaches to healthcare harm might be able to combine the dual needs of learning and improvement with the necessity for healing, as well as mitigating compounded harm and enhancing perceptions of organisational justice [13, 14].

Four foundational principles have been proposed for safer maternity care: dealing with structural problems, a real commitment to learning, learning from high performance, and facilitating system-wide improvements [15], but these general principles are out of the scope of this chapter that will focus on strategies to prevent intrapartum neurological injuries.

Training is a standard recommendation made to prevent intrapartum neurological injuries, and training is a feature of 'good maternity units' [16, 17], but not all training is equal or effective [18]. Effective training to prevent neurological injuries appears to have consistent principles: local, multi-professional and annual for all maternity staff [19]. This chapter will summarise the current strategies for prevention of intrapartum neonatal hypoxic-ischaemic brain injury, neonatal brachial plexus after shoulder dystocia, neonatal injuries after impacted foetal head (IFH) at caesarean birth and neonatal facial nerve palsy, including training.

19.2 Intrapartum Hypoxic-Ischaemic Brain Injury

Intrapartum hypoxic-ischaemic brain injury is one of the most severe neurological complications of childbirth. It occurs when the foetal brain is deprived of adequate oxygen and blood flow during labour and delivery, that results in permanent neurological damage, resulting in cerebral palsy and cognitive impairment. These brain injuries and associated cerebral palsy (CP) are the single largest contributors to litigation costs in England [20] and globally. Furthermore, the consequences for individuals and families can be devastating.

The two main MRI patterns of intrapartum hypoxic-ischaemic neonatal brain injury are chronic partial injury and acute profound injury [21], which have different intrapartum contributions. Approximately 10% of CP is thought to be related to intrapartum causes [22], and more recent exome sequencing studies have identified higher than average rates of pathogenic variants in infants with CP and perinatal asphyxia, suggesting that in this group of individuals with CP, perinatal asphyxia may be secondary to an underlying genetic aetiology [23].

19.2.1 Electronic Foetal Monitoring and Prevention

Although electronic foetal monitoring has been in clinical use for more than 30 years, its role in reducing hypoxic-ischaemic encephalopathy (HIE) and CP has been disappointing [21]. Computerised cardiotocographs (CTGs) have not improved outcomes [24], and neither has an increasing intrapartum intervention rate (▶ https://www.rcog.org.uk/about-us/quality-improvement-clinical-audit-and-research-projects/national-maternity-and-perinatal-audit-nmpa/). Finally, a population-level study in Norway concluded that there was no evidence that the introduction of STAN contributed to changes in the rates of stillbirths, neonatal deaths, intrapartum caesarean births, or instrumental vaginal deliveries, and there was an association between the introduction of STAN and a small increase in neonates with low Apgar scores [25].

However, new insights into intrapartum foetal monitoring may result in improved practice and outcomes. The impact of training for foetal monitoring on maternal and neonatal outcomes is limited with inconsistent effects [26], and a systems approach may be required [27] rather than the current focus on the CTG trace. CTG monitoring is an inherently collective and sociotechnical practice. Improving it will require accounting for complex system interdependencies, rather than focusing solely on discrete factors such as individual technical proficiency in interpreting trace [28].

Furthermore, there are four risk factors, including suspicion of foetal growth restriction, maternal pyrexia and presence of meconium, which are implicated in poor birth outcomes in addition to CTGs, and these risk factors should be included in the assessment of intrapartum foetal wellbeing [29]. This approach has been summarised by the Avoiding Brain Injury in Childbirth (ABC) collaboration and in the most recent NHS intrapartum foetal monitoring guidance. We should be asking the question 'is the baby OK', rather than 'is the CTG OK'? This approach has been incorporated into a new intrapartum tool for national implementation in England. Similar combined approaches have been proposed in the United States (US) [30].

19.3 Shoulder Dystocia and Associated Neurological Injuries

Shoulder dystocia is defined as a vaginal cephalic birth that requires additional obstetric manoeuvres to release the impacted shoulder after the head has been born, and routine traction employed to deliver a foetus without shoulder dystocia has failed [31]. An objective diagnosis of a prolonged head-to-body delivery time of more than 60 seconds has also been proposed [32, 33], but these data are often not routinely collected.

Neonatal hypoxic-ischaemic morbidity associated with shoulder dystocia is rare but increasingly being recognised [34]. The risk of hypoxia appears to be related to the duration of the head-body delivery interval (HBDI): the risk of HIE for HBDI less than 5 min was 0.5%, compared with 23.5% for HBDI more than 5 min ($P < 0.001$) [35].

Brachial plexus injury (BPI) refers to damage to a complex network of peripheral nerves located in the cervical neck, originating from spinal nerve roots C5 to T1, that innervate the muscles and skin of the shoulder, arm and hand. This results in disruption to the motor and sensory function of the affected limb. Injury to the upper trunk of the brachial plexus (C5-C6) can lead to Erb's palsy, which causes impaired functions of the muscles innervated by the roots.

BPI is one of the most important foetal complications of shoulder dystocia, complicating 2.3–16% of births complicated by [36–39]. Most cases resolve without permanent disability, with fewer than 10% resulting in permanent brachial plexus dysfunction [40]. A comprehensive summary of over 17 million births [41] demonstrated that the rate of neonatal BPI internationally was 1.4 per 1000 total births, and this rate has decreased to 0.5 per 1000 births for the most recent publications. The likelihood of permanent BPI (lasting more than 12 months) was 10–18% in the US-based reports and 19–23% in countries outside the US. A recent national study from Sweden reported a significant decrease in BPI from 3.1 per 1000 births in 1997 to 1.0 per 1000 births in 2019 despite an increase in the incidence of shoulder dystocia between 2005 and 2019 [42].

Neonatal BPI lasting more than 12 months has a significant effect on the affected individuals and their families: the overall mean utility scores, used to generate quality of life years (QALY) scores, for affected adults and parents of children with BPI were 0.56 and 0.80, respectively [43].

Neonatal BPI is the most common cause for litigation related to shoulder dystocia and one of the most frequently litigated obstetric-related complications in the UK [20].

19.3.1 Prevention of Shoulder Dystocia

Shoulder dystocia is difficult to predict and therefore difficult to prevent [31], and untargeted delivery by caesarean section is not a useful strategy to prevent shoulder dystocia [31].

However, foetal macrosomia (>4 kg) is associated with significantly increased risks of maternal and neonatal complications, including shoulder dystocia, brachial plexus injury and obstetric anal sphincter injury (OASI). Macrosomic babies are also at increased risk of perinatal hypoxia [44, 45].

After 37 weeks of gestation, the options available to prevent shoulder dystocia in infants with an EFW predicted to be more than 4000 g include early induction of labour (IOL) and planned caesarean birth, but these options have consequences and should be balanced against the current lack of accurate prediction of macrosomia in clinical practice, particularly the measurement of SFH [46].

There are differences between the options/modes of birth available for foetal macrosomia, and it is important to appreciate that a caesarean birth is not without consequence. The NICE caesarean guideline [47] reports the different risks and benefits of caesarean vs vaginal birth, and the risks of caesarean were identified in a national leaflet [48].

IOL prior to term for foetal macrosomia has been demonstrated to reduce the risk of shoulder dystocia by 40%, although no effect on neonatal outcomes was identified. There was a threefold increase in the rate of severe perineal tears in the IOL group in the last systematic review [49]. However, a recent UK study has reported no differences in perineal injury with early IOL, but again, there was no improvement in neonatal outcomes [50], and planned caesarean may be cost-saving [51].

19.3.2 Training

A reduction in injury rates has been associated with an increase in correctly managed cases of shoulder dystocia [39], ideally in the order of the RCOG algorithm [52].

Training for the management of shoulder dystocia has been associated with reductions in both HIE and BPI [39], and performance is improved for at least 12 months [53]. There were no permanent BPI at all after shoulder dystocia for more than 17,000 consecutive births (562 births complicated by shoulder dystocia) [54]. This improvement after training has been replicated in the USA [55, 56], Sweden [57], Finland [58], Germany [59, 60] and Spain [61].

NHS Resolution has published a small series of infants with hypoxic brain injuries following shoulder dystocia, with a median HBDI of seven minutes. It is likely that a more effective and efficient execution of the release manoeuvres would reduce the HBDI [31, 62], thereby reducing the risk of hypoxic brain injury.

Effective training for shoulder dystocia is cost-effective with cost savings of more than £1 million per quality-adjusted life year (QALY) saved [63].

Despite the similarity of the manoeuvres taught, not all training for shoulder dystocia is equal or effective in improving outcomes [18, 64–67]. A systematic review of interventions to decrease the complications after shoulder dystocia concluded that training was associated with decreases in the rate of BPI after shoulder dystocia [64].

The current RCOG guideline for shoulder dystocia [31] recommends that all staff should be trained locally and annually and provided with the opportunity to practice all the manoeuvres required to release the shoulder impaction using a high-fidelity model with a multi-professional team.

19.4 Impacted Foetal Head: Skull Fracture and Intracranial Haemorrhage

Impacted foetal head (IFH) at caesarean birth is an unpredictable and challenging obstetric emergency [68, 69] that most obstetricians, responding to a national survey, would define as 'the need for additional manoeuvres' at caesarean [4]. IFH has therefore been described as 'a caesarean birth where the obstetrician is unable to deliver the foetal head with their usual delivering hand, and additional manoeuvres and/or tocolysis are required to disimpact and deliver the head' [70].

IFH and its complications are being encountered more frequently by healthcare professionals [34, 69, 71]. Recent single-centre, UK studies estimate that IFH may complicate as many as 1 in 10 unplanned caesarean births (1.5% of all births) [69] and 16% of second stage caesarean births [72]. However, IFH is a more heterogeneous condition than previously thought, and >50% complicate caesareans in the first stage of labour [69].

19.4.1 Complications

IFH at caesarean is associated with potentially devastating consequences for both mother and baby. Difficulty disimpacting the foetal head, with a stretched and oedematous uterine lower segment, increases the risk of extension of the uterine incision, haemorrhage, bladder and ureteric injury [73].

Neonatal trauma includes skull fractures, subgaleal and intracranial haemorrhage, and/or delay in the birth of an already compromised foetus can result in hypoxic-ischaemic encephalopathy and, rarely, perinatal death [72, 74, 75].

There has been a sharp increase in reports of perinatal brain injury associated with IFH, prompting numerous coronial enquiries [17] and increased litigation both nationally [19] and internationally [21]. The NHS Resolution Early Notification Scheme identified IFH as a contributory factor in nearly 10% of potentially the most expensive maternity claims from 2018 [6], almost twice as common as those relating to shoulder dystocia [6].

19.4.2 Prevention

There is no useful prediction or prevention strategy for IFH at CS [69]. The foetal pillow has been proposed as an option to prevent IFH, but the foetal pillow is only licensed for caesarean at full cervical dilatation [68], and two of the largest randomised control trials reporting positive effects have recently been withdrawn by the publishing journals after concerns about scientific integrity were raised. A subsequent systematic review has concluded that a foetal pillow does not improve maternal or neonatal outcomes and should only be used in the context of a research trial [73].

19.4.3 Management

When an IFH is encountered, the obstetrician should first identify the lateral space to introduce their hand below the foetal head to flex and elevate it to the incision (abdominal cephalic disimpaction). This approach is likely to be effective in most cases [69].

The UK national Scientific Impact Paper (SIP) for IFH [70] and several other techniques are described to manage an IFH:

- Push technique: the assistant inserts a hand into the vagina to elevate the head [76].
- Pull technique, or reverse breech extraction: the operator grasps one or both foetal legs from the upper segment, delivering them through the uterine incision [77, 78].

A training programme has been developed by the PROMPT Maternity Foundation (▶ www.promptmaternity.org) with further materials and training developed by the ABC Collaboration (▶ https://www.gov.uk/government/news/new-nhs-programme-to-reduce-brain-injury-in-childbirth-trialled) for national implementation and evaluation using a dedicated core data set.

It is anticipated that this training will reduce neonatal neurological injury associated with IFH in a similar way that the introduction of training for shoulder dystocia has done.

19.5 Facial Nerve Palsy

Neonatal facial nerve palsy is a neurological condition characterised by partial or complete dysfunction of the facial nerve (cranial nerve VII) that impairs the muscles of facial expression and can also affect parasympathetic and sensory functions.

Facial nerve palsy can also occur during spontaneous vaginal birth, but this is less common than with forceps. Injury can occur when the forceps blade causes mechanical trauma to the nerve during passage through the birth canal, through compression or traction. The facial nerve exits through the stylomastoid foramen in the skull and passes over the parotid region, which is the region the forceps cover during assisted birth. Due to the lack of mature muscle development in the baby's face and minimal soft tissue protection, this means that the nerve is particularly vulnerable in neonates. Transient facial nerve palsy is a recognised complication of forceps application during assisted vaginal birth [79, 80].

19.5.1 Prevention

The facial nerve may be more susceptible to injury if the forceps blades are applied asymmetrically or with excessive pressure. Correct forceps application and technique are important to all forceps-expedited births; however, facial nerve palsies do not seem to be related to obstetric volume [81]. Therefore, it is unlikely that poor performance or inexperience significantly increases the risk of injury, and these neurological injuries may not be preventable despite optimal care.

19.6 Summary

This chapter discusses intrapartum neurological injuries that represent some of the most serious complications associated with childbirth. Such injuries can result in lifelong disability, placing significant emotional and financial burdens on families and healthcare systems as well as contributing significantly to litigation costs in England.

Although it is not always possible to predict or prevent injuries, all healthcare professionals involved in intrapartum care should understand the types of neurological injuries that may occur and ways to mitigate these where possible. Enhanced education for all maternity staff, including simulation-based training, may improve clinical performance and reduce injury rates.

Overall, the chapter highlights the complexities of intrapartum neurological injuries and that preventative measures may help to both safeguard outcomes for babies and their families and ensure the sustainability of maternity services.

Chapter Key Points

- Intrapartum neurological injuries contribute disproportionately to long-term morbidity and litigation.
- Effective prevention requires systems-based foetal monitoring and integration of additional risk factors beyond CTG.
- Shoulder dystocia-related neurological injury correlates strongly with head-to-body interval; efficient manoeuvres reduce risk.
- Impacted foetal head at caesarean is increasingly recognised and lacks reliable prediction; training improves safety.
- Simulation-based, local, multidisciplinary training significantly reduces HIE, BPI, and perinatal trauma.

Chapter-End Summary

Intrapartum neurological injuries such as HIE, BPI, and trauma from impacted foetal head remain major contributors to long-term disability and maternity litigation. Prevention depends on integrating foetal reserve and intrapartum risk factors, prompt recognition of emergencies, and execution of evidence-based manoeuvres. High-fidelity, multidisciplinary simulation training consistently reduces neurological injury rates. While some injuries cannot be predicted, systemic improvements in monitoring, early escalation, and structured team responses improve neonatal outcomes and maternity safety.

References

1. Kingdon C, Neilson J, Singleton V, Gyte G, Hart A, Gabbay M, Lavender T. Choice and birth method: mixed-method study of caesarean delivery for maternal request. British Journal of Obstetrics & Gynaecology. 2009;116(7):886–95.
2. NHS Litigation Authority. Ten years of maternity claims: an analysis of NHS litigation authority data. London: NHS Litigation Authority; 2012.
3. Kings Fund. Safe births: everybody's business. An independent inquiry into the safety of maternity services in England. London: Kings Fund; 2008.
4. CESDI. Confidential Enquiry into stillbirths and deaths in infancy, 7th annual report. London: CESDI; 2000. p. 106.
5. Ockenden D. Findings, conclusions and essential actions from the independent review of maternity services at the Shrewsbury and Telford Hospital NHS Trust 2022. Department of Health: Gov.UK. p. 1–235.
6. Allison Felker RP, Kotnis R, Kenyon S, Knight M, On behalf of MBRRACE-UK, editors. Saving lives, improving mothers' care compiled report – lessons learned to inform maternity care from the UK and Ireland confidential enquiries into maternal deaths and morbidity 2020–22. Oxford: National Perinatal Epidemiology Unit, University of Oxford; 2024.
7. McGowan J, et al. Quality and reporting of large-scale improvement programmes: a review of maternity initiatives in the English NHS, 2010–2023. BMJ Qual Saf. 2024;
8. Wears R, Sutcliffe K. Still not safe: Patient safety and the middle-managing of American medicine. New York: Oxford Press; 2019.

9. Macrae C. The problem with incident reporting. BMJ Qual Saf. 2015;25:71–5. https://doi.org/10.1136/bmjqs-2015-004732.
10. Walshe K, Higgins J. The use and impact of inquiries in the NHS. British Medical Journal. 2002;325:895–900.
11. Sibley M. Ockenden report: the refusal of our healthcare service to take patient experience seriously. BMJ. 2022;377:o875.
12. Wailling J, et al. Humanizing harm: using a restorative approach to heal and learn from adverse events. Health Expect. 2022;25(4):1192–9.
13. Mannat J, et al. Restorative just culture: a study of the practical and economic effects of implementing restorative justice in an NHS trust. MATEC Web Conf. 2019;273(01007)
14. Wailling J, Wilkinson J, Marshall C. Healing after harm: an evaluation of a restorative approach for addressing harm from surgical mesh. Kia ora te tangata: He arotakenga i te whakahaumanu. Wellington: The Diana Unwin Chair in Restorative Justice, Victoria University of Wellington; 2020.
15. Yau CWH, et al. Clinical negligence costs: taking action to safeguard NHS sustainability. BMJ. 2020;368:m552.
16. Liberati EG, et al. Seven features of safety in maternity units: a framework based on multisite ethnography and stakeholder consultation. BMJ Qual Saf; 2020.
17. Liberati EG, et al. How to be a very safe maternity unit: an ethnographic study. Soc Sci Med. 2019;223:64–72.
18. Draycott T. Not all training for obstetric emergencies is equal, or effective. BJOG. 2017;124(4):651.
19. Siassakos D, et al. The active components of effective training in obstetric emergencies. BJOG. 2009;116(8):1028–32.
20. Resolution N. Annual report and accounts 2020/21. London: NHS Resolution: HMSO; 2021. p. 1–168.
21. Leung TY, Chung TK. Severe chronic morbidity following childbirth. Best Pract Res Clin Obstet Gynaecol. 2009;23(3):401–23.
22. Cowan F, et al. Origin and timing of brain lesions in term infants with neonatal encephalopathy. Lancet. 2003;361(9359):736–42.
23. Wang Y, et al. Exome sequencing reveals genetic heterogeneity and clinically actionable findings in children with cerebral palsy. Nat Med. 2024;30(5):1395–405.
24. Brocklehurst P, et al. The INFANT trial. Lancet. 2017;390(10089):28.
25. Blix E, et al. The impact of the introduction of intrapartum fetal ECG ST segment analysis. A population study. Acta Obstet Gynecol Scand. 2022;101(7):809–18.
26. Kelly S, et al. Training in the use of intrapartum electronic fetal monitoring with cardiotocography: systematic review and meta-analysis. BJOG. 2021;
27. Kelly S, et al. Influences on safety of intrapartum electronic fetal heart rate monitoring practices: a scoping review. BMJ Open. 2024;14(12):e085827.
28. Lame G, et al. Why is safety in intrapartum electronic fetal monitoring so hard? A qualitative study combining human factors/ergonomics and social science analysis. BMJ Qual Saf. 2023;
29. Jindal S, et al. Risk factors for a serious adverse outcome in neonates: a retrospective cohort study of vaginal births. BJOG. 2023;130(12):1521–30.
30. Evans MI, et al. Improving the interpretation of electronic fetal monitoring: the fetal reserve index. Am J Obstet Gynecol. 2023;228(5S):S1129–43.
31. Crofts J, Fox R, Draycott T. Shoulder dystocia. In: RCOG, editor. Greentop guidelines. London: RCOG; 2012. p. 1–18.
32. Spong CY, et al. An objective definition of shoulder dystocia: prolonged head-to-body delivery intervals and/or the use of ancillary obstetric maneuvers. Obstet Gynecol. 1995;86(3):433–6.
33. Beall MH, et al. Objective definition of shoulder dystocia: a prospective evaluation. Am J Obstetr Gynecol. 1998;179(4):934–7.
34. Resolution N. Early notification scheme – year 1. London: NHS Resolution; 2019.
35. Leung TY, et al. Head-to-body delivery interval and risk of fetal acidosis and hypoxic ischaemic encephalopathy in shoulder dystocia: a retrospective review. BJOG. 2011;118(4):474–9.
36. Gherman RB, et al. The McRoberts' maneuver for the alleviation of shoulder dystocia: how successful is it? Am J Obstet Gynecol. 1997;176(3):656–61.
37. Gherman RB, Ouzounian JG, Goodwin TM. Obstetric maneuvers for shoulder dystocia and associated fetal morbidity. Am J Obstet Gynecol. 1998;178(6):1126–30.
38. Acker DB, Sachs BP, Friedman EA. Risk factors for shoulder dystocia. Obstet Gynecol. 1985;66(6):762–8.
39. Draycott TJ, et al. Improving neonatal outcome through practical shoulder dystocia training. Obstet Gynecol. 2008;112(1):14–20.
40. Gherman RB, et al. Spontaneous vaginal delivery: a risk factor for Erb's palsy? Am J Obstet Gynecol. 1998;178(3):423–7.
41. Chauhan SP, Blackwell SB, Ananth CV. Neonatal brachial plexus palsy: incidence, prevalence, and temporal trends. Semin Perinatol. 2014;38(4):210–8.
42. Mollberg M, et al. Increased incidence of shoulder dystocia but a declining incidence of obstetric brachial plexus palsy in vaginally delivered infants. Acta Obstet Gynecol Scand. 2023;102(1):76–81.
43. Yau CWH, et al. Obstetric brachial plexus injuries (OBPIs): health-related quality of life in affected adults and parents. Health Qual Life Outcomes. 2018;16(1):212.

44. Gillean JR, et al. Big infants in the neonatal intensive care unit. Am J Obstet Gynecol. 2005;192(6):1948–53. discussion 1953–5
45. Wang D, et al. Risk factors and outcomes of macrosomia in China: a multicentric survey based on birth data. J Matern Fetal Neonatal Med. 2017;30(5):623–7.
46. Sparks TN, et al. Fundal height: a useful screening tool for fetal growth? J Matern Fetal Neonatal Med. 2011;24(5):708–12.
47. NICE. Caesarean Section – clinical guideline. London: National Collaborating Centre for Women's and Children's Health; 2004. p. 1–98.
48. RCOG. Choosing to have a caesarean section. London: RCOG; 2015. p. 1–6.
49. Boulvain M, et al. Induction of labour at or near term for suspected fetal macrosomia. Cochrane Database Syst Rev (Online). 2016;5:CD000938.
50. Gardosi J, et al. Induction of labour versus standard care to prevent shoulder dystocia in fetuses suspected to be large for gestational age in the UK (the Big Baby trial): a multicentre, open-label, randomised controlled trial. Lancet. 2025;
51. Naghdi S, et al. Is it cost-effective to induce labour early to prevent shoulder dystocia? Evidence From the Big Baby Trial. BJOG; 2025.
52. Draycott T, Fox R, Montague I. RCOG Greentop guideline 42: shoulder dystocia. London: RCOG; 2005. p. 1–13.
53. Crofts JF, et al. Management of shoulder dystocia: skill retention 6 and 12 months after training. Obstet Gynecol. 2007;110(5):1069–74.
54. Crofts JF, et al. Prevention of brachial plexus injury-12 years of shoulder dystocia training: an interrupted time-series study. BJOG. 2016;123(1):111–8.
55. Weiner C, Samuelson L, Collins L. 61: 5-year experience with PROMP (PRactical Obstetric Multidisciplinary Training) reveals sustained and progressive improvements in obstetric outcomes at a US hospital. Am J Obstet Gynecol. 2014;210:S40.
56. Grunebaum A, Chervenak F, Skupski D. Effect of a comprehensive obstetric patient safety program on compensation payments and sentinel events. Am J Obstet Gynecol. 2011;204(2):97–105.
57. Dahlberg J, et al. Ten years of simulation-based shoulder dystocia training- impact on obstetric outcome, clinical management, staff confidence, and the pedagogical practice – a time series study. BMC Pregnancy Childbirth. 2018;18(1):1021–8.
58. Kaijomaa M, et al. Impact of simulation training on the management of shoulder dystocia and incidence of permanent brachial plexus birth injury: an observational study. BJOG. 2022;
59. Papageorgiou S, et al. Impact of introducing PROMPT on permanent brachial plexus injury and tears III degrees/IV degrees in shoulder dystocia: the Hanover Cohort Study. Obstet Gynecol Int. 2024;2024:8712553.
60. Sargut TA, Ferdowssian K, Mark-Sargut CS, Huscher D, Alsolivany J, Früh A, Bahm J, Thomale U, Dengler NF. Epidemiology and surgical management of obstetric brachial plexus injury: a national cohort study. J Neurosurg Pediatr. 2025;36(1):119–26.
61. López RS, et al. Incidencia de parálisis braquial obstétrica tras programa de entrenamiento en distocia de hombros. Anales de Pediatría; 2022.
62. Johansen LT, et al. How common is substandard obstetric care in adverse events of birth asphyxia, shoulder dystocia and postpartum hemorrhage? Findings from an external inspection of Norwegian maternity units. Acta Obstet Gynecol Scand. 2021;100(1):139–46.
63. Yau CWH, et al. A model-based cost-utility analysis of multi-professional simulation training in obstetric emergencies. PLoS One. 2021;16(3):e0249031.
64. Wagner SM, et al. Interventions to decrease complications after shoulder dystocia: a systematic review and Bayesian meta-analysis. Am J Obstet Gynecol. 2021;
65. MacKenzie IZ, et al. Management of shoulder dystocia: trends in incidence and maternal and neonatal morbidity. Obstet Gynecol. 2007;110(5):1059–68. https://doi.org/10.1097/01.AOG.0000287615.35425.5c.
66. Johnson GJ, et al. Pathophysiologic origins of brachial plexus injury. Obstet Gynecol. 2020;136(4):725–30.
67. Draycott T, et al. Myths and realities of training in obstetric emergencies. Best Pract Res Clin Obstet Gynaecol. 2015;29(8):1067–76.
68. Cornthwaite KR, et al. Management of impacted fetal head at cesarean delivery. Am J Obstet Gynecol. 2024;230(3S):S980–7.
69. Cornthwaite K, et al. Impacted fetal head: a retrospective cohort study of emergency caesarean section. Eur J Obstet Gynecol Reprod Biol. 2021;261:85–91.
70. Cornthwaite K, et al. Management of impacted fetal head at caesarean birth: scientific impact paper no. 73. BJOG. 2023;130(12):e40–64.
71. Rice A, et al. The impacted foetal head at caesarean section: incidence and techniques used in a single UK institution. J Obstetr Gynaecol. 2019;10:1–4.
72. Jones NW, et al. Impacted fetal head during second stage Caesarean birth: a prospective observational study. Eur J Obstetr Gynecol Reprod Biol. 2022;272:77–81.
73. Cornthwaite K, et al. Management of impacted fetal head at cesarean birth: a systematic review and meta-analysis. Acta Obstet Gynecol Scand. 2024;103(9):1702–13.
74. Steer PJ. Is a fractured skull discovered in the neonate after caesarean section delivery always evidence of negligence? BJOG. 2016;123(3):336.

75. Tan EK. Difficult caesarean delivery of an impacted head and neonatal skull fracture: can the morbidity be avoided? J Obstetr Gynaecol. 2007;27(4):427–8.
76. Landesman R, Graber EA. Abdominovaginal delivery: modification of the cesarean section operation to facilitate delivery of the impacted head. Am J Obstet Gynecol. 1984;148(6):707–10.
77. Berhan Y, Berhan A. A meta-analysis of reverse breech extraction to deliver a deeply impacted head during cesarean delivery. Int J Gynaecol Obstet. 2014;124(2):99–105.
78. Schwake D, Petchenkin L, Younis JS. Reverse breech extraction in cases of second stage caesarean section. J Obstet Gynaecol. 2012;32(6):548–51.
79. Murphy DJ, et al. Assisted vaginal birth: green-top guideline no. 26. BJOG. 2020;127(9):e70–e112.
80. Stock SJ, et al. Maternal and neonatal outcomes of successful Kielland's rotational forceps delivery. Obstetr Gynecol. 2013;121(5):1032–9.
81. Miller ES, et al. Association between obstetrician forceps volume and maternal and neonatal outcomes. Obstetr Gynecol. 2014:1.

AI and Big Data in Obstetrics

Lee Reicher, Liron Zahavi, and Eran Segal

Contents

Y. Yogev, A. Khalil (eds.), *Prevention of Complications in Obstetrics*,
https://doi.org/10.1007/978-3-032-23479-7_20

Learning Objectives

- Explain core AI concepts relevant to obstetrics (ML, DL, supervised/unsupervised).
- Identify major data sources used in perinatal big-data research.
- Describe AI applications in risk prediction, imaging, and fetal monitoring.
- Evaluate strengths and limitations of AI models in clinical obstetrics.
- Discuss ethical and regulatory considerations for AI deployment.

As part of this chapter, we explore how large datasets (often referred to as "big data") and artificial intelligence (AI) are revolutionizing the field of medicine and how increasingly important a role they will play within the specific context of perinatal care. As we stand on the threshold of a new era in healthcare, driven by technological innovation, this chapter aims to provide a comprehensive exploration of how these advancements are shaping perinatal medicine, enhancing outcomes for mothers and their newborns, and introducing new paradigms in obstetrics.

What You Will Learn in This Chapter

1. Introduction to AI and big data in healthcare: Understand the fundamental concepts of AI and big data analytics, their significance in healthcare, and how they're being utilized to interpret complex datasets, uncover hidden patterns, and inform clinical decisions with high precision.
2. Big data in perinatal medicine: The chapter covers the extensive variety of data generated during pregnancy—from genetics and ultrasound images to electronic health records and continuous monitoring during labor.
3. AI applications in perinatal medicine: Discover how AI and big data analytics are specifically applied in perinatal medicine, enhancing the ability to predict, diagnose, and manage pregnancy-related complications. Learn about the technologies enabling personalized care plans and how they contribute to the formulation of predictive, personalized, and preventative strategies.
4. Limitations and ethical considerations: Explore the challenges to the widespread adoption of these technologies, including data privacy concerns, the need for interoperability, and the ethical implications of AI in healthcare.

By the end of this chapter, readers will have a comprehensive overview of the current state and future potential of AI and big data in perinatal medicine. Equipped with this knowledge, healthcare professionals, researchers, and policymakers will be better positioned to navigate the challenges, leverage the opportunities, and contribute to the ongoing evolution of obstetrics in modern times.

20.1 Introduction to AI and Big Data in Healthcare

The term "big data" is often used to describe high volumes of data with complex relationships, which are not well-suited to traditional databases and analytic methods. PubMed searches on "big data" have revealed a rapid increase in articles in the field over the last decade, from nine articles in 2011 to over 5000 in 2023.

Big data in healthcare spans a diverse array of data types, each crucial for advancing medical research and improving patient care. Genomic data are essential for personalizing medicine by identifying genetic predispositions and tailoring treatments to individual genetic profiles [6]. Beyond genomics, omics sciences like proteomics, metabolomics, and transcriptomics provide insights at various molecular levels, supporting the development of specific medical interventions [17]. Electronic Health Records (EHRs) contain detailed records of patient encounters, including medical history and treatment outcomes, which are critical for clinical research and improving health services [11]. Physiological monitoring data from systems like electronic fetal monitors are vital for real-time decision-making in acute care [2]. Clinical laboratory quantification of biomarkers is essential for diagnosing conditions and monitoring treatments. Imaging data from techniques like X-rays and MRI scans are crucial for diagnostics and treatment planning [15]. Administrative and claims data from healthcare billing and logistics inform health services research and cost analysis [9]. Together, these data types are necessary for complex analyses that allow for more precise interventions and a deeper understanding of complex disorders [8]. The ability to aggregate and analyze these data with AI technologies can uncover hidden patterns, correlations, and insights that are otherwise unattainable.

The digitalization of healthcare and the rise of high-throughput omic technologies are generating a data avalanche in healthcare. As the amount of data collected and analyzed universally grows, researchers have developed improved tools to manage, store, and analyze data efficiently. These technologies are particularly important in medicine, where they help in the discovery of complex patterns and relationships in the vast amounts of data from various sources. Artificial intelligence (AI) is a broad field in computer science aimed at creating systems capable of performing tasks that would typically require human intelligence. These tasks include decision-making, pattern recognition, natural language understanding, and solving problems. In the context of healthcare, AI can be seen as the overarching technology that encompasses machine learning and deep learning.

Machine learning is a fundamental technology in data science that depends on having high-quality data, clearly defining the problem, and establishing methods for its evaluation. It uses computers to find patterns and relationships in data automatically. Instead of being programmed with specific instructions to perform a task, machine learning systems learn from the data they are given. This is like teaching the computer to recognize patterns by showing it many examples, rather than telling it what to specifically look for. Machine learning models can be divided into two main types: supervised and unsupervised learning. In supervised learning, the model is trained on data that is already labeled and is tested for its ability to assign the same types of labels to unseen samples. For example, it can be given X-rays that were interpreted by doctors along with the diagnosed diseases and learn to identify diseases in future X-rays on its own. Unsupervised learning, on the other hand, involves teaching the computer to find patterns and relationships in data without any preexisting labels. This could be like asking the computer to sort different types of imaging into groups without telling it what the groups represent. This can be useful, for example, to discover subtypes of a disease—without prior knowledge of what may characterize them.

Deep learning is a more advanced type of machine learning. Deep learning models, also termed “neural networks,” process data through algorithmic layers in a way that mimics how humans think and learn, making them particularly good at tasks such as recognizing speech, images, or complex patterns in data. The “depth” of these models, representing the numerous stages of computations applied to the data, requires more computational resources and bigger datasets to train and allows the discovery of more complex structures. For instance, deep learning has been used to automatically identify whether a tumor in a medical image is benign or malignant, based on many layers of processing.

These technologies, which are rapidly improving and becoming more prevalent and accessible, are transforming how medical research is done. They make it possible to handle and analyze the large volumes of data that modern healthcare generates, leading to better disease prediction, diagnosis, and treatment.

The integration of deep learning and AI into healthcare applications capitalizes on the extensive data related to medical conditions and diseases. This integration assists models in the crucial phases of execution or diagnosis, where precision and accuracy are paramount. For example, in the realm of cardiovascular care, the amalgamation of advanced imaging techniques with exhaustive eHealth records and pathology data facilitates a more detailed disease characterization [4]. This, in turn, leads to the formulation of personalized treatment plans tailored to the individual needs of patients. Similarly, the field of oncology has seen significant advancements through the application of AI and deep learning [7]. Enhanced understanding of tumor biology, achieved through state-of-the-art imaging and clinical research, supports the development of more effective precision medicine strategies. These strategies are revolutionizing cancer treatment, offering hope for better outcomes.

The transformation brought about by AI and big data in healthcare extends beyond mere technological advancement; it marks a paradigm shift towards more predictive, personalized, and preventative care. The potential of these technologies to analyze and interpret the complexities of vast datasets is not only optimizing treatment strategies but also redefining the possibilities within preventive medicine. As we delve into the specifics of perinatal medicine, the applications of AI and big data highlight a proactive approach to healthcare. By harnessing these technologies, the healthcare sector is moving towards a future where early detection, accurate diagnosis, and customized care plans become the standard, ensuring better health outcomes for mothers and their newborns.

20.2 Big Data in Perinatal Medicine

In the field of perinatal medicine, big data is becoming an invaluable resource for deepening our understanding of obstetric-related complications, many of which, like preeclampsia and spontaneous preterm birth, have complex and not fully understood causes. Perinatal medicine is particularly suited to leveraging big data, since a broad range of data types is generated during pregnancy and childbirth. Pregnant women undergo numerous screening tests, providing a wealth of data that can be analyzed for insights into maternal and fetal health. Genetic profiling can help identify markers associated with higher risks of certain pregnancy-related conditions, offering new insights into genetic predispositions for diseases like preeclampsia [18]. Ultrasound imaging is routinely performed at several stages of pregnancy, offering detailed visual data on fetal development and maternal health. These images can be analyzed to detect anomalies, track growth, and make informed predictions about potential complications [5]. Electronic Health Records (EHRs) are comprehensive sources that document every test, result, diagnosis, and treatment throughout pregnancy, creating a longitudinal health record for both mother and child [19]. The array of tests that pregnant women undergo—ranging from blood tests to glucose challenges and beyond—adds to this dataset, providing multiple points of data across the pregnancy timeline. During labor and delivery, the amount of data collected increases significantly. Every aspect of the delivery room is carefully recorded, from the length of labor to the specifics of medication administration and the monitoring of the mother's vital signs. Fetal monitoring provides continuous data streams during the later stages of pregnancy and labor, offering critical insights into the well-being of the fetus. Additionally, postnatal data continues to add to this rich dataset, including newborn screening results and postpartum health assessments of the mother. Finally, large-scale research databases and registries collect data on thousands of pregnancies, helping in the study of less common conditions and the effectiveness of different treatment approaches across diverse populations.

Traditionally, these types of data are used for immediate interpretation by physicians to make real-time decisions regarding the health of both mother and baby during labor and delivery. Historically, these valuable data streams—ranging from fetal heart rates to complex screening tests—were not systematically collected for any use beyond immediate clinical needs. However, there is a growing realization that these data can be preserved and analyzed later to extract deeper insights. With advancements in data analytics tools and increasing awareness of their potential, the practice of archiving and retrospectively analyzing data is becoming more common. This shift allows for the development of richer, data-driven understandings of labor patterns, complications, and outcomes.

Each type of data plays a crucial role in creating a detailed picture of maternal and child health. With the aggregation and analysis of these varied data types, researchers and clinicians can gain unprecedented insights into the complex dynamics of pregnancy and childbirth. This allows for enhanced predictive models, improved risk assessments, and more personalized approaches to care, ultimately leading to better outcomes for both mothers and their babies. Such extensive data collection and analysis underscore the unique position of perinatal medicine in the context of big data applications, highlighting its potential to transform maternal and fetal health outcomes significantly.

The vast array of data sources highlights the complexity and sheer volume of data collected, which requires sophisticated analytical tools for effective handling and interpretation. AI is particularly adept at managing these challenges, offering advanced data analysis capabilities that can identify patterns and insights beyond the reach of traditional methods.

20.3 AI Applications in Perinatal Medicine

The integration of AI into perinatal medicine is changing the landscape of maternal and fetal healthcare. Machine learning models are revolutionizing obstetric care, enhancing the ability of healthcare professionals to predict, diagnose, and manage pregnancy complications with unprecedented precision. There is a growing body of evidence that the application of machine learning in obstetrics has the potential to significantly enhance patient care.

20.3.1 AI for Risk Prediction in Pregnancy Complications

AI's capacity to detect hidden patterns in vast datasets has made it an invaluable tool for predicting pregnancy complications, offering a proactive approach to perinatal care. Early screening in pregnancy facilitates interventions that can reduce disease risks significantly [3]. Traditional scoring systems, which have not been regularly updated to reflect current research or population changes [13], are now being supplemented by machine learning algorithms. These algorithms utilize electronic health records and data from digital devices to better stratify patient risk.

A notable example involves a study on gestational diabetes mellitus (GDM) [1], typically diagnosed between 24 weeks and 28 weeks of gestation. Using a machine-learning approach to predict GDM on retrospective data of 588,622 pregnancies in Israel, the models predict GDM with high accuracy even at pregnancy initiation. Interrogating the model uncovered previously unreported risk factors, including results of previous pregnancy glucose challenge tests. This approach offers potential for early interventions and cost-effective screening to possibly bypass glucose tolerance tests for low-risk women.

Another example of leveraging big data and AI for risk prediction is a study focused on the early prediction of preeclampsia [12]. This study utilized data from 16,370 births at Lucile Packard Children's Hospital at Stanford, CA. Researchers employed two statistical learning algorithms, elastic net and gradient boosting, to develop predictive models for both general and early-onset preeclampsia (before 34 weeks of gestation). The models were built using data available before 16 weeks of gestation, which included 67 variables such as maternal characteristics, medical history, routine prenatal laboratory results, and medication intake. The results were promising: the elastic net algorithm produced a prediction model for preeclampsia with an area under the curve (AUC) of 0.79 and demonstrated a sensitivity of 45.2% with a false-positive rate of 8.1%. The model for early-onset preeclampsia performed even better, achieving an AUC of 0.89, with a true-positive rate of 72.3% and a false-positive rate of 8.8%. These models show that statistical learning methods can effectively use routine prenatal data to predict preeclampsia risk, offering a significant advance in early detection and potentially improving maternal and fetal outcomes by enabling timely interventions.

These predictive models enable early interventions that can mitigate the risk of complications, illustrating AI's pivotal role in enhancing maternal and fetal outcomes.

20.3.2 Utilizing AI in Diagnostic Imaging

Utilizing machine learning models in diagnostic imaging, particularly in obstetrics, has revolutionized how medical professionals monitor fetal health and manage pregnancy-related complications. Ultrasound, an essential tool used throughout pregnancy, plays a pivotal role in observing fetal growth and development as well as in diagnosing complications. It provides detailed information on fetal anatomy with high-quality images and improved diagnostic accuracy. The subjectivity of measurements and observations has also historically impacted the quality of ultrasound images, standard measurements, and precise diagnoses. Over the past decade, efforts to reduce intra- and inter-observer variability and enhance diagnostic accuracy have led to the introduction of automatic measurements and assessments using AI. The application of AI in obstetric ultrasound has improved accuracy in three key areas: structure identification, automated and standardized measurements, and classification diagnosis. Moreover, the integration of AI has the potential to reduce examination times and enhance workflow efficiency, although much of the AI-related research and commercial software development remains in the early stages.

The measurement of fetal nuchal translucency (NT) thickness is a critical parameter. A key step in accurately measuring NT is locating the mid-sagittal plane of the fetus using ultrasound imaging. Recent research has developed an innovative automatic method for detecting this plane using 3D ultrasound data, aimed at enhancing NT measurement precision and efficiency [14]. The approach taken in this study involves a strategic reduction of the massive search area typically required, which in turn decreases the computational load significantly. The method transforms the task of locating the sagittal plane into a problem of finding a symmetry plane and axis. This is facilitated by the use of a Deep Belief Network (DBN) and a modified circle detection method that leverages prior knowledge to guide the search process effectively. Experimental results from the study are promising. The method achieved high accuracy, with 88.6% of the detected planes having a distance error of less than 4 mm and 71.0% showing an angle error of less than 20 degrees.

Another example can be shown in a study aimed at assessing the accuracy of an automated three-dimensional (3D) ultrasound technology for fetal intracranial measurements [16]. The results of this automated method were compared with those obtained manually. The patients underwent two consecutive ultrasound examinations of the fetal head—one performed by a sonographer and the other by a physician. During each session, manual measurements of the biparietal diameter (BPD), head circumference (HC), transcerebellar diameter (TCD), cisterna magna (CM), and posterior horn of the lateral ventricle (Vp) were taken. These were followed by automated measurements using the AI-based tool. The study enrolled 143 women. Automated measurement acquisition rates were promising, with first-attempt success rates of 70% and 76% for sonographers and physicians, respectively. Reliability comparisons using intraclass correlation coefficients (ICC) showed good reliability for automated measurements of BPD and HC when compared to manual methods, with ICC values ranging from 0.80 to 0.88.

These studies demonstrate the effective application of AI in obstetric ultrasound, enhancing the precision of critical prenatal screenings. Such advancements not only save time for medical professionals but also boost diagnostic accuracy, facilitating earlier and more tailored interventions. Moreover, as these technologies advance, they are being integrated more seamlessly into real-time imaging processes. This allows obstetricians to perform instant analyses during patient exams, greatly improving decision-making and elevating the overall quality of prenatal care.

20.3.3 AI Applications in Fetal Monitoring and Assessment

The application of AI in fetal monitoring and assessment represents one of the most exciting advancements in perinatal medicine. AI models have been developed to analyze fetal heart rate patterns, predicting distress and other conditions that may necessitate intervention. Research in this area includes the use of machine learning to distinguish between normal and abnormal heart rate patterns, offering a powerful tool for early detection and prevention of fetal distress during labor.

Cardiotocography (CTG) is the most commonly used diagnostic tool for continuous fetal monitoring and assessing fetal distress. However, using current standards for interpretation, there is a significant amount of both inter- and intra-observer variation. The primary challenge in interpreting CTG data is its subjectivity, especially the notable variability between different observers and even the same observer at different times. AI has the potential to assist clinicians in interpreting CTG more objectively, enabling them to determine more accurately when medical interventions are necessary to prevent perinatal hypoxia and potentially fatal outcomes.

In a study conducted in a high-resource tertiary care university hospital, researchers evaluated the impact of implementing a central fetal monitoring system equipped with machine learning models of intrapartum CTG on the labor ward [10]. By integrating machine learning models, which aid in the quantification of challenging-to-assess parameters such as variability, and incorporating complex guidelines for CTG analysis, the system aimed to improve monitoring accuracy. It used visual and sound alerts to prompt healthcare professionals to reassess signs associated with fetal hypoxia. Results from 38,466 deliveries indicated significant improvements post-implementation. The incidence of hypoxic-ischemic encephalopathy per 1000 births notably decreased from 5.3% to 2.2%, and there was a modest reduction in overall cesarean delivery rates from 29.9% to 28.3% and in urgent cesarean deliveries from 21.6% to 19.2%. The study concluded that the introduction of a computerized analysis system for monitoring intrapartum CTG signals was associated with a significant reduction in the incidence of hypoxic-ischemic encephalopathy and a reduction in cesarean deliveries, underscoring the system's potential to enhance prenatal care and improve perinatal outcomes.

There are other data-driven systems that utilize deep learning and do not require the specification of features based on the CTG signals; they merely process the raw signals. By applying deep learning to CTG analysis, it is possible to improve the accuracy of fetal hypoxia detection, but it also requires a much larger database than previously used methods.

In a recent study [20], researchers employed an 8-layer deep convolutional neural network (CNN) to predict fetal acidemia. This system utilizes the continuous wavelet transform (CWT) to convert fetal heart rate signals into 2-dimensional images, capturing critical time and frequency domain characteristics without the need for complex feature engineering typically required in conventional machine learning approaches. The CNN model's ability to self-learn and retain informative features from these images represents a significant advantage over traditional methods. Using an open-access database for testing, the CNN demonstrated superior classification performance in comparison to other state-of-the-art methods. It achieved impressive results in a ten-fold cross-validation setup, with an accuracy of 98.34%, sensitivity of 98.22%, specificity of 94.87%, a quality index of 96.53%, and an area under the curve of 97.82%. These results suggest that once fully trained, this CNN could serve as a highly effective tool for objectively and accurately predicting fetal asphyxia, potentially improving outcomes by enabling earlier and more targeted interventions.

The integration of artificial intelligence into perinatal medicine holds immense promise for the future of maternal and fetal healthcare. Through applications in risk prediction, decision support, and fetal monitoring, AI is setting the stage for a new era of personalized, proactive, and efficient perinatal care. As research continues and these technologies become more deeply integrated into clinical practice, the potential for improving outcomes for mothers and their babies grows ever more significant. The examples and studies highlighted in this chapter are but a glimpse of AI's transformative impact, signaling a hopeful horizon for the field of perinatal medicine.

20.4 Limitations and Ethical Considerations

The advent of AI and big data in perinatal medicine is transforming the care provided to mothers and their unborn children. This technological revolution promises enhanced predictive capabilities, personalized treatments, and comprehensive monitoring. However, many studies require further development before transition to a clinical setting, and several limitations must be acknowledged and addressed to fully harness their potential.

The datasets used to train and test these AI models are often limited in scope and diversity. For instance, a model trained primarily on data from a specific demographic may not perform adequately when applied to a broader population. This necessitates comprehensive studies across varied populations to validate the clinical applicability of these AI tools and ensure they are robust and reliable across different clinical settings.

One notable challenge in the application of AI in healthcare is the "black box" nature of these systems, which is particularly problematic in medical settings. Deep learning models, while powerful, often do not provide insights into how decisions are derived, making it difficult for clinicians to interpret the results or trust them enough to make critical patient care decisions. This lack of transparency can hinder the adoption and effective use of AI in clinical environments where explainability is not just valuable but essential for patient safety and care. This issue becomes even more pronounced when considering the intricate requirements of medical professionals who must base their decisions on clear, understandable data. For example, while an AI system might excel in identifying patterns within complex data sets, such as subtle changes in fetal heart rate, these findings might not be presented in a way that is easily understandable to medical professionals without specialized training in data science. To bridge this gap, targeted educational programs and comprehensive training must be developed to equip healthcare providers with the necessary skills to effectively utilize these advanced technologies. An example of tackling this challenge is the application of explainable AI in the development of a preterm labor prediction tool. This tool not only predicts the likelihood of preterm labor but also explains the prediction by identifying specific health indicators and patterns in the patient's data. Such transparency builds trust among clinicians and patients, facilitating informed decision-making. Regulatory efforts, such as those proposed in the EU's Artificial Intelligence Act, which mandates transparency for high-risk AI applications, highlight the importance of accountability and could inspire similar regulations globally.

Ethical considerations also play a critical role in the deployment of AI in healthcare. Privacy concerns are at the forefront, as these systems often require extensive personal and sensitive data to train. An example of this could be the use of detailed patient histories and genetic information, which raises questions about how data is stored, protected, and potentially shared. Clear protocols and stringent data protection measures must be established to address these concerns.

Furthermore, the reliance on AI for health-related decisions introduces another layer of ethical complexity. While AI can support clinical decisions, the idea of completely substituting human judgment with machine intelligence is fraught with challenges. For instance, an algorithm might incorrectly diagnose a condition or fail to capture nuances in complex cases where human expertise and judgment are crucial. The consequences of such errors could be significant, emphasizing the need for AI systems to be used as aids in the decision-making process rather than as replacements for human expertise.

Currently, AI should be viewed as a supplementary tool that enhances the capabilities of obstetricians rather than replacing them. It is imperative to maintain a balanced approach where AI supports but does not overshadow the critical thinking and experiential knowledge of healthcare professionals. As AI technologies continue to evolve, ongoing evaluation, rigorous testing, and adaptation to clinical feedback will be essential to address these limitations and ethical concerns, ensuring that AI's integration into obstetrics maximizes benefits while minimizing risks.

20.5 Conclusions

This chapter has illustrated the transformative potential of these technologies in reshaping maternal and fetal healthcare. Through advanced data analysis and predictive modeling, AI and big data are enhancing the precision of diagnostics and the personalization of treatment strategies, paving the way for a new era in perinatal medicine. We have delved into the technological advancements that mark this era of healthcare, exploring how AI and big data analytics extend beyond their conventional roles to become central to predictive analytics, real-time monitoring, and the personalization of perinatal care.

Yet, these advancements are not without their challenges. The narrative acknowledges significant hurdles that temper the swift adoption and seamless integration of these technologies into perinatal care. Issues surrounding data privacy, the need for interoperability, and the quest for equitable access to these advanced technologies are dissected, underscoring the multifaceted challenges that lie ahead. These obstacles underscore the need for robust, innovative solutions that can harmonize the potential of AI and big data with the realities of healthcare delivery.

Looking forward, there are rich opportunities awaiting further research and collaboration in this field. It calls for a multidisciplinary approach, rallying experts from AI, data science, and clinical medicine to join forces. The development of ethical frameworks and the establishment of international regulatory standards are heralded as crucial steps toward guiding the responsible use of AI and big data in healthcare, ensuring that advancements in perinatal care are accessible and beneficial to all.

In conclusion, AI and big data hold remarkable promise for advancing preventive obstetrics, offering solutions that could lead to significant reductions in maternal and neonatal morbidity and mortality. With careful attention to the challenges and ethical implications discussed, we stand on the brink of a new frontier in healthcare, where data-driven insights and AI-augmented decision-making become cornerstones of prenatal care, heralding a safer, more effective era for expecting mothers and their children.

Chapter Key Points

- AI enables early prediction of pregnancy complications using large-scale EHR and multi-omic data.
- Deep learning improves diagnostic accuracy in obstetric ultrasound and reduces operator variability.
- AI-enhanced CTG interpretation can lower rates of HIE and unnecessary cesarean deliveries.
- Big data integrates genetics, imaging, labs, and monitoring to personalize perinatal care.
- Ethical safeguards—privacy, transparency, bias mitigation—are essential for responsible AI adoption.

Chapter-End Summary

AI and big data are reshaping obstetrics by enabling predictive, personalized, and data-driven care. Machine learning models improve early identification of gestational diabetes, preeclampsia, and fetal compromise. Deep learning supports automated ultrasound analysis and enhances fetal monitoring accuracy. Despite significant promise, challenges remain—model generalizability, explainability, privacy, and regulatory oversight. When integrated responsibly, AI has the potential to transform perinatal outcomes while augmenting, not replacing, clinical expertise.

References

1. Artzi NS, Shilo S, Hadar E, Rossman H, Barbash-Hazan S, Ben-Haroush A, et al. Prediction of gestational diabetes based on nationwide electronic health records. Nat Med. 2020;26:71–6.
2. Ben M'Barek I, Jauvion G, Ceccaldi P-F. Computerized cardiotocography analysis during labor – a state-of-the-art review. Acta Obstet Gynecol Scand. 2023;102:130–7.
3. Bertini A, Salas R, Chabert S, Sobrevia L, Pardo F. Using machine learning to predict complications in pregnancy: a systematic review. Front Bioeng Biotechnol. 2021;9:780389.
4. Dey D, Slomka PJ, Leeson P, Comaniciu D, Shrestha S, Sengupta PP, et al. Artificial intelligence in cardiovascular imaging: JACC state-of-the-art review. J Am Coll Cardiol. 2019;73:1317–35.
5. Gofer S, Haik O, Bardin R, Gilboa Y, Perlman S. Machine learning algorithms for classification of first-trimester fetal brain ultrasound images. J Ultrasound Med. 2022;41:1773–9.
6. Hassan M, Awan FM, Naz A, deAndrés-Galiana EJ, Alvarez O, Cernea A, et al. Innovations in genomics and big data analytics for personalized medicine and health care: a review. Int J Mol Sci. 2022;23
7. Kann BH, Hosny A, Aerts HJWL. Artificial intelligence for clinical oncology. Cancer Cell. 2021;39:916–27.
8. Khan ZF, Alotaibi SR. Applications of artificial intelligence and big data analytics in m-health: a healthcare system perspective. J Healthc Eng. 2020;2020:8894694.
9. Krefting J, Sen P, David-Rus D, Güldener U, Hawe JS, Cassese S, et al. Use of big data from health insurance for assessment of cardiovascular outcomes. Front Artif Intell. 2023;6:1155404.
10. Lopes-Pereira J, Costa A, Ayres-De-Campos D, Costa-Santos C, Amaral J, Bernardes J. Computerized analysis of cardiotocograms and ST signals is associated with significant reductions in hypoxic-ischemic encephalopathy and cesarean delivery: an observational study in 38,466 deliveries. Am J Obstet Gynecol. 2019;220(269):e1–269.e8.
11. Macias CG, Remy KE, Barda AJ. Utilizing big data from electronic health records in pediatric clinical care. Pediatr Res. 2023;93:382–9.
12. Marić I, Tsur A, Aghaeepour N, Montanari A, Stevenson DK, Shaw GM, et al. Early prediction of preeclampsia via machine learning. Am J Obstetr Gynecol MFM. 2020;2:100100.
13. Mateen BA, David AL, Denaxas S. Electronic health records to predict gestational diabetes risk. Trends Pharmacol Sci. 2020;41:301–4.
14. Nie S, Yu J, Chen P, Wang Y, Zhang JQ. Automatic detection of standard sagittal plane in the first trimester of pregnancy using 3-D ultrasound data. Ultrasound Med Biol. 2017;43:286–300.
15. Ontaneda D, Ross LA, Hohlfeld R. MRI, big data, and artificial intelligence: rewards vs risks. Neurology. 2021;97:975–6.
16. Pluym ID, Afshar Y, Holliman K, Kwan L, Bolagani A, Mok T, et al. Accuracy of automated three-dimensional ultrasound imaging technique for fetal head biometry. Ultrasound Obstet Gynecol. 2021;57:798–803.
17. Subramanian I, Verma S, Kumar S, Jere A, Anamika K. Multi-omics data integration, interpretation, and its application. Bioinform Biol Insights. 2020;14:1177932219899051.
18. Tyrmi JS, Kaartokallio T, Lokki AI, Jääskeläinen T, Kortelainen E, Ruotsalainen S, et al. Genetic risk factors associated with preeclampsia and hypertensive disorders of pregnancy. JAMA Cardiol. 2023;8:674–83.
19. Wing DA. The future of obstetrics and gynecology: MACRA, electronic health records, and more. Clin Obstet Gynecol. 2017;60:840–52.
20. Zhao Z, Deng Y, Zhang Y, Zhang Y, Zhang X, Shao L. DeepFHR: intelligent prediction of fetal Acidemia using fetal heart rate signals based on convolutional neural network. BMC Med Inform Decis Mak. 2019;19:286.

Intrapartum Care

Contents

Prevention of Intrapartum Caesarean Section

P. J. Steer

Contents

Y. Yogev, A. Khalil (eds.), *Prevention of Complications in Obstetrics*,
https://doi.org/10.1007/978-3-032-23479-7_21

Learning Objectives

- Understand historical and contemporary evidence on slow labour and oxytocin use.
- Describe best practices to minimise unnecessary intrapartum caesareans.
- Critically appraise the benefits and limitations of CTG versus intermittent auscultation.
- Identify clinical implications of epidural-associated pyrexia and appropriate management.
- Apply principles of individualised labour assessment to avoid unwarranted intervention.

What You Will Learn in This Chapter

The assumption in this chapter is that the pregnant person has made the choice, after appropriate counselling, to give birth to their baby vaginally, and that caesarean section (CS) is for them an undesirable option. The role of the birth attendants is therefore to facilitate this outcome and avoid interventions that will increase the risk of CS. The chapter will first assess attempts to optimise progress in labour and then suggest how to avoid the pitfalls of unnecessary or inappropriate intervention. The complications of the CS itself are covered in the chapters on neurological injury and postpartum haemorrhage.

Learning Objectives

To understand the effects of attempts to optimise progress in labour and to become aware of how some interventions can have undesirable side effects. The two major indications for intrapartum CS are inadequate progress or failure of progress in labour, and suspected foetal compromise.

21.1 Caesarean Section for Slow Progress in Labour

Labour is unusually slow in humans compared with other related species such as gorillas and chimpanzees, a phenomenon commonly attributed to the relatively small pelvis evolved in association with bipedalism (walking/running), and the relatively large foetal head associated with an increase in cognitive ability [1]. In a meta-analysis of the duration of the first (latent and active) and second stages of spontaneous labour in women without risk factors for complications and with good maternal and perinatal outcomes, Abalos et al. [2] found that among nulliparous women, the median duration of the active first stage (from the starting reference point of 4 cm cervical dilatation) ranged from 3.7 to 5.9 h (95th percentiles: 14.5–16.7 h). From 5 cm, the median duration was from 3.8 to 4.3 h (95th percentiles: 11.3–12.7 h). In nulliparous and parous women, respectively, the median duration of the second stage ranged from 14 to 66 min (95th percentiles: 65–138 min) and from 6 to 12 min (95th percentiles: 58–76 min). The 95th percentile of normal progress in nulliparae in the first stage of labour from 4 cm was 6 cm in 16.7 hours, approximately 0.36 cm per hour. Therefore, in modern practice, labour longer than 16 hours would generally be considered unduly prolonged, although traditionally, slow labour due to 'primary uterine inertia' was defined as a labour in which the first stage lasted longer than 48 hours (which led to the saying 'never let the sun set twice on a labouring woman'). In a report of 631 labourers with 'primary uterine inertia' (labour longer than 48 hours) published in 1949 from Queen Charlotte's Maternity Hospital in London, UK [3], the maternal mortality rate was 470 per 100,000, and the stillbirth rate attributed to the prolonged labour was 98 per 1000. Despite this, the CS rate was only 4.7% (the average in England and Wales in 1949 was 2%).

Figure 21.1 shows the change in total CS rates and perinatal mortality in England and Wales from 1947 to 2022. By 1968, the CS rate was still only 4%, with the intrapartum proportion about half that. But already there had been attempts to augment labour with oxytocin in order to limit the incidence of prolonged labour. Aleck Bourne in 1927 [4] reported that following the discovery of the uterotonic action of posterior pituitary extract by Sir Henry Dale in 1906 [5] 'It has been recognised for many years that while

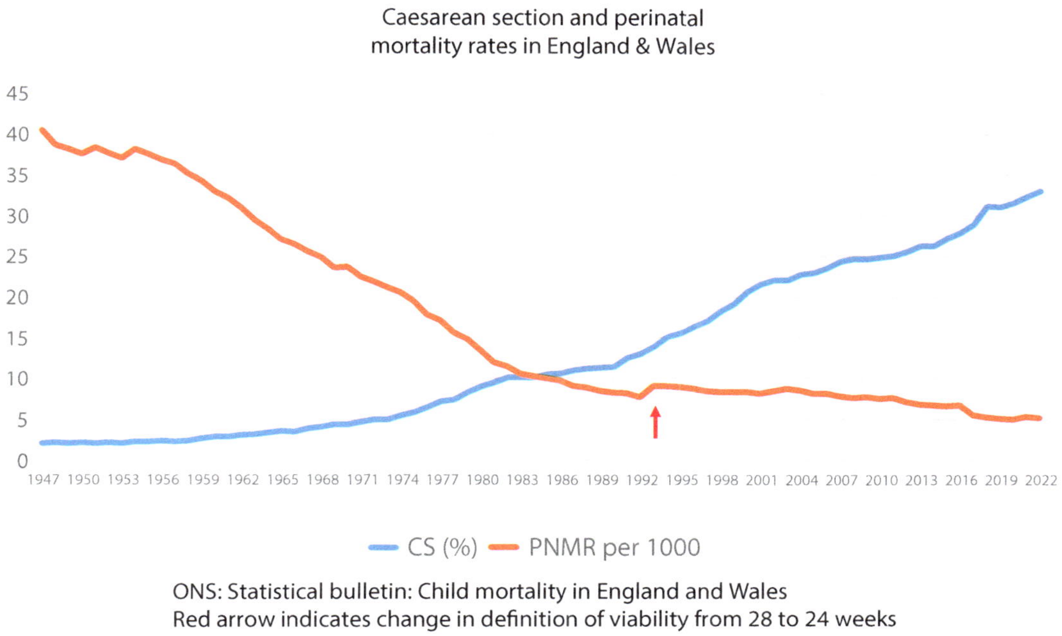

Fig. 21.1 Caesarean section and perinatal mortality rates in England & Wales. ONS: Statistical bulletin: Child mortality in England and Wales. The red arrow indicates a change in the definition of viability from 28 to 24 weeks

pituitary extract is of valuable assistance in midwifery (to augment contractions), there is a real danger in its indiscriminate use (with) reports from time to time of serious accidents such as lacerations of the cervix and perinaeum and even rupture of the uterus'. Such concerns limited the use of posterior pituitary extract, but the synthesis of oxytocin by Du Vigneaud in 1954 [6] made accurate dosing easier and in 1969 O'Driscoll et al. published from the National Maternity Hospital in Dublin the first of a series of reports regarding the 'prevention of prolonged labour' in nulliparae which led to the concept of 'the active management of labour' [7, 8]. This recommended the use of high dose rates of oxytocin (starting at 7 mU/min and increasing rapidly to 40 mU/min), limited only by evidence of 'foetal distress'. Importantly, the definition of 'prolonged labour' was a rate of cervical dilatation of <1 cm/hr., which was about the average for nullipara and therefore resulted in 55% of nullipara having their labour 'augmented'. By 1984, the active management of labour was credited by O'Driscoll et al. as the reason for the maintenance of a relatively low intrapartum CS rate at the National Maternity Hospital in Dublin (4.8%) [9]. The title of their paper was 'Active Management of Labor as an Alternative to Cesarean Section for Dystocia'.

Other maternity units attempted to replicate the active management of labour but reported higher CS rates—for example, Boyle et al. in Belfast reported in 1980 an augmentation rate in nullips of 42% but an intrapartum CS rate of 8.6% [10], and Cardozo et al. reported an augmentation rate of 36% but a CS rate of 8.7% [11]. Importantly, despite the widespread introduction of active management in England and Wales, the CS rate continued to climb inexorably (Fig. 21.1). By 1994, Thornton and Lilford wrote an editorial in the BMJ stating that 'Early amniotomy and early oxytocin do not reduce rates of caesarean sections and operative vaginal deliveries' [12], and Thornton went on to say in 1996 that 'Units should not introduce active management but should provide continuous support in labour. Units should perform amniotomy and oxytocin acceleration selectively, if at all' [13]. By 2007, the National Institute of Health and Clinical Excellence (UK NICE) guidelines stated in relation to delay in the established first stage of labour that 'The woman should be informed that the use of oxytocin following spontaneous or artificial rupture of the membranes will bring forward her time of birth but *will not influence the mode of birth* or other outcomes' (my italics) and recommended that active management should not be used routinely.

Despite these recommendations, high rates of oxytocin augmentation continued to be used. A Cochrane review in 2013 of 'Early amniotomy and early oxytocin for prevention of, or therapy for, delay in first stage spontaneous labour compared with routine care' reported that in 14 randomised trials including 8033 women, the rate of CS in labours actively managed was not significantly lower (Odds Ratio 0.89 (95% CI 0.79 to 1.01, $p = 0.06$); the CS rate was 11% with early oxytocin cf. 12.3% in controls [14]). In the same year a Cochrane review of oxytocin augmentation of established slow labour (as opposed to prophylactic augmentation) summarised the results of 5 trials including 1200 women and concluded that 'For women making slow progress in spontaneous labour, treatment with oxytocin as compared with no treatment or delayed oxytocin treatment did not result in any discernable difference in the number of caesarean sections performed' [15]. Both reviews did, however, report a labour shorter by 1.5–2 hours in the oxytocin group.

While there is clear empirical evidence that an infusion of oxytocin is necessary to 'kick-start' contractions in labours of spontaneous onset where contractions are infrequent (less than three per 10 min), and in induced labour using prostaglandins or cervical balloons where contractions do not commence or are similarly infrequent, in the last 20 years, accumulating evidence has suggested that continuing oxytocin infusion once labour is established is not only unnecessary but also might be harmful. In a 2017 meta-analysis of seven randomised controlled trials including 1307 parturients, Saccone et al. reported that the Caesarean section rate was significantly lower (9.3%) when oxytocin was discontinued in induced labour after the active phase had been established compared with controls (14.7%) [16]. The subsequent 'Condisox' double-blind randomised controlled trial of induced labour in 1200 women found no significant difference in Caesarean section rate when oxytocin was discontinued (16.6%) compared with when it was continued (14.2%), although the labour was 81 min longer in the discontinued group [17]. However, there were significantly ($p < 0.001$) fewer episodes of uterine hyperstimulation in the discontinued group (3.7%) compared with the continued group (12.9%), and this was associated with a lower rate of foetal heart rate abnormalities (27.9% versus 40.8%, $p < 0.001$). A secondary analysis of the trial showed that the lack of difference in the CS rate may have been in part due to the fact that in 42.4% of cases the birth attendants had switched from the study medication to open-label oxytocin, a rate that was particularly high in labours with evidence of a 'high resistance to progress' (unripe cervix, large babies, nulliparity) [18]. Despite the switch to open-label oxytocin, the Caesarean section rate was higher in such cases than in labourers where the study medication was continued. An important conclusion was that 'It may well be appropriate to have different norms for rates of cervical dilatation between nulliparous and parous women, and for those with ripe versus unripe cervices, so as to avoid unnecessary oxytocin infusion in labours that will be slower than average despite normal levels of uterine activity. Therefore, an individualised assessment of labour progress is needed'.

The 'STOPOXY' trial, an open-label multicentre randomised trial of discontinuing oxytocin in 2170 labours, was published in 2023 [19]. The authors highlighted the risks of tachysystole with oxytocin administration, which is associated with significant oxygen desaturation and non-reassuring foetal heart rate patterns, contributing to neonatal acidosis [20, 21]. It is also associated with higher rates of postpartum haemorrhage [22]. Although predominantly involving induced labour (81.0–83.1%), the study also included women receiving oxytocin in spontaneous labour. The primary outcome of the study was not caesarean section, but neonatal morbidity using a composite variable defined by an umbilical arterial pH at birth of less than 7·10, a base excess greater than 10 mmol/L, umbilical arterial lactate greater than 7 mmol/L, a 5-min Apgar score less than 7, or admission to the neonatal intensive care unit. There was no statistically significant difference in this outcome in a modified intention-to-treat analysis between the group where oxytocin was discontinued versus the group that continued (9.6% vs 9.2%, relative risk 1.0, 95% CI 0.8–1.4). Nor was there any statistically significant difference in Caesarean section rates, being 10.7% in the discontinued group and 9.9% in the continued group (relative risk 1.1, 95% confidence intervals 0.8–1.3). As with the CONDISOX trial, in the discontinued group, there was a high rate (40.5%) of oxytocin being restarted after discontinuation. Surprisingly, the only conclusion reached by the authors was 'discontinuing oxytocin when the active phase is reached did not show a reduction in neonatal morbidity compared to continuous oxytocin', when they might also have added that 'discontinuing oxytocin in 59.5% of labours had no effect on outcomes but was associated with a lower incidence of tachysystole (6.3% vs 10.4%)'. Thus, in cases where the labour ward is particularly busy, making it difficult to provide continuous supervision of oxytocin infusion by caregivers, parturients (and their babies) can be safeguarded by turning off oxytocin and reassured that discontinuation will not have an adverse effect on either mode of delivery or neonatal outcome, although they may take an hour or two longer to give birth.

If giving intravenous oxytocin has not been demonstrated to be beneficial other than by producing a slightly shorter labour, is there any harm in continuing it, as suggested by the authors of the STOPOXY trial? In a report from Sweden in 2007 on 77 cases of disciplinary action, 60 were related to intrapartum care. The authors reported that 'Injudicious use of oxytocin was common (68.5%), and was the primary reason for disciplinary action in 33% of the cases' [23]. A more extensive study of 472 cases, also in Sweden, published in 2008, reported that 'the most common events of malpractice in connection with delivery were neglecting to supervise fetal well-being in 173 cases, including incautious use of oxytocin in 126 cases (71%)' [24]. Searching the web for '10 years of maternity claims' brings up an analysis of NHS Litigation Authority data published in October 2012. Case study 2 describes the labour of a 31-year-old woman at 10 days post—due date. Despite an abnormal CTG, the registrar (resident obstetrician) prescribed Syntocinon, and this was subsequently increased several times by the midwife. This resulted in the birth of a baby in very poor condition who went on to have significant cognitive impairment, speech delay, microcephaly and complex febrile seizures. Similar cases were reported by the review team led by Donna Ockenden in relation to the maternity services at Shrewsbury and Telford Hospital NHS Trust. The emerging findings review published in 2020 [25] commented that 'Long labour exacerbated by use of oxytocin can result in an obstructed labour leading to fetal distress and also difficult caesarean delivery because the fetal head is deeply in the pelvis… The review team noted many examples where oxytocin was used injudiciously; these cases occurred across the time period of the 250 cases reviewed, which suggests a failure to learn from previous cases where the outcome was poor'. In her final report published in 2022 [26], Ms. Ockenden commented that 'A common theme identified by the review team was the inappropriate commencement and continuation of oxytocin despite evidence of deterioration of the baby's condition'. Similar comments have been made by coroners investigating perinatal deaths, in relation to which I have given expert evidence. There can be no doubt that the inappropriate use of oxytocin can cause perinatal asphyxia, leading to death or permanent disability. It therefore seems prudent not to give oxytocin to augment uterine contractions when there is no evidence for its use other than slow progress in labour with infrequent contractions (less than three contractions in 10 min). If the contractions are already three in 10 min or more, oxytocin should be given only with close and continuous personal supervision by an obstetrician or experienced midwife. If contractions are three in ten min or more, the only way to reliably assess their strength is to use an intrauterine catheter with an inbuilt pressure transducer or connected to an external pressure transducer. A 1996 study of 46 labourers showed that manual assessment of contractions as mild, moderate, or strong was incorrect in 51% of cases, and concerningly, 38% of strong contractions as measured by an intrauterine catheter were classified by the birthing attendant as moderate, and 6.5% of strong contractions were assessed as mild [27]. Assessment of contractions using external tocodynamometry can also be unreliable if the transducer is not correctly placed or if the mother is obese [28].

21.2 Caesarean Section for Foetal Compromise

21.2.1 Foetal Heart Rate Monitoring

The first person to make clear observations regarding the auscultation of the foetal heart during pregnancy was Viscomte Kergaradec, Jacques Alexandre Le Jumeau (1787–1877) in Paris. In 1821, he wrote 'One day whilst examining a patient near-term ..... with a stethoscope I was suddenly aware of the sound that I had not noticed before; it was like the ticking of a watch. At first I thought I was mistaken, but I was able to repeat the observation over and over again. On counting the beats I found that these occurred 143-148 times per minute, and the patient's pulse was only 72 per minute'. The stethoscope he used was based on that of Rene Laennec; although Adolf Pinard's name is usually attached to the traditional foetal stethoscope, he was, in fact, better known at the time for promoting external cephalic version to correct malpresentation.

Despite 200 years of the use of the Pinard stethoscope for intermittent auscultation, there is no scientific evidence of its value in preventing stillbirth. The foetal heart is often difficult to hear, especially if the mother is obese, and its use in the first stage of labour according to the NICE intrapartum care guidelines published in December 2022 was recommended as follows: 'carry out intermittent auscultation immediately after a palpated contraction for at least 1 minute, repeated at least once every 15 minutes, and record it as a single rate on a partogram and in the woman's notes; record accelerations and decelerations, if heard; palpate (and record on the partogram) the maternal pulse hourly, or more often if there are any concerns, to ensure differentiation between the maternal and fetal heartbeats'. The rationale given for using intermittent auscultation in this way is 'Explain to women that if there are no identified risk factors for foetal compromise, there is a risk of increased interventions with continuous CTG monitoring compared with intermittent auscultation, which may outweigh the benefits' [29].

So, does continuous electronic foetal heart rate monitoring reduce the rate of perinatal mortality and morbidity, and does this inevitably result in an increase in intervention? The steady improvement in perinatal mortality shown in Fig. 21.1 does not show any obvious change in trajectory following the widespread introduction of electronic foetal monitoring in the 1970s. During the 1980s and early 1990s, there was a series of randomised controlled trials of electronic foetal monitoring versus intermittent auscultation, of which the largest was carried out in Dublin [30]. A meta-analysis of nine trials was published by Vintzileos et al. in 1995 and reported that there was no statistically significant overall reduction in perinatal mortality (4.2 per thousand with electronic monitoring compared with 4.9 per thousand with intermittent auscultation) but there was a significant reduction in perinatal deaths attributed to hypoxia (0.7 per thousand with electronic monitoring and 1.8 per thousand with intermittent auscultation) [31]. There was, however, an increase in instrumental birth associated with electronic monitoring (12.2% versus 9.7%), and an increase in Caesarean section (5.2% versus 3.8%). In the same year, Thacker et al. performed a further meta-analysis including three additional trials and reported a statistically significant 50% reduction in neonatal seizures associated with the use of electronic foetal monitoring [32]. By 2017, the Cochrane review by Alfirevic et al. was able to include 13 trials involving over 37,000 women [33] (of which the largest was the Dublin trial, including almost 13,000). They concluded that continuous cardiotocography was not associated with a statistically significant improvement in the overall perinatal death rate (risk ratio 0.86, 95% confidence interval (CI) 0.59–1.23) but was associated with a halving of the neonatal seizure rate (RR 0.50, 95% CI 0.31 to 0.80). However, this was not associated with any significant difference in cerebral palsy rates (RR 1.75, 95% CI 0.84–3.63), which were in fact higher in the electronic monitoring group. The evidence on caesarean section and instrumental delivery rates was very limited, but although there was no statistically significant difference (CS RR 1.29, 95% CI 0.84–1.97, $N = 4044$, 1 trial, instrumental births RR 1.16, 95% CI 0.92–1.46, $N = 4044$, 1 trial), these data do give some support to the NICE recommendation that, to minimise operative intervention in low-risk labours, intermittent auscultation rather than continuous electronic foetal monitoring should be advised.

21.3 Other Methods of Foetal Assessment

For many years, rather than immediately expediting delivery when the foetal heart rate pattern deviated from normality, European obstetricians were recommended to take a foetal capillary blood sample (usually from the scalp, but also from the buttock with a breech presentation) and only proceed to delivery if the pH was unusually low. The technique was introduced by Saling in the 1960s, [34] before electronic foetal heart rate monitoring. The classic study by Beard and colleagues published in 1971 [35] showed that while a normal foetal heart rate pattern had a very high positive predictive value for a normal foetal capillary blood pH (only 2% were $\leq$7.25), even with the most abnormal pattern (a baseline tachycardia complicated by decelerations) almost 50% of the foetuses still had a pH $\geq$ 7.25 and therefore labour could be allowed to continue with close observation. Foetal blood sampling was never significantly adopted in the United States of America, and there remains a lack of evidence from trials of its value. As a result, the 'foetal monitoring in labour' NICE guideline published in December 2022 [29] stated at para 1.7.1 that 'NICE is unable to make a recommendation about fetal blood sampling because of limited evidence'. A 2002 meta-analysis of using foetal heart rate accelerations following digital intrapartum foetal scalp stimulation as a reassuring feature suggested that this might be of value [36] but it remains controversial.

Assessment of the foetal ECG using measurement of the ST segment of the foetal ECG was introduced in the 1980s as a potential way of assessing foetal acid-base status [37], and this was subsequently computerised as part of the 'STAN' system [38]. A 2013 Cochrane review [39] of six randomised trials (16,295 participants) reported that its findings 'provide some support for the use of foetal ST waveform analysis when a decision has been made to undertake continuous electronic foetal heart rate monitoring during labour. However, the advantages need to be considered along with the disadvantages of needing to use an internal scalp electrode, after membrane rupture, for ECG waveform recordings'. A large American multicentre study including 11,108 patients failed to find an advantage in its use [40], and an updated meta-analysis published in 2024 concluded that 'there is insufficient evidence to state that STAN as an adjunct to CTG leads to important clinical benefits compared with CTG alone' [41].

21.4 Pyrexia in Labour and Epidural Anaesthesia

Pyrexia in labour, traditionally attributed to chorioamnionitis, has long been known to be associated with poor outcomes in pregnancy. Large-scale studies report a ninefold increased risk of unexplained cerebral palsy [42] and an almost fourfold increased risk of neonatal encephalopathy [43]. Fusi et al. in 1989 drew attention to the association of epidural anaesthesia in labour with an increased rate of pyrexia [44]. An observational study in the USA reported that following the introduction of epidural anaesthesia on request, the incidence of intrapartum temperatures greater than 38 °C rose from 0.6% to 11% [45]. A study from Scotland reported that in women with epidural anaesthesia for pain relief in labour, maternal pyrexia rates were 11% compared with 0.8% in controls [46]. Corresponding rates of neonatal sepsis workup were 11.7% and 2.5%. A 2021 systematic review commented that while there is a known potential mechanism whereby pyrexia due to chorioamnionitis can cause foetal brain injury (abnormally elevated cytokine levels), whether hyperthermia due to epidural anaesthesia is benign remains uncertain [47]. What does seem clear, however, is that even if there is a clinical suspicion that pyrexia is associated with chorioamnionitis, because the duration of labour following the diagnosis does not correlate with adverse outcomes [48], correct management is to administer broad-spectrum antibiotic prophylaxis (usually with ampicillin and gentamicin) and there is no need to intervene with Caesarean section unless there are other specific foetal indications [49, 50].

21.5 Major Pitfalls to Be Avoided

The reasons for the inexorable rise in the incidence of caesarean section, illustrated in ■ Fig. 21.1, are difficult to define, but probably include an increasing intolerance of the pain of labour when this can be minimised by epidural anaesthesia and early recourse to delivery by Caesarean section. There may also be pressure to reduce the duration of labour to alleviate staffing shortages, and to avoid potential medicolegal litigation when things unexpectedly go wrong. However, if the birthing person's express wish is to avoid Caesarean section, then it is probably appropriate to advise minimum intervention. In particular, allowing labour to progress at its natural rate without oxytocin augmentation will avoid iatrogenic hyperstimulation, which can precipitate foetal decompensation requiring delivery by Caesarean section. Using intermittent auscultation rather than continuous electronic foetal monitoring will reduce the anxiety produced by non-reassuring foetal heart rate patterns, the great majority of which are associated with a normal outcome for the baby. Using nonpharmacological methods of pain relief such as birthing pools, hypnosis, the use of doulas and/or a supportive partner, and relaxation techniques, rather than epidural anaesthesia, will minimise the risk of precipitating caesarean section because of intrapartum pyrexia.

21.6 Summary

Increasing intolerance of slow labour, use of continuous electronic foetal heart rate monitoring, and the use of epidural anaesthesia for pain relief are associated with a progressive rise in intrapartum caesarean section seen in high-income countries. Avoiding oxytocin augmentation of labour, monitoring the foetus in low-risk labours by intermittent auscultation, and avoiding epidural anaesthesia for pain relief are the approaches most likely to result in a vaginal birth and minimise the incidence of unnecessary caesarean section.

Chapter Key Points

- Prolonged labour alone rarely indicates caesarean section; most slow labours progress normally with minimal intervention.
- Oxytocin shortens labour but does not reduce caesarean rates and may increase risks such as tachysystole and fetal compromise.
- Continuous CTG reduces neonatal seizures but increases operative births; intermittent auscultation is preferred for low-risk labours.
- Epidural analgesia markedly raises intrapartum pyrexia rates, often prompting unnecessary concern for chorioamnionitis.

- Individualised labour assessment is essential—norms differ by parity, cervical ripeness, and labour onset method.
- Avoiding unnecessary interventions (oxytocin, CTG, early epidurals) best supports vaginal birth when clinically safe.

Chapter-End Summary

Intrapartum caesarean section is most often driven by slow progress or suspected fetal compromise. Evidence shows that interventions such as prophylactic oxytocin, routine CTG use, and epidural analgesia can inadvertently increase caesarean rates without improving neonatal outcomes. Modern practice emphasises individualised assessment of labour progress, selective oxytocin uses only when contractions are inadequate, and preference for intermittent auscultation in low-risk settings. Appropriate management of intrapartum pyrexia and avoidance of unnecessary escalation help support physiologic labour and reduce iatrogenic pathways leading to caesarean birth.

References

1. Rosenberg K, Trevethan W. Bipedalism and human birth: the obstetrical dilemma revisited. Evol Anthropol. 1996;4:161–8.
2. Abalos E, Oladapo OT, Chamillard M, et al. Duration of spontaneous labour in 'low-risk' women with 'normal' perinatal outcomes: a systematic review. Eur J Obstet Gynecol Reprod Biol. 2018;223:123–32. https://doi.org/10.1016/j.ejogrb.2018.02.026.
3. MacRae DJ. Primary uterine inertia. J Obstet Gynaecol Br Emp. 1952;59:785–98.
4. Bourne A, Burn JH. The dosage and action of pituitary extract and the ergot alkaloids on the uterus in labour, with a note on the action of adrenalin. J Obstet Gynaecol Br Emp. 1927;34:249–72.
5. Dale HH. On some physiological actions of ergot. J Physiol. 1906;34:163–206.
6. Du Vigneau V, Ressler C, Swan JM, Roberts CW, Katsoyannis PG. The synthesis of oxytocin. J Am Chem Soc. 1954;76:3115–21.
7. O'Driscoll K, Jackson RJA, Gallagher JT. Prevention of prolonged labour. Br Med J. 1969;ii(5655):447–8.
8. O'Driscoll K, Stronge JM, Minogue M. Active management of labour. Br Med J. 1973;iii:135–7.
9. O'Driscoll K, Foley M, MacDonald D. Active management of labour as an alternative to cesarean section for dystocia. Obstet Gynecol. 1984;63:485–90.
10. Boyle DD, White RG, Ritchie JW. An assessment of active management of primigravid labour. Ir J Med Sci. 1980;149:465–8.
11. Cardozo L, Gibb DMF, Studd JWW, et al. Predictive value of cervimetric labour patterns in primigravidae. Br J Obstet Gynaecol. 1982;89:33–8.
12. Thornton JG, Lilford RJ. Active management of labour: current knowledge and research issues [published erratum appears in BMJ 1994 Sep 17;309(6956): 704] [see comments]. Br Med J. 1994;309:366–9.
13. Thornton JG. Active management of labour. Br Med J. 1996;313:378.
14. Wei S, Wo BL, Qi HP, et al. Early amniotomy and early oxytocin for prevention of, or therapy for, delay in first stage spontaneous labour compared with routine care. Cochrane Database Syst Rev. 2013;8:CD006794.
15. Bugg GJ, Siddiqui F, Thornton JG. Oxytocin versus no treatment or delayed treatment for slow progress in the first stage of spontaneous labour. Cochrane Database Syst Rev. 2013;6:CD007123.
16. Saccone G, Ciardulli A, Baxter JK, et al. Discontinuing oxytocin infusion in the active phase of labor: a systematic review and meta-analysis. Obstet Gynecol. 2017;130:1090–6.
17. Boie S, Glavind J, Uldbjerg N, et al. Continued versus discontinued oxytocin stimulation in the active phase of labour (CONDISOX): double blind randomised controlled trial. BMJ. 2021;373 https://doi.org/10.1136/bmj.n716.
18. Steer PJ, Glavind J, Uldbjerg N, et al. Continued versus discontinued oxytocin stimulation in the active phase of induced labour: factors associated with unexpectedly high rates of conversion to open label oxytocin in the CONDISOX trial. BJOG. 2023;130:636–42. https://doi.org/10.1111/1471-0528.17376.
19. Girault A, Sentilhes L, Desbrière R, et al. Impact of discontinuing oxytocin in active labour on neonatal morbidity: an open-label, multicentre, randomised trial. Lancet (London, England). 2023;402:2091–100. https://doi.org/10.1016/S0140-6736(23)01803-2.
20. Simpson KR, James DC. Effects of oxytocin-induced uterine hyperstimulation during labor on fetal oxygen status and fetal heart rate patterns. Am J Obstet Gynecol. 2008;199:34.e1–5. https://doi.org/10.1016/j.ajog.2007.12.015.
21. Bakker PCAM, Kurver PHJ, Kuik DJ, et al. Elevated uterine activity increases the risk of fetal aci-

dosis at birth. Am J Obstet Gynecol. 2007;196:313.e1–6. https://doi.org/10.1016/J.AJOG.2006.11.035.
22. Belghiti J, Kayem G, Dupont C, et al. Oxytocin during labour and risk of severe postpartum haemorrhage: a population-based, cohort-nested case-control study. BMJ Open. 2011;1 https://doi.org/10.1136/bmjopen-2011-000514.
23. Jonsson M, Norden SL, Hanson U. Analysis of malpractice claims with a focus on oxytocin use in labour. Acta Obs Gynecol Scand. 2007;86:315–9.
24. Berglund S, Grunewald C, Pettersson H, et al. Severe asphyxia due to delivery-related malpractice in Sweden 1990–2005. BJOG. 2008;115:316–23.
25. Ockenden D. Emerging findings and recommendations from the independent review of maternity services at the Shrewsbury and Telford NHS Trust. 2020. https://www.gov.uk/government/publications/ockenden-review-of-maternity-services-at-shrewsbury-and-telford-hospital-nhs-trust%0A. Accessed 3 Oct 2024.
26. The Ockenden Review. 2021. https://www.donnaockenden.com/the-ockenden-review-sath/. Accessed 10 May 2021.
27. Arrabal PP, Nagey DA. Is manual palpation of uterine contractions accurate? Am J Obstet Gynecol. 1996;174:217–9.
28. Miles AM, Monga M, Richeson KS. Correlation of external and internal monitoring of uterine activity in a cohort of term patients. Am J Perinatol. 2001;18:137–40.
29. National Institute for Health and Care Excellence. Fetal monitoring in labour NICE guideline [NG229] Published: 14 December 2022. 2022. https://www.nice.org.uk/guidance/ng229. Accessed 4 Oct 2024.
30. MacDonald D, Grant A, Sheridan-Pereira M, et al. The Dublin randomized controlled trial of intrapartum fetal heart rate monitoring. Am J Obstet Gynecol. 1985;152:524–39.
31. Vintzileos AM, Nochimson DJ, Guzman ER, et al. Intrapartum electronic fetal heart rate monitoring versus intermittent auscultation: a meta-analysis. Obstet Gynecol. 1995;85:149–55.
32. Thacker SB, Stroup DF, Peterson HB. Efficacy and safety of intrapartum electronic fetal monitoring: an update. Obstet Gynecol. 1995;86:613–20.
33. Alfirevic Z, Devane D, Gyte GM, et al. Continuous cardiotocography (CTG) as a form of electronic fetal monitoring (EFM) for fetal assessment during labour. Cochrane Database Syst Rev. 2017;2:CD006066.
34. Saling E. Neues Vorgehen zur Untersuchung des Kindes unter der Gehurt: Einführung, Technik und Grundlagen. Arch Gynakol. 1962;197:108–22. https://doi.org/10.1007/BF02590014.
35. Beard RW, Filshie GM, Knight CA, et al. The significance of the changes in the continuous foetal heart rate in the first stage of labour. J Obstet Gynaecol Br Commonw. 1971;78:865–81.
36. Skupski DW, Rosenberg CR, Eglinton GS. Intrapartum fetal stimulation tests: a meta-analysis. Obstet Gynecol. 2002;99:129–34. https://doi.org/10.1016/S0029-7844(01)01645-3.
37. Greene KR, Dawes GS, Lilja H, et al. Changes in the ST waveform of the fetal lamb electrocardiogram with hypoxemia. Am J Obstet Gynecol. 1982;144:950–8.
38. Rosen KG, Luzietti R. The fetal electrocardiogram: ST waveform analysis during labour. J Perinat Med. 1994;22:501–12.
39. Neilson JP. Fetal electrocardiogram (ECG) for fetal monitoring during labour. Cochrane Database Syst Rev. 2013;5:CD000116.
40. Belfort MA, Saade GR, Thom E, et al. A randomized trial of intrapartum fetal ECG ST-segment analysis. N Engl J Med. 2015;373:632–41.
41. Blix E, Brurberg KG, Reierth E, et al. ST waveform analysis vs cardiotocography alone for intrapartum fetal monitoring: an updated systematic review and meta-analysis of randomized trials. Acta Obstet Gynecol Scand. 2024;103:437–48. https://doi.org/10.1111/aogs.14752.
42. Grether JK, Nelson KB. Maternal infection and cerebral palsy in infants of normal birth weight. JAMA J Am Med Assoc. 1997;278:207–11.
43. Badawi N, Kurinczuk JJ, Keogh JM, et al. Antepartum risk factors for newborn encephalopathy: the Western Australian case-control study. Br Med J. 1998;317:1549–53.
44. Fusi L, Steer PJ, Maresh MJA, et al. Maternal pyrexia associated with the use of epidural anaesthesia in labour. Lancet. 1989;i:1250–2.
45. Yancey MK, Zhang J, Schwarz J, et al. Labor epidural analgesia and intrapartum maternal hyperthermia. Obstet Gynecol. 2001;98:763–70.
46. Agakidis C, Agakidou E, Philip TS, et al. Labor epidural analgesia is independent risk factor for neonatal pyrexia. J Matern Neonatal Med. 2011;24:1128–32.
47. Morton S, Kua J, Mullington CJ. Epidural analgesia, intrapartum hyperthermia, and neonatal brain injury: a systematic review and meta-analysis. Br J Anaesth. 2021;126:500–15. https://doi.org/10.1016/j.bja.2020.09.046.
48. Venkatesh KK, Glover AV, Vladutiu CJ, et al. Association of chorioamnionitis and its duration with adverse maternal outcomes by mode of delivery: a cohort study. BJOG An Int J Obstet Gynaecol. 2019;126:719–27. https://doi.org/10.1111/1471-0528.15565.
49. Jung E, Romero R, Suksai M, et al. Clinical chorioamnionitis at term: definition, pathogenesis, microbiology, diagnosis, and treatment. Am J Obstet Gynecol. 2024;230:S807–40. https://doi.org/10.1016/j.ajog.2023.02.002.
50. Goetzl L. Maternal fever in labor: etiologies, consequences, and clinical management. Am J Obstet Gynecol. 2023;228:S1274–82. https://doi.org/10.1016/j.ajog.2022.11.002.

Prevention of Postpartum Hemorrhage

Daniel Gabbai and Yariv Yogev

Contents

Y. Yogev, A. Khalil (eds.), *Prevention of Complications in Obstetrics*,
https://doi.org/10.1007/978-3-032-23479-7_22

Learning Objectives
- Identify major risk factors and pathophysiologic mechanisms of postpartum hemorrhage.
- Explain components of AMTSL and how they reduce PPH incidence.
- Compare pharmacologic agents used for PPH prevention, including indications and limitations.
- Describe non-pharmacologic techniques supporting PPH prevention (e.g., trauma avoidance, uterine tone monitoring).
- Recognize the importance of institutional preparedness, hemorrhage bundles, and QBL.

22.1 Epidemiology and Impact of Postpartum Hemorrhage

Postpartum hemorrhage (PPH) is classically defined as blood loss ≥500 mL after a vaginal birth or ≥1000 mL after a cesarean delivery [1]. It is a common obstetric emergency, with an estimated global prevalence of roughly 3–5% of all births, though rates vary widely by region [1]. PPH remains the leading cause of maternal mortality worldwide, responsible for approximately one-quarter of all maternal deaths [2]. Each year, about 14 million women experience PPH, resulting in around 70,000 maternal deaths globally [1]. This burden is disproportionately high in low-resource settings, particularly sub-Saharan Africa and South Asia, where two-thirds of the world's births occur and where the risk of death from PPH is highest [3]. Even when not fatal, severe hemorrhage can lead to serious morbidity—organ failure, emergency surgeries (such as hysterectomy), transfusion complications, and long-term health consequences [4]. Importantly, many of these deaths and complications are preventable with timely interventions [2].

In high-resource countries, maternal mortality from PPH has declined over the past decades, yet PPH still contributes significantly to morbidity. Notably, several developed regions have observed a rise in PPH incidence over time, possibly related to changes in obstetric practices and maternal characteristics [4]. In the United States, PPH accounts for ~11% of maternal deaths and is the leading cause of severe maternal morbidity on the day of birth [4]. Approximately 54–93% of hemorrhage-related maternal deaths are considered preventable with optimal care [5]. These statistics underscore the critical need for effective PPH prevention strategies in every setting. Comprehensive approaches—including risk assessment, prophylactic measures at every delivery, and system-wide protocols—are essential to reduce the incidence of PPH and improve maternal outcomes.

22.2 Risk Factors for Postpartum Hemorrhage

While PPH can occur unpredictably in any birth, several well-recognized risk factors predispose women to hemorrhage. It is useful to categorize causes of PPH by the "Four T's"—Tone, Tissue, Trauma, and Thrombin—and consider risk factors for each category [6]:
- Tone (Uterine Atony)—Uterine atony (failure of the uterus to contract effectively after birth) is by far the most common cause of PPH, accounting for about 70–80% of cases [4]. Conditions that overdistend or fatigue the uterus predispose to atony. These include multiple gestation, polyhydramnios, and fetal macrosomia (an overdistended uterus), high parity (grand multiparity with stretched uterine muscle), prolonged or rapid labor (uterine muscle exhaustion), intra-amniotic infection (chorioamnionitis) causing uterine inflammation, and uterine fibroids or anomalies that impair contractility [4]. Use of uterine relaxants (e.g., magnesium sulfate for preeclampsia, β-agonists like terbutaline for tocolysis, or general anesthesia agents) can also transiently predispose to atony [4]. A distended bladder postpartum may prevent the uterus from contracting well [6]. Notably, although

these factors increase risk, uterine atony and hemorrhage often occur with no identifiable risk factors, so vigilance is required for all births [4].

- Tissue (Retained Placental Tissue)—Incomplete delivery of the placenta or retained products can lead to hemorrhage by preventing effective uterine contraction. Retained placental lobules (succenturiate lobe), abnormally adherent placenta (placenta accreta spectrum), or retained blood clots can all cause persistent bleeding [4]. A prolonged third stage of labor or manual placenta removal in a previous birth raises suspicion for placental retention issues in subsequent deliveries [4]. Careful placental inspection for completeness after delivery is crucial to identify missing cotyledons.
- Trauma (Birth Canal or Uterine Injury)—Trauma to the genital tract can cause significant hemorrhage even with a well-contracted uterus. This category includes lacerations of the cervix, vagina, or perineum (often associated with precipitous labor or operative deliveries), vaginal hematomas (e.g., from forceps or vacuum delivery), uterine rupture (rare, but risk increased with previous uterine surgery such as a cesarean scar), and uterine inversion (collapse of the uterine fundus, associated with excessive cord traction or fundal pressure, especially in a relaxed uterus) [4]. An episiotomy can also contribute to blood loss; routine episiotomy is a risk factor for increased hemorrhage and anal tears and should be avoided unless clinically necessary [7]. Prompt recognition and repair of any tears is important to prevent ongoing hemorrhage from trauma sources.
- Thrombin (Coagulopathy)–Hemorrhage can be exacerbated by clotting abnormalities in the mother. Preexisting coagulation disorders (e.g., von Willebrand disease or other bleeding diathesis) and acquired coagulopathies can impair hemostasis [4]. Important acquired causes include severe preeclampsia with HELLP syndrome or disseminated intravascular coagulation (DIC), placental abruption leading to DIC, amniotic fluid embolism, and massive hemorrhage itself causing dilutional coagulopathy [4]. Women on therapeutic anticoagulation (e.g., for prosthetic valves or thrombosis) are also at higher risk of heavy bleeding [4]. In such cases, even modest bleeding can become life-threatening due to impaired clot formation. Correction of coagulopathies and involvement of transfusion medicine are key when hemorrhage occurs in these settings.

Other noteworthy risk factors include a history of prior PPH, which increases the risk of recurrence, and placenta previa (due to its associated risk of accreta and need for surgical delivery). However, it must be emphasized that PPH can occur without any known risk factors. Over half of women who hemorrhage have no high-risk indicators [4]. Therefore, while obstetric teams should identify and prepare for high-risk patients (e.g., deliver in a facility with blood transfusion capability for a woman with twins and placenta previa) [2], they must also maintain vigilance and apply preventive measures universally. Risk factor assessment (such as standardized hemorrhage risk scoring on admission) can help plan the level of precautions, but routine prophylaxis for all mothers in the third stage of labor is the cornerstone of PPH prevention.

22.3 Pathophysiology of Postpartum Hemorrhage

After delivery of the baby, the placenta shears off the uterine wall, leaving behind open uterine blood vessels that supplied the intervillous space. Under normal physiology, uterine contraction (myometrial contraction) is the critical mechanism that compresses these spiral arterioles and venous sinuses, effectively tamponading bleeding. This myometrial contraction, along with clot formation, usually keeps blood loss to a minimal, physiological amount. PPH occurs when this balance is disturbed—most commonly when the uterus fails to contract adequately (atony), or when an anatomical injury or retained tissue interferes with hemostasis.

Uterine atony represents the primary pathophysiologic cause in about 70–80% of PPH cases [4, 6]. In atony, the uterine muscle fibers do not shorten and compress the vessels, leading to unrestrained bleeding from the placental bed. Atony can result from overdistension (the muscle stretched too thin), muscle exhaustion (after very long labor or very rapid labor), infection, or use of uterine relaxant drugs, as noted above. At the molecular level, insufficient calcium influx or oxytocin receptor desensitization (from prolonged oxytocin infusion in labor) may contribute to poor uterine contractility in atony. Clinically, atony is manifested by a "boggy" enlarged uterus and excessive bleeding. Because atony is so common, first-line preventive and therapeutic measures target ensuring adequate uterine contraction (as described later).

Traumatic hemorrhage occurs when damage to the birth canal or uterus causes bleeding. A cervical or vaginal laceration, uterine rupture, or uterine inversion can each lead to rapid hemorrhage by opening arterial vessels. In these cases, even a firmly contracted uterus will not stop the hemorrhage until the tear is repaired or the inversion is corrected. Thus, identification of the source is key. Often trauma and atony coexist (e.g., atony leading to uterine inversion, or a big baby causing both a tear and atony), so parallel evaluation is needed.

Retained placental tissue causes hemorrhage through two mechanisms: It prevents full uterine contraction (contributing to atony), and it can cause persistent bleeding from the implantation site because a portion of the placenta remains attached and the uterus cannot involute. Small, retained fragments or clots can be enough to impede adequate contraction. In placenta accreta spectrum, where villi are abnormally invasive, the placenta does not separate cleanly, and massive hemorrhage can occur due to both atony and surgical bleeding from attempts to detach the placenta. Management often requires surgical intervention (e.g., manual extraction or hysterectomy in accreta) to remove the source of bleeding.

Coagulopathy (thrombin issues) in PPH is often secondary—extreme hemorrhage can consume clotting factors and platelets, leading to DIC, which in turn worsens bleeding in a vicious cycle. Additionally, obstetric conditions like severe preeclampsia, amniotic fluid embolism, or placental abruption can trigger DIC even before any blood loss, so that at delivery, the patient cannot clot properly and bleeds excessively. The pathophysiology here is a systemic failure of the clotting process. In these situations, uterotonics alone will not suffice; blood products and specific anticoagulation factor support (plasma, platelets, and fibrinogen) are required.

It is useful for clinicians to approach a hemorrhaging patient by simultaneously considering all Four T's (Tone, Trauma, Tissue, Thrombin) [4, 6]. Typically, uterine atony is assumed to be the culprit until proven otherwise, given its high incidence. However, one must quickly assess for lacerations or hematomas (if bleeding persists despite a firm fundus), ensure the placenta is complete, and evaluate if coagulopathy is present or developing. This comprehensive approach addresses the pathophysiologic pathways through which hemorrhage occurs. By understanding these mechanisms, specific preventive strategies can be employed to avert PPH—primarily focusing on maintaining uterine tone and avoiding trauma or retention of tissue, as detailed in subsequent sections.

22.4 Active Management of the Third Stage of Labor (AMTSL)

Active management of the third stage of labor is a proven strategy to prevent PPH. It entails a set of interventions performed after delivery of the fetus but before or just after expulsion of the placenta, aimed at facilitating placental delivery and promoting uterine contraction. The core components of AMTSL include administration of a prophylactic uterotonic, controlled cord traction, and uterine fundal massage after placental delivery (as needed). This approach contrasts with "expectant" or physiological management, where the placenta is delivered spontaneously without medical intervention, which is associated with a higher risk of hemorrhage.

Uterotonic Administration: The timely administration of a uterotonic drug is the cornerstone of AMTSL. Current guidelines uniformly recommend giving a uterotonic agent to every woman after the birth of the baby, preferably within one minute of delivery, to actively promote uterine contraction [2]. Oxytocin is the most-used agent (details in the next section). This prophylactic uterotonic greatly reduces the likelihood of uterine atony. Multiple studies and a Cochrane review have demonstrated that active management (primarily uterotonics) significantly decreases PPH rates and related morbidities compared to expectant management. In fact, it is estimated that proper use of AMTSL can prevent nearly 60% of hemorrhage cases [8]. Given this evidence, the World Health Organization (WHO) and International Federation of Gynecology and Obstetrics (FIGO) consider routine uterotonic use after birth as a standard of care for all deliveries [6].

Controlled Cord Traction (CCT): In AMTSL, the delivery provider does not wait passively for the placenta to expel. Instead, once signs of placental separation appear (gush of blood, cord lengthening, fundal rebound), the provider applies gentle traction on the umbilical cord with counter-pressure on the uterus (to prevent inversion) to assist delivery of the placenta. CCT helps expel the placenta more quickly and completely. It should be done by a trained provider to avoid complications. When done properly, CCT has not been shown to increase the risk of uterine inversion (a rare event in ~0.04% births) [9]. This step shortens the third stage of labor and reduces the incidence of retained placenta, thereby lowering PPH risk due to retained tissue. If the placenta does not deliver within the expected time frame (~30 minutes), preparations for manual removal should be made to prevent hemorrhage from a partial separation.

Uterine Massage and Tone Assessment: After the placenta is delivered, the uterine fundus is massaged to stimulate contraction and expel any clots. The uterus is palpated frequently in the first minutes to ensure it is firm. Uterine fundal massage has been a traditional component of AMTSL. However, evidence on routine, prolonged massage is mixed. The WHO specifically does not recommend continuous uterine massage as a standalone intervention to prevent PPH in women who have received prophylactic oxytocin, because routine massage beyond the initial assessment has not shown additional benefit and may cause discomfort. Instead, the recommendation is to monitor uterine tone and perform massage only as needed if the uterus is not firm [2]. Essentially, once a uterotonic has been given, the provider should check the fundus: if boggy, then massage (this is often referred to as "rub up a contraction"). Intermittent uterine tone assessment is important in the first 1–2 hours postpartum, as a soft uterus requires prompt intervention. In settings without uterotonics, massage has been shown to reduce blood loss, but with uterotonics on board, its role is adjunctive. Thus, the focus in AMTSL is uterotonic administration and delivering the placenta, with uterine massage as a follow-up measure to ensure contraction.

Umbilical Cord Clamping Timing: Historically, early cord clamping (within 30 seconds of birth) was part of active management protocols. However, modern evidence has confirmed that delayed cord clamping (waiting at least 1–3 minutes) improves neonatal outcomes (better newborn iron stores and reduced anemia) without significantly increasing maternal hemorrhage risk [10]. Professional guidelines, including WHO and American College of Obstetricians and Gynecologists (ACOG), now endorse delayed cord clamping for healthy term and preterm infants. Importantly, delayed cord clamping does not interfere with AMTSL; uterotonics can still be given immediately after birth, and one can wait ~60–120 seconds before clamping and then perform cord traction [2]. Studies show that delayed clamping does not increase PPH incidence [10]. Therefore, providers should integrate delayed cord clamping into the third stage, providing neonatal benefit while still performing the other active management steps in a timely manner.

In summary, active management of the third stage of labor is a critical, evidence-based practice that substantially reduces PPH. All women, regardless of risk factors, should receive active management unless a specific contraindication exists. Training birth attendants in AMTSL (particularly in the correct use of uterotonics and controlled cord traction) is a key intervention in both high- and low-resource settings. The widespread implementation of AMTSL—through initiatives by WHO, FIGO, the International Confederation of Midwives (ICM), and others—has been a cornerstone of global strategies to reduce maternal hemorrhage. Successful AMTSL requires coordination: having uterotonic drugs readily available in the delivery room, proper timing of administration (often as the newborn is being cared for), and careful delivery of the placenta. When performed consistently, AMTSL dramatically decreases the incidence of PPH and severe blood loss [8]. Thus, it forms the first line of defense in PPH prevention for every birth.

22.5 Pharmacologic Strategies for PPH Prevention

Pharmacologic prophylaxis—mainly the use of uterotonic medications—is the most effective approach to prevent PPH due to uterine atony. Uterotonics stimulate uterine muscle contraction, thereby accelerating placental separation and constricting the uterine blood vessels. Multiple uterotonic agents are available, and guidelines from WHO, FIGO, and ACOG provide recommendations on their use in the third stage of labor [2, 4]. Key pharmacologic options include:

- <u>Oxytocin (Pitocin)</u>: Oxytocin is the first-line uterotonic for PPH prevention in all births. It is a synthetic form of the natural hormone that induces uterine contractions. A dose of 10 International Units (IU) given intramuscularly (IM) or by slow intravenous (IV) is recommended soon after delivery of the baby [2]. Oxytocin has a rapid onset (within 2–3 minutes with IV, or a few minutes with IM) and effectively reduces hemorrhage risk. It has minimal side effects in most patients; transient hypotension or tachycardia can occur if given as an IV bolus, so it is often given as a short infusion. Oxytocin is safe in hypertensive women and can be used in almost all situations. WHO, FIGO, and ACOG all recommend oxytocin 10 IU as the uterotonic of choice for routine prophylaxis [2, 6]. In settings where IV access is available (e.g., during a cesarean), it may be given IV; otherwise, IM injection after birth is effective. Oxytocin should be available at every birth; its use is a major factor in the decline of PPH in facilities worldwide.
- <u>Carbetocin</u>: Carbetocin is a long-acting oxytocin analogue. A 100 µg IM or IV dose provides a prolonged uterotonic effect (about one hour of uterine contraction) from a single injection. Heat-stable carbetocin has gained attention for use in low-resource settings because, unlike oxytocin, it does not require refrigeration. A large WHO-led trial (the CHAMPION trial) in 2018 demonstrated that heat-stable carbetocin was non-inferior to oxytocin in preventing hemorrhage ≥500 mL or the need for additional uterotonics [2]. Based on this, the WHO updated its recommendations: carbetocin can be used for PPH prevention in all births if it is available at a similar cost to oxytocin [9]. Carbetocin is especially useful in settings where cold-chain storage for oxytocin is problematic or for cesarean deliveries (some obstetric guidelines prefer carbetocin at cesarean to ensure sustained uterine tone). Cost has been a barrier, but with the broader availability of generic and heat-stable formulations, carbetocin use is expected to increase. It has similar side effects to oxytocin (less risk of hypertension than ergometrine). In summary, carbetocin is an effective alternative to oxytocin, endorsed by FIGO/WHO, particularly in contexts where its storage and cost advantages come into play [9].
- <u>Ergometrine (Ergonovine) and Methylergometrine</u>: These ergot alkaloids cause tetanic uterine contractions. A typical dose is 0.2 mg IM after delivery. Ergomet-

rine is often combined with oxytocin in a single injection (e.g., "Syntometrine", which contains 5 IU oxytocin +0.5 mg ergometrine) for prophylaxis. Ergot alkaloids are very effective uterotonics, and some studies show the combination of oxytocin + ergometrine reduces PPH more than oxytocin alone. However, they have significant side effects: notably hypertension (by causing vasospasm) and nausea/vomiting. They are contraindicated in women with hypertensive disorders (preeclampsia) or cardiovascular disease. WHO suggests that ergometrine (alone or in combination) can be used for prevention only if oxytocin is unavailable or of uncertain quality, and only in women without high blood pressure [2]. Many low-resource hospitals still use the oxytocin/ergometrine combination routinely for added protection, but the trend is to use pure oxytocin first line and reserve ergometrine for backup or high-risk atony situations where blood pressure is normal. If used, careful attention to blood pressure and side effects is needed.

- **Misoprostol**: Misoprostol is a prostaglandin E1 analog available in tablet form. It has the advantage of being heat-stable, inexpensive, and can be given orally, sublingually, or rectally, making it extremely valuable in settings where injectables are not accessible. The recommended prophylactic dose is 400–600 µg orally (the common dose is 600 µg PO) after delivery of the baby [6]. Misoprostol is less effective than oxytocin (higher rates of PPH compared to oxytocin in head-to-head trials) but still significantly better than no uterotonic. WHO and FIGO endorse misoprostol use for PPH prevention in births attended by community health workers or in home births where oxytocin injection is not feasible [11]. For example, trained lay health workers have safely used 600 µg oral misoprostol for women delivering at home to reduce hemorrhage incidence. Misoprostol's side effects include fever, chills, and shivering (common but self-limited) and sometimes diarrhea. These are generally tolerable given the potentially lifesaving benefit. Misoprostol should only be administered by non-skilled personnel in such settings (to avoid misuse), whereas in hospitals, oxytocin remains preferred. Advance distribution of misoprostol to pregnant women (to self-administer immediately after birth if no skilled attendant is present) has been recommended by WHO in certain high-mortality regions as a harm-reduction strategy [2, 11]. In summary, misoprostol is a critical component of PPH prevention in low-resource and rural contexts; it fills the gap where oxytocin injections cannot reach, thereby extending prophylaxis to all birthing women.
- **Prostaglandin Analogs** (Carboprost, Dinoprost): Carboprost tromethamine (15-methyl $PGF_2\alpha$, brand Hemabate) 250 µg IM, or sulprostone (PGE2 analog used in some countries), are potent uterotonics mainly used for the treatment of atonic PPH unresponsive to first-line measures. They are not recommended for routine prophylaxis due to their side-effect profile [6]. Carboprost can cause significant bronchospasm (contraindicated in asthma), diarrhea, and fever. As prophylaxis, they offer no advantage over oxytocin/ergot and would subject women to unnecessary side effects. Therefore, guidelines advise against using injectable prostaglandins for primary prevention [2]. They should be reserved for therapeutic use if hemorrhage occurs despite prophylaxis.
- **Tranexamic Acid (TXA)**: Tranexamic acid is an antifibrinolytic that helps stabilize blood clots. It is not a uterotonic, but it has emerged as an important adjunct in PPH treatment. The landmark WOMAN trial (2017) [12] showed that IV TXA (1 g) given within 3 hours of PPH onset can reduce mortality from bleeding by about 30%, without increasing thrombotic risk. As a result, TXA is now recommended in the management of PPH, in addition to uterotonics, particularly for severe hemorrhage or suspected coagulopathy [13]. However, the role of TXA in PPH prevention has been under investigation. A recent large trial (WOMAN-2, published 2024)

[14] tested prophylactic TXA (1 g IV given immediately after vaginal birth) in women with anemia to see if it would prevent PPH. The outcome was negative—TXA given prophylactically did not significantly reduce PPH incidence (7.0% with TXA vs 6.6% with placebo) [14]. The trial's interpretation was that TXA shortly after birth did not reduce the risk of PPH in anemic women [14]. Therefore, routine prophylactic TXA is not currently recommended for PPH prevention in the general obstetric population. It may be considered in select high-risk cases (e.g., those with coagulopathies or planned cesarean in placenta accreta where massive hemorrhage is anticipated), but there is no guideline consensus for routine use in all women. TXA remains a critical medication to treat PPH once it is diagnosed, and every obstetric unit should have TXA available for that purpose [13]. For prevention, the focus remains on uterotonics as described above.

In practice, oxytocin is administered to virtually all women after childbirth as the primary prophylactic measure against hemorrhage [2]. The other pharmacologic agents serve as alternatives or additions based on specific contexts and risk factors. For example, in a high-risk delivery (e.g., twins with polyhydramnios in a remote clinic), one might give oxytocin and have misoprostol or ergometrine ready if the uterus remains soft. In a cesarean for placenta previa (high hemorrhage risk), some obstetricians might give IV oxytocin followed by IV TXA and even a dose of carboprost if uterine tone is suboptimal—essentially layering treatments to prevent hemorrhage. Generally, however, one effective uterotonic given prophylactically is sufficient for the majority of women, and additional doses or agents are used if bleeding ensues.

It is also important that infrastructure supports pharmacologic prevention: hospitals need policies to ensure uterotonics (oxytocin, especially) are stocked in delivery rooms and properly refrigerated, training for staff on correct administration, and policies allowing midwives to give uterotonics without waiting for a physician order in the moment of delivery (standing orders/protocols). In low-resource areas, making uterotonics available at the community level—via misoprostol distribution or oxytocin in Uniject devices—has been a major public health strategy to increase coverage of PPH prevention.

In summary, pharmacologic prophylaxis with uterotonics is the primary and most effective strategy to prevent postpartum hemorrhage. Oxytocin remains the gold standard for all births. Alternatives like carbetocin, ergometrine, and misoprostol play important roles when oxytocin is not available or additional support is needed. The use of these medications, guided by evidence-based protocols, has saved countless lives by preventing atony and reducing hemorrhage severity. Ongoing research continues to refine drug choices (e.g., heat-stable formulations, combination therapies), but the universal agreement is that every woman should receive a uterotonic in the third stage of labor to actively prevent PPH [6].

22.6 Non-pharmacologic Strategies and Supportive Measures

While uterotonic medications are central to PPH prevention, non-pharmacologic strategies also contribute significantly to reducing hemorrhage. These measures involve clinical techniques and supportive practices during and after birth that minimize bleeding and complement the action of drugs. Key non-pharmacologic approaches include:

- Proper Delivery Technique and Controlled Cord Traction: Gentle birthing techniques can prevent trauma. Avoiding undue fundal pressure on the uterus and waiting for signs of placental separation before applying cord traction reduces the risk of uterine inversion and ensures the placenta delivers intact. Controlled cord traction (as part of AMTSL) by an experienced provider helps prevent retained placenta and excessive bleeding. If resistance is met or the cord seems to be stretching, traction should be paused to avoid inversion [9]. Ensuring the uterus is slightly contracted (with a uterotonic) before applying traction also helps. In essence, skilled management of the third stage—not yanking on the cord too early, supporting the uterus—can prevent trauma and retention.

- Uterine Fundal Massage and Assessment: As discussed, routine continuous massage is not necessary if a uterotonic was given, but intermittent uterine assessment is crucial. The birth attendant should palpate the uterine fundus regularly (e.g., every 15 minutes in the first hour) to check that it is firm and contracted. If the uterus feels soft ("boggy"), immediate fundal massage is performed to stimulate contractions ("rubbing the fundus") [2]. Massage can express pooled blood and clots, helping the uterus contract better. This simple measure can often nip early atony in the bud before it progresses to hemorrhage. Uterine tone monitoring is recommended for all women postpartum [6]. In many hospitals, nurses are tasked with frequent uterine checks and massage PRN in the recovery period. This practice can be considered a preventive measure to detect and treat mild atony before it becomes a significant hemorrhage.
- Avoiding and Promptly Treating Genital Tract Trauma: Reducing unnecessary trauma at delivery can prevent hemorrhage from lacerations. Practitioners should avoid routine episiotomy, as it increases blood loss and the risk of severe perineal tears [7]. Episiotomy should only be done for specific indications (e.g., operative delivery, fetal distress) and in a controlled manner. Additionally, ensuring good perineal support in the second stage (for example, using warm compresses and controlled delivery of the head) may decrease the incidence of severe tears. If lacerations do occur, meticulous surgical repair of tears in the perineum, vagina, or cervix immediately after delivery is essential to prevent ongoing bleeding. Good lighting and anesthesia assist in thorough examination and repair. In the case of a suspected hematoma (e.g., the patient has severe pain or signs of blood loss with little visible bleeding), early evaluation and, if needed, surgical drainage of the hematoma can prevent escalation [4]. For cesarean deliveries or uterine surgery, careful surgical technique and securing uterine incision angles can prevent hemorrhage from uterine or broad ligament tears.
- Maintaining Bladder Emptiness: A distended bladder can impede effective uterine contraction by physically displacing the uterus. Immediately after delivery, especially if regional anesthesia was used, the patient often cannot feel bladder fullness. It is helpful to ensure the bladder is emptied (via straight catheterization or leaving an indwelling catheter for a short period if epidural/spinal anesthesia was used) during the immediate postpartum. An empty bladder allows the uterus to contract downward into the pelvis properly [6]. If the uterus is higher than expected or deviated, bladder distension should be suspected and addressed. This simple step can prevent atony that is easily reversible.
- Breastfeeding and Maternal–Infant Bonding: Early initiation of breastfeeding and skin-to-skin contact can augment uterine contraction through the release of endogenous oxytocin. Suckling triggers the mother's pituitary to secrete oxytocin, which helps contract the uterus (the same reflex that causes "afterpains" while breastfeeding). While the effect is mild compared to pharmacologic oxytocin, every bit helps in maintaining tone. Thus, from a prevention standpoint, encouraging the mother to breastfeed soon after birth benefits both the baby and may modestly support uterine involution.
- Thermal Care and Hydration: Keeping the mother warm and well-hydrated postpartum is a supportive measure to avoid exacerbating hemorrhage. Hypothermia and acidosis can worsen coagulopathy (the "lethal triad" in trauma)—although these are more concerns in massive hemorrhage situations, it is sensible to maintain normal temperature (using warm blankets, warmed IV fluids if needed) and adequate

volume status. These measures ensure optimal clotting function if any bleeding occurs.

- Recognition and Management of Retained Placenta: If the placenta does not deliver within 30 minutes of birth (or is incomplete), it is critical to intervene (through manual extraction by a skilled provider, with appropriate anesthesia and uterotonics) before hemorrhage becomes severe. A retained placenta can lead to sudden, significant bleeding once partial separation occurs. Thus, prompt manual removal of a retained placenta (and exploration of the uterus for additional fragments) is a preventive action to stop hemorrhage at its source. Following removal, inspecting the placenta to confirm it is complete is a standard step in the prevention of "tissue"-related hemorrhage.
- Special Prophylactic Measures in High-Risk Scenarios: In certain very high-risk obstetric situations (like placenta previa or placenta accreta spectrum), obstetric teams may employ specific prophylactic interventions. For example, in a placenta accreta case, a common strategy is to have blood products on hold and perhaps proceed directly to an operative management (such as cesarean hysterectomy) before catastrophic hemorrhage occurs. In cases of previa or anticipated atony (such as a uterus with fibroids or after multiple prior uterotonics), some centers may proactively insert a uterine tamponade balloon (Bakri balloon) after delivery/surgery as a preventive measure to compress the uterine vasculature. Similarly, interventional radiology can place balloon catheters in the internal iliac arteries predelivery in placenta accreta cases to occlude blood flow and reduce hemorrhage. These advanced measures are situation-specific and done in tertiary settings; while not routine, they illustrate how anticipating hemorrhage in high-risk patients can lead to proactive interventions that mitigate blood loss.
- Optimize Maternal Health (Indirect Prevention): While not a direct prevention of hemorrhage occurrence, improving a mother's health status can prevent hemorrhage from turning lethal. For instance, identifying and treating antenatal iron-deficiency anemia ensures the mother has better hemoglobin reserves if bleeding happens [4]. Proper management of pre-eclampsia (e.g., timely delivery in severe cases) can prevent coagulopathy that would worsen PPH. Infections should be treated early to avoid chorioamnionitis-related atony. Thus, broad prenatal care improvements and early risk management (like treating placenta previa with a planned delivery in a controlled setting) are part of a holistic PPH prevention strategy.

In combination, these non-pharmacologic strategies support the primary prevention efforts. They are often embedded in clinical protocols and training. For example, "rub the fundus, check the bladder, call for help, start massage" are immediate actions in a protocol when blood loss is noted to be more than normal. Many of these measures (uterine massage, empty bladder, etc.) appear in obstetric emergency checklists as first responses, which indeed are preventive steps to keep a developing hemorrhage from worsening. It is important to foster a practice environment where nurses and providers are vigilant in performing these tasks routinely (e.g., quantitative measurement of urine output to ensure bladder emptying, periodic uterine checks, etc.).

Ultimately, preventing PPH is not a single intervention but a bundle of practices. Uterotonics are chief among them, but the adjunct steps above further minimize risk. By delivering babies with care (avoiding trauma), actively managing the third stage, and promptly addressing any issues (like retained tissue or a full bladder), the obstetric team can often prevent a mild postpartum bleed from progressing to a hemorrhage emergency. In essence, attention to detail in the immediate postpartum period—examining the placenta, assessing the perineum, monitoring bleeding, and uterine tone—is a non-pharmacologic strategy that is just as vital as giving a dose of oxytocin.

22.7 Institutional Protocols and Systems for PPH Prevention

In addition to individual clinical practices, the establishment of institutional protocols and organized systems is a crucial aspect of preventing and managing postpartum hemorrhage. Obstetric hemorrhage emergencies unfold rapidly, and outcomes improve significantly when standardized protocols guide the team's response. Over the past decade, professional bodies like ACOG, the Joint Commission, and maternal safety organizations have championed the implementation of hemorrhage protocols in every birth facility [5]. Key elements of effective institutional preparedness include:

- Hospital-wide Hemorrhage Protocol: Every maternity unit should have a written protocol for obstetric hemorrhage that is readily accessible and rehearsed. ACOG recommends that all hospitals adopt organized, systematic processes to coordinate PPH response [4]. These protocols often stratify hemorrhage into stages (Stage 0: normal, Stage 1: >500 mL bleeding, Stage 2: continuing bleeding >1000 mL, Stage 3: massive hemorrhage) with checklists of actions for each. Stage-based management ensures a timely escalation of interventions (additional uterotonics, activating massive transfusion protocol, calling extra personnel) if bleeding progresses. Having this framework in place before an emergency occurs is preventive because it enables the team to act early and uniformly at the first sign of hemorrhage.
- Hemorrhage Cart and Supplies: Units should maintain a stocked obstetric hemorrhage cart or toolkit containing all needed supplies: uterotonic medications (with ready-to-use syringes), IV fluids and needles, a uterine tamponade balloon, sutures for uterine compression (e.g., for B-Lynch suture), and quick reference cards for the protocol. When hemorrhage is suspected, this cart is brought to the bedside. By having medications and tools immediately at hand, delays are reduced, and prophylactic measures (like second-line uterotonics or balloon insertion) can be instituted without searching for equipment. Many hospitals bundle these items in a tackle box or crash cart specifically for PPH.
- Massive Transfusion Protocol (MTP): For severe hemorrhages, rapid access to blood products is lifesaving. Institutions should have an MTP tailored to obstetrics, which might be activated at a certain estimated blood loss or clinical condition. This protocol usually ensures uncross-matched blood is available within minutes, and a balanced resuscitation with packed RBCs, plasma, platelets, and fibrinogen concentrate or cryoprecipitate is delivered to manage coagulopathy. Drills often include practice in activating MTP and coordinating with the blood bank. Preventive benefit comes from the speed at which bleeding patients receive blood—a prepared system can avert shock and DIC that would occur if transfusion were delayed.
- Team Communication and Escalation Plan: Protocols designate roles—who calls for extra help, who is responsible for uterotonics, who monitors vitals, who contacts the blood bank, etc. Multidisciplinary team training is emphasized [4]. For example, a hemorrhage response team might include an obstetrician, an anesthesiologist, a nursing lead, and a blood bank liaison. Regular simulation drills (e.g., simulating a PPH due to atony) improve team coordination and communication, so that in real events the team moves efficiently. ACOG highlights that drills and simulation-based training should be a part of preparedness [4]. This training means that when an actual PPH begins, the team recognizes it early and each member knows their tasks (one person massages the uterus and gives oxytocin, another prepares second-line meds like carboprost, another assesses for lacerations, etc.) without confusion. Early recognition and a rapid, organized response can prevent a moderate hemorrhage from escalating to a life-threatening one [4].

- Risk Assessment and Early Warning Systems: Many hospitals implement a PPH risk assessment tool on admission or intrapartum (scoring systems that assign low/medium/high risk based on factors like previa, anemia, labor duration). This can prompt preparations: for instance, a high-risk patient might have a type & crossmatch done in advance, an extra IV line placed, and uterotonics pre-drawn. Additionally, obstetric early warning criteria (vital sign triggers such as heart rate >110 or blood pressure dropping) can alert staff to possible occult hemorrhage. If such triggers are met, the protocol might call for immediate evaluation for bleeding. Using quantitative measurement of blood loss (QBL) for every delivery is increasingly standard [5]. Unlike visual estimation (which often underestimates high volumes) [5, 15], QBL involves weighing soaked pads and measuring blood in drapes to know the exact volume lost. This helps in early identification of hemorrhage—studies show QBL increases the likelihood of recognizing PPH promptly [16]. The AIM (Alliance for Innovation on Maternal Health) Obstetric Hemorrhage Bundle adopted in many US hospitals specifically includes quantitative cumulative blood loss as a key component [16]. Early recognition through these methods triggers the preventative actions sooner, thereby reducing progression to severe hemorrhage.
- Data Review and Continuous Improvement: Hospitals are encouraged to perform debriefs after hemorrhage events and regular audits of severe hemorrhage cases. By reviewing what went well or what could be improved (for example, a debrief might reveal a slight delay in uterotonic administration or an issue in blood release), the team refines the protocol. This continuous learning loop is part of institutional prevention—it helps close gaps in the system that may contribute to hemorrhage severity. Some hospitals have quality improvement projects aimed at reducing PPH rates or improving adherence to AMTSL, and they track metrics such as the percentage of women receiving uterotonics within 1 minute of birth or the incidence of transfusions over time.
- Outreach and Drills with Lower-Level Facilities: In regions where not all births occur in well-equipped hospitals, larger centers often work with smaller clinics to ensure they have basic hemorrhage protocols and resources (like a supply of misoprostol and a plan for transfer if hemorrhage occurs). This system-level preparation ensures that even at primary health centers, PPH prevention (uterotonics for all, etc.) is standard, and that there is a clear referral pathway for refractory cases.

The effectiveness of such institutional efforts is supported by evidence. For example, the implementation of the California Maternal Quality Care Collaborative (CMQCC) hemorrhage toolkit across numerous hospitals was associated with a significant reduction in severe maternal morbidity from hemorrhage [17]. Similarly, hospitals participating in the AIM hemorrhage bundle have reported improvements in early PPH recognition and reduced use of blood transfusions. ACOG's 2017 updated Practice Bulletin on PPH explicitly added recommendations for hospitals to establish protocols and drills as part of comprehensive hemorrhage prevention and management [4]. By having these systems in place, every team member knows that prevention of PPH is an ongoing process: from admission (risk assessment), during delivery (active management), and through the response (stage-based protocol if bleeding continues).

In summary, institutional readiness is a form of prevention. It ensures that prophylactic measures are reliably given to every patient (through checklist reminders and standing orders) and that any hemorrhage is met with a prepared, efficient response. This reduces the chance of an avoidable escalation. The motto is often "every birth, every time"—meaning every birth should have the necessary prevention (uterotonics, etc.), and every team should be ready to act at the slightest sign of trouble. Such preparedness ultimately saves lives and reduces complications by preventing delays and omissions in PPH care.

22.8 Global Guidelines and Recommendations

The prevention of postpartum hemorrhage is a priority in global maternal health, and leading organizations have published guidelines that converge on many key principles, with some variations to accommodate different contexts. Here we highlight recommendations from major authorities:

World Health Organization (WHO): WHO has issued evidence-based guidelines focused on both prevention and treatment of PPH, notably in its 2012 comprehensive guidelines and subsequent updates. WHO strongly recommends active management of the third stage of labor for all vaginal deliveries, with uterotonic prophylaxis for every birth as a top priority [2]. Oxytocin (10 IU IM/IV) is recommended as the first-line uterotonic for PPH prevention in all women [2]. In situations where oxytocin is unavailable or cannot be stored properly, WHO endorses alternative uterotonics: e.g., injectable ergometrine, oxytocin–ergometrine combination, or carbetocin (particularly heat-stable carbetocin where feasible) can be used, provided there are no contraindications (like hypertension for ergometrine) [13]. If no skilled provider is present to give injections, WHO supports the use of oral misoprostol (600 μg) by trained community health workers to prevent PPH in home births [2]. Indeed, WHO released a recommendation on advance distribution of misoprostol to pregnant women who may deliver without a skilled attendant, to ensure they have a uterotonic available immediately after birth [2]. Additionally, WHO emphasizes that delayed cord clamping (at least 1–3 minutes) should be practiced in conjunction with uterotonic use, as it benefits the infant and does not increase maternal hemorrhage risk. WHO guidelines advise against routine uterine massage after oxytocin for prevention, as no additional benefit was found [2]. In 2018, after the CHAMPION trial, the WHO included heat-stable carbetocin on its list of uterotonics for prevention in hospital settings, particularly in warm climates where oxytocin storage is challenging [18]. For treatment (beyond prevention), WHO (2017) added the recommendation of tranexamic acid within 3 hours of PPH onset as part of standard care, which underscores that prevention and treatment are part of a continuum of hemorrhage care [13]. Overall, WHO guidelines aim to be globally applicable—prioritizing uterotonics for all, encouraging task-shifting (misoprostol by lay health workers) where needed, and improving health system readiness. They also call for health facilities to have training and PPH protocols in place, aligning with broader quality of care initiatives.

International Federation of Gynecology and Obstetrics (FIGO) and International Confederation of Midwives (ICM): FIGO and ICM have actively collaborated to promote PPH prevention worldwide. They issued joint statements endorsing the WHO recommendations on PPH prevention and treatment [9]. FIGO's 2022 guidelines on PPH management reiterate that all women should receive a prophylactic uterotonic after delivery, as this practice has proven to reduce PPH rates [6]. FIGO specifically recommends oxytocin as the first choice and mirrors WHO in advising alternatives when oxytocin is not available (such as misoprostol in community settings, or an ergometrine combination) [6, 9]. FIGO and ICM have also been involved in initiatives like the FIGO PPH Prevention Champions and the Motherhood Initiative to implement training for AMTSL in resource-limited countries. They emphasize interdisciplinary teamwork—obstetricians and midwives working together—to ensure active management is performed consistently at every birth [6]. FIGO has published a postpartum hemorrhage clinical handbook (in 2012 and updated later), which provides algorithms and care pathways for prevention and management, aligned with WHO. This includes flowcharts for deciding which uterotonic to use depending on context (e.g., presence of a skilled provider, availability of oxytocin) [6, 9], reflecting a pragmatic approach: use oxytocin if you can, but if you can't, use the next best uterotonic rather than doing nothing. FIGO also underscores health system factors—ensuring availability of essential medicines (like including uterotonics and TXA in national Essential Medicine Lists) and advocating for governments to adopt these guidelines. In summary, FIGO/ICM guidance aligns closely with WHO, with a strong push for universal prophylaxis and capacity building for AMTSL across all birth settings.

American College of Obstetricians and Gynecologists (ACOG): ACOG's guidance (Practice Bulletin No. 183, 2017, and subsequent Committee Opinions) on PPH prevention and management is broadly consistent with WHO but tailored to higher-resource settings. ACOG recommends oxytocin after all deliveries as the standard for active management of the third stage [4]. Oxytocin infusion is routinely used after childbirth in US hospitals (often 10–20 U in IV fluid). ACOG acknowledges other uterotonics (methergine, carboprost, and misoprostol) as necessary agents if hemorrhage occurs, but for prevention, oxytocin is usually sufficient for routine cases. ACOG has focused heavily on institutional preparedness: it calls for every birth unit to have a hemorrhage protocol, ready access to medications, and to conduct drills [4, 5]. The College has partnered in national initiatives like the AIM Safety Bundle for hemorrhage [4]. ACOG also emphasizes quantification of blood loss and the use of early warning criteria as best practices in obstetric care to catch hemorrhage early [5]. In terms of pharmacologic updates, after the WOMAN trial, ACOG incorporated tranexamic acid as a consideration in PPH management (especially if uterotonics and massage are not rapidly effective) [4], but it does not recommend TXA for routine prophylaxis (consistent with the WOMAN-2 findings). ACOG's guidelines also mention specific risk mitigation: for example, women with known coagulopathies or placenta accreta should be managed in centers with appropriate resources. While ACOG doesn't have a separate category of community-level prophylaxis (since most US births are in facilities), it does strongly promote patient blood management—optimizing hemoglobin antenatally, autologous blood donation considered in rare cases, etc., to improve outcomes if hemorrhage happens. Overall, ACOG's stance is very much in line with global principles: active management for all, and preparedness. The main difference is context—ACOG assumes availability of IV oxytocin and surgical resources, whereas WHO/FIGO also provides guidance for when those are lacking.

Royal College of Obstetricians and Gynecologists (RCOG) and Others: In the UK, the RCOG Green-top Guideline No. 52 on PPH (2016, updated 2023) similarly advocates for active management of the third stage to prevent PPH. NICE guidelines advise offering active management to all women, while respecting that a woman may choose the physiological third stage, but she should be informed that this doubles the risk of PPH and blood transfusion. If physiological management is attempted and bleeding is more than normal or the placenta is delayed, conversion to active management (giving a uterotonic) is indicated. RCOG's guidance on prevention aligns with using oxytocin 10 IU IM as standard, and ergometrine-oxytocin for higher risk cases if there are no contraindications. Like ACOG, RCOG emphasizes readiness: they have introduced obstetric hemorrhage bundles in the UK's Each Baby Counts initiative. Other organizations, like the International Confederation of Midwives (ICM), have worked on training midwives in AMTSL and postpartum monitoring, which is crucial for prevention, especially in out-of-hospital births.

Global Initiatives and Goals: Recognizing that PPH remains the leading cause of maternal death, WHO and partners launched in 2023 a "Roadmap to Combat PPH 2023–2030" [1]. This global plan aims to ensure 100% coverage of uterotonics at birth, improve access to newer interventions (like TXA and carbetocin), and improve accountability for maternal bleeding outcomes. There is also an increased push for innovation (for example, non-injectable oxytocin formulations, improved blood loss measurement tools) to aid prevention. The collective global target is to reduce maternal mortality further and specifically to drastically cut deaths from hemorrhage, which are seen as largely preventable with the tools now available.

In conclusion, despite slight differences in emphasis or context, the global guidelines from WHO, FIGO/ICM, ACOG, RCOG, and others uniformly underscore a few fundamental practices for PPH prevention: routine active management of the third stage with a uterotonic for every birth; readiness to use additional uterotonics or interventions if needed; careful monitoring in the immediate postpartum; and having system-level protocols to support the obstetric team. They also highlight that no single strategy is enough—success requires combining prophylactic medications, clinical skills, and institutional preparedness. The ongoing collaboration between international agencies means that messages are consistent worldwide, which helps standardize training: for example, a trainee obstetrician or midwife will hear the same guidance on AMTSL whether they are in a low-income country or a high-income hospital, merely adapted to the resources available. By adhering to these guidelines and continuously updating them with emerging evidence (such as new trial results), the medical community moves closer to the goal of making PPH a rare and well-managed event, rather than a leading killer of mothers.

Chapter Key Points

- PPH remains the leading cause of preventable maternal mortality worldwide.
- Most PPH cases are due to uterine atony; universal uterotonic prophylaxis is the most effective preventive measure.
- Active management of the third stage of labor (AMTSL) can prevent ~60% of PPH cases.
- Oxytocin 10 IU IM/IV is the gold-standard uterotonic; alternatives exist when oxytocin is unavailable.
- Risk assessment is valuable, but over half of PPH occurs without risk factors—prevention must be universal.
- Institutional protocols, QBL, and rapid-response systems are essential to reduce morbidity and mortality.

Chapter-End Summary

Postpartum hemorrhage remains a major cause of preventable maternal morbidity and mortality. Because many cases occur without identifiable risk factors, universal prophylaxis—especially AMTSL with timely uterotonic administration—is essential. Oxytocin remains first-line, with misoprostol, ergometrine, and carbetocin as context-specific alternatives. Prevention also relies on non-pharmacologic vigilance, trauma minimization, and prompt management of retained tissue. At the systems level, standardized protocols, hemorrhage carts, quantitative blood loss, and simulation training dramatically improve early recognition and response. When combined, these strategies substantially reduce the incidence and severity of PPH and improve maternal outcomes.

References

1. World Health Organization. A roadmap to combat postpartum haemorrhage between 2023 and 2030. 2023.
2. World Health Organization. WHO recommendations for the prevention and treatment of postpartum Haemorrhage. Geneva, Switzerland; 2012.
3. Say L, Chou D, Gemmill A, Tunçalp Ö, Moller AB, Daniels J, et al. Global causes of maternal death: a WHO systematic analysis. Lancet Glob Health. 2014 Jun;2(6):e323–33.
4. Committee on Practice Bulletins-Obstetrics. Practice Bulletin No. 183: Postpartum Hemorrhage. Obstet Gynecol. 2017;130(4):e168–86.
5. Quantitative Blood Loss in Obstetric Hemorrhage: ACOG COMMITTEE OPINION, Number 794. Obstet Gynecol. 2019;134(6):e150–6.
6. Escobar MF, Nassar AH, Theron G, Barnea ER, Nicholson W, Ramasauskaite D, et al. FIGO recommendations on the management of postpartum hemorrhage 2022. Int J Gynecol Obstet. 2022;157(S1):3–50.
7. Prevention and Management of Postpartum Haemorrhage: Green-top Guideline No. 52. BJOG. 2017;124(5):e106–49.
8. Fissahaye B, Dheresa M, Assefa N, Tesfaye D, Eyeberu A, Balis B, et al. Active management of the third stage of labor and associated factors among maternity care providers in public health

facilities in Eastern Ethiopia: a multi-center study. BMC Pregnancy Childbirth. 2023;23(1):701.
9. Begum F, Beyeza J, Burke T, Evans C, Hanson C, Lalonde A, et al. FIGO and the International Confederation of Midwives endorse WHO guidelines on prevention and treatment of postpartum hemorrhage. Int J Gynecol Obstet. 2022;158(S1):6–10.
10. Rabe H, Gyte GM, Díaz-Rossello JL, Duley L. Effect of timing of umbilical cord clamping and other strategies to influence placental transfusion at preterm birth on maternal and infant outcomes. Cochrane Database Syst Rev. 2019;9(9):CD003248.
11. Langenbach C. Misoprostol in preventing postpartum hemorrhage: a meta-analysis. Int J Gynaecol Obstet. 2006;92(1):10–8.
12. WOMAN Trial Collaborators. Effect of early tranexamic acid administration on mortality, hysterectomy, and other morbidities in women with post-partum haemorrhage (WOMAN): an international, randomised, double-blind, placebo-controlled trial. Lancet. 2017;389(10084):2105–16.
13. Vogel JP, Oladapo OT, Dowswell T, Gülmezoglu AM. Updated WHO recommendation on intravenous tranexamic acid for the treatment of post-partum haemorrhage. Lancet Glob Health. 2018;6(1):e18–9.
14. WOMAN-2 Trial Collaborators. The effect of tranexamic acid on postpartum bleeding in women with moderate and severe anaemia (WOMAN-2): an international, randomised, double-blind, placebo-controlled trial. Lancet. 2024;404(10463):1645–56.
15. Ayala M, Nookala V, Fogel J, Fatehi M. Visual estimation of blood loss versus quantitative blood loss for maternal outcomes related to obstetrical hemorrhage. Proc (Bayl Univ Med Cent). 2023;36(3):341–5.
16. Atallah F, Goffman D. Bundles for maternal safety: promises and challenges of bundle implementation: the case of obstetric hemorrhage. Clin Obstet Gynecol. 2019;62(3):539–49.
17. Main EK, Cape V, Abreo A, Vasher J, Woods A, Carpenter A, et al. Reduction of severe maternal morbidity from hemorrhage using a state perinatal quality collaborative. Am J Obstet Gynecol. 2017;216(3):298.e1–298.e11.
18. Widmer M, Piaggio G, Nguyen TMH, Osoti A, Owa OO, Misra S, et al. Heat-stable Carbetocin versus oxytocin to prevent hemorrhage after vaginal birth. N Engl J Med. 2018;379(8):743–52.

Prevention of Obstetric Anal Sphincter Injuries (OASIs)

Nicola Adanna Okeahialam, Ranee Thakar, and Abdul H. Sultan

Contents

Y. Yogev, A. Khalil (eds.), *Prevention of Complications in Obstetrics*,
https://doi.org/10.1007/978-3-032-23479-7_23

23

Learning Objectives

- Recognise modifiable and non-modifiable OASI risk factors.
- Interpret evidence on episiotomy type, instrument choice, and preventative intrapartum practices.
- Explain prediction models and their current limitations.
- Describe antenatal and intrapartum interventions proven to reduce OASI risk.
- Understand the role of care bundles and patient-centred counselling.

Learning Objectives

- Understand risk factors associated with OASIs.
- Learn about risk models described to predict OASIs.
- Learn about antenatal and intrapartum interventions known to reduce the risk of OASIs.

23.1 Introduction

Obstetric anal sphincter injuries (OASIs) are defined as injuries sustained to the anal sphincter during vaginal birth. These injuries are classified anatomically using the Sultan classification, which is based on the extent of injury to the external anal sphincter (EAS), internal anal sphincter (IAS) and anal mucosa (Table 23.1) [1].

A meta-analysis has demonstrated that the incidence of OASI globally is 2.4–6.5%, with the highest rate occurring in North America (Fig. 23.1) [2]. In the United Kingdom (UK), a national survey of 215 maternity units found the incidence of OASI to be 2.9% (6.1% and 1.7% in primiparous and multiparous, respectively) [3]. However, population-based studies in the UK, Australia, Denmark, Norway, Sweden, Finland, China and Canada have shown that the incidence of OASIs is increasing [4–8]. These injuries are significant risk factors for the development of anal incontinence, with a meta-analysis demonstrating that approximately 18% of women develop symptoms up to 2 years following vaginal birth [9, 10]. Other long-term sequelae include urinary incontinence, chronic pelvic pain and dyspareunia [11]. Moreover, women with OASI are more likely to report their birth as traumatic and demonstrate birth-related avoidance symptoms and post-traumatic stress disorder up to 6–10 months following birth [12]. Due to the significant physical, psychological and social impact of OASIs, prevention of these injuries is imperative.

Table 23.1 Perineal trauma classification recommended by the Royal College of Obstetricians and Gynaecologists

Degree	Injury
Intact	No visible tear
First	Perineal skin only
Second	Perineal muscles but not involving the anal sphincter
Third	Anal sphincter complex 3a- less than 50% of the EAS thickness torn 3b- greater than 50% of the EAS thickness torn 3c- both EAS and IAS torn
Fourth	Anal sphincter complex and anal mucosa
Rectal buttonhole tear	Rectal mucosa (with or without injury to the anal sphincter complex)

The prevention of OASI would not only benefit women but also the attributed healthcare costs. For example, in the UK, between 2000 and 2010, the NHS Litigation Authority reported that the total cost of claims following OASIs, including both damages and legal costs, was estimated to be £31 million [13]. In addition, in 2013/14, the economic burden of OASI was estimated to be £3.7 million (for assisted vaginal birth) and £9.8 million (for spontaneous vaginal birth) due to the length of hospital stay and postnatal symptom management [14].

In this chapter, we will assess the current evidence-based approach to preventing OASIs by describing the associated risk factors,

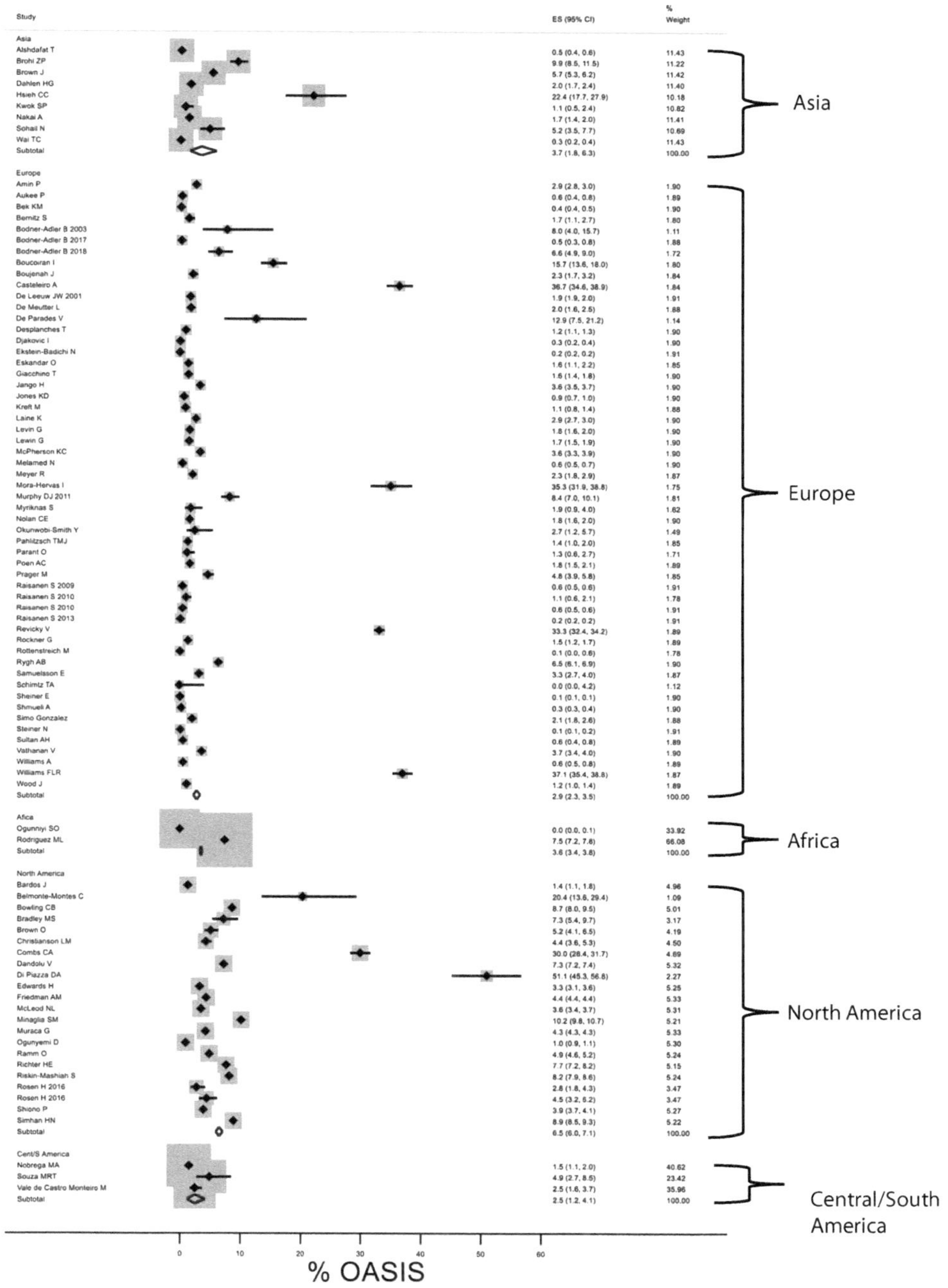

Continent	Number of studies	OASI incidence (95%CI)	Comparison (p-value)
Asia	9	3.7% (1.8%-6.3%)	<0.001
Europe	55	2.9% (2.3%-3.5%)	
Africa	2	3.6% (3.4%-3.8%)	
North America	22	6.5% (6.0%-7.1%)	
Central/South America	3	2.4% (1.2%-4.1%)	

Fig. 23.1 Incidence of OASI by continent. (Reproduced with permission [15])

prediction models, and interventions that can be implemented to prevent these injuries.

23.2 Risk Factors

Risk factors associated with OASI can be divided into modifiable and non-modifiable risks. A meta-analysis by Hu et al. [16, 17] identified seven modifiable and eight non-modifiable independent risk factors related to OASI from 47 studies. These risk factors are described in ◘ Table 23.2. It is important to note that 4 (57.1%) modifiable and 6 (75.0%) non-modifiable risk factors had evidence of substantial heterogeneity. Therefore, the summary estimates should be interpreted with caution.

To reduce the risk of OASI, modifiable risk factors should be addressed, as measures can be taken to address them. Forceps-assisted birth without episiotomy is associated with a ninefold increase in OASI, and vacuum-assisted birth without episiotomy is associated with a threefold increase in OASI [16]. However, the evidence surrounding this effect differs between nulliparous and multiparous women. In addition, the type of episiotomy performed is of significant importance. Traditionally, midline episiotomy is preferred in the United States of America (USA), and mediolateral episiotomy (MLE) in the UK and Europe [19, 20]. However, the quasi-randomised controlled trial (RCT) performed by Coats et al., including 407 nulliparous women randomised to

◘ Table 23.2 Independent modifiable and non-modifiable risk factors associated with OASI (Reproduced with permissions [16])

Risk factor	Number of studies	Adjusted OR (95% CI)	*p*-value	I^2 (%)
Modifiable				
Epidural analgesia	18	0.89 (0.81–0.97)	0.01	92
Labour induction	6	1.05 (1.01–1.09)	0.02	0
Labour augmentation	9	1.19 (1.06–1.35)	0.004	86
Forceps delivery without episiotomy	4	8.89 (7.77–10.40)	<0.001	0
Forceps delivery with episiotomy	4	5.43 (1.42–20.76)	0.01	99
Vacuum delivery without episiotomy	3	3.17 (3.00–3.36)	<0.001	0
Vacuum delivery with episiotomy	4	2.52 (1.05–6.05)	0.01	100
Non-modifiable				
Maternal age ≥35 years	3	1.22 (1.09–1.36)	<0.001	0
Asian ethnicity	8	2.06 (1.74–2.45)	<0.001	94
Nulliparity	14	2.39 (1.93–2.96)	<0.001	76
VBAC	4	1.23 (1.07–1.41)	0.003	69
BMI ≤18.5 kg/m^2	2	1.31 (1.22–1.41)	<0.001	0
Estimated birthweight ≥3500 g	6	1.74 (1.58–1.92)	<0.001	46
Foetal malposition	13	1.64 (1.41–1.91)	<0.001	57
Gestational age ≥40 weeks	5	1.18 (1.11–1.26)	<0.001	10

OR Odds ratio
CI Confidence interval
I^2 >50% = substantial heterogeneity [18]

either MLE or midline episiotomy, found that midline episiotomy significantly increased the incidence of OASI by 10% (12% vs 2%, $p < 0.001$) [21]. Midline episiotomies are performed in the midline through the central tendon of the perineal body [20]. Whilst MLEs are performed at a lateral angle of 60 degrees from the midline at the crowning of the foetal head [22]. An angle of 60° has been shown to result in a post-delivery angle of 45°, whilst an angle of 45° results in a post-delivery angle of 23° [22]. This is important, as the incidence of OASI following episiotomy is reduced by 50% for every six degrees of the angle away from the midline [22]. Lateral episiotomies (LE) are also described in the literature as being used and are performed two centimetres away from the midline [20]. This type of episiotomy has been shown not to differ significantly from MLE with respect to the incidence of OASI [20, 22]. Whilst episiotomy should be considered with assisted vaginal births, with unassisted vaginal births, routine episiotomy is not recommended, as selective episiotomy in comparison to routine episiotomy reduces the incidence of OASI by 30% (RR 0.70 [95% CI 0.52–0.94]) (Fig. 23.2) [15].

One meta-analysis has been performed to evaluate the effect of MLE/LE on OASI rates with both vacuum- and forceps-assisted births [23]. The meta-analysis by Okeahialam et al. [23] included 703,977 women and demonstrated that, in nulliparous women undergoing a vacuum-assisted birth, the use of an MLE/LE reduced the rate of OASI by 43%, with a number needed to treat (NNT) of 28 women to prevent one additional OASI. However, multiparous women had no significant reduction (Fig. 23.3).

With nulliparous women undergoing a forceps-assisted birth, the use of an MLE/LE reduced the rate of OASI by 68%, with an NNT to prevent one additional OASI of eight women. However, there was no significant reduction in multiparous women (Fig. 23.4).

However, a limitation of this meta-analysis is that it included non-randomised studies with the presence of significant heterogeneity and a high risk of bias across studies. Therefore, these findings should be interpreted with caution, as routine episiotomy is associated with increased blood loss, perineal pain, dyspareunia and pelvic floor dysfunction [24]. However, when this meta-analysis

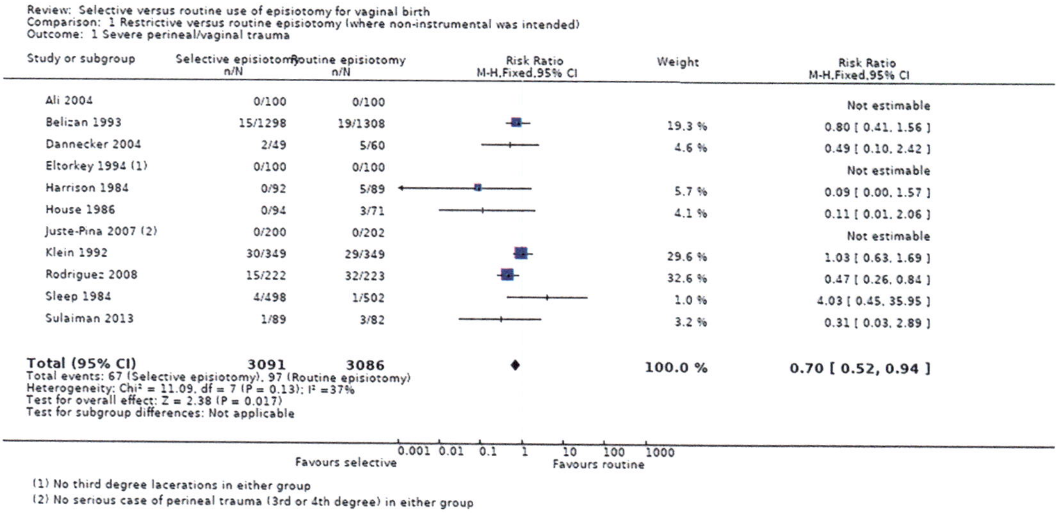

Fig. 23.2 The incidence of OASI with selective episiotomy in comparison to routine episiotomy. (Reproduced with permission [15])

Study or Subgroup	Episiotomy Events	Episiotomy Total	No Episiotomy Events	No Episiotomy Total	Weight	Odds Ratio M-H, Random, 95% CI
1.6.1 Nulliparous Ventouse						
Van Bavel 2018	2830	113619	2317	16538	4.5%	0.16 [0.15, 0.17]
Shmueli 2017	52	2681	16	1088	3.9%	1.33 [0.75, 2.33]
Schmitz 2014	0	157	5	79	0.9%	0.04 [0.00, 0.79]
Sagi-Dain 2020	2	67	3	68	1.8%	0.67 [0.11, 4.12]
Rognant 2012	33	1665	3	296	2.7%	1.97 [0.60, 6.48]
Raisanen 2012	349	11031	84	1954	4.4%	0.73 [0.57, 0.93]
Raisanen 2009	242	17564	56	1955	4.3%	0.47 [0.35, 0.64]
Parnell 2001	26	140	29	123	3.9%	0.74 [0.41, 1.34]
Murphy 2008	2	25	0	22	0.8%	4.79 [0.22, 105.30]
Marschalek 2018	863	19168	470	7230	4.5%	0.68 [0.60, 0.76]
Macleod 2008	11	256	11	200	3.3%	0.77 [0.33, 1.82]
Levin 2020	47	2427	27	795	4.1%	0.56 [0.35, 0.91]
Jango 2014	1180	11178	4143	27810	4.5%	0.67 [0.63, 0.72]
I Gurol-Urganci 2013	2667	115948	3114	48657	4.5%	0.34 [0.33, 0.36]
Gachon 2019	2	145	26	493	2.3%	0.25 [0.06, 1.07]
de Vogel 2012	63	1750	64	383	4.2%	0.19 [0.13, 0.27]
De Leeuw 2008	197	14350	321	2913	4.4%	0.11 [0.09, 0.13]
Boujenah 2019	2	238	4	156	1.9%	0.32 [0.06, 1.78]
Bodner-Adler 2018	21	372	18	200	3.7%	0.60 [0.31, 1.16]
Baghurst 2012	136	2381	151	2255	4.4%	0.84 [0.66, 1.07]
Ampt 2013	1219	19661	1262	19415	4.5%	0.95 [0.88, 1.03]
Subtotal (95% CI)		**334823**		**132630**	**73.3%**	**0.51 [0.35, 0.73]**
Total events	9944		12124			
Heterogeneity: Tau² = 0.57; Chi² = 2113.74, df = 20 (P < 0.00001); I² = 99%						
Test for overall effect: Z = 3.63 (P = 0.0003)						
1.6.2 Multiparous Ventouse						
Van Bavel 2018	416	20246	667	8937	4.4%	0.26 [0.23, 0.29]
Shmueli 2017	1	397	0	509	0.8%	3.85 [0.16, 94.88]
Raisanen 2012	29	1332	12	1448	3.7%	2.66 [1.35, 5.24]
Gachon 2019	0	31	12	200	0.9%	0.24 [0.01, 4.15]
de Vogel 2012	7	244	14	139	3.2%	0.26 [0.10, 0.67]
De Leeuw 2008	31	2430	97	1561	4.2%	0.20 [0.13, 0.29]
D'Souza 2020	1	32	3	12	1.2%	0.10 [0.01, 1.05]
Baghurst 2012	15	430	32	1272	3.8%	1.40 [0.75, 2.61]
Ampt 2013	146	3743	286	9225	4.4%	1.27 [1.04, 1.55]
Subtotal (95% CI)		**28885**		**23303**	**26.7%**	**0.58 [0.26, 1.27]**
Total events	646		1123			
Heterogeneity: Tau² = 1.09; Chi² = 231.03, df = 8 (P < 0.00001); I² = 97%						
Test for overall effect: Z = 1.37 (P = 0.17)						
Total (95% CI)		**363708**		**155933**	**100.0%**	**0.53 [0.39, 0.72]**
Total events	10590		13247			
Heterogeneity: Tau² = 0.57; Chi² = 2345.42, df = 29 (P < 0.00001); I² = 99%						
Test for overall effect: Z = 4.02 (P < 0.0001)						
Test for subgroup differences: Chi² = 0.08, df = 1 (P = 0.78), I² = 0%						

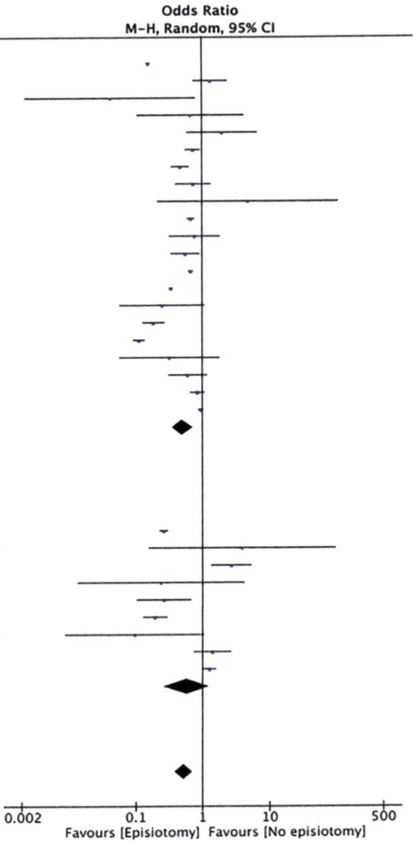

Fig. 23.3 The incidence of obstetric anal sphincter injury with mediolateral/lateral episiotomy and ventouse-assisted births in nulliparous and multiparous women. (Reproduced with permission [23])

was performed, only two RCTs were published: one evaluating the effect of selective MLE in vacuum-assisted births alone and the other, which evaluated the effect in nulliparous women alone undergoing a vacuum or forceps, did not reach adequate statistical power [25, 26]. In Sweden, the "Lateral episiotomy versus no episiotomy to reduce obstetric anal sphincter injury in vacuum-assisted delivery (EVA)" study in 714 nulliparous women demonstrated that LE reduced the rate of OASIs by 57% (RR 0.47 [96% CI 0.23–0.97]), with a number needed to treat (NNT) of 14 women to prevent one additional OASI [27]. Therefore, as LE does not differ significantly from MLE with respect to the incidence of OASI, the findings by Bergendahl can be extrapolated to apply to MLE also [20, 22, 28]. Hopefully, this new study can be used to inform future practice and policy.

Instrument choice is important with regard to the risk of OASI. However, selecting the most appropriate instrument requires accurate clinical assessment, clinician experience/skill and supported decision-making, considering the woman's preferences. However, the use of the vacuum rather than forceps for assisted birth appears to reduce maternal morbidity with regard to OASI, as forceps-assisted birth has been shown to double the risk of anal sphincter trauma (RR 1.83 [95% CI 1.32–2.55]) [29] (Fig. 23.5).

Study or Subgroup	Episiotomy Events	Episiotomy Total	No Episiotomy Events	No Episiotomy Total	Weight	Odds Ratio M-H, Random, 95% CI
1.4.1 Nulliparous Forceps						
De Parades 2004	11	89	1	4	1.5%	0.42 [0.04, 4.43]
de Vogel 2012	3	254	4	16	2.6%	0.04 [0.01, 0.18]
Meyer 2020	15	508	3	154	3.5%	1.53 [0.44, 5.36]
Boujenah 2019	19	793	12	155	5.5%	0.29 [0.14, 0.62]
Macleod 2008	95	810	10	94	5.7%	1.12 [0.56, 2.22]
Marschalek 2018	33	336	21	168	6.2%	0.76 [0.43, 1.36]
Gachon 2019	29	649	89	584	6.8%	0.26 [0.17, 0.40]
De Leeuw 2008	147	5808	141	600	7.4%	0.08 [0.07, 0.11]
Baghurst 2012	230	2068	122	569	7.4%	0.46 [0.36, 0.58]
Van Bavel 2018	314	9204	174	651	7.5%	0.10 [0.08, 0.12]
Ampt 2013	1633	16663	728	4333	7.7%	0.54 [0.49, 0.59]
I Gurol-Urganci 2013	9942	101456	4465	19670	7.7%	0.37 [0.36, 0.38]
Subtotal (95% CI)		**138638**		**26998**	**69.3%**	**0.32 [0.22, 0.46]**
Total events	12471		5770			
Heterogeneity: Tau² = 0.32; Chi² = 391.82, df = 11 (P < 0.00001); I² = 97%						
Test for overall effect: Z = 6.00 (P < 0.00001)						
1.4.2 Multiparous Forceps						
Meyer 2020	1	58	0	44	0.9%	2.32 [0.09, 58.37]
D'Souza 2020	1	34	1	3	0.9%	0.06 [0.00, 1.37]
de Vogel 2012	1	41	2	5	1.2%	0.04 [0.00, 0.54]
Baghurst 2012	35	397	2	232	3.0%	11.12 [2.65, 46.67]
Gachon 2019	6	119	9	151	4.2%	0.84 [0.29, 2.42]
De Leeuw 2008	26	849	34	221	6.4%	0.17 [0.10, 0.30]
Van Bavel 2018	38	1470	43	304	6.7%	0.16 [0.10, 0.25]
Ampt 2013	156	2600	120	1690	7.4%	0.84 [0.65, 1.07]
Subtotal (95% CI)		**5568**		**2650**	**30.7%**	**0.48 [0.18, 1.25]**
Total events	264		211			
Heterogeneity: Tau² = 1.34; Chi² = 83.38, df = 7 (P < 0.00001); I² = 92%						
Test for overall effect: Z = 1.50 (P = 0.13)						
Total (95% CI)		**144206**		**29648**	**100.0%**	**0.36 [0.26, 0.49]**
Total events	12735		5981			
Heterogeneity: Tau² = 0.35; Chi² = 485.34, df = 19 (P < 0.00001); I² = 96%						
Test for overall effect: Z = 6.30 (P < 0.00001)						
Test for subgroup differences: Chi² = 0.59, df = 1 (P = 0.44), I² = 0%						

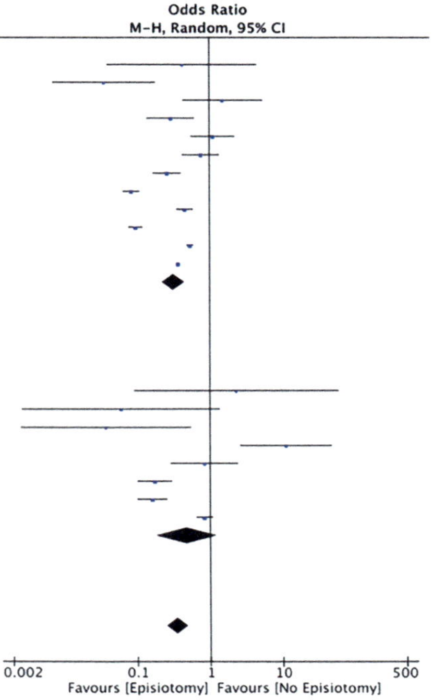

Fig. 23.4 The incidence of obstetric anal sphincter injury with mediolateral/lateral episiotomy and forceps-assisted births in nulliparous and multiparous women. (Reproduced with permission [23])

Study or Subgroup	Any forceps Events	Any forceps Total	Any vacuum cup Events	Any vacuum cup Total	Weight	Risk Ratio M-H, Random, 95% CI
Bofill 1996a	90	315	38	322	24.4%	2.42 [1.71 , 3.42]
Dell 1985	10	45	18	73	13.8%	0.90 [0.46 , 1.78]
Fitzpatrick 2003	10	61	5	69	8.0%	2.26 [0.82 , 6.25]
Johanson 1989	16	132	6	132	9.5%	2.67 [1.08 , 6.60]
Johanson 1993	25	311	15	296	15.3%	1.59 [0.85 , 2.95]
Lasbrey 1964	2	131	0	121	1.1%	4.62 [0.22 , 95.30]
Shekhar 2013	2	50	0	50	1.2%	5.00 [0.25 , 101.58]
Vacca 1983	26	152	9	152	12.8%	2.89 [1.40 , 5.96]
Williams 1991	12	40	12	41	14.0%	1.02 [0.52 , 2.01]
Total (95% CI)		**1237**		**1256**	**100.0%**	**1.83 [1.32 , 2.55]**
Total events:	193		103			
Heterogeneity: Tau² = 0.08; Chi² = 12.88, df = 8 (P = 0.12); I² = 38%						
Test for overall effect: Z = 3.60 (P = 0.0003)						
Test for subgroup differences: Not applicable						

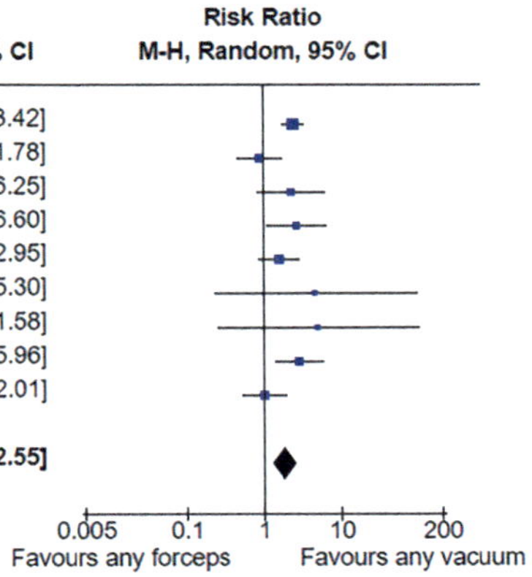

Fig. 23.5 Forest plot of the incidence of severe perineal trauma in women undergoing a vacuum or forceps-assisted birth. (Reproduced with permission [29])

23.3 Prediction Models

Nine studies have created prediction models using risk factors highlighted in the literature that can be used to reduce the rate of OASI [16, 30–36]. Prediction models are useful if they can guide antenatal counselling regarding a woman's specific risk of OASI. However, the difficulty is that many of the modifiable risk factors associated with OASI occur in labour or at the time of birth. Table 23.3 describes the prediction models published in the literature.

Table 23.3 Summary of OASI prediction models and their performance

Author (year)	Study design	Factors	AUC
Cochrane (2024) [30][d]	Retrospective cohort	Nulliparity Ethnicity Episiotomy status BMI Advanced maternal age Length of second stage	0.79
Hu (2023) [16]	Meta-analysis	Model 1: ***Antenatal variables*** Maternal age Parity VBAC BMI Gestational age Estimated birthweight Foetal position	[c]
		Model 2: ***Intrapartum variables*** Epidural analgesia Labour induction Labour augmentation Episiotomy Assisted vaginal birth	[c]
Chill (2021) [31]	Retrospective cohort	Nulliparity Low BMI Advanced gestational age Maternal age	0.76
Luchristt (2021) [32][a]	Prospective cohort	Advanced maternal age Low BMI No previous vaginal birth Nonsmoker Assisted vaginal birth	0.79
Gilchrist-Scott (2020) [33]	Prospective cohort	Assisted vaginal birth VBAC Ethnicity Smoking	0.79
McPherson (2014) [34]	Retrospective cohort	Nulliparity Ethnicity (African-Caribbean) Nonsmoker Birth in hospital Water birth Assisted vaginal birth	0.64
Meister (2016) [35]	Retrospective cohort	Nulliparity Ethnicity (non-African American) Prolonged second stage Nonsmoker Infant birthweight ≥3500 g Assisted vaginal birth	0.83

(continued)

Table 23.3 (continued)

Author (year)	Study design	Factors	AUC
Webb (2017) [37]	Retrospective cohort	Nulliparity Induction/augmentation of labour Prolonged second stage Prolonged active second stage Head circumference ≥37 cm Increased birthweight (per unit (kg)) *Mediolateral episiotomy*[b]	0.77
		Prebirth variables Advanced maternal age Foetal malposition (occipito-posterior) Induction/augmentation of labour Infant birthweight ≥4000 g	0.71
Woo (2020) [36]	Retrospective cohort	Advanced maternal age Advanced gestational age Ethnicity (Asian) Prolonged second stage Assisted vaginal birth Previous OASI	[c]

Reproduced with permission [38]

AUC Area under the curve (on receiver operator curve analysis), which represented the percentage of the time the prediction model would correctly assign a randomly selected patient

[a]Study population = vaginal birth after previous caesarean section

[b]Mediolateral episiotomy = protective variable

[c]These studies created a risk stratification tool and did not report the model AUC

[d]Forceps-assisted births only

Chill et al. addressed this difficulty with their prediction model, which included factors known prior to birth [31]. This retrospective study performed in Israel included 98,463 women, with an OASI rate of 0.3%. Risk factors in the prediction model included lower gravidity, lower parity, lower maternal BMI, increased maternal age and increased gestational age. This model had acceptable performance; 76% of the time, it would correctly assign a randomly selected patient. However, as the OASI rate was so low, their findings may not be generalisable. Further research is required to create a clinically useful prediction model that can be used in the antenatal period to identify women at increased risk of OASI and appropriately counsel them.

23.4 Interventions That Can Be Implemented to Prevent OASIs

23.4.1 Antenatal

23.4.1.1 Perineal Massage

Third-trimester antenatal perineal massage before vaginal birth may be useful to prevent perineal tears. Lubricants such as vitamin E oil, almond oil or olive oil can be used. Figure 23.6 shows a "how-to-guide" of performing perineal massage. Seven published RCTs have evaluated the effectiveness of perineal massage [39]. Pooling of these results

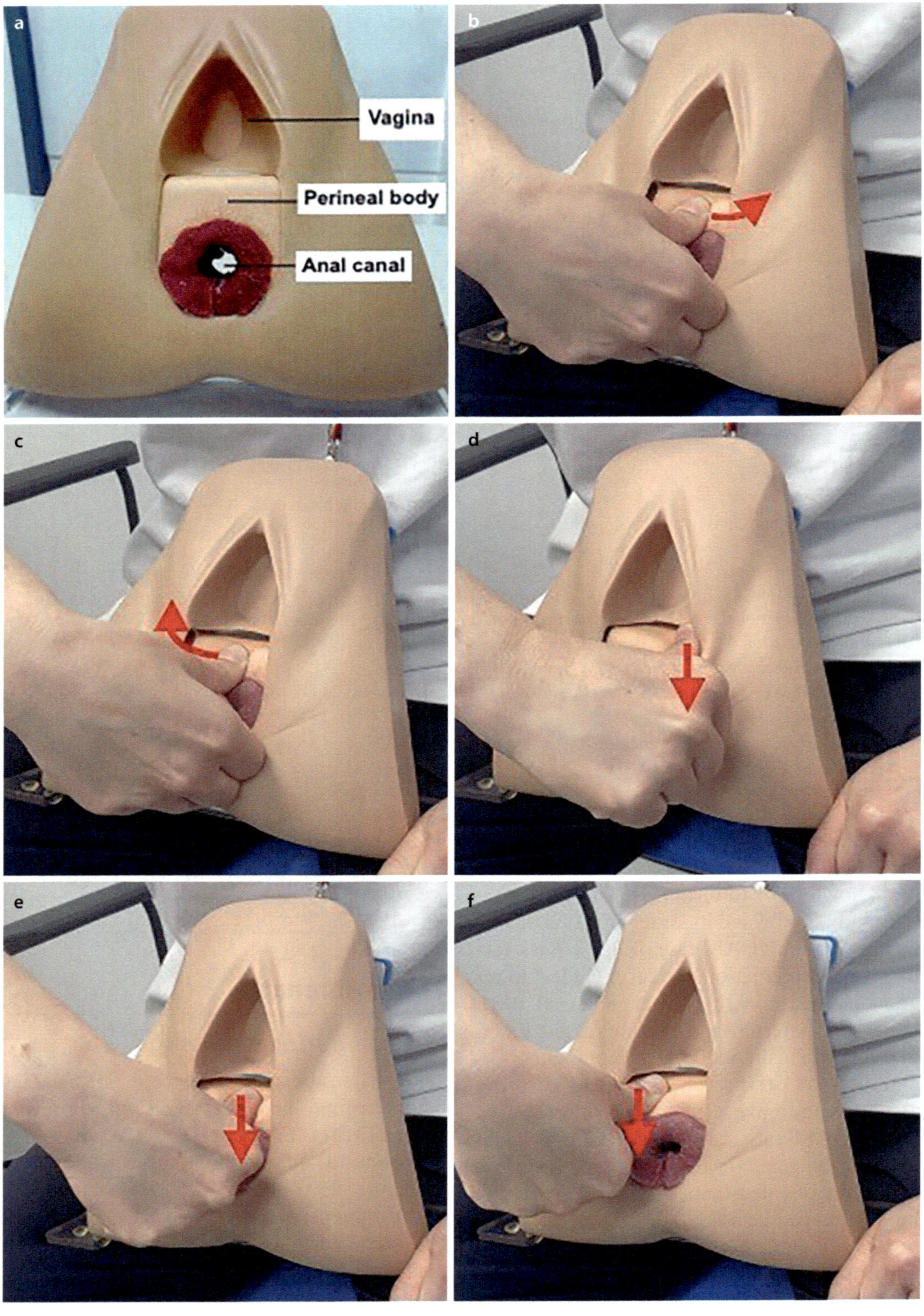

Fig. 23.6 How-to-guide image of the antenatal perineal massage technique using a model **a**. Massage can be performed by applying pressure in a U-shape from left **b** to right **c** and in a downward direction on the left **d**, mid **e** and right **f** aspect of the posterior fourchette (arrowed)

showed that perineal massage reduced the incidence of OASI by 64% (RR 0.36 [95% CI 0.14–0.89]) [40]. However, the previously published Cochrane review [40], which included four studies, analysed nulliparous and parous women separately and showed no significant difference with regard to OASI rate, but a 9% reduction in the incidence of perineal trauma requiring suturing in nulliparous women (RR 0.91 [95% CI 0.83–1.08]) and a 16% reduction in the incidence of episiotomy in nulliparous women (RR 0.84 [95% CI 0.74–0.95]). Unlike the Cochrane review, in the meta-analysis by Abdelhakim et al., subgroup analysis based on parity was not performed [39].

23.4.2 Intrapartum

23.4.2.1 Second-Stage Perineal Massage

Perineal massage in the second stage of labour can be performed using two gloved fingers (index and middle fingers or thumbs) inserted inside the vagina and moved laterally and carefully, with simultaneous downward pressure towards the rectum, using a water-based lubricant [41, 42]. A meta-analysis has shown that the use of perineal massage in the second stage reduces the risk of OASI by 51% (RR 0.49 [95% CI 0.25–0.94]) (◘ Fig. 23.7). It can also reduce the incidence of episiotomy by 44% (RR 0.56 [95% CI 0.38–0.82]) and increase the incidence of an intact perineum by 40% (RR 1.40 [95% CI 1.01–1.93]) [42]. Moreover, there was no significant increase in the incidence of labial, vaginal, clitoral or peri-urethral tears. Perineal massage was usually performed by the clinician between and during pushing for between 5 and 15 min [42].

The meta-analysis by Aquino et al. performed subgroup analysis based on parity and found that in nulliparous women, the risk of OASI was reduced by 91% (RR 0.09 [95% CI 0.01–1.62]), the incidence of episiotomy by 56% (RR 0.44 [95% CI 0.23–0.83]) and the incidence of an intact perineum increased twofold (RR 2.41 [95% CI 1.09–5.35]). However, no differences were seen in multiparous women [42].

23.4.2.2 Second-Stage Perineal Warm Compress

Using a warm compress on the perineum during the second stage of labour can improve the stretch and elasticity of the perineal muscles by increasing blood flow and encouraging relaxation [43]. A meta-analysis has shown that this can reduce the risk of OASI by 66% (RR 0.34 [95% CI 0.20–0.57]) (◘ Fig. 23.8). The incidence of second-degree tears was also reduced by 60% (RR 0.40 [95% CI 0.27–0.59]). An improvement was also seen in the incidence of episiotomy (RR 0.69 [95% CI 0.58–0.83]) (◘ Fig. 23.9) [44].

Careful attention should be paid to the temperature of the compress to avoid inadvertent injury. The reported technique in the literature involves soaking the compress in tap water boiled at a temperature of 45–59 °C. The compress was then wrung out and used for a maximum of 15 minutes then rewarmed [45]. This technique may be difficult to apply in clinical practice.

Study or Subgroup	Massage Events	Massage Total	Control Events	Control Total	Weight	Risk Ratio M-H, Random, 95% CI
Albers 2005	5	403	6	404	27.6%	0.84 [0.26, 2.72]
Attarha 2009	0	85	5	85	5.1%	0.09 [0.01, 1.62]
Geranmayer 2011	0	45	0	45		Not estimable
Sohrabi 2012	0	40	0	40		Not estimable
Stamp 2001	12	708	24	632	67.2%	0.45 [0.23, 0.89]
Total (95% CI)		**1281**		**1206**	**100.0%**	**0.49 [0.25, 0.94]**
Total events	17		35			

Heterogeneity: $Tau^2 = 0.05$; $Chi^2 = 2.22$, df = 2 (P = 0.33); $I^2 = 10\%$
Test for overall effect: Z = 2.13 (P = 0.03)

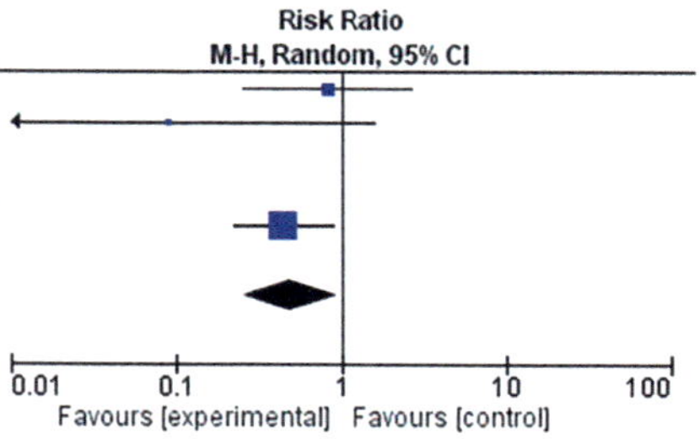

◘ **Fig. 23.7** Forest plot of the risk of OASI with second-stage perineal massage. (Reproduced with permission [42])

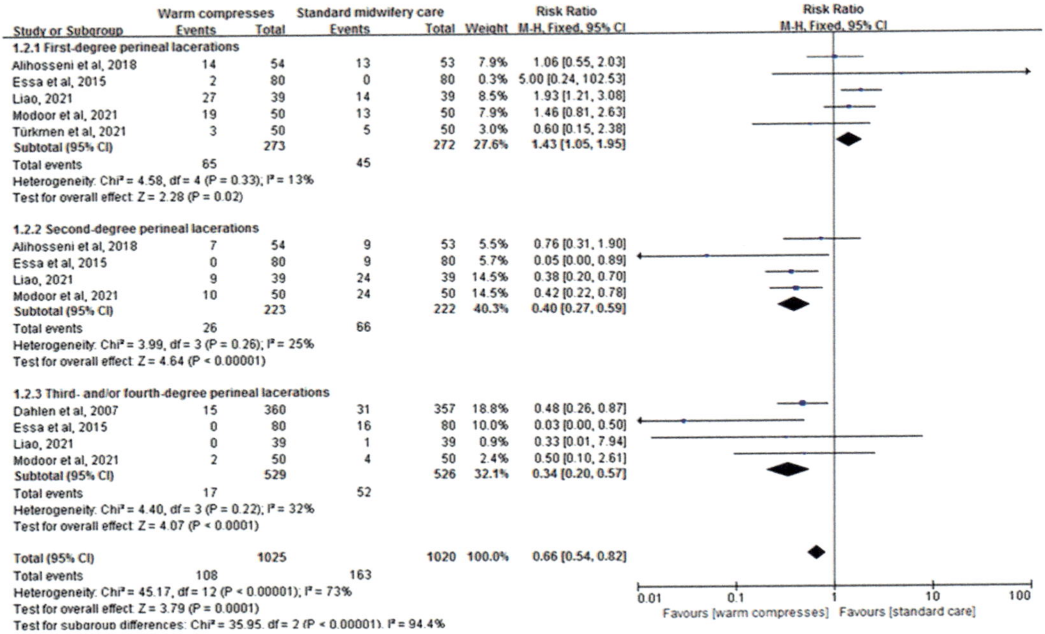

Fig. 23.8 Forest plot of the risk of perineal trauma with second-stage perineal warm compress. (Reproduced with permission [44])

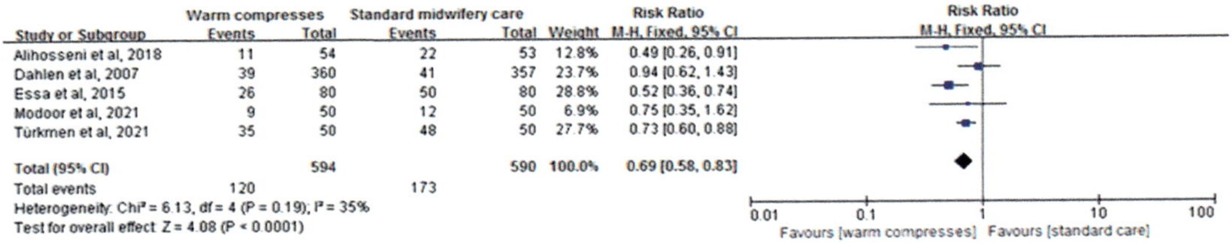

Fig. 23.9 Forest plot of the risk of episiotomy with second-stage perineal warm compress. (Reproduced with permission [44])

23.4.2.3 Manual Perineal Protection

Manual perineal protection aims to reduce perineal muscular tension and disperse the highest tension across a wider surface area. This technique has been shown to reduce tension in the perineal muscles by 40% [46]. There are two techniques described in the literature; the Finnish and Viennese [47]. The Finnish manual perineal protection involves using the technique shown in the "how-to-guide" in Figs. 23.10 and 23.11. This technique can be used in several birthing positions, including during water birth.

> **Worked-out Examples- Manual Perineal Protection Tips**
>
> *Edqvist* et al. [48]
>
> - Good communication with the woman
> - Visualise the perineum throughout the delivery
> - Consider a second clinician for support:
>   - Can reduce the rate of OASI 31%

However, a survey of 124 clinicians found that there was a significant variation in practice

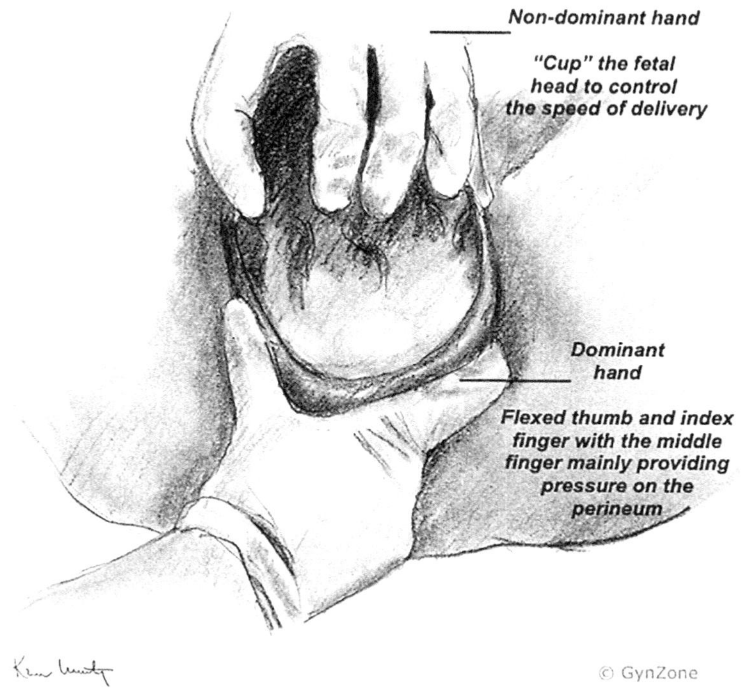

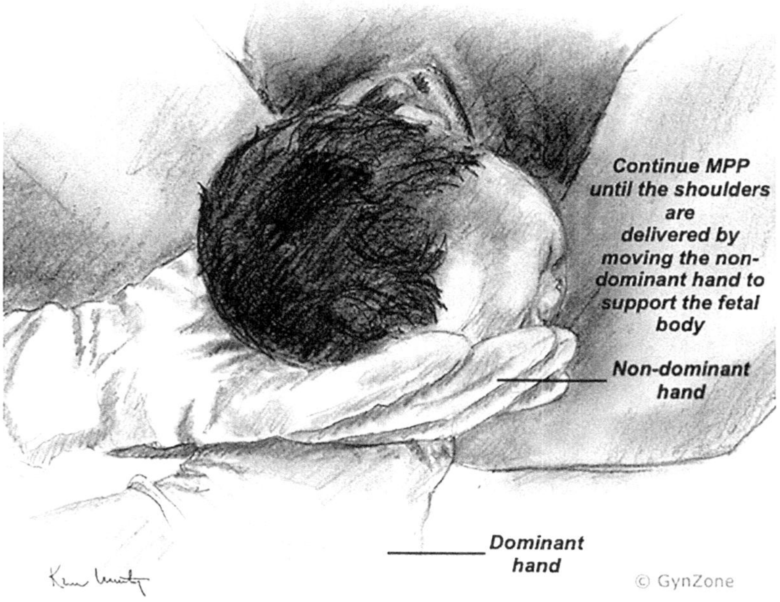

Fig. 23.10 How to guide image for manual perineal protection (MPP) shown with spontaneous vaginal birth. (Illustrations are courtesy of © Gynzone)

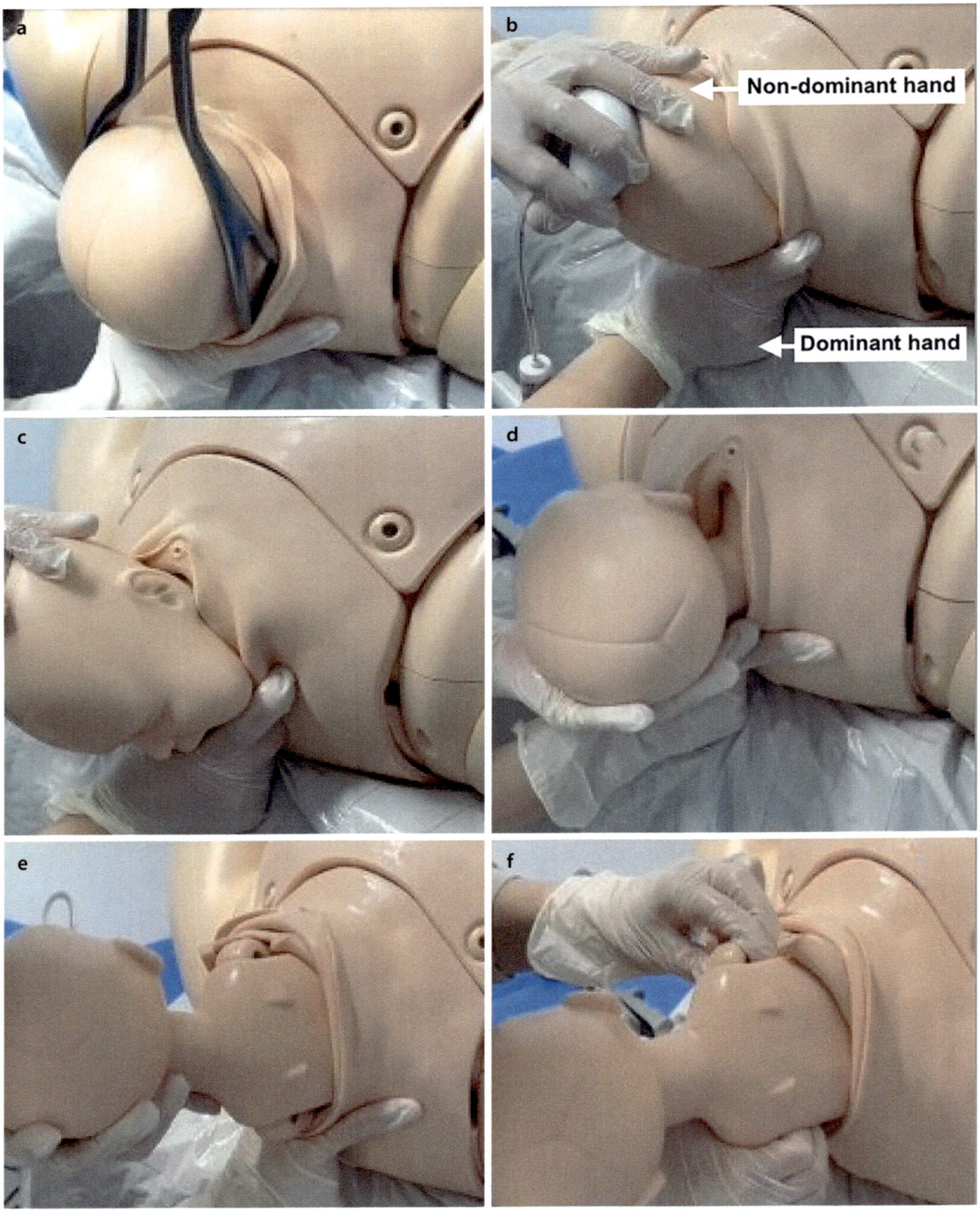

Fig. 23.11 How to guide for manual perineal protection (MPP) shown with forceps **a** and vacuum **b** on a birthing simulator. **b** The dominant hand flexes the thumb and index finger, with the middle finger mainly providing pressure on the perineum. The non-dominant hand "cups" the foetal head to control the speed of delivery and facilitate head extension. **c** MPP supports the delivery of the foetal chin. **d** The non-dominant hand is moved to support the foetal body and provide axial traction to aid delivery. **e** MPP is continued until the shoulders are delivered. **f** Once the shoulders are delivered, the hands can be moved to deliver the foetal body

with regard to manual perineal protection, as only 5.6% were able to describe the technique correctly [47]. This lack of knowledge and standardised technique is a likely reason why the meta-analysis by Bulchandani et al. found that although within the three included non-randomised studies manual perineal protection was associated with a 55% reduction in severe perineal trauma (RR 0.45 [95% CI 0.40–0.50]), no difference was seen in the three included RCTs [49].

Manual perineal protection has been incorporated into a number of care bundles, which have been introduced in the UK and Australia [50, 51]. Figure 23.12 highlights the components of the OASI Care Bundle introduced in the UK in collaboration with the Royal College of Obstetricians and Gynaecologists and the Royal College of Midwives. Implementation of this intervention was found to reduce the risk of OASIs by 20% (aOR) 0.80 [95% CI 0.65–0.98]) with no effect on caesarean birth or episiotomy rates [50].

A qualitative study including 19 women evaluating the impact of the OASI Care Bundle highlighted three main themes from their semi-structured interviews. This included "memories of touch", where manual perineal protection was described as a positive experience; "midwife as a supportive guide", where good communication between the women and midwife improved the birth experience; and "education", which highlighted that women need more information regarding perineal trauma. Figure 23.13 highlights some of the comments from each theme. With regard to education, ensuring women are well informed is essential, as without this, women feel disempowered, excluded and disconnected from their birth experience [53].

To enhance the patient experience, the needs of all must be met, including our diverse group of patients and service users. For example, a cohort study by Sørby et al. [54] demonstrated that increased residence time in a more resourced country reduces the rate of OASI. Therefore, migrant women need to be empowered early in the antenatal periods with information about maternity services and labour care [55].

1. From 32 weeks in the antenatal period, the midwife or doctor will **discuss OASI with the woman**, including her personal risk factors and ways to minimize her risk, including the three subsequent components of the care bundle. An information leaflet (now referred to as a 'discussion guide' to highlight women's active participation) was developed with women's feedback to support this component.
2. At the time of birth and with the woman's consent, the midwife or doctor use their hands to support both the perineum and baby's head (known as **manual perineal protection, or MPP**) while communicating with the woman to encourage a slow and guided birth.
    - For spontaneous vaginal births, MPP should be used unless the woman's chosen birth position (i.e. water births) doesn't enable MPP to be used or she declines this technique.
    - For assisted vaginal births (i.e. forceps, ventouse), MPP should always be used unless the woman declines this technique.
3. *If clinically indicated* and with the woman's consent, a **mediolateral episiotomy** should be done at an angle of 60 degrees from the midline at crowning.
4. Following all vaginal births, **a systematic examination of the vagina and ano-rectum** should be offered to immediately assess whether there has been any damage to the external or internal anal sphincter and genitalia so that treatment options can be discussed and implemented as necessary. Prior discussion about the risks and benefits supports women to make an informed decision. Any tears are graded in accordance with RCOG Green-top guidelines.

Fig. 23.12 The OASI Care Bundle. (Reproduced with permission [52])

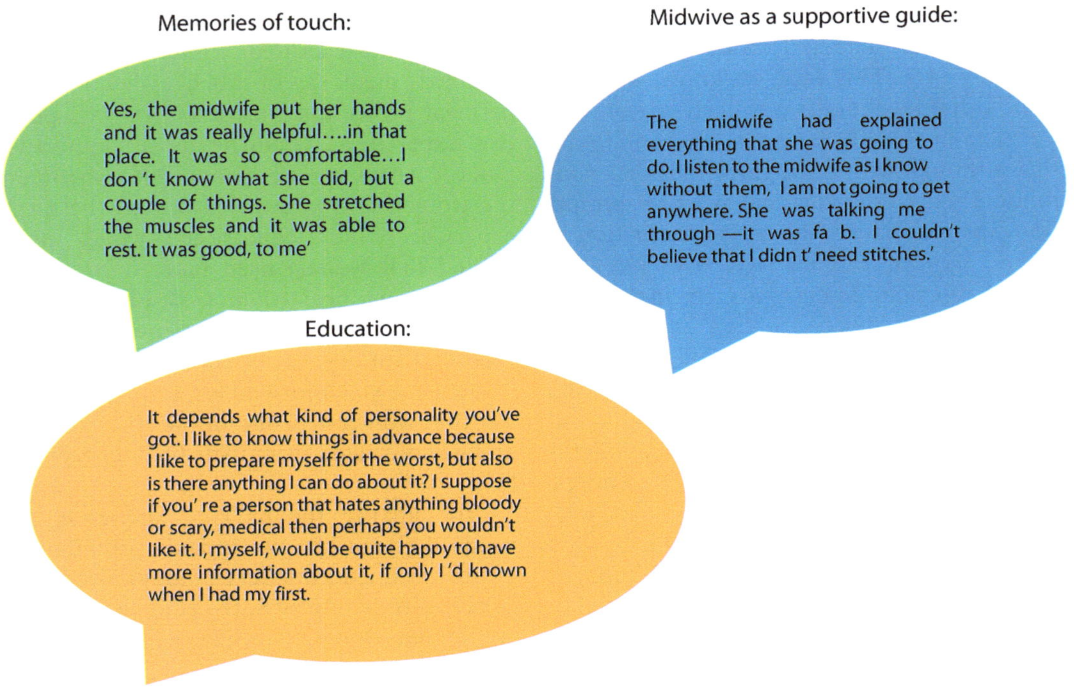

Fig. 23.13 Case studies of women's experiences with the OASI Care Bundle. (Reproduced with permission [56])

23.5 Chapter-End Summaries

OASIs are associated with significant maternal morbidity and long-term sequelae. In order to alleviate the potential consequences of these injuries, preventative methods must be used in the antenatal and intrapartum periods. This chapter describes the associated risk factors and interventions that can be implemented to reduce the risk of OASI. Care bundles can also be utilised to educate and empower women in the antenatal period and provide clinicians with tools to reduce these injuries.

Major Pearls/*Pitfalls*

- Independent risk factors for OASI include:
  - Non-modifiable: Maternal age, Asian ethnicity, nulliparity, VBAC, low BMI, large-for-gestational-age foetus, foetal malposition, gestational age ≥40 weeks.
  - Modifiable: Epidural anaesthesia, labour induction, labour augmentation, assisted vaginal birth.
  - *All risk factors that can be modified occur during labour and birth, meaning that counselling with regard to risk prediction is difficult in the antenatal period.*
- Episiotomy should be considered with assisted vaginal births, particularly with nulliparous women.
- If able, consider having a second clinician to provide support with manual perineal protection, as this support can further reduce the risk of OASI.

Chapter Key Points

- OASIs carry major long-term morbidity, including anal incontinence, sexual dysfunction, and psychological trauma.
- Risk is highest with forceps births, midline episiotomy, foetal malposition, high birthweight, and nulliparity.
- Mediolateral/lateral episiotomy significantly reduces OASI risk in nulliparous assisted births.

- Antenatal and intrapartum perineal massage, warm compresses, and manual perineal protection all reduce OASI risk.
- Care bundles standardise prevention and reduce OASI by ~20% without increasing CS rates.

Chapter-End Summary

Obstetric anal sphincter injuries remain a major source of maternal morbidity worldwide. Prevention requires addressing modifiable labour-related risks, optimising instrument and episiotomy choices, and applying evidence-based techniques such as mediolateral/lateral episiotomy in assisted births, perineal massage, warm compresses, and manual perineal protection. Whilst prediction models offer emerging tools, most OASI risks arise intrapartum, highlighting the need for intrapartum vigilance and skilled care. Implementation of standardised prevention bundles—such as the OASI Care Bundle—improves outcomes, enhances communication, and supports shared decision-making, reducing severe perineal trauma without increasing operative birth rates.

References

1. Sultan AH. Obstetric perineal injury and anal incontinence. Clin Risk. 1999;5(6):193–6.
2. Orlando A, Thomas G, Murphy J, Hotouras A, Bassett P, Vaizey C. A systematic review and a meta-analysis on the incidence of obstetric anal sphincter injuries during vaginal delivery. Color Dis. 2024;26(2):227–42.
3. Thiagamoorthy G, Johnson A, Thakar R, Sultan AH. National survey of perineal trauma and its subsequent management in the United Kingdom. Int Urogynecol J. 2014;25(12):1621–7.
4. Laine K, Gissler M, Pirhonen J. Changing incidence of anal sphincter tears in four Nordic countries through the last decades. Eur J Obstet Gynecol Reprod Biol. 2009;146(1):71–5.
5. Ampt AJ, Ford JB, Roberts CL, Morris JM. Trends in obstetric anal sphincter injuries and associated risk factors for vaginal singleton term births in New South Wales 2001–2009. Aust N Z J Obstet Gynaecol. 2013;53(1):9–16.
6. Gurol-Urganci I, Cromwell D, Edozien L, Mahmood T, Adams E, Richmond D, et al. Third- and fourth-degree perineal tears among primiparous women in England between 2000 and 2012: time trends and risk factors. BJOG: Int J Obstet Gy. 2013;120(12):1516–25.
7. Chi Wai T, Cecilia CW, Anny TWM, Hau Yee L. Incidence and risk factors of obstetric anal sphincter injuries after various modes of vaginal deliveries in Chinese women. Chin Med J. 2015;128(18):2420–5.
8. McLeod NL, Gilmour DT, Joseph KS, Farrell SA, Luther ER. Trends in major risk factors for anal sphincter lacerations: a 10-year study. J Obstet Gynaecol Can. 2003;25(7):586–93.
9. Okeahialam NA, Taithongchai A, Thakar R, Sultan AH. Corrigendum to 'The incidence of anal incontinence following obstetric anal sphincter injury graded using the Sultan classification: a network meta-analysis'. Am J Obstet Gynecol. 2023;228(6):675–88. Am J Obstet Gynecol 2024 S000293782400070X.
10. Okeahialam NA, Taithongchai A, Thakar R, Sultan AH. The incidence of anal incontinence following obstetric anal sphincter injury (OASI) graded using the Sultan classification: a network meta-analysis. Am J Obstet Gynecol. 2022;228:675–88. S0002937822021676.
11. Desseauve D, Proust S, Carlier-Guerin C, Rutten C, Pierre F, Fritel X. Evaluation of long-term pelvic floor symptoms after an obstetric anal sphincter injury (OASI) at least one year after delivery: a retrospective cohort study of 159 cases. Gynecol Obstet Fertil. 2016;44(7–8):385–90.
12. Molyneux R, Fowler G, Slade P. The postnatal effects of perineal trauma on maternal psychological and emotional wellbeing: a longitudinal study. Eur J Obstet Gynecol Reprod Biol. 2024;294:238–44.
13. NHS Litigation Authority. Ten years of maternity claims: an analysis of NHS litigation authority data. NHSLA; 2012. p. 49–60.
14. Orlovic M, Carter AW, Marti J, Mossialos E. Estimating the incidence and the economic burden of third and fourth-degree obstetric tears in the English NHS: an observational study using propensity score matching. BMJ Open. 2017;7(6):e015463.
15. Jiang H, Qian X, Carroli G, Garner P. Selective versus routine use of episiotomy for vaginal birth. Cochrane Database Syst Rev [Internet]. 2017. [cited 2021 Dec 26];2017(2):CD000081. Available from: http://doi.wiley.com/10.1002/14651858.CD000081.pub3.
16. Hu Y, Lu H, Zhang J, Ren L, Yang M. Predicting obstetric anal sphincter injuries among laboring women: 2 prediction models and 1 risk calculator. Interdiscip Nurs Res. 2023;2(1):13–8.

17. Hu Y, Lu H, Huang Q, Ren L, Wang N, Huang J, et al. Risk factors for severe perineal lacerations during childbirth: a systematic review and meta-analysis of cohort studies. J Clin Nurs. 2023;32(13–14):3248–65.
18. Deeks J, Higgins J, Altman D. Chapter 10: Analysing data and undertaking meta-analyses. In: Higgins J, Thomas J, Chandler J, Cumpston M, Li T, Page M, et al., editors. Cochrane handbook for systematic reviews of interventions version 64 [Internet]. Cochrane; 2023. Available from: www.training.cochrane.org/handbook.
19. Thacker SB. Midline versus mediolateral episiotomy. BMJ. 2000;320(7250):1615–6.
20. Kalis V, Laine K, de Leeuw J, Ismail K, Tincello D. Classification of episiotomy: towards a standardisation of terminology: international classification of episiotomy. BJOG Int J Obstet Gynaecol. 2012;119(5):522–6.
21. Coats PM, Chan KK, Wilkins M, Beard RJ. A comparison between midline and mediolateral episiotomies. BJOG. 1980;87(5):408–12.
22. Kalis V, Landsmanova J, Bednarova B, Karbanova J, Laine K, Rokyta Z. Evaluation of the incision angle of mediolateral episiotomy at 60 degrees. Int J Gynaecol Obstet. 2011;112(3):220–4.
23. Okeahialam NA, Wong KW, Jha S, Sultan AH, Thakar R. Mediolateral/lateral episiotomy with operative vaginal delivery and the risk reduction of obstetric anal sphincter injury (OASI): a systematic review and meta-analysis. Int Urogynecol J. 2022;33(6):1393–405.
24. Seijmonsbergen-Schermers AE, Geerts CC, Prins M, van Diem MT, Klomp T, Lagro-Janssen ALM, et al. The use of episiotomy in a low-risk population in The Netherlands: a secondary analysis. Birth. 2013 Dec;40(4):247–55.
25. Sagi-Dain L, Kreinin-Bleicher I, Bahous R, Gur Arye N, Shema T, Eshel A, et al. Is it time to abandon episiotomy use? A randomized controlled trial (EPITRIAL). Int Urogynecol J. 2020;31(11):2377–85.
26. Murphy D, Macleod M, Bahl R, Goyder K, Howarth L, Strachan B. A randomised controlled trial of routine versus restrictive use of episiotomy at operative vaginal delivery: a multicentre pilot study. BJOG Int J Obstet Gynaecol. 2008;115(13):1695–703.
27. Bergendahl S, Jonsson M, Hesselman S, Ankarcrona V, Leijonhufvud Å, Wihlbäck AC, et al. Lateral episiotomy or no episiotomy in vacuum assisted delivery in nulliparous women (EVA): multicentre, open label, randomised controlled trial. BMJ. 2024;385:e079014.
28. Thakar R, Sultan AH. Lateral episiotomy during vacuum assisted childbirth. BMJ. 2024 Jun;385:q1287.
29. Verma GL, Spalding JJ, Wilkinson MD, Hofmeyr GJ, Vannevel V, O'Mahony F. Instruments for assisted vaginal birth. Cochrane Pregnancy and Childbirth Group, editor. Cochrane Database Syst Rev [Internet]. 2021. [cited 2021 Dec 26];2021(9). Available from: http://doi.wiley.com/10.1002/14651858.CD005455.pub3.
30. Cochrane E, Getradjman C, Doctor T, Roger S, Stratis C, Wang K, et al. Adjusting models to better predict obstetric anal sphincter injury (OASIS) in forceps-assisted vaginal deliveries: a retrospective cross-sectional trial. Int J Gynaecol Obstet. 2024;167(1):383–8. ijgo.15574.
31. Chill HH, Guedalia J, Lipschuetz M, Shimonovitz T, Unger R, Shveiky D, et al. Prediction model for obstetric anal sphincter injury using machine learning. Int Urogynecol J. 2021;32(9):2393–9.
32. Luchristt D, Brown O, Pidaparti M, Kenton K, Lewicky-Gaupp C, Miller ES. Predicting obstetrical anal sphincter injuries in patients who undergo vaginal birth after cesarean delivery. Am J Obstet Gynecol. 2021;225(2):173.e1–8.
33. Gilchrist-Scott D, Brown O, Lewicky-Gaupp C, Miller ES, Mueller M, Kenton K. Predicting obstetric anal sphincter injury (OASIS) in women undergoing trial of labor after cesarean (TOLAC) [25L]. Obstet Gynecol. 2020;135(1):130S.
34. McPherson KC, Beggs AD, Sultan AH, Thakar R. Can the risk of obstetric anal sphincter injuries (OASIs) be predicted using a risk-scoring system? BMC Res Notes. 2014;7(1):471.
35. Meister MRL, Cahill AG, Conner SN, Woolfolk CL, Lowder JL. Predicting obstetric anal sphincter injuries in a modern obstetric population. Am J Obstet Gynecol. 2016;215(3):310.e1–7.
36. Woo VG, Hung YY, Ritterman-Weintraub ML, Painter CE, Ramm O. A clinical risk model to predict obstetric anal sphincter injuries in laboring patients. Female Pelvic Med Reconstr Surg. 2020;26(8):520–5.
37. Webb SS, Hemming K, Khalfaoui MY, Henriksen TB, Kindberg S, Stensgaard S, et al. An obstetric sphincter injury risk identification system (OSIRIS): is this a clinically useful tool? Int Urogynecol J. 2017;28(3):367–74.
38. Okeahialam NA, Draycott TJ, Thakar R. Prevention of perineal trauma. In: Sultan AH, Thakar R, Lewicky-Gaupp C, editors. Pelvic floor, perineal, and anal sphincter trauma during childbirth: diagnosis, management and prevention [Internet]. Cham: Springer International Publishing; 2024. p. 191–208. Available from: https://doi.org/10.1007/978-3-031-43095-4_12.
39. Abdelhakim AM, Eldesouky E, Elmagd IA, Mohammed A, Farag EA, Mohammed AE, et al. Antenatal perineal massage benefits in reducing perineal trauma and postpartum morbidities: a systematic review and meta-analysis of randomized controlled trials. Int Urogynecol J. 2020;31(9):1735–45.
40. Beckmann MM, Stock OM. Antenatal perineal massage for reducing perineal trauma. Cochrane

Pregnancy and Childbirth Group, editor. Cochrane Database Syst Rev [Internet]. 2013. [cited 2021 Dec 20]. Available from: https://doi.wiley.com/10.1002/14651858.CD005123.pub3
41. Albers LL, Sedler KD, Bedrick EJ, Teaf D, Peralta P. Midwifery care measures in the second stage of labor and reduction of genital tract trauma at birth: a randomized trial. J Midwifery Womens Health. 2005;50(5):365–72.
42. Aquino CI, Guida M, Saccone G, Cruz Y, Vitagliano A, Zullo F, et al. Perineal massage during labor: a systematic review and meta-analysis of randomized controlled trials. J Matern Fetal Neonatal Med. 2020;33(6):1051–63.
43. Nakano J, Yamabayashi C, Scott A, Reid WD. The effect of heat applied with stretch to increase range of motion: a systematic review. Phys Ther Sport. 2012;13(3):180–8.
44. Sun R, Huang J, Zhu X, Hou R, Zang Y, Li Y, et al. Effects of perineal warm compresses during the second stage of labor on reducing perineal trauma and relieving postpartum perineal pain in Primiparous women: a systematic review and meta-analyses. Healthcare. 2024;12(7):702.
45. Dahlen HG, Homer CSE, Cooke M, Upton AM, Nunn R, Brodrick B. Perineal outcomes and maternal comfort related to the application of perineal warm packs in the second stage of labor: a randomized controlled trial. Birth. 2007;34(4):282–90.
46. Jansova M, Kalis V, Rusavy Z, Zemcik R, Lobovsky L, Laine K. Modeling manual perineal protection during vaginal delivery. Int Urogynecol J. 2014;25(1):65–71.
47. Kleprlikova H, Kalis V, Lucovnik M, Rusavy Z, Blaganje M, Thakar R, et al. Manual perineal protection: the know-how and the know-why. Acta Obstet Gynecol Scand. 2020;99(4):445–50.
48. Edqvist M, Dahlen HG, Häggsgård C, Tern H, Ängeby K, Teleman P, et al. The effect of two midwives during the second stage of labour to reduce severe perineal trauma (Oneplus): a multicentre, randomised controlled trial in Sweden. Lancet. 2022;399:S014067362200188X.
49. Bulchandani S, Watts E, Sucharitha A, Yates D, Ismail K. Manual perineal support at the time of childbirth: a systematic review and meta-analysis. BJOG: Int J Obstet Gy. 2015;122(9):1157–65.
50. Gurol-Urganci I, Bidwell P, Sevdalis N, Silverton L, Novis V, Freeman R, et al. Impact of a quality improvement project to reduce the rate of obstetric anal sphincter injury: a multicentre study with a stepped-wedge design. BJOG: Int J Obstet Gy. 2021;128(3):584–92.
51. Women's Healthcare Australasia. The how to guide: WHA CEC perineal protection bundle. [Internet]. 2019. Available from: https://women.wcha.asn.au/collaborative/intervention-bundle.
52. Jurczuk M, Bidwell P, Gurol-Urganci I, van der Meulen J, Sevdalis N, Silverton L, et al. The OASI care bundle quality improvement project: lessons learned and future direction. Int Urogynecol J. 2021;32(7):1989–95.
53. Koster D, Romijn C, Sakko E, Stam C, Steenhuis N, De Vries D, et al. Traumatic childbirth experiences: practice-based implications for maternity care professionals from the woman's perspective. Scand Caring Sci. 2020;34(3):792–9.
54. Sørbye I, Bains S, Vangen S, Sundby J, Lindskog B, Owe K. Obstetric anal sphincter injury by maternal origin and length of residence: a nationwide cohort study. BJOG. 2022;129(3):423–31.
55. Higginbottom GMA, Evans C, Morgan M, Bharj KK, Eldridge J, Hussain B. Experience of and access to maternity care in the UK by immigrant women: a narrative synthesis systematic review. BMJ Open. 2019;9(12):e029478.
56. Bidwell P, Sevdalis N, Silverton L, Harris J, Gurol-Urganci I, Hellyer A, et al. Women's experiences of the OASI care bundle; a package of care to reduce severe perineal trauma. Int Urogynecol J. 2021;32(7):1807–16.

Further Reading

Gurol-Urganci I, Bidwell P, Sevdalis N, Silverton L, Novis V, Freeman R, et al. Impact of a quality improvement project to reduce the rate of obstetric anal sphincter injury: a multicentre study with a stepped-wedge design. BJOG. 2020;128(3):584–92.

Okeahialam NA, Sultan AH, Thakar R. The prevention of perineal trauma during vaginal birth. Am J Obstet Gynecol. 2024;230(3S):S991–S1004.

Sultan AH, Thakar R, Lewicky-Gaupp C, editors. Pelvic floor, perineal, and anal sphincter trauma during childbirth: diagnosis, management and prevention. Cham: Springer International Publishing; 2024.

Prevention of Uterine Rupture After Prior Cesarean Delivery

Yannay Khaikin and Amir Aviram

Contents

Y. Yogev, A. Khalil (eds.), *Prevention of Complications in Obstetrics*,
https://doi.org/10.1007/978-3-032-23479-7_24

Learning Objectives

After reviewing this chapter, the reader will be able to:

- Define uterine rupture, as well as describe its epidemiology and associated risk factors.
- Understand the key components of the diagnosis and management of uterine rupture.
- Appreciate the currently available and potential future prevention strategies for uterine rupture, using prevention categories as a framework.
- Identify major epidemiologic patterns and risk factors for uterine rupture during TOLAC.
- Explain how candidate selection for TOLAC affects rupture risk.
- Describe intrapartum factors influencing risk, including induction and augmentation methods.
- Understand the prevention framework (primordial → quaternary) as applied to uterine rupture.
- Recognize clinical signs requiring urgent evaluation and intervention.

24.1 Introduction

Uterine rupture during a trial of labor after cesarean delivery (TOLAC) is one of the most significant and frightening obstetrical complications, with the potential to cause serious maternal and fetal morbidity and sometimes mortality. With the worldwide rise in the rates of cesarean deliveries (CD), there is evidence that more patients are seeking TOLAC and are at risk of uterine rupture [1, 2]. Strategies aimed at preventing uterine rupture and its associated complications are of great importance for obstetrical providers and their patients. This chapter will review the definitions, epidemiology, and risk factors for uterine rupture and explore the available risk-reduction strategies.

24.2 Case Example

Eboh et al. described the following case of uterine rupture in their manuscript from 2022 [3]. A 32-year-old pregnant individual at 36 weeks of gestation presented to the labor and delivery unit with 48 hours of mild abdominal pain, vaginal bleeding, and no sensation of fetal movements. Her previous delivery was by cesarean section at 39 weeks for breech presentation. Prior to her visit to the unit, she was attempting a home birth with a doula and no other medical personnel. Obstetrical care had been limited in this pregnancy and included only an ultrasound at 20 weeks that showed normal anatomy and appropriate fetal size for gestational age (GA). An ultrasound examination was done, revealing an empty uterus, and a demised fetus was identified in the abdominal cavity. An emergency exploratory laparotomy was performed, where the deceased fetus was found, approximately term size, floating in the abdominal cavity "en caul". The membranes were intact, with the placenta attached. The anterior uterine wall was ruptured in the lower segment through the previous hysterotomy scar. Fortunately, the uterus was not actively bleeding and was repaired with two layers using an absorbable suture, avoiding the need for a hysterectomy. The total blood loss of the procedure was estimated at 1.2 L. The patient had an otherwise normal postoperative recovery without complications.

This case report demonstrates a clear example of uterine rupture in which the diagnosis took place after a fetal demise. Importantly, significant maternal complications were avoided, including severe hemorrhage, hysterectomy, or maternal death. One should also remember that while the uterine rupture and subsequent fetal death likely occurred outside the hospital, these events can also happen in a supervised environment.

24.3 Definition of Uterine Rupture

The terminology surrounding uterine rupture varies in the literature. The diagnosis can be categorized into either complete vs. incomplete disruption of the uterine layers, leading to either clinical or subclinical syndromes in the mother and fetus. Definitions can be further subdivided based on whether the uterus is previously scarred or unscarred. Rupture in an unscarred uterus is much less common, is more likely to occur in the context of trauma or obstructed labor and has a higher incidence in less developed countries [4]. Alternatively, the categories may be broken down by the timing at which the rupture occurs during pregnancy (i.e., 1st, 2nd, or 3rd trimester). For the purpose of this chapter, *uterine rupture* is defined as the complete disruption of all uterine layers, including the serosa (also known as the visceral peritoneum), typically resulting in clinically meaningful changes, such as maternal abdominal pain, signs of hemorrhagic shock, or a change in the fetal heart rate. If the serosa is intact but there is a disruption in the underlying myometrium, the term incomplete uterine rupture or *uterine scar dehiscence* is used. Uterine scar dehiscence is typically found incidentally during CD and is often not associated with clinically significant fetal or maternal changes. A 2004 meta-analysis of ten prospective trials found the pooled rate of symptomatic rupture to be 3.8 (95% CI 1.3–6.2) per 1000 trials of labor (0.38%) [5]. In the same analysis, among studies that routinely examined the uterus after successful TOLAC, the average rate of asymptomatic rupture or dehiscence was 13 (range 5–20) per 1000 trials of labor (1.3%). The remainder of the chapter will focus on complete uterine rupture in the context of a previous CD.

24.4 Epidemiology

Cesarean delivery rates are increasing worldwide, with some regions having rates as high as 42% [2]. Consequently, more patients are facing a choice about whether to attempt TOLAC or have a repeat CD in a subsequent pregnancy. A recent national cross-sectional survey of American births found an increase in the incidence of TOLAC from 2015 to 2020, with an annual percent increase of 4.25% (95% CI 2.9–5.6%) [1].

The incidence of uterine rupture during TOLAC is challenging to measure. Firstly, rupture rates depend on several factors and vary both locally and globally. Additionally, many studies measure different health outcomes. For example, some do not make a distinction between *complete* and *incomplete* rupture or between the *actual* and the *intended* routes of delivery [6]. A 2009 meta-analysis, including 17 studies, estimated an incidence of uterine rupture among patients undergoing TOLAC of 0.72% after one previous CD and 1.59% after two CDs [7]. More recently, a secondary analysis of the World Health Organization Multicountry Survey on Maternal and Newborn Health, which included data on deliveries from 359 facilities in 29 countries, found an incidence of uterine rupture among women with at least one prior CD of 0.5%, ranging from 0.2% in high Human Development Index (HDI) countries to 1.0% in low HDI countries [8]. The authors noted, however, that these rates should be compared with caution, as the numbers of observed uterine rupture events were very few in some countries, a distinction between dehiscence and rupture was not made, and the survey did not collect information on whether patients were attempting TOLAC.

24.5 Choosing the Right Candidate for TOLAC

Uterine rupture risk is significantly greater during a TOLAC compared to a repeat elective CD [6, 9]. A report by the Oregon Evidence-based Practice Center in 2010 found that the risk of uterine rupture was 18 times higher during TOLAC compared to elective repeat CD (0.47% vs. 0.02%, respectively) [6]. Among the four studies included in that analysis ($n = 47{,}202$), 96% of uterine rupture cases occurred in the TOLAC group. However, many of the factors associated with uterine rupture are non-modifiable when it comes time to decide whether to proceed with a TOLAC. Thus, choosing the right candidates for TOLAC is probably the most important step in minimizing uterine rupture risk. Decision-making should incorporate information about the patient, the previous pregnancy history, and features of the current pregnancy.

24.5.1 Patient Factors

Increasing maternal age appears to convey a modest increase in the risk of uterine rupture. Several studies have reported on this factor but with variable age categories [6]. For example, a population-based study from Norway found that maternal age greater than 35 was associated with an adjusted odds ratio of 2.5 (95% CI 1.3–4.9) for rupture compared to patients with maternal age less than 35 years [9]. Obesity, as well as lower maternal education level and socio-economic status, has been associated with uterine rupture, but there are currently insufficient data to make strong conclusions [8, 10, 11]. Finally, uterine anomalies can also be associated with uterine rupture. A 2005 review of the literature found that most functional noncommunicating uterine horns are first diagnosed during or after the third decade of life in the context of obstetrical uterine rupture [12]. Rates of prerupture diagnosis were low at just 15%. The key to successful management of noncommunicating rudimentary horns, the authors of the review conclude, is early diagnosis and surgical removal before pregnancy.

24.5.2 Previous Pregnancy

The events and outcomes of previous pregnancies can influence the risk of uterine rupture in the current pregnancy. These include the presence of a previous successful vaginal birth, the number of previous CDs, and surgical techniques used during the previous CD. Previous vaginal birth has been consistently associated with lower rates of uterine rupture (aOR 0.26–0.62) [6, 13]. Inversely, two or more CDs have been shown across several studies to increase the risk of a uterine rupture (aOR 1.36–5.3) [6, 7, 11].

Many studies have evaluated surgical techniques at CD and the risk of uterine rupture in a future pregnancy. A 2019 systematic review summarized 14 available studies on single- vs. double-layer closure and the risk of uterine rupture [14]. The authors reported that half of the studies favored double-layer closure. However, a more recent meta-analysis of 18 randomized controlled trials found no significant difference in dehiscence or uterine rupture risk (RR 1.88; 95% CI 0.63–5.62; $p = 0.26$), despite pooled results favoring double-layer closure for the outcome of residual greater myometrial thickness [15]. With respect to the anatomic location of the previous hysterotomy, three obstetrical societies: the Royal College of Obstetricians and Gynecologists (RCOG), the American College of Obstetricians and Gynecologists (ACOG), and the Society for Obstetrician and Gynecologist of Canada (SOGC) report transverse lower-segment scars as lowest risk, with fundal, classical, or T-shaped scars incurring higher risk [14]. In a prospective National Institutes of Health (NIH) study of almost 46,000 patients undergoing TOLAC, the uterine rupture rate was 1.9% in those with a prior classical, inverted T, or J incision who either presented in advanced labor or refused a repeat cesarean birth vs. 0.7% in those with a prior low transverse incision [16]. A more recent cross-sectional analysis in the USA of over 25,000 patients with prior classical cesarean delivery found that, among patients with classical incisions, uterine rupture occurred in 10.6% of those who underwent labor compared with 0.3% of those who did not [17].

24.5.3 Current Pregnancy

Factors in the current pregnancy have also been associated with uterine rupture risk. For example, measurement of uterine scar thickness near term has been studied as a predictor of uterine rupture. A systematic review of 12 studies concluded that lower uterine segment scar thickness is a strong predictor of uterine scar defect; however, due to study heterogeneity, a single thickness cutoff has not yet been determined [18]. The risk of uterine rupture appears to be minimized at a scar thickness of 4.5 mm or greater [6]. A uterine scar niche, or isthmocele, is a pouchlike defect in the anterior uterine wall at the site of a prior CD scar that is associated with a thin residual myometrium [19]. Surgical repair of uterine scar niche has been reported with some mixed results regarding the optimal approach to surgical repair (hysteroscopic, laparoscopic, or vaginal) and a myometrial thickness cutoff for which to recommend surgical intervention [19]. Surgical management shows promise in the preservation of the uterus, symptom management (e.g., bleeding or pain), and infertility [19], but there are currently no long-term studies available that assess whether these techniques alter the risk of uterine rupture in a subsequent pregnancy.

The impact of multiple pregnancy was evaluated against singleton pregnancies in a case-control study involving 19 academic hospitals in the USA between 1999 and 2002, including more than 550 multiple pregnancies and close to 14,000 singleton pregnancies [20]. The study found that in the context of TOLAC, multiple pregnancies did not increase the risk of uterine rupture (aOR 1.19; 95% CI 0.43–3.30), blood product transfusion, or maternal intensive care unit (ICU) admission. A more recent case-control study compared cases of reported uterine rupture vs. matched nonuterine rupture controls between 2011 and 2012 [10]. This analysis found that multiple pregnancy was associated with uterine rupture risk only in patients without a previous CD (aOR 2.49; 95% CI 1.66–3.75). Although not a contraindication for TOLAC, the RCOG recommends a cautious approach in the context of twin gestation [21].

The inter-delivery interval is another factor to consider. Several studies have evaluated its effect on uterine rupture risk [6, 14]. Variable interval cutoffs have been studied, including <18 months (aOR 2.5; 95% CI 1.0–5.6), ≤24 months (aOR 2.05–2.65), and ≤37 months (aOR 1.00; 95% CI 0.99–1.00) [6, 10]. One retrospective study in the USA assessed patients with at least one prior CD undergoing TOLAC between 1995 and 2000 [22]. The study included 128 cases of uterine rupture (0.9%), as well as patients in five categories of inter-delivery interval duration (6, 6–11, 12–17, 18–59 and ≥60 months). Multivariable analysis showed that an inter-delivery interval less than 6 months (vs. 18–59 months) was the only category that significantly increased the odds of uterine rupture (aOR 3.05; 95% CI 1.36–6.87), blood transfusion (aOR 3.55; 95% CI 1.56–8.10), or composite morbidity, including uterine rupture, bladder or bowel injury, and uterine artery laceration (aOR 1.92; 95% CI 1.01–3.62). Overall, a longer inter-delivery interval appears to be protective against uterine rupture, but a clear cutoff has not been determined.

Finally, high fetal birthweight may also increase uterine rupture risk, suggesting that risk stratification may be achieved using ultrasound-estimated fetal weight. However, results are mixed, and definitive conclusions cannot be made with the available evidence [6, 9]. As with several other factors, including maternal age and multiple gestation, the RCOG advises a cautious approach in cases of suspected fetal macrosomia [21].

24.6 Optimizing Intrapartum Management

Once a decision is made to proceed with a TOLAC, several intrapartum factors influence the risk of uterine rupture. Factors to consider include induction and augmentation of labor and timing of delivery.

Compared with spontaneous onset of labor, induction of labor increases the risk of uterine rupture [6, 9, 10]. Interestingly, in a meta-analysis, Guise et al. found that within the trial of labor studies, the pooled risk of uterine rupture for the *spontaneous labor* group was 0.8% (95% CI 0.7–1.1), which was higher than the pooled estimates from all TOLAC studies (0.47%; 95% CI 0.28–0.77), suggesting that the baseline risk is higher in the induction studies [6]. Further sub-analysis showed a statistically significant difference between induction vs. spontaneous labor only in the ≥40 weeks of gestation group (risk difference 1.8%; 95% CI 0.1–3.5), but not in earlier gestational ages (GA). Additionally, we cannot assume that all induction techniques impose an equal risk, and there are clinical scenarios where delivery, whether by induction or repeat CD, is indicated for other reasons. The same meta-analysis from 2010 reported that the lowest rates of uterine rupture given induction of labor occur with oxytocin use (1.1%), followed by prostaglandin E2 (2%), and misoprostol (6%); however, the authors caution against extrapolation of these findings because of imprecision and inconsistencies among the results of the included studies [6]. A 2017 Cochrane review of induction of labor methods for patients with prior CD concluded that there is insufficient high-quality evidence to make conclusions about methods of induction [6, 23]. A Norwegian cohort study discussed earlier reported a similar increase in odds of rupture with both prostaglandins and oxytocin vs. spontaneous labor (aOR 2.5 and 2.8, respectively) [9]. Oxytocin use for augmentation of labor was also associated with rupture in that study (aOR 4.4; 95% CI 2.9–6.6). Concerning mechanical methods of induction, there is currently insufficient evidence to guide clinical recommendations [23]. A secondary analysis of a prospective trial published in 2019 evaluated the safety of a transcervical Foley catheter for cervical ripening during a TOLAC [24]. The study compared 323 patients who received a Foley catheter as part of their induction protocol with 2240 patients who underwent induction without a Foley catheter. After adjusting for several factors, a Foley catheter was found not to be associated with an increased risk of uterine rupture (aOR 2.02; 95% CI 0.71–5.78) or uterine scar dehiscence (aOR 1.32; 95% CI 0.37–4.72).

As mentioned, increasing GA at the time of TOLAC may increase the risk of uterine rupture. In the Norwegian cohort study, among patients undergoing TOLAC with a previous CD ($n = 57{,}859$), GA ≥ 41 weeks (vs. 37–40 weeks) had a modest increase in the odds of rupture after adjusting for demographic factors and the presence of a previous miscarriage (aOR 1.6; 95% CI 1.1–2.3) [9]. Preterm delivery (<36 weeks vs. 37–40 weeks) was not demonstrated to increase the risk of uterine rupture. Importantly, the effect of GA in this analysis was not controlled for whether labor was spontaneous or induced. A cohort study published in 2004 looking at GA found similarly that GA ≥ 41 weeks (vs. 37–40 weeks) increased the odds of uterine rupture (aOR 2.85; 95% CI 1.27–6.42) [25]. In keeping with these findings, a 2005 cohort study suggested that preterm delivery (average GA 33.9 weeks) vs. term (average GA 39.2 weeks) was protective; however, that result was not statistically significant (aOR 0.28; 95% CI 0.07–1.17) [26]. The evidence supporting the notion that higher GA imposes a greater risk of rupture is inconsistent. For example, in a nested case-control study published in 2003, the authors found that GA ≥ 40 weeks (vs. <40 weeks) appeared to be protective, but these results were based on a small sample (21 cases and 84 controls) without statistical significance (aOR 0.24; 95% CI 0.04–1.43) [27].

24.7 Models for Prediction of Uterine Rupture Risk

Attempts have been made to create prediction models for uterine rupture risk during TOLAC based on some of the risk factors discussed above [6]. It was argued that although consideration of risk factors is important to decision-making, the infrequency of uterine rupture, coupled with relatively weak associations for rupture risk, prevents the development of an accurate prediction tool [28]. However, the incorporation of new parameters, such as uterine scar thickness, may improve model performance. A recent attempt included a model developed using a large cross-sectional survey between 2015 and 2016 of patients with a previous uterine scar across 96 hospitals China ($n = 74{,}180$) [11]. The authors created three models using multivariable logistic regression and identified the best model based on receiver operating characteristic curves. The best model (area under the curve 0.81) included eight variables that had an OR >1.5 for uterine rupture in their analysis: maternal age, prepregnancy BMI, number of previous CD, number of previous abortions, presence of anemia, gestational diabetes, placenta previa, and hospital level (secondary vs. tertiary). The optimal cutoff score for this model was 6.5 points, putting patients into either a low-risk group (uterine rupture risk of 0.21%) or a high-risk group (uterine rupture risk of 2.83%). The study results have some limitations, as the outcome included both dehiscence and complete rupture, and despite this, the rate of the primary outcome of 0.18% (95% CI 0.05–0.23%) was low compared to other estimates. Additionally, the study did not differentiate between patients who attempted TOLAC vs. elective CD, which further complicates generalizability. Finally, the model required external validation in another cohort.

24.8 Predicting Successful Vaginal Birth After Cesarean Section (VBAC)

An important consideration for patient counseling is the likelihood of successful VBAC. A 2019 guideline from the SOGC summarizes the evidence on the likelihood of successful vaginal birth [29]. Factors that increase the chances of vaginal birth include younger maternal age (<30 years), lower BMI (<30 kg/m^2), previous vaginal birth, a previous indication for CD that is not labor dystocia (e.g., breech presentation, abnormal fetal heart rate), spontaneous labor, and a birthweight <4000 g. Factors that reduce the likelihood include GA > 40 weeks and preeclampsia. Similarly to uterine rupture, there are efforts to create prediction tools for successful VBAC. One example is a calculator developed by the Maternal–Fetal Medicine Units Network, which is freely available online (► https://mfmunetwork.bsc.gwu.edu/web/mfmunetwork/vaginal-birth-after-cesarean-calculator) [30, 31]. This calculator was developed based on a multivariable logistic regression model and can be applied in early pregnancy or at the time of delivery admission. The latest versions of the calculators, with race and ethnicity parameters removed, have areas under the curve of 0.75 (95% CI 0.74–0.77) for early pregnancy and 0.78 (95% CI 0.77–0.79) at the end of pregnancy. These new models have not yet been validated in other populations.

24.9 Clinical Presentation

Uterine rupture can present at any time: before, during, or even after labor and delivery. None of the symptoms or signs of rupture are pathognomonic, and many can be misleading. Some patients can be completely asymptomatic without significant maternal or fetal signs, although this is more common in cases of incomplete rupture, as discussed earlier. It is essential to keep the diagnosis in mind and continuously monitor patients undergoing TOLAC for signs or symptoms of uterine rupture.

Patients with uterine rupture may describe abdominal pain on a wide spectrum, from minimal to severe. For patients admitted in labor, pain may be partially or completely by neuraxial analgesia. The pain may also be inappropriately disregarded as normal labor pains. Surprisingly, detectable uterine contractions are not essential, especially for patients whose previous uterine scar is high on the uterus or in whom the pregnancy is at an earlier GA [32]. When present, there are several types of uterine contraction patterns associated with uterine rupture (e.g., hyperstimulation, loss of activity, and increasing baseline tone), with some studies showing no change in uterine activity between cases and controls [33]. Although an intrauterine pressure catheter (IUPC) may identify more subtle changes compared to more commonly used tocodynamometry (e.g., contraction amplitude and increasing baseline), there is insufficient evidence to recommend routine IUPC use in TOLAC [33]. Vaginal bleeding is another important sign, but bleeding from the site of rupture can be entirely intraperitoneal. As with the pain, bleeding can also be disregarded as part of the normal cervical changes of labor.

On physical examination, it is essential to identify signs of maternal hemorrhagic shock (hypotension, tachycardia, and low urine output). Abdominal tenderness may be present, especially if uterine contents or blood have spread to the rest of the abdomen. Tenderness over the previous uterine scar, palpable fetal parts, or an abnormal uterine shape, although intuitive considerations, are not reliable signs of rupture [32]. Finally, there may be evidence of fetal distress or fetal death on cardiotocography. Importantly, with modern trends in labor analgesia, fetal heart rate abnormality has become the most common sign of uterine rupture in labor [34]. There does not appear to be a single type of fetal heart rate abnormality that is common to all uterine rupture cases, but fetal bradycardia is an important sign [35, 36].

Point-of-care ultrasound (POCUS) has growing applications in the labor and delivery unit, including labor monitoring, determination of fetal presentation, and placental location. Rapid POCUS visualization may be of crucial value in the diagnosis of uterine rupture; however, only a small number of case reports exist on its use in this context, and no formal measurement validation or guidance on its use currently exists [37–39].

24.10 Diagnosis

If uterine rupture is suspected, urgent diagnosis and management are essential to prevent complications. The diagnosis is made by emergency exploratory laparotomy. In cases without labor or where maternal and fetal status is stable, ultrasound imaging may be considered. Diagnostic imaging features include disruption of the myometrium, an extra-uterine hematoma, hemoperitoneum, protruding extra-uterine membranes or fetal parts, or an empty uterus [40]. Additional imaging performed in the setting of maternal trauma as part of a trauma workup, including computed tomography or magnetic resonance imaging, may also support the diagnosis [40, 41].

24.11 Management

In the event that uterine rupture is suspected, urgent management is required. Initial steps involve resuscitation of the mother when there is evidence of maternal hemorrhagic shock, and urgent delivery of the fetus [4, 32]. Once the fetus and placenta are delivered, control of hemorrhage becomes the priority. The pelvic anatomy needs to be carefully examined to identify all sources of bleeding. Rupture can distort anatomy, and involvement of the bladder, broad ligament, or uterine sites other than the previous uterine incision has been reported [32]. The surgical team must then determine if the uterus can be repaired or if a hysterectomy is needed to minimize maternal complications. Subtotal hysterectomy may be technically easier and the preferred option; however, when the placenta is in the lower segment, a total hysterectomy may be necessary to prevent bleeding from the placental attachment site [32].

24.12 Clinical Outcomes

Uterine rupture can result in severe adverse outcomes for the mother and the fetus/neonate. For the mother, significant hemorrhage may lead to hemorrhagic shock, the need for hysterectomy, and potentially death. Maternal mortality in the context of uterine rupture is fortunately very rare, with most studies reporting no cases [6]. A retrospective study of maternal deaths in Canada from 1991 to 2001 detected four deaths (0.2%) out of 1898 cases of uterine rupture during the study period [42]. In general, hysterectomy is rare among patients having a repeat CD or TOLAC, occurring in less than 3% of patients who had a previous CD, with no significant difference between routes of delivery among patients at term [6]. Hysterectomy rates specifically among patients with rupture are estimated at 13% (95% CI 4–27%) based on pooled data from five cohort studies [5]. Transfusion is another important complication that gives insight into the amount of maternal hemorrhage. Most studies measuring this outcome do not report rates specific to patients who have a diagnosis of uterine rupture. From nine cohort studies, there was no significant difference in transfusion rates between TOLAC (0.9%; 95% CI 0.4–2.0%) and elective repeat CD (1.2%; 95% CI 0.5–2.6%) [6].

For the fetus/neonate, adverse outcomes include hypoxia, ischemic encephalopathy, and death. The rate of perinatal mortality ranges widely from 0% to 20%, with a pooled risk of 6.2% (95%CI 1.8–18.8% from six studies across all GA categories [6]. The rate is lower (0–2.8%) when considering only the two studies that reported term patients, specifically [6]. More recently, a Norwegian population-based study reported on neonatal outcomes with complete uterine rupture [43]. Of the 244 births involving uterine rupture, 64 (26.2%) had intrapartum or neonatal death, 56 (23%) required neonatal intensive care admission, and 15 (6.1%) had hypoxic ischemic encephalopathy. This analysis also found that the mortality rate decreased with time, with higher rates from 1967 to 1977 (51.6%) compared to 2000–2008 (15.0%). Diagnosis of fetal extrusion and/or placental separation incurred the highest odds of intrapartum/neonatal mortality (OR 18.9; 95% CI 7.5–42.4). Overall, 109 (44.7%) neonates were classified as healthy.

If uterine rupture occurs, does the location of birth influence the presence or extent of maternal and neonatal complications? An argument can be made that delivering in a hospital setting with close monitoring and nearby surgical capabilities could increase early detection and rapid surgical management. A 2004 prospective cohort study in 41 US out-of-hospital birthing centers aimed to test this hypothesis [44]. Of the 1453 included patients undergoing TOLAC in a birthing center, 24% were transferred to hospital during labor, 6 (0.4%) had a diagnosis of uterine rupture, 15 infants (1%) had a 5-minute Apgar score less than 7, and there were 7 (0.5%) fetal/neonatal deaths, with most of the fetal deaths (5/7) occurring in the absence of uterine rupture. The authors concluded that because of the increased risk of complications requiring hospital management during TOLAC, birthing centers should refer patients with a previous CD to hospitals for delivery. Indeed, the Norwegian cohort study investigating neonatal outcomes found that timing of delivery from the moment of clinical suspicion was associated with fetal/neonatal mortality: >30 vs. <20 minutes increased the odds of death (aOR 16.7; 95% CI 6.4–43.5), although 2 of the 64 recorded deaths occurred within just 10 minutes of diagnostic suspicion, and the number of patients in each category was relatively small [43]. A 2005 commentary in The *Lancet* challenged the purported superiority of in-hospital management, citing a wide variation in hospital response times, along with the high rates of successful TOLAC and low rates of uterine rupture in the birthing center data [45]. The author urged future initiatives to examine, "strategies of combining the strengths of these apparently opposed philosophies of maternity service to provide safe intrapartum care with high levels of maternal satisfaction and low intervention." A retrospective cohort study of over three hundred thousand Canadian patients with previous CD may give some further insight into this debate [46]. The authors found that a higher risk of adverse outcomes like uterine rupture was associated with low-volume birthing units (<500 births per year vs. ≥500 births per year). For example, the adjusted odds ratios for uterine rupture were 4.02 (95% CI 2.48–6.51) and 2.30 (95% CI 2.04–2.59), respectively.

24.13 Review of Prevention Strategies

Prevention strategies have been classified into five stages: primordial, primary, secondary, tertiary, and quaternary prevention [47]. ◘ Table 24.1 outlines each prevention stage and the associated possible strategies to prevent uterine rupture. In this case, the "disease" we are aiming to prevent is *clinically significant uterine rupture*.

An opportunity for prevention of uterine rupture can occur at four instances in a patient's clinical trajectory. The earliest instance is at the first CD, which includes the decision to deliver a CD in the first place, as

Table 24.1 Prevention strategies [48] for clinically significant uterine rupture as the target of prevention

Prevention stage	Prevention strategy	Opportunities for innovation/improvement
Primordial Factors to target the population as a whole, social and environmental conditions, laws and national policy	Minimize unplanned/unwanted pregnancy Minimize short inter-pregnancy interval Avoid primary CD	Access to contraception Access to safe abortion Access to obstetrical care See safe prevention of the primary cesarean delivery [49]
Primary Prevent disease from ever occurring, risk reduction in susceptible populations	Optimize surgical techniques during primary CD Repair of thin uterine myometrium (scar) Choosing the right candidate for TOLAC based on maternal and pregnancy factors Optimize labor management	More high-quality research (see *Guise 2010* [6]) Standardization of outcomes Standards for reference predictors Hospital vs. out-of-hospital RCTs for induction methods vs. expectant management Optimization of predictive models Novel predictive factors
Secondary Early disease detection before the onset of clinical signs and symptoms	Skilled birth attendant Risk stratification for birthing centers IUPC Continuous fetal monitoring POCUS in labor? Computerized cardiotocography (cCTG)?	Research on hospital vs. out-of-hospital detection Strategies to combine strengths of hospital- and community-based obstetrical care [45] Research on novel detection methods: POCUS and cCTG as detection tools
Clinically significant uterine rupture Complete uterine rupture causes: abnormal fetal heart rate, severe maternal abdominal pain or bleeding, hemodynamic instability, fetal death, maternal death		
Tertiary Symptomatic patients, aim to reduce the severity of the disease and associated sequelae	Skilled birth attendant Patient education Availability of urgent transfer to hospital Availability of blood products	More research on time-to-delivery to cutoffs Quality control and institutional protocolization of intervention strategies
Quaternary Prevention of medical interventions that are likely to cause more harm than good	Limited data	Studies of long-term outcomes (e.g., guidance on repair vs. hysterectomy for the preservation of fertility)

RCT randomized controlled trial, *IUPC* intrauterine pressure catheter, *POCUS* point-of-care ultrasound

well as the technical aspects of the operation. Between pregnancies, there may be an opportunity to further minimize rupture risk with the repair of a thin uterine scar. Next, risk reduction can occur in the subsequent pregnancy when a decision is being made about TOLAC vs. repeat elective CD. Statistical models have the potential at this stage to assist in risk stratification, decision-making, and patient counseling (MFMU VBAC Calculator). The last opportunity is during the trial of labor itself, at which point choices can be made about induction methods. Once uterine rupture occurs (either complete or incomplete), the focus then shifts to early disease detection (secondary prevention) and early intervention to prevent complications (tertiary prevention).

Uterine rupture is a challenging outcome to study—and therefore predict—for several reasons: it is relatively uncommon, many individual factors have a relatively small influence on risk, and existing data is often heterogeneous in the reporting of health outcomes, making pooled analysis and generalizability challenging [6, 28]. Without good predictive models, obstetrical providers and policymakers must consider a variety of individual factors when counseling patients, making clinical decisions, or developing risk-reducing policies.

24.14 Prevention in the Case Example

At the beginning of this chapter, a case report of uterine rupture was introduced from a manuscript by Eboh et al. [3] To summarize, the authors describe a case of uterine rupture during a TOLAC at home without medical personnel. How could the events in that case have been optimized to prevent uterine rupture and, subsequently, fetal death? Consider prevention strategies using the framework in ◘ Table 24.1:

- *Primordial Prevention*: The first CD for breech presentation could have potentially been prevented with a trial of an external cephalic version. The inter-pregnancy interval could also be increased with good counseling and the availability of contraceptive options.
- *Primary Prevention*: Before pregnancy, uterine scar thickness could have been measured, with the opportunity for repair of an isthmocele or thin residual myometrium, if present. During pregnancy, the intervention likely of the highest value to the patient is increased interaction with obstetrical care. Obstetrical providers have an opportunity to counsel patients on individualized risks based on a variety of characteristics discussed in this chapter (e.g., age, previous vaginal birth, quality of previous uterine incision, etc.). In the setting of uncertainty, shared decision-making must account for the patient's values and objectives.
- *Secondary Prevention*: Unfortunately, there is no singular reliable clinical sign or symptom for the early detection of uterine rupture, and our patient had relatively mild symptoms. In this case, patient counseling could have been used to emphasize the patient's baseline risk and review concerning signs or symptoms that warrant earlier assessment by a skilled obstetrical provider. Developing hospital-based labor units that prioritize patient values and minimize unnecessary interventions is also essential to creating trusting relationships.
- *Tertiary Prevention*: A skilled birth attendant who can recognize concerning signs in labor, or who has training in fetal heart rate monitoring might not have prevented the uterine rupture event but may have facilitated urgent transfer to the hospital, potentially minimizing complications.

The prevention framework described in the previous section is not intended to, or capable of, preventing any *individual* uterine rupture event. Binary prediction of rupture for an individual patient is impossible, and prediction, especially of an uncommon event, comes with significant uncertainty [28]. What prevention strategies offer is an opportunity for large-scale changes that can minimize uterine rupture rates and associated complications in the aggregate.

Chapter Key Points

- Uterine rupture is rare but potentially catastrophic, most commonly occurring during TOLAC.
- Risk varies widely based on prior cesarean type, inter-delivery interval, induction method, and labor management.
- Lower uterine segment scar thickness >4.5 mm is associated with reduced rupture risk.
- Primary prevention begins with avoiding the first cesarean and optimizing surgical technique.
- Intrapartum vigilance—continuous fetal monitoring, cautious induction, timely recognition—is central to prevention.

Chapter-End Summary

Uterine rupture is a significant complication of TOLAC. The overall risk of uterine rupture is relatively low, but the consequences can be grave, including maternal hemorrhage and the need for hysterectomy, as well as neonatal hypoxia or death. This chapter reviewed the currently known factors associated with uterine rupture and incorporated them into a prevention strategy framework. Strategies to prevent uterine rupture can be implemented in four instances in a patient's care: (1) during the first CD, (2) between pregnancies, (3) during delivery planning in the current pregnancy, and (4) during the trial of labor itself. Uterine rupture is impossible to predict on an individual basis, and it is essential to counsel patients on their delivery options, integrating patient factors, preferences, and risk tolerance. However, the obstetrical community has an opportunity to reduce the uterine rupture incidence and associated complications for populations as a whole. Important steps to achieving this objective include lowering the CD rate, standardizing the reporting of health outcomes in research to allow for better aggregate analysis, and developing novel clinical tools for risk stratification and early disease detection.

Chapter-End Summary

Uterine rupture remains an uncommon but severe complication, most often arising during TOLAC. Prevention involves a multilayered strategy across the reproductive continuum: minimizing primary cesarean deliveries, optimizing closure techniques, assessing scar thickness, careful candidate selection, and evidence-based intrapartum management. Although no single sign reliably predicts rupture, continuous monitoring and prompt recognition of fetal heart rate abnormalities remain critical. When rupture occurs, rapid surgical intervention mitigates maternal morbidity and improves neonatal outcomes.

References

1. Bruno AM, Allshouse AA, Metz TD. Trends in attempted and successful trial of labor after cesarean delivery in the United States from 2010 to 2020. Obstet Gynecol. 2023;141:173–5. https://doi.org/10.1097/AOG.0000000000004998.
2. Betran AP, Ye J, Moller AB, Souza JP, Zhang J. Trends and projections of caesarean section rates: global and regional estimates. BMJ Glob Health. 2021;6:e005671. https://doi.org/10.1136/BMJGH-2021-005671.
3. Eboh S, Burghul S, Galloway M, Sanchez A, Ventolini G. Preterm complete uterine rupture with en caul expulsion. Clin Med Insights Case Rep. 2022;15:11795476221112376. https://doi.org/10.1177/11795476221112376.
4. Murphy DJ. Uterine rupture. Curr Opin Obstet Gynecol. 2006;18:135–40. https://doi.org/10.1097/01.GCO.0000192989.45589.57.
5. Guise JM, McDonagh MS, Osterweil P, Nygren P, Chan BKS, Helfand M. Systematic review of the incidence and consequences of uterine rupture in women with previous caesarean section. BMJ. 2004;329:19–23. https://doi.org/10.1136/BMJ.329.7456.19.
6. Guise JM, Eden K, Emeis C, Denman MA, Marshall N, Fu RR, et al. Vaginal birth after cesarean: new insights. Evid Rep Technol Assess (Full Rep). 2010;191:1.
7. Tahseen S, Griffiths M. Vaginal birth after two caesarean sections (VBAC-2)-a systematic review with meta-analysis of success rate and adverse outcomes of VBAC-2 versus VBAC-1 and repeat (third) caesarean sections. BJOG. 2010;117:5–19. https://doi.org/10.1111/J.1471-0528.2009.02351.X.
8. Motomura K, Ganchimeg T, Nagata C, Ota E, Vogel JP, Betran AP, et al. Incidence and outcomes of uterine rupture among women with prior caesarean section: WHO Multicountry Survey on Maternal and Newborn Health. Sci Rep. 2017;7:44093. https://doi.org/10.1038/SREP44093.
9. Al-Zirqi I, Daltveit AK, Forsén L, Stray-Pedersen B, Vangen S. Risk factors for complete uterine rupture. Am J Obstet Gynecol. 2017;216:165.e1–8. https://doi.org/10.1016/J.AJOG.2016.10.017.
10. Vilchez G, Nazeer S, Kumar K, Warren M, Dai J, Sokol RJ. Contemporary epidemiology and novel predictors of uterine rupture: a nationwide population-based study. Arch Gynecol Obstet. 2017;296:869–75. https://doi.org/10.1007/S00404-017-4508-4/TABLES/4.
11. Zhan W, Zhu J, Hua X, Ye J, Chen Q, Zhang J. Epidemiology of uterine rupture among pregnant women in China and development of a risk prediction model: analysis of data from a multicentre, cross-sectional study. BMJ Open. 2021;11:e054540. https://doi.org/10.1136/BMJOPEN-2021-054540.

12. Jayasinghe Y, Rane A, Stalewski H, Grover S. The presentation and early diagnosis of the rudimentary uterine horn. Obstet Gynecol. 2005;105:1456–67. https://doi.org/10.1097/01.AOG.0000161321.94364.56.
13. Smith GCS, Pell JP, Pasupathy D, Dobbie R. Factors predisposing to perinatal death related to uterine rupture during attempted vaginal birth after caesarean section: retrospective cohort study. BMJ. 2004;329:375–7. https://doi.org/10.1136/BMJ.38160.634352.55.
14. Tanos V, Toney ZA. Uterine scar rupture – prediction, prevention, diagnosis, and management. Best Pract Res Clin Obstet Gynaecol. 2019;59:115–31. https://doi.org/10.1016/J.BPOBGYN.2019.01.009.
15. Qayum K, Kar I, Sofi J, Panneerselvam H. Single-versus double-layer uterine closure after cesarean section delivery: a systematic review and meta-analysis. Cureus. 2021;13:e18405. https://doi.org/10.7759/CUREUS.18405.
16. Landon MB, Hauth JC, Leveno KJ, Spong CY, Leindecker S, Varner MW, et al. Maternal and perinatal outcomes associated with a trial of labor after prior cesarean delivery. N Engl J Med. 2004;351:2581–9. https://doi.org/10.1056/NEJMOA040405.
17. Thompson BB, Reddy UM, Burn M, Abdel-Razeq S, Xu X. Maternal outcomes in subsequent pregnancies after classical cesarean delivery. Obstet Gynecol. 2022;140:212–9. https://doi.org/10.1097/AOG.0000000000004869.
18. Jastrow N, Chaillet N, Roberge S, Morency AM, Lacasse Y, Bujold E. Sonographic lower uterine segment thickness and risk of uterine scar defect: a systematic review. J Obstet Gynaecol Can. 2010;32:321–7. https://doi.org/10.1016/S1701-2163(16)34475-9.
19. Setubal A, Alves J, Osório F, Guerra A, Fernandes R, Albornoz J, et al. Treatment for uterine isthmocele, a pouchlike defect at the site of a cesarean section scar. J Minim Invasive Gynecol. 2018;25:38–46. https://doi.org/10.1016/J.JMIG.2017.09.022.
20. Varner MW, Thom E, Spong CY, Landon MB, Leveno KJ, Rouse DJ, et al. Trial of labor after one previous cesarean delivery for multifetal gestation. Obstet Gynecol. 2007;110:814–9. https://doi.org/10.1097/01.AOG.0000280586.05350.9E.
21. Gupta JR, Smith G, Chodankar R. Birth after previous cesarean birth (Green-top guideline No. 45). Royal College of Obstetricians and Gynaecologists; 2015.
22. Stamilio DM, Defranco E, Paré E, Odibo AO, Peipert JF, Allsworth JE, et al. Short interpregnancy interval: risk of uterine rupture and complications of vaginal birth after cesarean delivery. Obstet Gynecol. 2007;110:1075–82. https://doi.org/10.1097/01.AOG.0000286759.49895.46.
23. West HM, Jozwiak M, Dodd JM. Methods of term labour induction for women with a previous caesarean section. Cochrane Database Syst Rev. 2017;6:CD009792. https://doi.org/10.1002/14651858.CD009792.PUB3.
24. Katz Eriksen JL, Chandrasekaran S, Delaney SS. Is Foley catheter use during a trial of labor after cesarean associated with uterine rupture? Am J Perinatol. 2019;36:1431–6. https://doi.org/10.1055/S-0039-1691766.
25. Hammoud A, Hendler I, Gauthier RJ, Berman S, Sansregret A, Bujold E. The effect of gestational age on trial of labor after cesarean section. J Matern Fetal Neonatal Med. 2004;15:202–6. https://doi.org/10.1080/14767050410001668329.
26. Quiñones JN, Stamilio DM, Paré E, Peipert JF, Stevens E, Macones GA. The effect of prematurity on vaginal birth after cesarean delivery: success and maternal morbidity. Obstet Gynecol. 2005;105:519–24. https://doi.org/10.1097/01.AOG.0000153493.15922.85.
27. Shipp TD, Zelop C, Cohen A, Repke JT, Lieberman E. Post-cesarean delivery fever and uterine rupture in a subsequent trial of labor. Obstet Gynecol. 2003;101:136–9. https://doi.org/10.1016/S0029-7844(02)02319-0.
28. Landon MB. Predicting uterine rupture in women undergoing trial of labor after prior cesarean delivery. Semin Perinatol. 2010;34:267–71. https://doi.org/10.1053/J.SEMPERI.2010.03.005.
29. Dy J, DeMeester S, Lipworth H, Barrett J. No. 382-trial of labour after caesarean. J Obstet Gynaecol Can. 2019;41:992–1011. https://doi.org/10.1016/J.JOGC.2018.11.008.
30. Grobman WA, Sandoval GJ, Rice MM, Chauhan SP, Clifton RG, Costantine MM, et al. Prediction of vaginal birth after cesarean using information at admission for delivery: a calculator without race or ethnicity. Am J Obstet Gynecol. 2023;230:S804. https://doi.org/10.1016/J.AJOG.2023.02.008.
31. Grobman WA, Sandoval G, Rice MM, Bailit JL, Chauhan SP, Costantine MM, et al. Prediction of vaginal birth after cesarean delivery in term gestations: a calculator without race and ethnicity. Am J Obstet Gynecol. 2021;225:664.e1–7. https://doi.org/10.1016/J.AJOG.2021.05.021.
32. Turner MJ. Uterine rupture. Best Pract Res Clin Obstet Gynaecol. 2002;16:69–79. https://doi.org/10.1053/beog.2001.0256.
33. Vlemminx MWC, de Lau H, Oei SG. Tocogram characteristics of uterine rupture: a systematic review. Arch Gynecol Obstet. 2017;295:17–26. https://doi.org/10.1007/S00404-016-4214-7/FIGURES/2.
34. Kieser KE, Baskett TF. A 10-year population-based study of uterine rupture. Obstet Gynecol. 2002;100:749–53. https://doi.org/10.1016/S0029-7844(02)02161-0.
35. Menihan CA. Uterine rupture in women attempting a vaginal birth following prior cesarean birth. J Perinatol. 1998;18:440–3.
36. Ridgeway JJ, Weyrich DL, Benedetti TJ. Fetal heart rate changes associated with uterine rupture.

Obstet Gynecol. 2004;103:506–12. https://doi.org/10.1097/01.AOG.0000113619.67704.99.
37. Weissmann-Brenner A, Gilboa Y, Yerushalmi GM, Achiron R, Schiff E. Sonographic presentations of uterine rupture following vaginal birth after cesarean – report of two cases 12 h apart. Case Rep Perinat Med. 2012;1:3–5. https://doi.org/10.1515/CRPM-2011-0001.
38. Matsubara S, Shimada K, Kuwata T, Usui R, Suzuki M. Thin anterior uterine wall with incomplete uterine rupture in a primigravida detected by palpation and ultrasound: a case report. J Med Case Rep. 2011;5:1–4. https://doi.org/10.1186/1752-1947-5-14/FIGURES/2.
39. van Alphen M, van Vugt JMG, Hummel P, van Geijn HP. Recurrent uterine rupture diagnosed by ultrasound. Ultrasound Obstet Gynecol. 1995;5:419–21. https://doi.org/10.1046/J.1469-0705.1995.05060419.X.
40. Kaakaji Y, Nghiem HV, Nodell C, Winter TC. Sonography of obstetric and gynecologic emergencies: part I, Obstetric emergencies. AJR Am J Roentgenol. 2000;174:641–9. https://doi.org/10.2214/AJR.174.3.1740641.
41. Eller AG, Fisher B. Images in clinical medicine. Diagnosis of uterine rupture on CT. N Engl J Med. 2009;360:170. https://doi.org/10.1056/NEJMICM075079.
42. Wen SW, Huang L, Liston R, Heaman M, Baskett T, Rusen ID, et al. Severe maternal morbidity in Canada, 1991–2001. CMAJ. 2005;173:759–64. https://doi.org/10.1503/CMAJ.045156.
43. Al-Zirqi I, Daltveit AK, Vangen S. Infant outcome after complete uterine rupture. Am J Obstet Gynecol. 2018;219:109.e1–8. https://doi.org/10.1016/J.AJOG.2018.04.010.
44. Lieberman E, Ernst EK, Rooks JP, Stapleton S, Flamm B. Results of the national study of vaginal birth after cesarean in birth centers. Obstet Gynecol. 2004;104:933–42. https://doi.org/10.1097/01.AOG.0000143257.29471.82.
45. Windrim R. Vaginal delivery in birth centre after previous caesarean section. Lancet. 2005;365:106–7. https://doi.org/10.1016/S0140-6736(05)17719-8.
46. Wen SW, Rusen ID, Walker M, Liston R, Kramer MS, Baskett T, et al. Comparison of maternal mortality and morbidity between trial of labor and elective cesarean section among women with previous cesarean delivery. Am J Obstet Gynecol. 2004;191:1263–9. https://doi.org/10.1016/j.ajog.2004.03.022.
47. Kisling LA, Das JM. Prevention strategies. StatPearls Publishing; 2023. p. 1–4. https://www.ncbi.nlm.nih.gov/books/NBK537222/. Accessed 12 Jan 2024.
48. Leavell HR, Clark GE. The science and art of preventing disease, prolonging life, and promoting physical and mental health and efficiency. In: Leavell HR, Clark GE, editors. Preventive medicine for the doctor in his community. 3rd ed. New York: Robert E. Krieger Publishing Company; 1979.
49. Spong CY, Berghella V, Wenstrom KD, Mercer BM, Saade GR. Preventing the first cesarean delivery: summary of a Joint Eunice Kennedy Shriver National Institute of Child Health and Human Development, Society for Maternal-Fetal Medicine, and American College of Obstetricians and Gynecologists workshop. Obstet Gynecol. 2012;120:1181. https://doi.org/10.1097/AOG.0B013E3182704880.

Further Reading

Guise JM, Eden K, Emeis C, Denman MA, Marshall N, Fu RR, et al. Vaginal birth after cesarean: new insights. Evid Rep Technol Assess (Full Rep). 2010;191:1. *The most comprehensive systematic review and meta-analysis on TOLAC to date.*

Murphy DJ. Uterine rupture. Curr Opin Obstet Gynecol. 2006;18:135–40. https://doi.org/10.1097/01.GCO.0000192989.45589.57. *Another chapter that covers uterine rupture more holistically, including rupture in an unscarred uterus and low-resource settings.*

Perdue M, Felder L, Berghella V. First-trimester uterine rupture: a case report and systematic review of the literature. Am J Obstet Gynecol. 2022;227:209–17. https://doi.org/10.1016/J.AJOG.2022.04.035. *A systematic review of the literature of first-trimester uterine rupture.*

Neonatal Care

Contents

Prevention of Intracranial Hemorrhage in Neonates

Sharon Morag and Dror Mandel

Contents

Y. Yogev, A. Khalil (eds.), *Prevention of Complications in Obstetrics*,
https://doi.org/10.1007/978-3-032-23479-7_25

Learning Objectives

- Understand the pathophysiology of intraventricular hemorrhage (IVH) in preterm infants.
- Discuss methods for the prevention and reduction of severity of the IVH and the importance of adherence to intraventricular hemorrhage prevention bundles (IVHPBs).
  - I. Prenatal interventions for preventing IVH
    1. Prevention of preterm birth
    2. Antenatal corticosteroids
    3. Other pharmacologic agents
    4. Maternal transport
  - II. Perinatal and postnatal interventions for preventing IVH
    1. Delayed cord clamping (DCC)
    2. Minimizing Fluctuations in Cerebral Blood Flow:
       - (a) Minimal handling of preterm infants
       - (b) Reducing painful or stressful procedures
       - (c) The use of indomethacin
       - (d) Ensuring cerebral autoregulation
       - (e) Optimizing respiratory support

Learning Objectives

- Explain the pathophysiology of IVH and vulnerability of the germinal matrix.
- Identify prenatal, perinatal, and postnatal interventions that reduce IVH incidence.
- Describe the role of ACS, magnesium sulfate, and maternal transport in IVH prevention.
- Discuss hemodynamic, respiratory, and handling strategies that stabilize cerebral blood flow.
- Recognize the impact of structured IVH prevention bundles on neonatal outcomes.

25.1 Introduction

Intracranial hemorrhage (ICH) in neonates is a significant concern in Neonatology. It can manifest in various forms, each with distinct characteristics and clinical implications.

There are several types of ICH: (1) intraventricular hemorrhage (IVH): Intraventricular hemorrhage is one of the most common types of ICH observed in neonates, particularly in those with gestational ages less than 30 weeks. This type of hemorrhage is characterized by bleeding into the ventricles of the brain, which can lead to major complications such as hydrocephalus; (2) subdural hemorrhage (SDH): Subdural hemorrhage occurs between the dura mater and the surface of the brain. It is the second most common type of hemorrhage and can result from birth trauma or may be spontaneous, with varying clinical manifestations ranging from asymptomatic to severe; (3) intra-parenchymal hemorrhage (IPH): Intraparenchymal hemorrhage refers to bleeding within the brain tissue itself. This type of hemorrhage can be associated with neurological deficits depending on the affected area of the brain and the volume of bleeding; (4) subpial hemorrhage: subpial hemorrhage occurs just beneath the pia mater. Similar to other forms of ICH, it can have a range of clinical presentations and may be associated with underlying conditions that predispose the infant to bleeding; (5) Other: additional types of hemorrhage include subarachnoid hemorrhage and epidural hemorrhage. These forms of hemorrhage may arise from various etiologies, including traumatic delivery or congenital vascular malformations.

In this chapter, we will focus only on the prevention of Intraventricular Hemorrhage (IVH) in preterm neonates. IVH is the most common neurological complication in preterm infants, with a reported prevalence of 20–59% of all preterm infants [1–7], an incidence that is inversely proportional to gestational age. This condition can lead to severe neurological impairments and mortality. Understanding the mechanisms, risk factors, and preventive strategies for IVH is crucial in neonatal care to improve outcomes for these vulnerable infants.

25.2 Pathophysiology of IVH

The pathophysiology of IVH in preterm infants is multifaceted, involving the fragility of the germinal matrix, fluctuating cerebral blood flow, and impaired autoregulation of cerebral circulation. The germinal matrix (HM) is a site for the production of neural precursors and glial cell production, located in the subdependable regions of the caudothalamic groove. As such, this area is called GM/subependymal hemorrhage. The blood in the GM can expand to the lateral ventricles and form IVH. Since the GM is an embryonic structure, which begins to develop around 24 weeks of pregnancy and disappears around 34 weeks of pregnancy, GM matrix or IVH is an almost exclusive complication of premature infants and is rarely seen in babies born at term. Breakage of blood vessels in the GM can result from blood clotting disorders or cerebral blood flow (CBF) disorders. Premature infants are much more sensitive to changes in CBF flow because they have pressure-passive circulation, i.e., changes in systemic blood flow pass directly to CBF without autoregulation, which does not exist as a physiological mechanism in term neonates. Hence, small preterm infants cannot control their CBF to protect against fluctuations. Such fluctuations in CBF can be caused by various factors, such as respiratory distress, hypotension, rapid volume expansion, mechanical ventilation, and others.

Stabilizing CBF in the first days of life, especially during the first 24 hours after birth, will lower the risk of developing GM-IVH. Fifty percent of IVH cases will occur in the first day of life, 90 percent of cases will occur in the first 72 hours after birth [8], and 100 percent of cases will occur by 1 week of age [9]. In view of the severe consequences that intraventricular bleeding can cause to the developing brain of preterm infants that can lead to long-term neurological complications [10, 11], it is necessary to reduce as much as possible the incidence of intraventricular bleeding in preterm infants through quality processes based on evidence from the neonatal medical literature.

Prevention or reduction of the severity of IVH is a mandatory tool in every NICU, and many quality improvement (QI) tools have been published in the literature, including a systematic review on QI interventions that aimed to prevent or reduce the severity of intraventricular hemorrhage [12]. Such QI tools and adherence to intraventricular hemorrhage prevention bundles (IVHPBs) can guide and assist NICU teams in better practice. These bundles consist of a series of best-practice interventions aimed at minimizing the risk of IVH in preterm infants. In a study where adherence to these bundles was poor (24%), a significant rate of severe IVH (9.8%) was reported, highlighting the necessity for targeted improvement initiatives [13].

Implementation of IVHPBs has been shown to decrease the incidence of IVH, particularly when tailored to address the specific needs of neonates born at extremely low birth weights or at a very early gestational age infants. Primary prevention effective strategies are crucial in reducing the incidence of intracranial hemorrhage in preterm neonates. Key methods include controlling risk factors and educating healthcare providers and parents about the signs of potential complications. Moreover, a multidisciplinary approach is essential in the management and prevention of IVH in NICUs. Collaborative efforts among neonatologists, nursing staff, and other healthcare professionals have shown promising results in promoting adherence to best practices [14]. This approach includes the education of NICU staff regarding the importance of early interventions and sustained adherence to the IVH bundle protocols, which are critical to mitigating risks associated with brain injuries in extremely preterm infants.

The purpose of this chapter is to describe the preventable risk factors for IVH in premature infants, by dividing them into prenatal factors, factors during the labor process, and postnatal factors.

25.2.1 Prenatal Interventions for Preventing IVH

1. **Prevention of Preterm Birth:**
   Preventing preterm birth is a key element in reducing all-cause morbidities in general and IVH in particular, but this critical issue is not within the scope of this chapter and is discussed in detail in ▶ Chaps. 7 and 8.
2. **Antenatal Corticosteroids:**
   Antenatal corticosteroids (ACS) administration to women at risk for preterm labor has emerged as a cornerstone intervention for improving outcomes in preterm infants. The benefits of ACS arise primarily from their ability to cross the placenta, promoting the maturation of key structures in the embryonic lungs and other organs essential for neonatal health [15, 16]. This mechanism is particularly critical as preterm infants are often born with underdeveloped lungs, leading to significant respiratory complications, in particular respiratory distress syndrome (RDS) and pneumothorax, that are associated both with increased risk for IVH [17, 18].

   The 2020 Cochrane review on the effectiveness of ACS [19] concluded that the use of antenatal corticosteroids probably reduces the risk of GMH-IVH (RR 0.58, 95% CI 0.45–0.75; 8475 infants; 12 studies) with moderate-certainty. Additionally, the administration of ACS has been associated with a probable decrease in the risk of intraventricular hemorrhage (IVH) and developmental delays in childhood, underscoring the long-term benefits of timely corticosteroid therapy.

   The physiological effects of glucocorticoids on lung development are well-documented. They stimulate the production of surfactant, a substance critical for reducing surface tension in the alveoli, which enhances lung compliance [15]. Moreover, glucocorticoids influence the structural development of the lungs, promoting alveolar growth and vascularization, which are vital for optimal respiratory function in preterm infants. This multifaceted impact of ACS extends beyond the lungs, as studies indicate that these corticosteroids can also positively affect other organ systems, such as the gastrointestinal tract (e.g., a reduction in the incidence of necrotizing enterocolitis (NEC)), contributing to a more favorable overall developmental trajectory [16].

   The World Health Organization (WHO) and the American College of Obstetricians and Gynecologists (ACOG) have recognized the importance of ACS in prenatal care and currently recommend their administration to mothers between 24 and 34 weeks of gestation who are at risk of imminent preterm birth, provided that specific criteria related to maternal and newborn care are met [20, 21]. This guideline reflects a consensus in the medical community regarding the evidence-based benefits of ACS in preventing preterm birth complications. In a prospective, randomized controlled trial Ment et al. found that there was less antenatal steroid treatment (19% vs 32%, $p = 0.03$) and more vaginal deliveries (71% vs 45%, $p < 0.0001$) in the group with early intraventricular hemorrhage and that in those who received ACS, those. This was the first data to suggest that antenatal steroids have an important roll in decreasing the risk of IVH [22]. Additional studies have demonstrated similar results. For example, Wei et al. showed that administering a course of corticosteroids to women before their expected preterm birth reduced the occurrence of IVH in all grades and particularly reduced the occurrence of severe IVH in premature infants born at a gestational age of 22–29 weeks [23]. Antenatal steroids are most effective in decreasing the risk of developing IVH when administered 7–24 days prior to birth [24]. In addition, antenatal steroids can lower the risk of IVH indirectly by enhancing outcomes in RDS and reducing the need for prolonged mechanical ventilation [25]. While the precise mechanism for this effect remains unclear, it is probably linked to the suppression of cerebral angiogenesis [26].

3. **Other Pharmacologic Agents:**
From a pharmacological perspective, several studies have proposed that magnesium sulfate, vitamin K, and phenobarbital given before birth may serve as preventive measures against GMH-IVH. Although some studies have shown that antenatal administration of magnesium sulfate substantially reduced the risk of CP (RR 0.69; 95% CI 0.54–0.87), there was no difference in rates of IVH between groups [27, 28]. A recent Cochrane review [29] has found that magnesium sulfate administration in women at risk of preterm birth may potentially reduce the risk of severe IVH in neonates. Specifically, it may decrease the incidence of severe IVH (grade 3 or 4) by 24%, as reflected in a relative risk of 0.76 in the moderate-certainty evidence from five randomized controlled trials (RCTs) involving 5885 infants. However, no significant difference was observed between C and the placebo groups in less severe IVH grades. This suggests that magnesium sulfate's neuroprotective benefits may specifically target more severe forms of IVH in preterm infants. Research on the effects of phenobarbital and vitamin K administration in preventing GMH-IVH does not support their use as effective measures [30, 31].
4. **Maternal Transport:**
Maternal transport to specialized care centers is an important strategy in the prevention of IVH, improving both short- and long-term neurological outcomes for preterm infants. A key advantage of maternal transport is the ability to provide specialized perinatal care, which can stabilize both the mother and the fetus [32–35]. This includes the capacity for careful monitoring and the application of pre- and postnatal interventions, such as ACS administration, delayed cord clamping, and precision in ventilation management at birth, which are known to reduce hemodynamic fluctuations in preterm infants and decrease the risk of IVH. Maternal transport also minimizes the physiological stresses associated with neonatal transport, which can contribute to fluctuations in cerebral blood flow and pressure that are risk factors for IVH [32–35]. These interventions will be discussed in detail in the next paragraph. It was demonstrated that infants born outside a specialized facility who require transport have a significantly higher risk of developing IVH compared to those born within such centers. This elevated risk persists regardless of the mode of transport, the distance traveled, or the experience level of the transport team [35].

25.2.2 Perinatal and Postnatal Interventions for Preventing IVH

1. **Delayed Cord Clamping (DCC):**
Placental transfusion during DCC can provide up to 80 mL of blood in a term infant in 1 minute and up to 40–50 mg/kg of iron, immunoglobulins, and stem cells [36]. It has become the accepted standard in newborn care, with benefits to the neonate, including decreased mortality in preterm infants [37], increased hematocrit, decreased need for postnatal blood transfusions, stabilization of postnatal blood pressure, and improved intravascular volume, all factors believed to lower the risk of IVH.

While previous studies have reported a reduced incidence of IVH in infants receiving placental transfusions [38], a 2012 Cochrane review [39] revealed no significant difference in IVH rates between infants with early versus delayed cord clamping (DCC). However, only three out of the 18 included RCTs have specifically assessed IVH as an outcome in infants under 28 weeks of gestation [39, 40]. Delayed cord clamping (DCC) has been recommended by ACOG and the American Academy of Pediatrics for 30–60 seconds in vigorous term and preterm infants [41, 42].

Studies have suggested that umbilical cord milking (UCM), in which blood is stripped from an unclamped umbilical cord 2–3 times before clamping, is associated with an increased risk of IVH in preterm infants. A retrospective study of 1834 infants <29 weeks' gestation has found that infants receiving UCM had a higher odds ratio of severe IVH compared with those who received DCC (aOR 1.70 95% CI 1.20, 2.43) [43]. Indeed, the PREMOD-2 trial, which compared DCC to UCM, was prematurely halted due to a signal of harm in the cord milking group. Although there was no difference in the composite outcome of death and severe IVH between the groups, infants in the UCM group had a significantly increased risk of severe IVH (8% vs 3%, $p = 0.02$) and this difference was greater in infants of a lower gestational age, i.e., infants born at 23–27 weeks' gestation ($p = 0.002$) [44]. For this reason, the majority of institutional guidelines recommend DCC as the preferred method of placental transfusion in preterm infants.

2. **Minimizing Fluctuations in Cerebral Blood Flow:**
   Stabilizing the infant's hemodynamic status by maintaining adequate blood pressure and avoiding rapid volume expansion is crucial. Continuous monitoring and minimal handling can help prevent sudden changes in cerebral perfusion.
   (a) Minimal handling during care and medical procedures is believed to promote autonomic stability in preterm infants. While not conclusively proven, this approach is logical and carries no apparent negative effects [45, 46]. Reducing trauma during delivery by using gentle handling techniques and avoiding abrupt movements of the infant's head can help lower the risk of intraventricular hemorrhage (IVH). Maintaining the head in a midline (neutral) position is believed to optimize cerebral venous drainage through the internal jugular veins, which serve as the primary outflow routes for cranial blood. Rotating the head to either side can potentially obstruct or compress the jugular veins on that side, impairing proper venous drainage and increasing the risk of cerebral complications such as IVH.
   (b) Reducing painful or stressful procedures can also positively impact brain development, as repeated exposure to pain may adversely affect the development of white matter and subcortical gray matter. Avoiding frequent interventions like heel sticks, venous blood draws, routine tracheal suctioning, lumbar punctures, ambient noise, alarm noise, and avoidance of rapid volume infusions and infusions of sodium bicarbonate is of great benefit for preterm infants. Utilizing umbilical arterial catheters for blood sampling can further aid in maintaining hemodynamic stability while minimizing painful stimuli. This approach not only reduces unnecessary discomfort but also protects the infant's fragile brain vessels. Even seemingly routine procedures, such as diaper changes, may introduce stress that leads to autonomic instability, making it beneficial to reduce stimulation whenever possible. The cumulative effect of minimizing these disturbances is likely to contribute to better cerebral and overall development, as it provides the infant with a more stable and less stressful environment during a critical period of brain maturation. Overall, this gentle care approach, paired with other neuroprotective measures, could contribute to improved outcomes in preterm infants.
   (c) Indomethacin, a nonsteroidal anti-inflammatory drug (NSAID), has been explored for its potential role in reducing the risk of intraventricular hemorrhage in preterm infants, particularly those born at very low birth weights (VLBW). Several quality improvement initiatives and studies have focused on the incorporation of indomethacin as part of broader strategies aimed at preventing severe brain injury, including IVH. Carteaux et al. [32] and McLendon et al. [33] both emphasize the development and implementation

of potentially better practices (PBPs) for the prevention of brain hemorrhage and ischemic injury in VLBW infants, which often include the careful use of indomethacin. Kramer et al. [47] demonstrated a reduction in severe IVH in preterm infants through a quality improvement project that likely included pharmacological interventions like indomethacin. Similarly, Persad et al. [48] discussed the effectiveness of a "brain protection bundle" in reducing severe IVH, highlighting the importance of combining various preventive measures, including indomethacin, in infants less than 30 weeks' gestational age. Shukla et al. [49] further supported the role of pharmacological and non-pharmacological interventions in reducing brain injury through a quality improvement initiative, with indomethacin playing a crucial role in such interventions. Finally, Travers et al. [50] described a quality improvement bundle targeting extremely preterm infants in the first week of life, where indomethacin is commonly included as a prophylactic measure to prevent IVH. These studies collectively underscore the significance of indomethacin within a multidisciplinary approach to reducing IVH and improving neurological outcomes in preterm infants.

(d) Ensuring cerebral autoregulation and thus stability and reducing fluctuations in cerebral blood flow are essential components of neonatal care bundles aimed at reducing the risk of IVH, as highlighted by several studies. Al-Haddad et al. [51] highlighted the effectiveness of a care bundle that includes careful monitoring and adjustment of blood pressure, fluid balance, and electrolytes to reduce IVH in high-risk neonates. Similarly, Carteaux et al. [32] and McLendon et al. [33] emphasize the importance of potentially better practices (PBPs) that focus on stabilizing hemodynamics and maintaining proper electrolyte balance in very low birth weight (VLBW) infants to prevent brain injury. Other studies, such as those by Chiriboga et al. [52] and de Bijl-Marcus et al. [53], have demonstrated the success of comprehensive neonatal care bundles that incorporate fluid and electrolyte management, alongside other interventions, in reducing severe IVH rates. Chiruvolu et al. [54] also explored the positive effects of delayed cord clamping on hemodynamic stability in preterm infants, further contributing to the prevention of IVH. Kramer et al. [47] reinforced the significance of hemodynamic management within quality improvement initiatives, where maintaining stable blood pressure and fluid homeostasis is crucial for neuroprotection in preterm infants. Overall, these studies underscore the importance of integrated hemodynamic and electrolyte management within care bundles to mitigate the risk of IVH and improve neonatal outcomes.

(e) Optimizing respiratory support plays a crucial role in the prevention of IVH in preterm infants, as evidenced by several studies emphasizing the importance of optimized respiratory management within neuroprotective care bundles. Carteaux et al. [32] and McLendon et al. [33] both highlighted the role of respiratory care as part of potentially better practices (PBPs) aimed at reducing brain hemorrhage in very low birth weight infants by minimizing fluctuations in blood oxygen levels and maintaining stable ventilation strategies. Respiratory distress and the use of invasive ventilation can increase the risk of IVH, which has led to the development of noninvasive ventilation techniques and careful monitoring of respiratory parameters to reduce these risks. Murthy et al. [55] reinforced the inclusion of respiratory care within a neuroprotection care bundle, showing that meticulous respiratory management can decrease the incidence of acute brain injury in pre-

25

term infants. Schmid et al. [56] demonstrated that prospective risk monitoring, including respiratory factors, was associated with reduced IVH rates in preterm neonates. Shukla et al. [49] and Travers et al. [50] also emphasized the need for quality improvement bundles that incorporate respiratory stabilization, including optimal oxygenation and ventilation strategies, to prevent IVH. Gross et al. [57] and Saxton et al. [58] provided further evidence on how the implementation of specialized neonatal care bundles, including respiratory care protocols, effectively reduced the rates of severe IVH by addressing key respiratory risk factors in the early care of preterm infants. Collectively, these studies highlight the critical role of respiratory care in preventing IVH through careful management of ventilation, oxygenation, and respiratory support in preterm infants.

25.3 Summary

In this chapter we focused on the prevention of intraventricular hemorrhage (IVH) in preterm infants, a critical aspect of neonatal care. We discussed the pathophysiology and risk factors associated with IVH and emphasized the importance of early and effective prevention strategies, highlighting the importance of the first 24–72 hours of life care, success of bundle care approaches and multidisciplinary care, prenatal and postnatal interventions.

By understanding and applying these principles, healthcare providers can significantly reduce the incidence of IVH and improve outcomes for preterm infants.

Chapter Key Points

- IVH is most common in preterm infants <30 weeks due to germinal matrix fragility and impaired cerebral autoregulation.
- Most IVH occurs within the first 24–72 hours, highlighting the need for early stabilization.
- Antenatal corticosteroids reduce IVH risk and improve neonatal outcomes.
- Delayed cord clamping and avoidance of umbilical cord milking reduce severe IVH risk.
- IVH prevention bundles and minimal-handling protocols significantly reduce severe IVH rates in NICUs.

Chapter-End Summary

Intraventricular hemorrhage remains a major morbidity in extremely preterm infants, arising primarily from germinal matrix fragility and fluctuations in cerebral blood flow. Prevention requires a continuum of interventions: prenatal strategies such as antenatal corticosteroids and maternal transport; delivery-room measures including delayed cord clamping; and NICU practices focused on hemodynamic stability, minimal handling, respiratory optimization, and adherence to evidence-based IVH prevention bundles. When implemented consistently, these approaches significantly reduce the incidence and severity of IVH and improve long-term neurodevelopmental outcomes.

References

1. Harke HT, Haeye RI, Storch A, et al. Perinatal cerebral hemorrhage. J Pediatr. 1972;37:80.
2. Jaeger M, Grussner SE, Omwandho CO, Klein K, Tinneberg HR, Klingmuller V. Cranial sonography for newborn screening: a 10-year retrospective study in 11,887 newborns. Rofo. 2004;176(6):852–8.
3. Leech RW, Kohnen P. Subependymal and intraventricular hemorrhages in the newborn. Am J Pathol. 1974;77(3):465–75.
4. Papile LA, Burstein J, Burstein R, Koffler H. Incidence and evolution of subependymal and intraventricular hemorrhage: a study of infants with birth weights less than 1,500 gm. J Pediatr. 1978;92(4):529–34.

5. Philip AG, Allan WC, Tito AM, Wheeler LR. Intraventricular hemorrhage in preterm infants: declining incidence in the 1980's. Pediatrics. 1989;84(5):797–801.
6. Takashima S, Becker LE. Intraventricular and subependymal hemorrhage in infants dying within 10 hours of birth. Brain Dev. 1983;5(1):9–13.
7. Kadri H, Mawla AA, Kazah J. The incidence, timing, and predisposing factors of germinal matrix and intraventricular hemorrhage (GMH/IVH) in preterm neonates. Childs Nerv Syst. 2006;22(9):1086–90.
8. Perlman JM, Volpe JJ. Intraventricular hemorrhage in extremely small premature infants. Am J Dis Child. 1986;140(11):1122–4.
9. Paneth N, Pinto-Martin J, Gardiner J, Wallenstein S, Katsikiotis V, Hegyi T, Hiatt IM, Susser M. Incidence and timing of germinal matrix/intraventricular hemorrhage in low birth weight infants. Am J Epidemiol. 1993;137(11):1167–76.
10. Inder T, Perlman JM, Volpe JJ. Preterm intraventricular hemorrhage/post-hemorrhagic hydrocephalus. In: Volpe's neurology of the newborn. 6th ed. Elsevier; 2017.
11. Inder TE, Volpe JJ, Anderson PJ. Defining the neurologic consequences of preterm birth. N Engl J Med. 2023;389(5):441–53.
12. Edwards EM, Ehret DEY, Cohen H, Zayack D, Soll RF, Horbar JD. Quality improvement interventions to prevent intraventricular hemorrhage: a systematic review. Pediatrics. 2024;154(2):e2023064431.
13. Kolnik SE, Upadhyay K, Wood TR, Juul SE, Valentine GC. Reducing severe intraventricular hemorrhage in preterm infants with improved care bundle adherence. Pediatrics. 2023;152(3):e2021056104.
14. Kramer KP, Minot K, Butler C, Haynes K, Mason A, Nguyen L, Wynn S, Liebowitz M, Rogers EE. Reduction of severe intraventricular hemorrhage in preterm infants: a quality improvement project. Pediatrics. 2022;149(3):e2021050652.
15. Bird AD, McDougall AR, Seow B, Hooper SB, Cole TJ. Glucocorticoid regulation of lung development: lessons learned from conditional GR knockout mice. Mol Endocrinol. 2015;29(2):158–71.
16. Bolt RJ, van Weissenbruch MM, Lafeber HN, Delemarre-van de Waal HA. Glucocorticoids and lung development in the fetus and preterm infant. Pediatr Pulmonol. 2001;32(1):76–91.
17. Bada HS. Prevention of intracranial hemorrhage. NeoReviews. 2000;1(3):e48–52.
18. Pishva N, Parsa G, Saki F, Saki M, Saki MR. Intraventricular hemorrhage in premature infants and its association with pneumothorax. Acta Med Iran. 2012;50:473–6.
19. McGoldrick E, Stewart F, Parker R, Dalziel SR. Antenatal corticosteroids for accelerating fetal lung maturation for women at risk of preterm birth. Cochrane Database Syst Rev. 2020;12:CD004454.
20. WHO Guidelines Approved by the Guidelines Review Committee. WHO recommendations on interventions to improve preterm birth outcomes: evidence base. Geneva: World Health Organization; 2015.
21. Committee on Obstetric Practice. Committee Opinion No. 713: antenatal corticosteroid therapy for fetal maturation. Obstet Gynecol. 2017;130(2):e102–9.
22. Ment LR, Oh W, Ehrenkranz RA, Philip AG, Duncan CC, Makuch RW. Antenatal steroids, delivery mode, and intraventricular hemorrhage in preterm infants. Am J Obstet Gynecol. 1995;172:795–800.
23. Wei JC, Catalano R, Profit J, Gould JB, Lee HC. Impact of antenatal steroids on intraventricular hemorrhage in very-low-birth weight infants. J Perinatol. 2016;36:352–6.
24. Fortmann I, Mertens L, Boeckel H, Gruttner B, Humberg A, Astiz M, et al. A timely administration of antenatal steroids is highly protective against intraventricular hemorrhage: an observational multicenter cohort study of very low birth weight infants. Front Pediatr. 2022;10:721355.
25. Helwich E, Rutkowska M, Bokiniec R, Gulczynska E, Hozejowski R. Intraventricular hemorrhage in premature infants with Respiratory Distress Syndrome treated with surfactant: incidence and risk factors in the prospective cohort study. Dev Period Med. 2017;21:328–35.
26. Vinukonda G, Dummula K, Malik S, Hu F, Thompson CI, Csiszar A, et al. Effect of prenatal glucocorticoids on cerebral vasculature of the developing brain. Stroke. 2010;41:1766–73.
27. Doyle LW, Crowther CA, Middleton P, Marret S. Antenatal magnesium sulfate and neurologic outcome in preterm infants: a systematic review. Obstet Gynecol. 2009;113:1327–33.
28. Rouse DJ, Hirtz DG, Thom E, et al. A randomized, controlled trial of magnesium sulfate for the prevention of cerebral palsy. N Engl J Med. 2008;359:895–905.
29. Shepherd ES, Goldsmith S, Doyle LW, Middleton P, Marret S, Rouse DJ, Pryde P, Wolf HT, Crowther CA. Magnesium sulphate for women at risk of preterm birth for neuroprotection of the fetus. Cochrane Database Syst Rev. 2024;5(5):CD004661.
30. Crowther CA, Crosby DD, Henderson-Smart DJ. Phenobarbital prior to preterm birth for preventing neonatal periventricular haemorrhage. Cochrane Database Syst Rev. 2010;1:CD000164.
31. Crowther CA, Crosby DD, Henderson-Smart DJ. Vitamin K prior to preterm birth for preventing neonatal periventricular haemorrhage. Cochrane Database Syst Rev. 2010;1:CD000229.
32. Carteaux P, Cohen H, Check J, et al. Evaluation and development of potentially better practices for the prevention of brain hemorrhage and ischemic

brain injury in very low birth weight infants. Pediatrics. 2003;111(4 Pt 2):e489–96.
33. McLendon D, Check J, Carteaux P, et al. Implementation of potentially better practices for the prevention of brain hemorrhage and ischemic brain injury in very low birth weight infants. Pediatrics. 2003;111(4 Pt 2):e497–503.
34. Synnes AR, Macnab YC, Qiu Z, et al. Neonatal intensive care unit characteristics affect the incidence of severe intraventricular hemorrhage. Med Care. 2006;44(8):754–9.
35. Morris H, Magers N, Saunders S, Vesoulis Z. Potential risk modifiers for severe intraventricular hemorrhage in very low birthweight infants requiring transport. J Matern Fetal Neonatal Med. 2020:1–4.
36. Lim J, Hagen E. Reducing germinal matrix-intraventricular hemorrhage: perinatal and delivery room factors. NeoReviews. 2019;20(8):e452–63.
37. Tarnow-Mordi W, Morris J, Kirby A, et al., Australian Placental Transfusion Study Collaborative Group. Delayed versus immediate cord clamping in preterm infants. N Engl J Med. 2017;377(25):2445–55.
38. Backes CH, Rivera BK, Haque U, et al. Placental transfusion strategies in very preterm neonates: a systematic review and meta-analysis. Obstet Gynecol. 2014;124(1):47–56.
39. Rabe H, Diaz-Rossello JL, Duley L, Dowswell T. Effect of timing of umbilical cord clamping and other strategies to influence placental transfusion at preterm birth on maternal and infant outcomes. Cochrane Database Syst Rev. 2012;(8):CD003248.
40. Fogarty M, Osborn DA, Askie L, et al. Delayed vs early umbilical cord clamping for preterm infants: a systematic review and meta-analysis. Am J Obstetr Gynecol. 2018;218(1):1–18.
41. Committee on Obstetric Practice. Committee Opinion No. 684: delayed umbilical cord clamping after birth. Obstet Gynecol. 2017;129(1):e5–e10.
42. American Academy of Pediatrics Statement of Endorsement. Delayed umbilical cord clamping after birth. Pediatrics. 2017;139(6):e20170957.
43. Kumbhat N, Eggleston B, Davis AS, DeMauro SB, Van Meurs KP, Foglia EE, Lakshminrusimha S, Walsh MC, Watterberg KL, Wyckoff MH, Das A, Handley SC, Generic Database Subcommittee of the National Institute of Child Health and Human Development Neonatal Research Network. Umbilical cord milking vs delayed cord clamping and associations with in-hospital outcomes among extremely premature infants. J Pediatr. 2021;232:87–94.e4.
44. Katheria A, Reister F, Essers J, et al. Association of umbilical cord milking vs delayed umbilical cord clamping with death or severe intraventricular hemorrhage among preterm infants. JAMA. 2019;322(19):1877–86.
45. Bada HS, Korones SB, Perry EH, et al. Frequent handling in the neonatal intensive care unit and intraventricular hemorrhage. J Pediatr. 1990;117:126–31.
46. Lea CL, Smith-Collins A, Luyt K. Protecting the premature brain: current evidence-based strategies for minimising perinatal brain injury in preterm infants. Arch Dis Child Fetal Neonatal Ed. 2017;102:F176–82.
47. Kramer KP, Minot K, Butler C, et al. Reduction of severe intraventricular hemorrhage in preterm infants: a quality improvement project. Pediatrics. 2022;149(3):e2021050652.
48. Persad N, Kelly E, Amaral N, et al. Impact of a "brain protection bundle" in reducing severe intraventricular hemorrhage in preterm infants <30 weeks GA: a retrospective single centre study. Children (Basel). 2021;8(11):983.
49. Shukla VV, Klinger A, Yazdi S, et al. Prevention of severe brain injury in very preterm neonates: a quality improvement initiative. J Perinatol. 2022;42(10):1417–23.
50. Travers CP, Gentle S, Freeman AE, et al. A quality improvement bundle to improve outcomes in extremely preterm infants in the first week. Pediatrics. 2022;149(2):e2020037341.
51. Al-Haddad BJS, Bergam B, Johnson A, et al. Effectiveness of a care bundle for primary prevention of intraventricular hemorrhage in high-risk neonates: a Bayesian analysis. J Perinatol. 2023;43(6):722–7.
52. Chiriboga N, Cortez J, Pena-Ariet A, et al. Successful implementation of an intracranial hemorrhage (ICH) bundle in reducing severe ICH: a quality improvement project. J Perinatol. 2019;39(1):143–51.
53. De Bijl-Marcus K, Brouwer AJ, De Vries LS, Groenendaal F, Wezel-Meijler GV. Neonatal care bundles are associated with a reduction in the incidence of intraventricular haemorrhage in preterm infants: a multicentre cohort study. Arch Dis Child Fetal Neonatal Ed. 2020;105(4):419–24.
54. Chiruvolu A, Tolia VN, Qin H, et al. Effect of delayed cord clamping on very preterm infants. Am J Obstet Gynecol. 2015;213(5):676.e1–7.
55. Murthy P, Zein H, Thomas S, et al. Neuroprotection care bundle implementation to decrease acute brain injury in preterm infants. Pediatr Neurol. 2020;110:42–8.
56. Schmid MB, Reister F, Mayer B, Hopfner RJ, Fuchs H, Hummler HD. Prospective risk factor monitoring reduces intracranial hemorrhage rates in preterm infants. Dtsch Arztebl Int. 2013;110(29–30):489–96.
57. Gross M, Engel C, Trotter A. Evaluating the effect of a neonatal care bundle for the prevention of intraventricular hemorrhage in preterm infants. Children (Basel). 2021;8(4):2570.
58. Saxton SN, Evered J, McCoy K, Atkins K. Effects of a small-baby protocol on early and long-term outcomes in extremely preterm infants: a quality improvement study. Early Hum Dev. 2023;179:105733.

Prevention of Hypoglycemia

Rafael Mendelsohn

Contents

Y. Yogev, A. Khalil (eds.), *Prevention of Complications in Obstetrics*,
https://doi.org/10.1007/978-3-032-23479-7_26

Learning Objectives

- Understanding basic concepts in glucose regulation in the newborn
- Understanding risk factors for hypoglycemia in the newborn population
- Learning measures to prevent hypoglycemia in the newborn population
  - **Case Studies**
    Examples to illustrate topics, principles, theories, and methods, and how they are applied in the real world
  - **Highlight Major Pearls/Pitfalls**
    Understand the mechanism of glucose metabolism.
    Educate parents and the team regarding the importance of glucose metabolism.
    Educate the team and the parents regarding the ways to prevent hypoglycemia.
    Educate the team and the parents regarding the clinical signs and symptoms of hypoglycemia for early recognition.
    Have local protocols for recognition of the at-risk population and for close monitoring and prevention of hypoglycemia.
  - **How-to-Guides/Recipes for a Method or Tool** (again not sure what fits here)
    Shows how to apply a tool, method, or theory
  - **Worked-Out Examples** (again not sure what fits here) Demonstrating solution techniques to problems to help readers understand how to apply a theory or method
- Explain the physiology of neonatal glucose regulation.
- Identify major maternal and neonatal risk factors for hypoglycemia.
- Apply evidence-based preventive strategies including feeding, thermal care, and early screening.
- Recognize signs of symptomatic and asymptomatic hypoglycemia.
- Understand management pathways including feeding, dextrose gel, IV glucose, and medications.

26.1 Introduction

Neonatal hypoglycemia is one of the most frequently encountered issues in newborn care and is a leading cause of admission to neonatal units. Literature discussing newborn hypoglycemia, its causes, and significance goes back to more than 75 years ago, yet the definition of hypoglycemia in the neonatal population is a controversial issue as asymptomatic transient hypoglycemia is part of the normal adaptation of a newborn after delivery.

Early detection and treatment of hypoglycemia are extremely important, as a delay in the diagnosis of hypoglycemia in the newborn may lead to irreversible neurologic damage and neurodevelopmental impairment in later stages of life.

Early diagnosis of hypoglycemia may be challenging as some of the hypoglycemic newborns will show no symptoms, while others will show nonspecific signs and symptoms (that may be attributed to other causes).

The combination of absent clinical signs or nonspecific presentation, with the potential irreversible future damage requires clinicians to be aware of risk factors for hypoglycemia, to have an effective screening workflow for this population, and to have a high index of suspicion for early detection and treatment of newborns with hypoglycemia.

In this chapter, we will discuss the physiology of glucose regulation in the newborn, the normal values of glucose in this population as well as the risk factors for hypoglycemia in the newborn, the clinical signs and symptoms of hypoglycemia as well as the ways to prevent hypoglycemia in the newborn population [1–3].

26.2 Physiology of Glucose Regulation

26.2.1 Metabolic Transition at Birth

The newborn infant has a glucose utilization of 4–6 mg/kg/min, which is two- to threefold

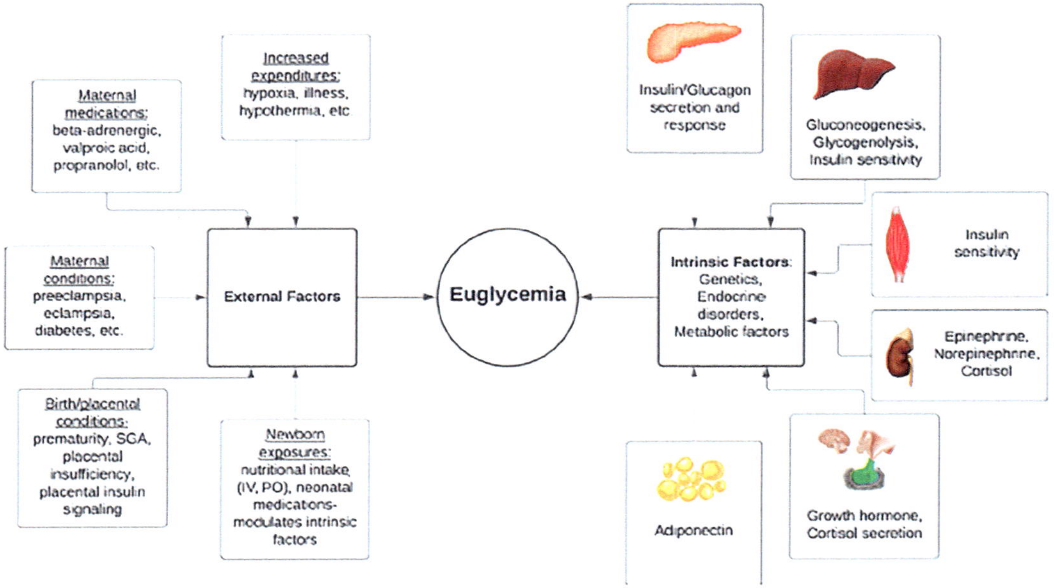

Fig. 26.1 Extrinsic and intrinsic factors modulating glucose control in newborns. (Image from Blanco and Kim [7])

higher than that of an adult, mainly due to the proportionally large brain, which consumes more than half of the total glucose consumption of the body.

While in utero, the fetus depends on maternal blood glucose and maintains a glucose level, which is about 70% of the maternal level. Once the cord is clamped, the newborn must adapt to maintaining their own glucose levels.

As in all mammals, the human infant experiences a sharp drop in blood glucose levels right after delivery, with the nadir arriving at about 2–4 hours of age at an estimated level of 20–25 mg/dL. This drop is considered a physiologic hypoglycemia that seems to play an important role in the adaptation of the infant, which will eventually lead to normal glucose homeostasis. The initial hypoglycemia is corrected by the production of energy from ketone bodies released from fat, and after a few hours, glycogenosis and gluconeogenesis kick in, mediated by insulin secretion, and contribute to the increase in blood levels. And within a few hours—the glucose-stimulated insulin secretion mechanisms mature, infant feeding begins, and the blood glucose levels of the newborn at age 72 hours and beyond are similar to those of children [1, 4–7] (Fig. 26.1).

26.3 Normal Blood Glucose

Hypoglycemia cannot be defined as a specific blood glucose concentration, as:

- Thresholds for specific brain responses to hypoglycemia occur across different glucose levels.
- A single value of blood glucose leading to brain injury could not be found.
- The extent of injury is influenced not only by the level of blood glucose but also by factors such as duration and degree of hypoglycemia.
- Potential artifacts and technical factors may influence the interpretation of any single blood glucose value (blood glucose measurement will be discussed later in this chapter).

Basing the diagnosis on clinical signs is not sufficient, as clinical hypoglycemia is defined as a low enough plasma glucose to cause symptoms of impaired brain function, but the signs and symptoms of hypoglycemia are nonspecific.

In adult-guidelines emphasize the value of Whipple's triad for confirming hypoglycemia: the combination of a documented low blood glucose level, that is associated with symptoms of hypoglycemia and relief of signs/symptoms when glucose concentration is restored to normal.

In the newborn population, signs and symptoms are not always communicated and may be nonspecific, with the symptoms often seen as a result of other causes not associated with hypoglycemia, thus recognition of hypoglycemia may require confirmation by repeated measurements, and suspected hypoglycemia should be treated promptly to avoid potential adverse consequences.

Symptomatic hypoglycemia in a newborn is present when the newborn is found to have symptoms associated with hypoglycemia, and a low blood glucose level is found. These infants require immediate attention and correction of the glucose level, as the symptoms may represent the effect of the low glucose level (especially if those resolve after correction, as described by Whipple's triad).

As mentioned previously, after delivery, the newborn experiences a physiologic drop in blood glucose levels, which in turn initiates processes that are important for the development of a functioning mechanism for blood glucose homeostasis, and within the first 72 hours of life, the infant establishes the complex hormonal and neurogenic responses for maintaining normal blood glucose.

In recent years, several papers have tried to assess what the normal glucose values of blood glucose in the newborn infant are but have yet to arrive at shared consensus.

A few guidelines and recommendations were published in the last few years, including ones from the American Association of Pediatrics (AAP), the Pediatric Endocrine Society (PES), the British Association of Perinatal Medicine (BAPM), the European Foundation of Care for the Newborn Infant (EFCNI), and the Canadian Pediatric Society (CPS), all are based on similar literature, yet they have adopted different recommendations regarding several parameters: diagnostic measures: whether to follow the value of blood or plasma glucose for diagnosis, what the risk factors for hypoglycemia are, the recommended screening, what the normal values are, and what the recommended interventions for an asymptomatic or a symptomatic newborn are.

The different accepted levels of glucose according to the age of the newborn are described in the table below. More than the value itself, clear guidelines and accepted pathways of screening and managing newborn hypoglycemia will be discussed further in this chapter [1, 4, 6, 8].

26.3.1 Glucose Measurements

Not only is the value of glucose levels debatable but the measurement method as well. There are various ways to measure blood glucose.

When measuring glucose levels using whole blood glucose, the value might be lower 15% than the plasma glucose, as the sample examination is usually delayed, and RBCs may consume the glucose within the sample.

Point-of-care devices are recommended screening tools for hypoglycemia, have limited accuracy for lower glucose levels, and may have a range of 10–15 mg/dL, which might represent a significant inaccuracy. Low plasma glucose can be confirmed with a specific laboratory exam, but it requires larger volumes of blood, and the result is often delayed—hence, this method is not routinely used for the diagnosis of hypoglycemia in the newborn infant.

Blood gas analysis is considered a reliable exam, with an immediate result, and thus is very frequently used to follow and diagnose hypoglycemia.

High-accuracy devices, using small volumes of blood and providing a quick result, were recently developed and might be the future of glucose monitoring in this population. Some papers describing continuous glucose monitoring for term and preterm infant have been published recently and might hold a promising direction to control and monitor blood glucose for the high-risk population, without the need to repeatedly poke the newborn for blood samples [1, 4–6].

26.3.2 Persistent Hypoglycemia

While transient neonatal hypoglycemia in the first 48–72 hours of life is a relatively common finding and is correlated to physiologic changes in the newborn, hypoglycemia that persists beyond the initial 72 hours of life is considered persistent hypoglycemia and should be further assessed.

Family history and newborn risk factors for hypoglycemia should be assessed, as well as signs suggestive of medical conditions associated with persistent hypoglycemia. Hypopituitarism may be evident by cleft lip or palate, micropenis, and other midline anomalies, adrenal insufficiency can be evident with electrolyte imbalance, low blood pressure, and skin pigmentation, hepatomegaly can be found in some metabolic diseases associated with abnormal glucose metabolism, and other genetic conditions that may affect the glucose homeostasis such as Beckwith–Wiedemann (presented with macroglossia, hemihypertrophy, and omphalocele) should be sought.

Lab work should be sent according to clinical signs and symptoms, with a critical sample as an important assessment of many components that contribute to the glucose homeostasis. Critical sample should be sent in cases of spontaneous hypoglycemia (usually later than 48–72 hours) and includes glucose, bicarbonate, beta-hydroxy-butyrate and a lactate (some recommendations include cortisol as well). The Pediatric Endocrine Society further recommends keeping plasma in reserve for further possible tests such as plasma insulin, FFA, and C-peptide, and total and free carnitine and acyl-carnitine [1, 4].

26.4 Clinical Signs and Symptoms and Long-Term Outcomes of Hypoglycemia

26.4.1 Clinical Signs and Symptoms

The symptoms of hypoglycemia may not correlate with the level of blood glucose, as some newborns may show clinical signs and symptoms of variant significance, at blood glucose levels at which other newborns will show no clinical signs.

The clinical signs and symptoms may be divided into two main groups:

1. Neurogenic (autonomic) symptoms result from the increased sympathetic nervous tone that may be triggered by the hypoglycemia.
   Adrenergic responses may lead to tachypnea and tachycardia, tremor, and anxiety, while cholinergic responses may lead to excessive sweating and paresthesia.
2. Neuroglycopenic signs are caused by the lack of sufficient glucose supply to the brain, affecting its metabolism and energy utilization. These may result in an altered level of consciousness, jitteriness, apneic events, low muscular tone, lethargy, poor feeding, and eventually if prolonged and significant-coma, and seizures [1, 4].

26.4.2 Neurodevelopmental Outcome

Hypoglycemia has short-term signs and symptoms that represent the acute response of the body systems to the low blood glucose levels and may alert the caring team to treat and prevent and correct the blood glucose.

If low blood glucose persists long term, damage might develop and neurodevelopmental effects might be evident.

While in adults, a level of 50 mg/dL is associated with neuroglycopenia—level at which there is an inadequate supply of glucose for the brain, the critical threshold of glucose levels associated with brain injury is not clear, and further, it is believed that not only a single low level is responsible for long-term outcomes but also the period of low glucose might have an effect.

One study suggested that the critical glucose concentration, <47 mg/dL, would reliably predict adverse outcomes. It found that the number of days on which these infants experienced moderate hypoglycemia (<47 mg/dL) was strongly related to reduced scores for mental and motor development at 18 months of corrected age. The study did have some weak points, and later studies did not show the same association, and more so, later data suggest that the danger threshold must be lower than many had come to think it was, but the value of "47" mg/dL became the worldwide standard and was applied to other newborn populations, and was the number used in further later studies.

Magnetic resonance imaging of the brain in humans suggests that the occipital lobe may be vulnerable to injury caused by neonatal hypoglycemia, and a link between hypoglycemia and visual impairment has been previously reported.

Neurologic dysfunction is a significant pathology that can occur due to persistent hypoglycemia, and although defining the exact level or extent of what is considered significant, it is clear that monitoring for, preventing, and treating newborn hypoglycemia, though remains largely empirical, is highly important for preventing future pathology. It is also noted that repeated and prolonged very low blood glucose concentrations (persistent hypoglycemia), may be associated with conditions of excessive insulin secretion that have been associated with abnormal neurologic outcomes and should be investigated and treated [5, 6].

26.5 Risk Factors for Neonatal Hypoglycemia

As in many other systems, the newborn glycemic system is affected both by maternal and neonatal elements, and thus, the factors for hypoglycemia are affected by both. It is important to know and define the risk factors for hypoglycemia, as those with these risk factors will be the ones screened for glucose levels.

A. Maternal Risk Factors
   - Diabetes (gestational, preexisting)—maternal elevated glucose levels (that cross the placenta to the fetal side) lead to fetal hyperinsulinism. After delivery and clamping of the cord, maternal glucose transfer to the newborn is discontinued abruptly, while the hyperinsulinism may persist for a few more days, leading to low blood glucose levels.
   - Medications (e.g., beta-blockers, antenatal steroids)—some medications used by the pregnant women may affect the newborn physiology and lead to low glucose levels.

B. Neonatal Factors
   - Symptoms of hypoglycemia: Any infant with symptoms that might be associated with hypoglycemia should be assessed for blood glucose levels.
   - Prematurity: Greater than 50% will develop hypoglycemia. Abnormal glucose metabolism as well as low glycogen storage in this population may lead to hypoglycemic events.
   - Small for Gestational Age (SGA), Intra-Uterine Growth Restrictions (IUGR): This population is exposed to hypoglycemia due to inadequate glycogen and substrates for gluconeogenesis. Irregular insulin secretion may also be present in this population and contribute to a more persistent hypoglycemia.
   - Large for Gestational Age (LGA): It is not fully understood if nonsyndromic LGA non-IDM infants are truly at risk for hypoglycemia, but as these often coexist, LGA infants are recommended for blood glucose screening as per most protocols.
   - Perinatal Stress, Infections and Metabolic Disorders: Both increased consumption and decreased ability of the body to produce glucose may lead to its low levels.
   - Congenital syndromes (e.g., Beckwith–Wiedemann) are associated with hyperinsulinemic hypoglycemia as well as with other abnormal physical features (e.g., midline facial malformations, microphallus) [5, 7].

26.6 Prevention: Screening and Early Detection of Hypoglycemia

As neonatal hypoglycemia is a common diagnosis that might have long-term effects on neurodevelopment, it is highly important to prevent and treat infants with hypoglycemia.

The different guidelines share the same principles when it comes to the prevention recommendations: these include

1. Prenatal Care

Prenatal care and follow-up lead to optimizing maternal glucose levels, especially in diabetic mothers—one of the main risk groups for neonatal hypoglycemia.

Monitoring maternal medications impacting fetal glucose metabolism and close follow-up of fetal growth and development may facilitate better fetal glucose balance and help identify some congenital conditions associated with hypoglycemia.

2. Immediate Identification of At-Risk Population

The risk factors for hypoglycemia should be assessed prenatally as well as immediately postnatally to identify the population at risk for close monitoring of blood glucose and early follow-up, recognition, and family education regarding hypoglycemia and its consequences.

Having local guidelines and protocols for screening the at-risk population as well as defining targets of glucose thresholds for treating asymptomatic and symptomatic newborns facilitates better recognition and treatment of this population.

3. Prevention of Hypothermia

Hypothermia can lead to hypoglycemia and metabolic acidosis. Normothermia is a crucial topic in the newborn population (as discussed in ► Chap. 6) and as among other organ systems, it can contribute to the development of hypoglycemia, the at-risk population should be closely monitored, parents should be educated, and the care team should place emphasis on routes to prevent, monitor, and if needed, treat hypothermia.

Whether using a hat, warmth of the ambient temperature, or skin-to-skin contact with the mother—maintaining normal body temperature has a significant role in the prevention of hypoglycemia in the newborn population.

4. Timely Feeding

Clear instructions for families regarding feeding times and feeding volume expectations should be performed and closely monitored, and abnormal feeding behavior (not waking up for feeds, latching issues, or ineffective sucking) should prompt a response from the caring team.

Infants as a general population and more so infants at risk for hypoglycemia depend on feeds for maintaining normal blood glucose levels and thus require timely feeding with proper volumes.

5. Regular Monitoring of Blood Glucose Levels (Using Reliable Instruments)

At times, even if care team and family education is performed well, newborns at-risk might suffer from hypoglycemic events.

As mentioned before, these events might be asymptomatic thus regular monitoring for infants at risk (and blood glucose measurements of infants with clinical signs that might be associated with hypoglycemia) is highly important.

As mentioned previously, some inconsistencies regarding the exact blood value to be considered as a cutoff for hypoglycemia are still to be found, yet it is recommended for each unit to adopt its local recommendations and have clear guidelines for normal values accepted for blood glucose.

6. Identification of Signs and Symptoms of Hypoglycemia

As the clinical signs and symptoms of hypoglycemia might be non-specific, team education for subtle signs is important as well as maintaining a high index of suspicion toward this entity. Family education regarding the signs and red flags is highly important, as well as often they will be the ones to identify clinical signs.

Due to the nonspecific nature of the symptoms associated with hypoglycemia, whenever a clinical sign suggesting hypoglycemia is present, a blood glucose level should be taken to rule out the presence of hypoglycemia.

7. Prevention of Reccurrence

It is important to keep in mind that even if hypoglycemia has developed, it is important to prevent its reccurrence as recurrent events may increase the risk for neurological consequences later in life.

Immediate treatment of hypoglycemia and maintaining recurrent blood glucose measurements are recommended until the newborn maintains normal blood glucose values based on feeding at regular volumes and intervals [1, 5].

26.7 Management of Hypoglycemia

Once diagnosed, neonatal hypoglycemia should be immediately addressed and treated. Whether symptomatic or not, glucose delivery to the tissues is essential, and should be promptly renewed at a rate that will compensate for the low level and maintain the newborn's glucose use.

As described earlier, different societies' guidelines differ from one another. In ◘ Fig. 26.2 is the 2011 American Academy of Pediatrics (AAP) recommendations flowchart, for follow-up, diagnosis, and treatment (@Screening and management of postnatal glucose homeostasis: Image from Adamkin DH. Neonatal hypoglycemia. *Semin Fetal Neonatal Med.* 2017) [6].

When discussing glucose tissue delivery, glucose infusion rate (GIR) is the key element; it represents the glucose delivery in mg per kg (of infant weight) per minute.

As mentioned earlier in this chapter, a newborn infant has a glucose utilization of 4–6 mg/kg/min; this range might change according to the clinical situation and reach significantly higher values in babies with higher metabolic needs, or with hyperinsulinism.

The treatment of hypoglycemia is based on simple principles of maintaining GIR according to the newborn's needs and once achieving normal blood glucose levels, trying to wean support until the newborn's glucose values are normal when based solely on regu-

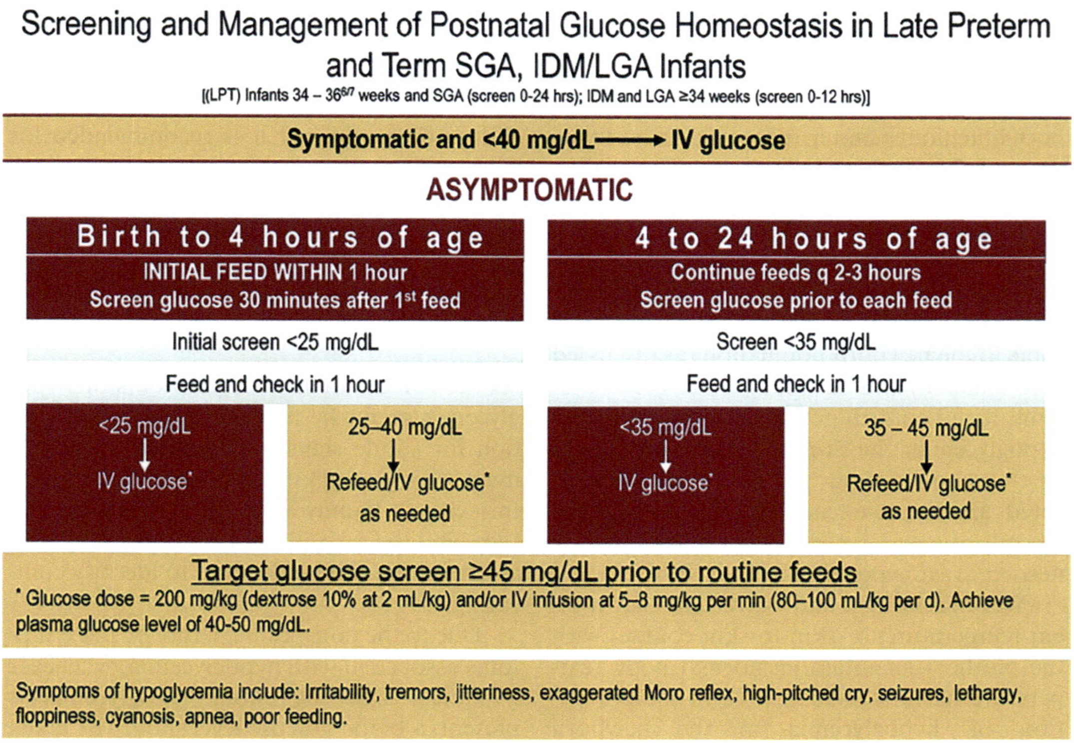

◘ **Fig. 26.2** Suggested algorithm for the management of neonatal hypoglycemia lar feeding (i.e., non-IV fluid support and no glycemic fortification of feeds).

Newborn glucose delivery can be achieved by feeding or by IV infusion, and in some cases, medications may be used to facilitate achieving a euglycemic state.

The treatment of hypoglycemia is based on these principles:

26.7.1 Feeding

Feeding is the most common form of support for maintaining a euglycemic state, for babies with or without risk for hypoglycemia.

Whether breastfeeding or formula-fed, frequency, timing, and volume of feeding as well as infants' clinical state and glucose requirements need to be taken into account to maintain euglycemia.

Breastfeeding has been associated with a reduced need for the treatment of hypoglycemia—in a study of the prevention of neonatal hypoglycemia, the change in plasma glucose concentration after breastfeeding was similar to the use of formula or Dextrose Gel. However, breastfeeding was associated with a reduced need for a second treatment, independent of the initial blood glucose concentration.

Infants of diabetic mothers who were breastfed within 30 minutes had higher blood glucose concentrations than a similar population that was not fed or that received infant formula.

Nevertheless, in some situations, breastfeeding is not available or not effective and when balancing the decision for IV dextrose and the separation of the mother–infant dyad—formula feeds are warranted.

26.7.2 Dextrose Oral Gel

In 2013, 200 mg 40% dextrose gel was examined versus placebo in at-risk infants with a GA of 35–42 weeks and found that the use of oral dextrose gel decreased NICU admission for hypoglycemia. Further studies showed that the use of dextrose gel appears to be safe and may reduce other risks related to treatment of hypoglycemia, such as decreasing breastfeeding, and decreasing health care costs. Dextrose gel has since been widely accepted as part of the treatment for newborn hypoglycemia and has been incorporated into many societies' recommendations and hospital guidelines.

26.7.3 Fortification of Oral Feeding

In some cases, in order to prevent the need to treat the infant with IV infusion, or to facilitate weaning of IV infusion, oral feeds may be fortified with policose (which is added to the bottled feed) in order to provide a higher glucose delivery rate.

Once euglycemia is achieved, this supplementation can be gradually weaned.

26.7.4 IV Infusion

If oral supplementation of glucose is insufficient or glucose values and the clinical state require, an infant may be treated with IV glucose; the initial treatment consists of 200 mg/kg (2 mL/kg) of 10% dextrose in water administered over 1 minute, followed by a continuous glucose infusion at 6–8 mg/kg/min and titrated up by 1–2 mg/kg/min every 4–6 hours until euglycemia is achieved, after which titration down can occur.

The glucose infusion rate may be increased or decreased by changing either the rate of infusion or its glucose concentration, according to local guidelines and the clinical state of the newborn.

Some data suggest that a steeper rise in blood glucose may be associated with adverse long-term outcomes, thus avoiding boluses while providing a continuous infusion in asymptomatic neonates might be preferred.

26.7.5 Medication

When GIR exceeds 10–14 mg/kg/hour, other intervention are considered: these include

- Steroids: Hydrocortisone reduces the peripheral utilization of glucose and enhances the effects of glucagon and gluconeogenesis; it can be given as a stress dose.

- Glucagon: If hyperinsulinism is suspected, glucagon may be used. Glucagon counteracts the effects of insulin. Administering a single glucagon bolus and monitoring its effect on glucose levels may be both a clinical tool to detect and prove the presence of hyperinsulinism and at the same time may be a route to treat a hypoglycemia. Glucagon may also be given as a continuous IV infusion (parallel to an IV dextrose infusion) to suppress the insulin effect and maintain euglycemia in a hyperinsulimenic patient.
- Diazoxide: If hyperinsulinism is suspected or proved as the mechanism for hypoglycemia, diazoxide may be used as it inhibits insulin secretion by the beta cells in the pancreas, by opening ATP-sensitive potassium channels. It might be associated with fluid retention, pulmonary hypertension, and some other possible adverse effects.
- Somatostatin: Somatostatin can be used alone or in conjunction with glucagon therapy to suppress both insulin and glucagon output. An alternative to somatostatin is its analog, octreotide.
- Partial Pancreatectomy: In rare and particular subset of infants with adenomatous pancreatic hyperplasia, a partial pancreatectomy may be needed [1, 5–7].

26.8 Conclusion

Hypoglycemia is a common issue within the newborn population.

Though there is no clear consensus regarding the threshold value for diagnosis of hypoglycemia, the level beyond which hypoglycemia may have long-term consequences, and there are inconsistencies in the different protocols for treating hypoglycemia, medical teams treating the newborn population encounter this entity frequently and need to have a good understanding of the mechanisms contributing to its development, the risk factors for the population that need to be followed up, the signs and symptoms of hypoglycemia and the interventions required to treating those with hypoglycemia.

Many medical societies underline the need to prevent and to identify early neonates with hypoglycemia in order to treat it early and prevent long-term brain injury.

It is crucial for teams to educate caregivers regarding this topic and have local protocols and guidelines for the prevention, recognition, and treatment of hypoglycemia.

Chapter Key Points

- Neonatal hypoglycemia is common, often asymptomatic, and may lead to long-term neurodevelopmental injury if unrecognized.
- Early feeding, normothermia, and rapid identification of at-risk infants are the cornerstone of prevention.
- Screening protocols differ among societies, but all emphasize monitoring infants with maternal or neonatal risk factors.
- Dextrose gel is an effective first-line therapy that reduces NICU admissions and supports breastfeeding.
- Persistent hypoglycemia (>72 hours) requires evaluation for endocrine/metabolic disease.

Chapter-End Summary

Neonatal hypoglycemia is a frequent metabolic problem during the transition from intra- to extra-uterine life. While physiologic hypoglycemia is expected in the first hours, prolonged or severe hypoglycemia may cause long-term neurologic injury. Prevention relies on risk identification, early feeding, maintenance of normothermia, parental and staff education, and standardized screening protocols. Dextrose gel and structured approaches to feeding help reduce interventions and NICU admissions. Persistent hypoglycemia warrants evaluation for endocrine or metabolic disease. Consistent preventive practice and early recognition substantially improve neonatal outcomes.

References

1. Giouleka S, Gkiouleka M, Tsakiridis I, Daniilidou A, Mamopoulos A, Athanasiadis A, Dagklis T. Diagnosis and management of neonatal hypoglycemia: a comprehensive review of guidelines. Children (Basel). 2023;10(7):1220. https://doi.org/10.3390/children10071220. PMID: 37508719; PMCID: PMC10378472.
2. Norval MA, Kennedy RLJ, Berkson J. Blood sugar in newborn infants. J Pediatr. 1949;34(3):342–51. ISSN 0022-3476.
3. Hartmann AF, Jaudon JC, Morton M. Hypoglycemia. J Pediatr. 1937;11(1):1–36. ISSN 0022-3476.
4. Thornton PS, Stanley CA, De Leon DD, Harris D, Haymond MW, Hussain K, Levitsky LL, Murad MH, Rozance PJ, Simmons RA, Sperling MA, Weinstein DA, White NH, Wolfsdorf JI, Pediatric Endocrine Society. Recommendations from the Pediatric Endocrine Society for evaluation and management of persistent hypoglycemia in neonates, infants, and children. J Pediatr. 2015;167(2):238–45. https://doi.org/10.1016/j.jpeds.2015.03.057. Epub 2015 May 6. PMID: 25957977.
5. Rozance PJ, Wolfsdorf JI. Hypoglycemia in the newborn. Pediatr Clin N Am. 2019;66(2):333–42. https://doi.org/10.1016/j.pcl.2018.12.004. Epub 2019 Feb 1. PMID: 30819340.
6. Adamkin DH. Neonatal hypoglycemia. Semin Fetal Neonatal Med. 2017;22(1):36–41. https://doi.org/10.1016/j.siny.2016.08.007. Epub 2016 Sep 4. PMID: 27605513.
7. Blanco CL, Kim J. Neonatal glucose homeostasis. Clin Perinatol. 2022;49(2):393–404. https://doi.org/10.1016/j.clp.2022.02.003. Epub 2022 Apr 21. PMID: 35659093.
8. Adamkin DH, Committee on Fetus and Newborn. Postnatal glucose homeostasis in late-preterm and term infants. Pediatrics. 2011;127(3):e20103851. https://doi.org/10.1542/peds.2010-3851.

Prevention of Neonatal Respiratory Complications

Chris Dewhurst, Violeta Torres-Sanchez, and Daniel Crankshaw

Contents

Y. Yogev, A. Khalil (eds.), *Prevention of Complications in Obstetrics*,
https://doi.org/10.1007/978-3-032-23479-7_27

Learning Objectives

- Understand major neonatal respiratory disorders and their pathophysiology.
- Recognize antenatal, perinatal, and postnatal risk factors contributing to respiratory morbidity.
- Apply evidence-based antenatal prevention strategies (ACS, infection prevention, preterm birth reduction).
- Identify key neonatal interventions that prevent progression of respiratory distress.
- Describe long-term management strategies including BPD prevention and infection reduction.

27.1 Introduction

Neonatal respiratory disorders represent a significant cause of morbidity and mortality among newborns, particularly in preterm infants. Globally, respiratory issues are amongst the most common causes of neonatal mortality and for survivors can result in long-term health complications, including chronic lung disease and impaired neurodevelopment. The prevention of neonatal respiratory disorders is therefore a critical goal for both clinicians and public health systems. Effective prevention requires a comprehensive understanding of the risk factors, medical interventions, and socio-environmental conditions that contribute to the onset of respiratory disorders in newborns. Preventive strategies must target various stages of infant development, from preconception and pregnancy to labour and postnatal care.

This chapter explores the preventive measures for neonatal respiratory disorders by examining the causes, risk factors, and medical interventions available for both preterm and full-term infants. From improving maternal health to adopting advanced neonatal care strategies, this paper addresses the multidisciplinary efforts needed to prevent neonatal respiratory disorders. The aim is to provide a thorough exploration of prevention methods and future research possibilities that could significantly reduce neonatal respiratory morbidity and mortality.

Despite improvements in perinatal and neonatal care in the last 30 years, respiratory disorders remain a significant cause of morbidity and mortality in newborns and in later childhood. Many of the crucial stages in lung development occur in utero and the factors that affect this environment influence the respiratory system at birth as well as in later childhood. Understanding these factors can assist in preventing or minimising respiratory complications that occur in the neonatal period as well as in later childhood. This chapter aims to provide an extensive overview of the prevention strategies for neonatal respiratory disorders, examining risk factors, preventive measures, and the importance of a multi-faceted approach involving healthcare professionals, parents, and communities.

27.1.1 Overview of Lung Development

Lung development is a complex, highly regulated process that begins in the early embryonic life from continues through pregnancy, infancy and into childhood. This intricate development involves multiple stages of morphogenesis, cellular differentiation, and structural maturation that are described below.

Embryonic stage (3–8 weeks gestation)	Pseudoglandular stage (5–17 weeks' gestation)	Canalicular stage (16–26 weeks' gestation)	Saccular stage (24 weeks-birth):	Alveolar stage (36 weeks–8 years)
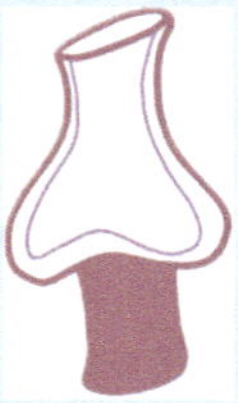	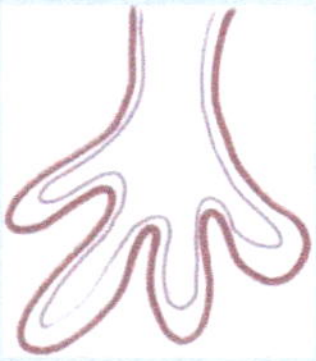	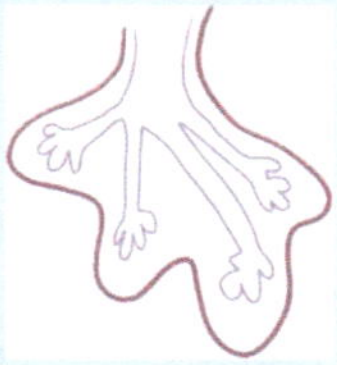	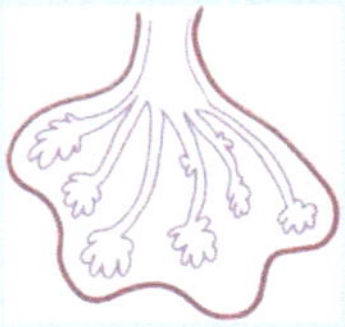	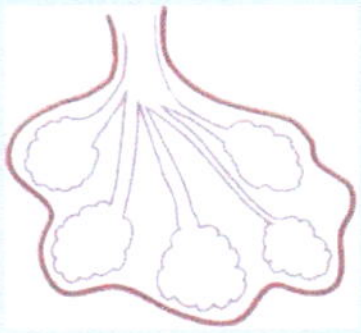
Primitive gut tube → laryngotracheal groove → trachea + two lung buds → L and R primary bronchi → bronchial tree	Bronchial tree → terminal bronchioles No gas exchange	Vascularisation and alveolar ducts formation Type I and II alveolar cells differentiation	Terminal airways → saccules (alveoli precursor) Type II alveolar cells increase surfactant production	Alveoli maturation Septation divides saccules into smaller alveoli Thinning of alveolar-capillary barrier

Disruption in lung development can lead to a range of congenital and neonatal conditions. For example, early delivery results in an underdeveloped respiratory system being used for ventilation and gas exchange. This results in interruption to the usual lung development and results in lung injury.

27.2 Understanding Neonatal Respiratory Disorders

27.2.1 An Overview of Neonatal Respiratory Disorders

Neonatal respiratory disorders encompass a wide range of conditions that impact on a newborn's ability to breathe effectively. These disorders can arise from congenital lung malformations, pulmonary hypoplasia, premature delivery, infection, or other complications during birth and early postnatal life.

27.2.1.1 Respiratory Distress Syndrome (RDS)

Respiratory distress syndrome, also known as RDS, hyaline membrane disease or surfactant deficient lung disease, is the most common respiratory disorder in premature infants but can also occur in term babies.

The primary cause of RDS is surfactant deficiency. Surfactant is a complex mixture of lipids, proteins, and carbohydrates that is produced by Type II pneumocytes. Surfactant lines the alveoli of the lungs, reducing surface tension and preventing alveoli collapse. Surfactant production begins between 24 and 28 weeks gestational age but is not produced in sufficient quantities to prevent alveoli collapse until usually around 32 weeks. This is why the disorder is predominantly a disease of preterm infants with its incidence being inversely related to gestational age (see ◻ Fig. 27.1). RDS can, however, also occur in more mature infants particularly those whose mothers are diabetic when high glucose levels inhibit the production of surfactant.

After birth, neonates with RDS present with respiratory distress manifested by tachypnoea and increased work of breathing. In developed countries, the management consists of early intervention with respiratory support, exogenous surfactant administration, and monitoring of physiological parameters and blood gas analysis. Surfactant administration significantly improves outcomes in neonates with RDS [24]. Without treatment, RDS can lead to severe complications, including respiratory failure, pneumothorax, chronic lung disease, and death.

Include x-ray of dense RDS.

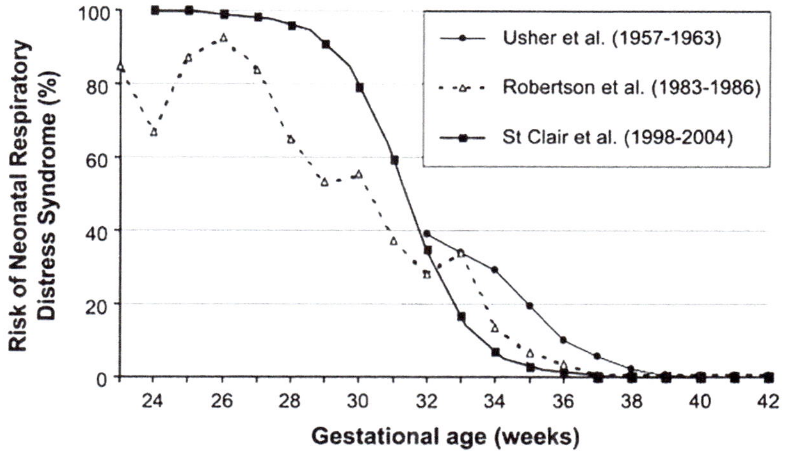

Fig. 27.1 The risk of neonatal respiratory distress syndrome in relation to gestational age St. Clair et al. [30]

27.2.1.2 Transient Tachypnoea of the Newborn (TTN)

TTN is a self-limiting condition characterised by tachypnoea in the first hours of life. It occurs when residual foetal lung fluid is not adequately cleared during birth, leading to temporary respiratory distress.

TTN is more common in full-term or late-preterm infants and those born via caesarean section, where the combination of loss of the natural expulsion of foetal lung fluid during birth is bypassed and lack of foetal stress with catecholamine release results in retention of foetal lung fluid.

Newborns with TTN exhibit tachypnoea, mild cyanosis, and sometimes mild increased work of breathing. Symptoms usually resolve within 48–72 hours as the fluid is absorbed and most newborns do not require any additional ventilatory support. More severe cases may require respiratory support with either non-invasive methods such as continuous positive airway pressure (CPAP) or high flow nasal cannula oxygen and/or mechanical ventilation.

Include x-ray of TTN.

27.2.1.3 Meconium Aspiration Syndrome (MAS)

MAS occurs when a newborn inhales meconium-stained amniotic fluid before, during, or immediately after birth. The passage of meconium perinatally can be a physiological event in term/post-term babies. Meconium-stained amniotic fluid (MSAF) occurs in 4–22% of all births, with higher incidence (23–52%) in infants born >42 weeks' gestation. From these babies, 3–12% will develop MAS [8].

MAS presents with signs of respiratory distress, including tachypnoea, grunting, cyanosis, and coarse breath sounds due to meconium obstructing the airways.

MAS can cause severe lung disease with inflammation, airway blockage, persistent pulmonary hypertension of the newborn (PPHN), which can lead to significant morbidity and mortality in very severe cases.

In the most severe cases, these infants may require mechanical ventilation, surfactant therapy, and management of persistent pulmonary hypertension (PPHN), with extracorporeal membrane oxygenation (ECMO) being necessary in the most critical situations.

Include x-ray of MAS.

27.2.1.4 Neonatal Pneumonia

Neonatal pneumonia can present at or shortly after birth due to either infection in utero or during labour. It is more common in preterm infants and those with compromised immune systems or underlying respiratory conditions. Symptoms include respiratory distress, fever, lethargy, poor feeding, and, in severe cases, septic shock. If not treated promptly with IV antibiotics and appropriate respiratory support, it can lead to serious complications, including respiratory failure, sepsis, and death.

27.2.1.5 Persistent Pulmonary Hypertension of the Newborn (PPHN)

Persistent pulmonary hypertension of the newborn (PPHN) is the result of a persistent increase in the pulmonary vascular resistance (PVR), resulting in right-to-left shunt, which can lead to hypoxic respiratory failure. Symptoms include respiratory distress and cyanosis. PPHN can be associated with meconium aspiration syndrome, sepsis, pneumonia, RDS, congenital diaphragmatic hernia, and perinatal asphyxia.

Treatment of PPHN will invariably require addressing the underlying condition. In severe cases, these infants will require mechanical ventilation and pharmacological treatment to overcome PVR, including inotropes. In critical cases, extracorporeal membrane oxygenation (ECMO) may be necessary.

27.2.1.6 Congenital Diaphragmatic Hernia (CDH)

Congenital diaphragmatic hernia is the herniation of abdominal content into the chest, caused by a developmental defect of the diaphragm. Incidence is 1 in 3000 live births. CDH is commonly associated with lung hypoplasia and immaturity, and pulmonary hypertension. Severity and prognosis will depend mostly on the location, gestation, and extent of lung hypoplasia. Left-sided defects are by far most common but right-sided carry a poorer prognosis. Most CDH will be diagnosed antenatally, though some can present postnatally. Antenatal diagnosis is crucial for optimising management, as CDH babies will routinely be intubated immediately after delivery. Ultimately, the treatment is surgical, but the aim is to stabilise them prior to the intervention [28].

Include x-ray of CDH.

27.2.1.7 Congenital Lung Malformations (CLM)

Congenital lung malformations (CLMs) are a collection of rare developmental anomalies of the lung. Main types are congenital pulmonary airway malformations (CPAM), bronchopulmonary sequestration (BPS), congenital lobar overinflation, bronchogenic cyst, and bronchial atresia. CLMs occur in around 1 out of 10,000 live births [5]. They are typically diagnosed antenatally and confirmed by chest CT angiography in the first few months of life. Severity and prognosis are dependent on the lesion size, abnormal development of lung tissue and vasculature, and presence of hydrops fetalis.

Antenatal diagnosis is crucial in the presence of hydrops fetalis, as in utero treatment might be an option. Options for in utero treatment would depend on gestational age and extent of the lesions. Options range from maternal steroids to intra-utero surgery in specialist centres [4].

Surgical treatment is the gold standard for symptomatic CLMs, but a consensus on asymptomatic cases has not been reached [19]. More recently, a watch and wait approach has been followed with positive outcomes. In summary, antenatal diagnosis is essential for the optimal management of CLM.

27.2.1.8 Bronchopulmonary Dysplasia/Chronic Lung Disease

BPD/chronic lung disease is a chronic lung condition that usually results following premature birth and neonatal intensive care. The babies have ongoing respiratory distress and reduced lung function that can continue into childhood and late adulthood. In more severe cases, there can be an ongoing oxygen requirement that persists through the first few years of life. BPD results from interruption to the normal lung development of alveolarisation and microvascular development that ensues from being born prematurely. Neonatal care with mechanical ventilation also causes lung injury from direct mechanical trauma, lung inflammation, and oxygen toxicity. BPD is most common in extremely premature infants (less-than-32-weeks' gestation) who require respiratory support for extended periods. In childhood they exhibit symptoms of chronic respiratory distress, including respiratory distress, frequent respiratory infections, asthma-type symptoms, and the need for prolonged oxygen support. Due to the increased metabolic demands of chronic respiratory distress, poor growth can occur during infancy and childhood.

(CXR of BPD).

27.2.2 Prevalence and Statistics

Neonatal respiratory disorders remain a major cause of neonatal morbidity and mortality worldwide, particularly in preterm infants. Prematurity rates range from 4% to 16%, depending on the country. In the UK, around 7–8% of all babies are born premature [14]. According to the World Health Organisation (WHO), complications from preterm birth, including respiratory disorders, account for nearly 35% of all neonatal deaths globally. It is estimated that 15 million babies are born preterm each year, and nearly one million die from related complications, with respiratory distress being a leading factor [34].

In high-income countries with advanced neonatal care, the survival rate for preterm infants with respiratory disorders has improved dramatically. However, with increased survival there are more survivors of extreme prematurity into later childhood with respiratory and neurological problems.

27.2.3 Long-Term Impact on Infant Health and Development

Neonatal respiratory disorders, particularly those affecting preterm infants, can have lasting effects on an infant's health and development. These disorders often lead to:

- **Chronic Lung Disease**: Conditions such as BPD can result in chronic lung disease, where infants experience long-term breathing difficulties, recurrent respiratory infections, and impaired lung function throughout childhood and adulthood.
- **Neurodevelopmental Delays**: The hypoxia associated with severe respiratory disorders can affect brain development, leading to cognitive delays, motor impairments, and developmental disabilities in later life.
- **Increased Risk of Asthma**: Infants who experience neonatal respiratory disorders, particularly those with a history of BPD or MAS, have a higher risk of developing asthma and other respiratory conditions during childhood.
- **Growth Impairments**: Chronic respiratory issues can interfere with an infant's ability to feed and grow properly, leading to poor weight gain, failure to thrive, and stunted growth.

The prevention of neonatal respiratory disorders is therefore critical not only for reducing neonatal mortality but also for improving long-term health outcomes for infants.

27.3 Risk Factors Contributing to Neonatal Respiratory Disorders

The development of neonatal respiratory disorders is multifactorial, arising from a combination of biological, environmental, and social determinants. Understanding the key risk factors is essential for the implementation of preventive strategies that can mitigate or reduce the incidence of these disorders. The risk factors can be broadly categorised into maternal, foetal, environmental, and healthcare-related contributors.

27.3.1 Preterm Birth

One of the most significant risk factors for neonatal respiratory disorders is **preterm birth**, defined as delivery before 37 weeks of gestation. The earlier a baby is born, the higher the risk of respiratory problems due to the underdevelopment of the lungs.

- **Immature Lungs**: In preterm infants, the lungs may not have developed sufficiently to support effective gas exchange. The production of surfactant, a critical substance for preventing the collapse of alveoli, typically begins around 24–28 weeks of gestation and reaches adequate levels by around 34 weeks. Infants born before this time often experience surfactant deficiency, leading to conditions such as **respiratory distress syndrome (RDS)**.
- **Incomplete Alveolarisation**: Preterm infants often have underdeveloped alveoli, the small air sacs responsible for gas exchange in the lungs. The alveolar stage of lung development continues well into childhood, but premature birth can interrupt this process, resulting in fewer, less functional alveoli at birth.
- **Associated Complications**: Preterm birth is often associated with other complications that can exacerbate respiratory issues, including intraventricular haemorrhage, patent ductus arteriosus, and neonatal infections, all of which increase the risk of developing respiratory disorders like **bronchopulmonary dysplasia (BPD)**.

Contributing Factors to Preterm Birth

- **Maternal Infections**: Maternal infections, including urinary tract infections, bacterial vaginosis, or intra-amniotic infections, can trigger preterm labour. These infections can induce an inflammatory response that contributes to premature rupture of membranes or preterm contractions.
- **Multiple Pregnancies**: Twin, triplet, or higher-order pregnancies are more likely to result in preterm birth. The increased pressure on the uterus from multiple foetuses can lead to preterm labour, and infants born prematurely from multiple pregnancies often experience respiratory complications.
- **Pre-eclampsia and Other Maternal Conditions**: Pre-eclampsia, characterised by high blood pressure and damage to organ systems, often necessitates early delivery to protect both the mother and infant. This can lead to respiratory complications if the infant is born too early.

27.3.2 Maternal Health Factors

Maternal health and lifestyle play a crucial role in the risk of neonatal respiratory disorders. Conditions such as diabetes, infections, poor nutrition, and substance abuse can all increase the likelihood of complications during pregnancy and childbirth that lead to respiratory problems in the newborn.

- **Maternal Diabetes**:
  - **Gestational diabetes (GDM)** and **pre-existing diabetes** (Type 1 or Type 2) are significant risk factors for neonatal respiratory disorders. Infants born to mothers with poorly controlled diabetes are at increased risk for **RDS** even at term. Elevated glucose levels can delay the maturation of foetal lungs and inhibit surfactant production, resulting in immature lung function at birth.
  - Diabetic pregnancies are also associated with larger-than-average infants (macrosomia), which can complicate delivery and increase the risk of birth-related trauma and subsequent respiratory distress.
  - Early maternal diabetes control, especially GDM, reduces the risk of neonatal respiratory distress [27].
- **Maternal Infections**:
  - **Chorioamnionitis**, an infection of the placental tissues and amniotic fluid, can induce premature labour and result in preterm birth. Intrauterine infections also increase the risk of neonatal pneumonia, which can complicate breathing at birth.
  - Viral infections, such as **cytomegalovirus (CMV)**, **rubella**, or **herpes simplex virus**, can directly affect foetal lung development, increasing the risk of respiratory disorders.
- **Maternal Asthma**:
  - **Maternal asthma** is a risk factor in the development of neonatal respiratory distress. Maternal asthma control might improve neonatal lung function and reduce the incidence of respiratory problems [22].
- **Substance Use (Tobacco, Alcohol, Drugs)**:
  - **Smoking**: Maternal smoking during pregnancy is a significant contributor to neonatal respiratory issues. The harm-

ful substances in cigarettes, including nicotine and carbon monoxide, restrict oxygen supply to the foetus, impair lung development, and increase the likelihood of preterm birth [11]. Smoking is associated with a higher incidence of low birth weight (LBW), prematurity, and RDS in newborns. Smoking cessation preconception reduces rates of low birth weight to a similar incidence than non-smokers. Incidence of LBW increases with continued smoking throughout pregnancy [20].
  - **Alcohol and Drug Use**: Maternal alcohol consumption during pregnancy can lead to **foetal alcohol syndrome**, which is associated with respiratory difficulties. The use of illicit drugs, such as cocaine or opioids, can also lead to preterm labour, placental abruption, and poor foetal oxygenation, increasing the risk of respiratory disorders.
- **Obesity**: Maternal obesity increases the risk of complications during pregnancy, such as gestational diabetes and pre-eclampsia, are linked to preterm birth and neonatal respiratory problems. Obesity can also lead to obstructed labour, increasing the chances of caesarean section, which has been associated with an increased risk of **Transient Tachypnoea of the Newborn (TTN)**. Maternal obesity not only increases the incidence of respiratory illness but also the risk of childhood and adult obesity in their offspring [16].

27.3.3 Genetic Predispositions

- **Family History of Respiratory Conditions**: A family history of asthma increases the likelihood that a newborn will experience respiratory problems and childhood asthma.
- Genetic factors that influence lung development, immune responses, or surfactant production can predispose some infants to neonatal respiratory disorders [26].
- Other genetic disorders, such as **cystic fibrosis**, may impair airway function and increase the risk of lung infections and respiratory failure.

27.3.4 Environmental Factors

- **Air Pollution**: Exposure to high levels of environmental pollution, both before and during pregnancy, has been linked to poor lung development and increased respiratory distress in newborns. Pollutants such as particulate matter (PM2.5), nitrogen dioxide (NO2), and sulphur dioxide (SO2) can impair foetal lung development and increase the risk of respiratory disorders such as **BPD** and asthma later in life [3, 25].

27.3.5 Inadequate Antenatal Care

Access to quality antenatal care is essential for early detection and management of risk factors associated with neonatal respiratory disorders. Inadequate or delayed prenatal care can lead to untreated maternal health conditions and missed opportunities for early intervention.

- **Missed Congenital Abnormalities**: As discussed in the overview of neonatal respiratory conditions, certain lung pathologies, when identified antenatally, allow for more effective care and, consequently, a better prognosis.
- **Delayed Diagnosis of Preterm Labour**: Without adequate antenatal monitoring, signs of preterm labour may go unnoticed, and crucial interventions, such as antenatal corticosteroid administration, may be delayed.
- **Missed Infections**: Untreated maternal infections, such as urinary tract infections or sexually transmitted infections (e.g. syphilis or chlamydia), can lead to preterm birth or intrauterine infections that affect neonatal respiratory health.
- **Lack of Nutritional Support**: Proper maternal nutrition is vital for foetal lung development. Inadequate nutrition, particularly deficiencies in essential nutrients like vitamins A, C, D, and E, can compromise lung maturation and increase the risk of respiratory problems at birth.

27

27.3.6 Birth-Related Factors

The mode of delivery and the conditions surrounding birth also play an essential role in the development of neonatal respiratory disorders. Birth-related factors that can contribute to respiratory issues include:

- **Caesarean Section**:
  - Infants born via caesarean section (C-section) are at a higher risk of developing **Transient Tachypnoea of the Newborn (TTN)**. During vaginal delivery, the baby's chest is compressed, helping to expel fluid from the lungs. In C-section deliveries, especially elective ones before labour begins, this fluid clearance process is incomplete, leading to respiratory difficulties.
- **Birth Asphyxia**:
  - **Perinatal asphyxia**, where the baby does not receive enough oxygen during the birth process, can result in significant respiratory challenges at birth. Birth asphyxia can lead to conditions like **meconium aspiration syndrome (MAS)**, where the baby inhales meconium-stained amniotic fluid into the lungs, causing obstruction and inflammation. In severe cases, birth asphyxia can lead to hypoxic-ischaemic encephalopathy (HIE). These babies often require mechanical ventilation.

27.3.7 Conclusion of Risk Factors

Neonatal respiratory disorders are the result of a complex interplay between maternal, foetal, environmental, and birth-related factors. Preterm birth remains the most significant risk factor, but maternal health conditions, genetic predispositions, and environmental influences also contribute substantially to the development of respiratory issues in newborns. By understanding these risk factors, healthcare providers and public health systems can take proactive measures to mitigate the risk, ensuring better neonatal outcomes and healthier long-term outcomes.

27.4 Preventive Strategies Before Birth

The prevention of neonatal respiratory disorders begins before birth through a combination of maternal health optimisation, appropriate antenatal care, and proactive interventions. These strategies are designed to address the underlying risk factors that contribute to respiratory disorders, such as preterm birth, maternal infections, and genetic predispositions. By focusing on prevention during pregnancy, the risk of complications that lead to respiratory distress at birth can be significantly reduced.

27.4.1 Antenatal Corticosteroids

One of the most critical interventions to reduce the risk of respiratory distress in preterm infants is the administration of **antenatal corticosteroids**. Steroids, such as betamethasone or dexamethasone, help accelerate foetal lung maturation and promote the production of surfactant, reducing the risk of neonatal RDS and mortality [17].

Indications Antenatal corticosteroids are administered to pregnant women at risk of preterm labour between 24 and 34 weeks of gestation. In some cases, they may also be used up to 36 weeks if early delivery is anticipated. Women who are at risk for conditions like pre-eclampsia, preterm premature rupture of membranes (PPROM), or multiple pregnancies are candidates for this intervention.

Mechanism of Action Corticosteroids stimulate the foetal lungs to produce surfactant, which reduces surface tension in the alveoli and prevents their collapse during exhalation.

Timing Antenatal steroids are most effective if given 24 hours to 7 days prior to the baby's delivery.

Effectiveness Studies have shown that antenatal corticosteroid treatment can reduce the risk of neonatal death, RDS, and other complications like intraventricular haemorrhage by approximately 40–50%. In resource-limited settings where access to mechanical ventilation and surfactant therapy is restricted, antenatal corticosteroids are particularly crucial for improving neonatal outcomes.

Limitations Mainly relies upon the timing of corticosteroid administration and delivery. Anticipating preterm deliveries and predicting the optimal window for corticosteroid administration can be challenging [31].

27.4.2 Tocolysis for Preterm Labour

Tocolysis refers to the use of medications to delay preterm labour. While tocolytic drugs do not prevent preterm birth indefinitely, they can provide a critical window of time to administer antenatal corticosteroids and transfer the mother to a facility equipped to handle preterm deliveries.

- **Common Tocolytic Agents**:
  - **Beta-adrenergic agonists** (e.g. terbutaline) work by relaxing the smooth muscles of the uterus to delay contractions.
  - **Calcium channel blockers** (e.g. nifedipine) inhibit calcium influx into muscle cells, reducing uterine contractions.
  - **Nonsteroidal anti-inflammatory drugs (NSAIDs)** (e.g. indomethacin) can block the production of prostaglandins, which play a role in triggering labour.
- **Timing**: Tocolytic therapy is generally administered when labour begins before 34 weeks of gestation. Delaying birth by 24–48 hours can allow time for antenatal corticosteroids to take effect, improving lung maturity in the foetus.
- **Limitations**: While tocolysis can help delay preterm labour, it is not always successful, and its use is typically limited to short-term interventions. The primary goal is to optimise the timing of delivery to improve neonatal outcomes, rather than to prevent preterm birth entirely [6].

27.4.3 Infection Prevention and Management

Maternal infections, particularly **intrauterine infections** like chorioamnionitis, are significant contributors to preterm birth and neonatal respiratory disorders. Effective prevention and management of infections during pregnancy can reduce the risk of respiratory complications in newborns.

- **Screening and Treatment**:
  - **Group B Streptococcus (GBS)**: If positive, intrapartum antibiotic prophylaxis is administered during labour to prevent the transmission of GBS to the newborn, which can cause neonatal pneumonia and sepsis. Identification and intrapartum prophylaxis treatment for GBS reduces the incidence of early onset GBS sepsis [15].
  - **Urinary Tract Infections (UTIs)**: UTIs during pregnancy are associated with an increased risk of preterm labour. Early diagnosis and treatment with appropriate antibiotics are essential to prevent complications.
  - **Sexually Transmitted Infections (STIs)**: Untreated STIs, such as syphilis, gonorrhoea, and chlamydia, can lead to preterm birth and neonatal infections. Routine prenatal screening and treatment of STIs are important for preventing these outcomes.
- **Vaccination**:
  - **Influenza** and **pertussis (whooping cough)** vaccinations are recommended during pregnancy to protect both the mother and the newborn. Influenza can lead to preterm labour and respiratory complications in newborns, while pertussis poses a direct risk of respiratory failure in infants.
  - **COVID-19**: Pregnant women are at increased risk of severe illness from COVID-19, which can also lead to preterm birth. Vaccination against COVID-19 during pregnancy has been shown to protect both the mother and newborn, reducing the risk of respiratory complications at birth.

- **Infection Control in Healthcare Settings**: In resource-limited settings or overcrowded healthcare facilities, the risk of nosocomial infections (hospital-acquired infections) increases, particularly for preterm infants. Strict infection control measures, including hand hygiene, use of personal protective equipment, and proper neonatal isolation protocols, are essential to prevent the transmission of infections that could complicate neonatal respiratory health.

27.4.4 Nutrition and Maternal Health Optimisation

Proper nutrition and management of maternal health conditions during pregnancy are crucial for supporting foetal lung development and preventing respiratory disorders in newborns.

- **Nutritional Supplements**:
  - **Folic Acid**: Adequate folic acid intake before and during pregnancy helps prevent neural tube defects and supports overall foetal growth. While its direct impact on respiratory disorders is limited, optimal foetal development reduces the risk of complications that could affect lung function [35].
  - **Vitamin D**: Vitamin D plays a role in immune system function and lung development. Deficiencies in Vitamin D during pregnancy have been associated with an increased maternal morbidity, including conditions like pre-eclampsia and gestational diabetes, as well as adverse neonatal outcomes such as preterm birth and low birth weight. These factors can directly impact neonatal respiratory outcomes [2].
  - **Omega-3 Fatty Acids**: Omega-3 fatty acids, found in fish oil, may help reduce the risk of pre-eclampsia, low birth weight, and preterm birth—all of which increase the risk of neonatal respiratory complications [9].
- **Management of Maternal Conditions**:
  - **Diabetes**: Proper management of gestational diabetes or pre-existing diabetes is essential for preventing complications such as macrosomia (large for gestational age infants), which can increase the risk of birth-related trauma and respiratory distress. Tight blood sugar control can also reduce the risk of delayed lung maturation and RDS.
  - **Hypertension and Pre-eclampsia**: Hypertension and pre-eclampsia can result in poor placental function, leading to intrauterine growth restriction (IUGR) and preterm birth. Managing these conditions through medications, regular monitoring, and lifestyle modifications can reduce the risk of respiratory complications in newborns.
- **Weight Management**: Maternal obesity increases the risk of preterm birth, gestational diabetes, and hypertensive disorders, all of which can contribute to neonatal respiratory issues. Maintaining a healthy weight before and during pregnancy through proper diet and physical activity is key to preventing complications.
- **Smoking cessation**: Smoking cessation support is a powerful preventive measure that can decrease the risk of prematurity and low birth weight babies.

27.4.5 Genetic Counselling and Prenatal Diagnosis

For families with a history of genetic conditions that affect lung development or respiratory function, such as **cystic fibrosis, congenital diaphragmatic hernia, or congenital lung malformations** prenatal genetic counselling and testing can help identify potential risks and guide decision-making during pregnancy and delivery.

- **Carrier Screening**: Couples planning to conceive may undergo carrier screening for conditions like cystic fibrosis. If both parents are carriers, genetic counselling can provide information about the likelihood of the baby inheriting the disorder and the implications for respiratory health.

- **Prenatal Imaging and Diagnosis**:
  - **Ultrasound**: Detailed ultrasounds can detect congenital abnormalities such as diaphragmatic hernias or lung masses (e.g. congenital pulmonary airway malformation) that could cause respiratory distress at birth. Early diagnosis allows for careful planning of delivery in a specialised facility where immediate surgical intervention or respiratory support is available.
  - **Amniocentesis**: In cases where a genetic disorder is suspected, amniocentesis can be performed to diagnose conditions that might lead to respiratory complications. This information helps in preparing for the appropriate level of neonatal care at birth.

27.4.6 Preventing Preterm Birth

Since preterm birth is the leading risk factor for neonatal respiratory disorders, preventing preterm birth is a key preventive strategy. Several approaches are used to reduce the likelihood of preterm labour and delivery.

- **Progesterone Therapy**: For women with a history of preterm birth or a short cervix (measured by ultrasound), **progesterone** supplementation can help reduce the risk of preterm labour. Progesterone, a hormone that supports pregnancy, is administered either via injection or vaginal suppositories to help maintain cervical length and prevent early contractions [13].
- **Cervical Cerclage**: For women with cervical insufficiency, where the cervix shortens or opens prematurely, a surgical procedure known as **cervical cerclage** may be performed. This involves stitching the cervix closed to prevent early dilation and labour. Cerclage can reduce the risk of preterm birth in women with a history of second-trimester losses or a short cervix detected by ultrasound [32].
- **Lifestyle Modifications**: Lifestyle changes, such as avoiding smoking, reducing physical stress, and attending regular prenatal care visits, can help lower the risk of preterm labour. Pregnant women at risk of preterm birth may also be advised to limit physical activity and avoid heavy lifting to reduce pressure on the cervix.

27.4.7 Optimal Timing and Mode of Delivery

The timing and mode of delivery play a crucial role in reducing the risk of neonatal respiratory disorders. Planned early deliveries, whether via caesarean section or induction of labour, should be carefully considered to avoid unnecessary respiratory complications.

- **Avoiding Elective Early Deliveries**: Elective inductions or caesarean sections before 39 weeks of gestation are associated with an increased risk of **Transient Tachypnoea of the Newborn (TTN)** and **RDS** due to incomplete lung maturation. Unless there are clear medical indications, delaying delivery until 39 weeks allows the foetal lungs to mature fully.
- **Caesarean Section Considerations**: For infants at high risk of respiratory distress, such as those with congenital abnormalities or growth restriction, caesarean delivery may be planned to ensure safe delivery and immediate access to neonatal care. However, in low-risk pregnancies, vaginal delivery is generally preferred to promote fluid clearance from the lungs during birth. The role of antenatal corticosteroids prior to an elective caesarean section at term has been explored, which has been linked to reduced admission to neonatal intensive care units (NICU) with respiratory morbidity; however, this is not current practice and further evidence would need to be found. [29].

27.4.8 Conclusion of Preventive Strategies Before Birth

The prevention of neonatal respiratory disorders relies heavily on proactive maternal and antenatal care. Through interventions like antenatal corticosteroids, tocolysis, infection prevention, and proper management of maternal health conditions, the risk of respiratory distress at birth can be significantly reduced. Preventive measures targeting preterm birth, genetic counselling, and optimal delivery planning further enhance neonatal outcomes. By focusing on prevention before birth, healthcare providers can help ensure that newborns enter the world with healthier lungs and a lower risk of respiratory complications.

27.5 Preventive Strategies After Birth

Once a newborn is delivered, particularly if born preterm or with known risk factors, immediate steps must be taken to mitigate the risk of respiratory complications. The window after birth is critical, as many neonatal respiratory disorders manifest within minutes to hours of delivery. The interventions in this phase focus on stabilising the infant, ensuring optimal respiratory function, and preventing complications. Below are key preventive strategies after birth to reduce the incidence and severity of neonatal respiratory disorders.

27.5.1 Surfactant Therapy

Surfactant therapy is one of the cornerstone treatments for newborns, particularly preterm infants, at risk of **respiratory distress syndrome (RDS)**. This therapy can be both preventive and therapeutic, depending on the infant's condition at birth.

- **Function of Surfactant**: Surfactant is a naturally occurring substance in the lungs that reduces surface tension in the alveoli, preventing their collapse and facilitating proper gas exchange. In preterm infants, surfactant production is often insufficient, leading to RDS.
- **Prophylactic vs rescue Surfactant Administration**: There has been no clear evidence to back the use of routine surfactant in infants at risk of developing RDS [23]. However, there is strong evidence to suggest that rescue surfactant administration decreases mortality, risk of pneumothorax and development of PPHN [21].
- **Methods of Administration**: Surfactant is delivered directly into the infant's lungs through an endotracheal tube. Newer techniques, such as **less invasive surfactant administration (LISA)**, which uses a thin catheter to administer surfactant, have shown reduced risk of intubation in the first 3 days, mortality, and development of BPD [1].

27.5.2 Non-invasive Respiratory Support (CPAP and HFNC)

Continuous positive airway pressure (CPAP) is a non-invasive ventilation strategy used to prevent and treat respiratory distress in newborns. It helps keep the airways and alveoli open by delivering a constant flow of air or oxygen through nasal prongs or a mask. Nasal CPAP has been shown to reduce the need for intubation and development of BPD [33].

High flow nasal cannula (HFNC) ensures the delivery of humidified, heated oxygen at higher flow rates. In preterm infants, HFNC has shown higher treatment failure in the first 3/7, compared to CPAP [12].

Limitations: Babies with severe lung pathology may need additional support, requiring escalation to mechanical ventilation. Non-invasive respiratory support has been linked to complications such as gut distension and feeding intolerance.

27.5.3 Mechanical Ventilation and Advanced Respiratory Support

For infants with severe respiratory distress or failure, **mechanical ventilation** may be required. While it is a life-saving intervention, the goal is to minimise its use and duration to reduce the risk of lung injury, which can lead to **Bronchopulmonary Dysplasia (BPD)**.

- **Indications for Mechanical Ventilation**: Primary management or infants who do not respond adequately to CPAP or who have severe respiratory failure, as indicated by blood gas measurements, will require mechanical ventilation. Conditions like severe **RDS**, **MAS**, or **persistent pulmonary hypertension of the newborn (PPHN)** may necessitate this intervention.

- **Ventilation Strategies**:
  - **Gentle Ventilation**: Modern ventilators are designed to use low pressure and minimal tidal volumes to reduce the risk of lung injury, a practice known as **gentle ventilation** or **lung-protective strategies**.
  - **High-Frequency Ventilation (HFV)**: In some cases, particularly with conditions like **BPD** or **MAS**, **high-frequency ventilation** may be used. This technique delivers very small volumes of air at a rapid rate to avoid overinflating the lungs and causing injury.
- **Weaning from Ventilation**: The goal of mechanical ventilation is to support the infant until their lungs are mature enough to function independently. As soon as the infant's condition stabilises, efforts are made to wean them from mechanical ventilation to less invasive forms of respiratory support, such as CPAP or **nasal intermittent positive pressure ventilation (NIPPV)**.

27.5.4 Oxygen Therapy and Avoiding Hyperoxia

Oxygen therapy is frequently required for neonates with respiratory distress, but careful management of oxygen levels is crucial to avoid both hypoxia (low oxygen levels) and hyperoxia (excessive oxygen levels), both of which can cause significant harm.

- **Avoiding Oxygen Toxicity**: Excessive oxygen exposure can lead to **retinopathy of prematurity (ROP)**, a condition that can cause blindness, and **BPD**, a chronic lung disease. Careful titration of oxygen to the lowest effective dose is essential to avoid these complications.
- **Weaning from Oxygen**: As the infant's respiratory condition improves, efforts are made to reduce and eventually discontinue supplemental oxygen to minimise the risk of oxygen-related complications. Some infants, who develop BPD, might require oxygen long term and can be discharged with home oxygen.

27.5.5 Thermoregulation and Energy Conservation

Maintaining an optimal body temperature is essential for newborns, particularly preterm infants, who have difficulty regulating their own body temperature. Hypothermia can exacerbate respiratory distress by increasing the infant's metabolic demands and impairing lung function.

- **Incubators and Radiant Warmers**: Infants at risk of respiratory disorders are often placed in incubators or under radiant warmers immediately after birth to maintain a stable body temperature. These devices provide controlled warmth to prevent hypothermia while allowing easy access for respiratory support and monitoring.
- **Skin-to-Skin Care (Kangaroo Care)**: For stable preterm and term infants, **skin-to-skin care** or **kangaroo care** (where the baby is placed on the mother's chest) helps maintain body temperature and has been shown to improve respiratory stability. This practice also promotes bonding and can improve breastfeeding success.

27.5.6 Nutritional Support for Preterm Infants

Adequate nutrition is critical for the growth and lung development of preterm infants, who are at high risk for respiratory disorders. Ensuring proper caloric intake and nutrient supplementation is essential for recovery and long-term lung health.

- **Breast Milk Feeding**: Breast milk is the ideal source of nutrition for preterm infants as it provides essential nutrients, growth factors, and antibodies that support lung development and protect against infections. **Fortified breast milk** may be necessary for very preterm infants to meet their increased nutritional needs.

- **Parenteral Nutrition**: For extremely preterm infants or those unable to tolerate enteral feeding (feeding through the digestive tract), **parenteral nutrition** (intravenous feeding) is initiated to ensure they receive the necessary calories, protein, and micronutrients to support their growth and respiratory function.
- **Vitamin A Supplementation**: Vitamin A plays a crucial role in lung development and immune function. Preterm infants are often given vitamin A supplementation which can reduce the risk of **bronchopulmonary dysplasia (BPD)** and support overall respiratory health [7].

27.5.7 Prevention of Nosocomial Infections

Preterm infants and those with respiratory disorders are at high risk for hospital-acquired infections (nosocomial infections), which can worsen respiratory outcomes. Preventing these infections is essential for improving long-term respiratory health.

- **Infection Control Practices**: Strict hand hygiene, use of personal protective equipment, and proper disinfection of medical equipment are critical to preventing infections in neonatal intensive care units (NICUs). Limiting visitors and isolating infants with known infections also helps reduce the risk of cross-infection.
- **Early Antibiotic Use**: In some cases, antibiotics may be administered prophylactically to infants at high risk for infection, such as those born after prolonged rupture of membranes or with signs of infection at birth. However, antibiotic use is carefully monitored to avoid the development of antibiotic resistance. Studies have shown that antibiotic use in the first year of life can be linked to atopy development in childhood [10].
- **Immunisations**: Vaccinations, such as those for respiratory syncytial virus (RSV) and influenza, play a critical role in preventing respiratory infections in high-risk infants. **Palivizumab**, a monoclonal antibody, is used to prevent severe RSV infection in preterm infants and those with chronic lung disease.

27.5.8 Conclusion of Preventive Strategies After Birth

The immediate postnatal period is crucial for preventing and managing neonatal respiratory disorders. Early interventions such as surfactant therapy, CPAP, and careful oxygen management significantly improve outcomes for at-risk infants. Other measures, including infection prevention, nutritional support, and temperature regulation, further contribute to optimising respiratory health. By providing comprehensive care in the early hours and days of life, healthcare providers can significantly reduce the risk of respiratory complications and improve long-term outcomes for newborns.

27.6 Long-Term Prevention and Management of Respiratory Disorders

Neonatal respiratory disorders often have long-lasting impacts on a child's health, particularly in preterm infants or those who experienced severe respiratory distress at birth. Long-term management strategies focus on mitigating chronic respiratory conditions, promoting lung development, and improving overall health to prevent recurrent respiratory issues. Additionally, healthcare providers and caregivers must ensure continuous monitoring and provide interventions that support long-term lung health. Below are key strategies for the long-term prevention and management of respiratory disorders in neonates.

27.6.1 Management of Bronchopulmonary Dysplasia (BPD)

- **Ongoing Respiratory Support**: Infants with BPD may require long-term supplemental oxygen even after discharge from the hospital to ensure adequate oxygenation and prevent further lung damage. Oxygen weaning is gradual, guided by regular monitoring of oxygen saturation levels and blood gases.

- **Diuretic Therapy**: Diuretics are widely used in infants with BPD, but their effectiveness remains uncertain [18].
- **Nutrition for Lung Growth**: Proper nutrition is essential for lung repair and growth in infants with BPD. High-calorie diets, fortified breast milk, or specialised formulas are often required to support growth, as these infants typically have higher energy demands due to their increased work of breathing.
- **Long-Term Monitoring**: Children with BPD require long-term follow-up to monitor lung function, growth, and development. Respiratory function tests, chest X-rays, and echocardiograms may be performed regularly to assess lung health and detect complications such as pulmonary hypertension.

27.6.2 Prevention of Respiratory Infections

Respiratory infections pose a significant threat to infants who have experienced neonatal respiratory disorders, as their lungs may be more vulnerable to damage from infections. Preventing respiratory infections is a critical component of long-term respiratory health management.

- **Vaccinations**: Ensuring that infants receive all recommended vaccinations is essential for preventing respiratory infections. This includes routine childhood immunisations, as well as vaccines for **influenza** and **respiratory syncytial virus (RSV)**, which can cause severe respiratory illness in young children.
- **Breastfeeding**: Breastfeeding has been shown to reduce the risk of respiratory infections in infants due to the presence of antibodies and other immune-protective factors in breast milk. Exclusive breastfeeding for the first 6 months of life is recommended to strengthen the infant's immune system.
- **Limiting Exposure to Second-hand Smoke and Environmental Pollutants**: Exposure to second-hand smoke and other environmental pollutants can exacerbate respiratory conditions and increase the risk of infections. Parents and caregivers are advised to create a smoke-free environment and minimise exposure to indoor and outdoor pollutants.
- **Hand Hygiene and Infection Control**: Practicing good hygiene, such as frequent handwashing and limiting contact with sick individuals, is critical in preventing respiratory infections. Caregivers should be particularly vigilant during cold and flu season, as infants with compromised lung health are more susceptible to severe illness.

27.6.3 Respiratory Rehabilitation and Physical Therapy

Infants and children who have experienced significant neonatal respiratory issues may benefit from **respiratory rehabilitation** and **physical therapy** to improve lung function and overall physical development.

- **Pulmonary Rehabilitation Programmes**: For children with chronic lung disease, pulmonary rehabilitation programmes can help improve breathing patterns, increase exercise tolerance, and promote lung function. These programmes often include breathing exercises, physical activity, and education for caregivers on managing respiratory conditions.
- **Physical Therapy**: Physical therapy helps improve overall strength and mobility, particularly in children who have experienced long hospital stays or developmental delays due to prolonged respiratory support. Therapy may focus on building endurance, improving posture and chest mobility, and encouraging physical activity to enhance lung capacity.
- **Speech and Feeding Therapy**: Some infants who have experienced neonatal respiratory distress may have difficulty with feeding and swallowing due to oral-motor dysfunction or prolonged intubation. **Speech-**

language Therapists may provide help to improve feeding skills and support oral development.

27.6.4 Long-Term Follow-Up for Preterm Infants

Infants born prematurely, especially those who experienced respiratory distress or required intensive respiratory support, require long-term follow-up to monitor for potential complications.

- **Regular Pulmonary Evaluations**: Regular assessments of lung function are essential for preterm infants who have had RDS, BPD, or other respiratory conditions. Pulmonary function tests and imaging studies are used to detect long-term lung damage and monitor for conditions like asthma or airway obstruction.
- **Neurodevelopmental Follow-Up**: Preterm infants, particularly those with respiratory complications, are at increased risk for neurodevelopmental delays and disabilities. Multidisciplinary follow-up programmes that include paediatricians, neurologists, and developmental specialists can help identify and address any developmental concerns early on.
- **Growth and Nutrition Monitoring**: Preterm infants often have difficulty gaining weight and maintaining proper growth due to increased energy demands from chronic respiratory conditions. Close monitoring of weight gain, growth charts, and nutritional intake is crucial to ensure adequate lung and overall development.

27.6.5 Asthma Management in Children with a History of Neonatal Respiratory Disorders

Children who experience neonatal respiratory distress, particularly those with **RDS** or **BPD**, are at increased risk of developing **asthma** or asthma-like symptoms later in life. Managing asthma effectively is important for preventing exacerbations and promoting healthy lung function.

- **Early Diagnosis and Monitoring**: Children with a history of neonatal respiratory issues should be monitored for signs of asthma, including recurrent wheezing, coughing, and shortness of breath. Early diagnosis allows for prompt intervention and better long-term control of the condition.
- **Preventive Asthma Medications**: Inhaled corticosteroids and bronchodilators may be prescribed to children with persistent asthma symptoms to reduce airway inflammation and prevent asthma attacks. Long-term use of these medications is tailored to the child's needs and monitored regularly by healthcare providers.
- **Avoiding Asthma Triggers**: Identifying and avoiding asthma triggers, such as allergens, smoke, and respiratory infections, is crucial for preventing asthma exacerbations. Parents and caregivers are educated on how to manage environmental triggers and recognise early signs of an asthma attack.

27.6.6 Parental Education and Support

The involvement of parents and caregivers is critical to the long-term management of neonatal respiratory disorders. Educating parents about the signs of respiratory distress, infection prevention, and proper use of medications is essential for maintaining the child's respiratory health.

- **Recognising Early Signs of Respiratory Issues**: Parents are trained to recognise early warning signs of respiratory distress, which can prevent respiratory complications from becoming life-threatening.
- **Administering Medications and Oxygen**: For infants and children requiring long-term oxygen therapy or medications like bronchodilators, parents are educated on how to administer these treatments at home. This includes proper use of inhalers, nebulisers, and oxygen tanks or concentrators.

- **Support Groups and Resources**: Parents of children with chronic respiratory conditions may benefit from joining support groups or accessing resources from organisations that provide information on managing neonatal respiratory disorders. Connecting with other families facing similar challenges can offer emotional support and practical advice.

27.6.7 Conclusion of Long-Term Prevention and Management of Respiratory Disorders

Long-term prevention and management of neonatal respiratory disorders require a comprehensive approach that includes ongoing medical care, parental education, and preventive measures to protect the child from infections and environmental risks. For children with chronic lung conditions such as BPD or asthma, early interventions and continuous monitoring are key to improving respiratory function and overall quality of life. By supporting lung development through proper nutrition, respiratory therapy, and preventive care, healthcare providers can help minimise the long-term impacts of neonatal respiratory disorders and ensure healthier outcomes as the child grows.

27.7 Conclusion on Prevention of Neonatal Respiratory Disorders

Neonatal respiratory disorders present significant challenges to the health and survival of newborns, particularly those born prematurely. However, advances in maternal care, neonatal interventions, and long-term management strategies have greatly improved outcomes for these vulnerable infants. From the use of antenatal corticosteroids and surfactant therapy to non-invasive respiratory support and nutritional optimisation, a variety of preventive measures are available to reduce the incidence and severity of respiratory distress in neonates.

Preventive strategies must begin before birth, with attention to maternal health, infection prevention, and proper timing of delivery. After birth, prompt interventions such as CPAP, oxygen therapy, and surfactant administration are crucial for stabilising at-risk infants. Long-term management, including pulmonary rehabilitation, infection prevention, and careful monitoring, ensures that children who experience neonatal respiratory disorders can lead healthy lives with minimal respiratory complications.

Through continued research and innovations in neonatal care, healthcare providers can further reduce the burden of respiratory disorders and improve the quality of life for countless newborns and their families. The key to success lies in a proactive, multidisciplinary approach that addresses both the short-term and long-term needs of these infants.

Chapter Key Points

- Neonatal respiratory disorders are a leading cause of neonatal morbidity and mortality worldwide.
- Prevention must begin antenatally: maternal optimisation, infection control, preterm birth prevention, corticosteroids.
- Postnatal strategies include surfactant therapy, CPAP, oxygen management, thermoregulation, and nutritional support.
- Risk identification (maternal, fetal, environmental, birth-related) is critical for targeted prevention.
- Long-term follow-up and prevention strategies reduce chronic lung disease, infections, and developmental complications.

Chapter-End Summary

Neonatal respiratory disorders remain a major contributor to neonatal morbidity and mortality. Prevention requires coordinated antenatal interventions—such as optimal maternal health, infection prevention, and avoiding early elective delivery—combined with evidence-based postnatal practices including surfactant therapy, CPAP, oxygen titration, thermoregulation, and nutrition. Long-term prevention focuses on reducing chronic respiratory sequelae through monitoring, infection prevention, parental education, and early rehabilitation. A multidisciplinary approach across the perinatal continuum is essential for reducing respiratory complications and improving outcomes.

27

References

1. Abdel-Latif ME, Davis PG, Wheeler KI, et al. Surfactant therapy via thin catheter in preterm infants with or at risk of respiratory distress syndrome. Cochrane Database Syst Rev. 2021. https://doi.org/10.1002/14651858.CD011672.pub2.
2. Agarwal S, Kovilam O, Agrawal DK. Vitamin D and its impact on maternal-fetal outcomes in pregnancy: a critical review. Crit Rev Food Sci Nutr. 2018;58:755–69. https://doi.org/10.1080/10408398.2016.1220915.
3. Aguilera J, Konvinse K, Lee A, et al. Air pollution and pregnancy. Semin Perinatol. 2023;47:151838. https://doi.org/10.1016/j.semperi.2023.151838.
4. Alexia Egloff M, Dorothy I, Bulas M. Congenital pulmonary airway malformation: prenatal diagnosis and management. UpToDate; 2024.
5. Barazzone-Argiroffo C, Lascano Maillard J, Vidal I, et al. New insights on congenital pulmonary airways malformations revealed by proteomic analyses. Orphanet J Rare Dis. 2019;14:272. https://doi.org/10.1186/s13023-019-1192-4.
6. Di Renzo G, Al Saleh E, Mattei A, et al. Use of tocolytics: what is the benefit of gaining 48 hours for the fetus? BJOG. 2006;113:72–7. https://doi.org/10.1111/j.1471-0528.2006.01127.x.
7. Ding Y, Chen Z, Lu Y. Vitamin A supplementation prevents the bronchopulmonary dysplasia in premature infants. Medicine. 2021;100:e23101. https://doi.org/10.1097/MD.0000000000023101.
8. Dini G, Ceccarelli S, Celi F, et al. Meconium aspiration syndrome: from pathophysiology to treatment. Ann Med Surg. 2024;86:2023–31. https://doi.org/10.1097/MS9.0000000000001835.
9. Firouzabadi FD, Shab-Bidar S, Jayedi A. The effects of omega-3 polyunsaturated fatty acids supplementation in pregnancy, lactation, and infancy: an umbrella review of meta-analyses of randomized trials. Pharmacol Res. 2022;177:106100. https://doi.org/10.1016/j.phrs.2022.106100.
10. Foliaki S, Pearce N, Björkstén B, et al. Antibiotic use in infancy and symptoms of asthma, rhinoconjunctivitis, and eczema in children 6 and 7 years old: International Study of Asthma and Allergies in Childhood Phase III. J Allergy Clin Immunol. 2009;124:982–9. https://doi.org/10.1016/j.jaci.2009.08.017.
11. Gibbs K, Collaco JM, McGrath-Morrow SA. Impact of tobacco smoke and nicotine exposure on lung development. Chest. 2016;149:552–61. https://doi.org/10.1378/chest.15-1858.
12. Hodgson KA, Wilkinson D, De Paoli AG, Manley BJ. Nasal high flow therapy for primary respiratory support in preterm infants. Cochrane Database Syst Rev. 2023. https://doi.org/10.1002/14651858.CD006405.pub4.
13. Jarde A, Lutsiv O, Beyene J, McDonald S. Vaginal progesterone, oral progesterone, 17-OHPC, cerclage, and pessary for preventing preterm birth in at-risk singleton pregnancies: an updated systematic review and network meta-analysis. BJOG. 2019;126:556–67. https://doi.org/10.1111/1471-0528.15566.
14. Kayode G, Howell A, Burden C, et al. Socioeconomic and ethnic disparities in preterm births in an English maternity setting: a population-based study of 1.3 million births. BMC Med. 2024;22:371. https://doi.org/10.1186/s12916-024-03493-x.
15. Lin FYC, Brenner RA, Johnson YR, et al. The effectiveness of risk-based intrapartum chemoprophylaxis for the prevention of early-onset neonatal group B streptococcal disease. Am J Obstet Gynecol. 2001;184:1204–10. https://doi.org/10.1067/mob.2001.113875.
16. McGillick EV, Lock MC, Orgeig S, Morrison JL. Maternal obesity mediated predisposition to respiratory complications at birth and in later life: understanding the implications of the obesogenic intrauterine environment. Paediatr Respir Rev. 2017;21:11–8. https://doi.org/10.1016/j.prrv.2016.10.003.
17. McGoldrick E, Stewart F, Parker R, Dalziel SR. Antenatal corticosteroids for accelerating fetal lung maturation for women at risk of preterm birth. Cochrane Database Syst Rev. 2020. https://doi.org/10.1002/14651858.CD004454.pub4.
18. Ó Briain E, Byrne AO, Dowling J, et al. Diuretics use in the management of bronchopulmonary dysplasia in preterm infants: a systematic review. Acta Paediatr. 2024;113:394–402. https://doi.org/10.1111/apa.17093.
19. Pederiva F, Rothenberg SS, Hall N, et al. Congenital lung malformations. Nat Rev Dis Primers. 2023;9:60. https://doi.org/10.1038/s41572-023-00470-1.
20. Polakowski LL, Akinbami LJ, Mendola P. Prenatal smoking cessation and the risk of delivering preterm and small-for-gestational-age newborns.

Obstet Gynecol. 2009;114:318–25. https://doi.org/10.1097/AOG.0b013e3181ae9e9c.
21. Ramaswamy VV, Abiramalatha T, Bandyopadhyay T, et al. Surfactant therapy in late preterm and term neonates with respiratory distress syndrome: a systematic review and meta-analysis. Arch Dis Child Fetal Neonatal Ed. 2022;107:393–7. https://doi.org/10.1136/archdischild-2021-322890.
22. Robinson JL, Gatford KL, Clifton VL, et al. The impact of maternal asthma on the fetal lung: outcomes, mechanisms and interventions. Paediatr Respir Rev. 2024;51:38–45. https://doi.org/10.1016/j.prrv.2023.12.004.
23. Rojas-Reyes MX, Morley CJ, Soll R. Prophylactic versus selective use of surfactant in preventing morbidity and mortality in preterm infants. Cochrane Database Syst Rev. 2012. https://doi.org/10.1002/14651858.CD000510.pub2.
24. Sardesai S, Biniwale M, Wertheimer F, et al. Evolution of surfactant therapy for respiratory distress syndrome: past, present, and future. Pediatr Res. 2017;81:240–8. https://doi.org/10.1038/pr.2016.203.
25. Seeni I, Ha S, Nobles C, et al. Air pollution exposure during pregnancy: maternal asthma and neonatal respiratory outcomes. Ann Epidemiol. 2018;28:612–618.e4. https://doi.org/10.1016/j.annepidem.2018.06.003.
26. Shen CL, Zhang Q, Meyer Hudson J, et al. Genetic factors contribute to risk for neonatal respiratory distress syndrome among moderately preterm, late preterm, and term infants. J Pediatr. 2016;172:69–74.e2. https://doi.org/10.1016/j.jpeds.2016.01.031.
27. Simmons D, Immanuel J, Hague WM, et al. Effect of treatment for early gestational diabetes mellitus on neonatal respiratory distress: a secondary analysis of the TOBOGM study. BJOG. 2024. https://doi.org/10.1111/1471-0528.17938.
28. Snoek KG, Reiss IKM, Greenough A, et al. Standardized postnatal management of infants with congenital diaphragmatic hernia in Europe: the CDH EURO consortium consensus – 2015 update. Neonatology. 2016;110:66–74. https://doi.org/10.1159/000444210.
29. Sotiriadis A, McGoldrick E, Makrydimas G, et al. Antenatal corticosteroids prior to planned caesarean at term for improving neonatal outcomes. Cochrane Database Syst Rev. 2021. https://doi.org/10.1002/14651858.CD006614.pub4.
30. St. Clair C, Norwitz E, Woensdregt K, et al. The probability of neonatal respiratory distress syndrome as a function of gestational age and lecithin/sphingomyelin ratio. Am J Perinatol. 2008;25:473–80. https://doi.org/10.1055/s-0028-1085066.
31. Stock S, Thomson A, Papworth S. Antenatal corticosteroids to reduce neonatal morbidity and mortality. BJOG. 2022;129:e35–60. https://doi.org/10.1111/1471-0528.17027.
32. Story L, Shennan A. Cervical cerclage: an evolving evidence base. BJOG. 2024;131:1579–86. https://doi.org/10.1111/1471-0528.17905.
33. Subramaniam P, Ho JJ, Davis PG. Prophylactic or very early initiation of continuous positive airway pressure (CPAP) for preterm infants. Cochrane Database Syst Rev. 2021. https://doi.org/10.1002/14651858.CD001243.pub4.
34. The World Health Organisation (WHO). Preterm birth. 2023. https://www.who.int/news-room/fact-sheets/detail/preterm-birth.
35. Viswanathan M, Urrutia RP, Hudson KN, et al. Folic acid supplementation to prevent neural tube defects. JAMA. 2023;330:460. https://doi.org/10.1001/jama.2023.9864.

GPSR Compliance

The European Union's (EU) General Product Safety Regulation (GPSR) is a set of rules that requires consumer products to be safe and our obligations to ensure this.

If you have any concerns about our products, you can contact us on ProductSafety@springernature.com

In case Publisher is established outside the EU, the EU authorized representative is:

Springer Nature Customer Service Center GmbH
Europaplatz 3
69115 Heidelberg, Germany

Batch number: 10731383

Printed by Printforce, the Netherlands